Second Edition

Nutrition in
PUBLIC
HEALTH

Principles, Policies, and Practice

Arlene Spark
Lauren M. Dinour
Janel Obenchain

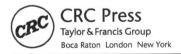

CRC Press
Taylor & Francis Group
Boca Raton London New York

CRC Press is an imprint of the
Taylor & Francis Group, an **informa** business

CRC Press
Taylor & Francis Group
6000 Broken Sound Parkway NW, Suite 300
Boca Raton, FL 33487-2742

First issued in paperback 2021

© 2016 by Taylor & Francis Group, LLC
CRC Press is an imprint of Taylor & Francis Group, an Informa business

No claim to original U.S. Government works

ISBN 13: 978-1-03-209828-9 (pbk)
ISBN 13: 978-1-4665-8994-0 (hbk)

To the memory of my hero, A. Daniel Ochs, MD.

Arlene Spark

To Itai for his endless support and patience,
and to Orli and Talia for their unconditional love and continuous inspiration.

Lauren M. Dinour

Mom and Dad—This one's for you.

Janel Obenchain

Contents

Preface to the Second Edition

Soon after publication of the first edition of this book, Jose Vazquez, PhD, then master teacher of science in the Liberal Studies Program at New York University, wrote to me to say that he enjoyed reading *Nutrition in Public Health*, but had found two typos in the Cultural Competence chapter that "could be fixed for the second edition." Dried salt cod, he wrote, should be spelled *bacalao*, and rice and beans should be *arroz con gandules*. I thanked Dr. Vazquez for his kind words, printed out his message, and tucked it into my copy of the book.

In addition to correcting the spelling of some Spanish dishes, the second edition of *Nutrition in Public Health* contains revisions of features found in the first edition. For example, chapters have been extensively revised to reflect new research; new topics such as the use of social media in health communications and the need for cultural competency around gender identity and gender expression; new programs and initiatives; updated URLs; and the most recent government guidance, including a preview of anticipated changes in the 2015 edition of the *Dietary Guidelines for Americans.**

There are, however, aspects of *Nutrition in Public Health* that are totally new to the second edition. Two of my former graduate students in the CUNY School of Public Health, Lauren M. Dinour, DPH, RD, and Janel Obenchain, MPH, assumed primary responsibility for not only revising the book but also refocusing it from primarily a reference book to a book suitable for the classroom.

The addition of such ancillaries as critical thinking questions and PowerPoint presentations makes this edition suitable for instruction in advanced-level undergraduate nutrition courses and graduate-level courses in both public health and public health nutrition, in social work, and in myriad other courses in the social sciences. We strived to retain the reference value of the book, which makes this volume useful not only for researchers but also for public health practitioners in state and local health departments, health and human services agencies, cooperative extension offices, research foundations, and health-related components in the private sector.

We've corrected spelling mistakes and typos we found in the first edition of this book, some brought to our attention by users of the book and others we found during the revision process. Nevertheless, I assume full responsibility for any errors that appear in the current edition. I would appreciate your calling to my attention any errors you find, which I will tuck into my copy of this book so the errors are not repeated in future editions.

Arlene Spark

---

* PowerPoint slides regarding the 2015 edition of the *Dietary Guidelines for Americans* are available for textbook adopters. Current information is also available at the *Dietary Guidelines* home page: http://health.gov/dietaryguidelines/.

Preface to the First Edition

Immediately after deciding to embark on writing this book, I did exactly what any other public health nutritionist in the Internet age would do—a Google search to determine the availability of other books, and also journals, dedicated to nutrition in public health. I identified six books with "community nutrition" in the title but only two books and a single journal devoted exclusively to public health nutrition. I found myself asking why I should not be reticent to add yet another book to what already seemed like a crowded field. Are nutrition and public health sufficiently mature for three new books in that many years? I believe the answer to that question is a resounding, unequivocal "yes!" Three books and a journal dedicated to a topic that unarguably holds the key to the primary and secondary prevention of some of the major causes of premature death in the United States must still be considered woefully inadequate.

The purpose of *Nutrition in Public Health: Principles, Policies, and Practice* is to provide public health professionals with an overview of the field, with a focus on the federal government's role in determining nutrition policy and practice. The book was written with the conviction that an understanding of government and a familiarity with the demographic profile of the United States population are necessary in order to appreciate nutrition in public health today.

The principles of public health nutrition are presented in the first half of the book. These eight chapters examine the population of the United States, nutritional epidemiology, food and nutrition surveys for monitoring the public's health, programs to reduce disparities in the prevalence of diet-related chronic disease, weight control challenges and solutions, and an examination of special populations—breastfeeding mothers, people with HIV and AIDS, and prison inmates.

The nutrition policy of the United States is addressed in the two chapters that deal with food and nutrition politics and dietary advice.

The last third of the book deals with practicing public health nutrition. These five chapters present the tools for conducting a food and nutrition assessment of a community, designing and carrying out a social marketing campaign, and writing a grant proposal. Programs to promote food security and to ensure the safety of the food supply are also discussed.

Arlene Spark

Acknowledgments

Hunter College President Jennifer Raab, LLB and Provost Vita Rabinowitz, PhD, provided summer 2015 financial support through the Presidential Fund for Faculty Advancement. My family has always stood by me, although Danielle Bier, Barbara and Brian Wachs, and Jayne Workman told me countless times that this is the last book they have the energy to support me through. My mentor, hero, and life partner, Daniel Ochs, MD (1928–2013), saw me through the first edition of this book and part of the second edition. His memory sustains me.

Once, Lauren M. Dinour, DPH, RD, and Janel Obenchain, MPH, were my students. Now they're my colleagues and coauthors. Lauren and Janel are in large part responsible for the second edition of this book.

Arlene Spark

Like any good nutrition policy or practice, the writing of this book took a significant amount of time, effort, and collaboration. My sincerest thanks to those who assisted and supported me through its completion. First and foremost, I am indebted to Arlene Spark, EdD, RD, FADA, FACN, for taking me with her on this journey. Arlene has graciously served as my teacher and trusted advisor throughout my graduate education and beyond, and has continuously stressed that I "can have it all." Indeed, I feel as if I do. My heartfelt gratitude to Janel Obenchain, MPH, who joined our team when we needed her the most and kept us moving forward.

Montclair State University graduate students Kaitlyn O'Connor and Megan Trusdell deserve my deep appreciation for providing valuable research, writing assistance, and PowerPoint development, particularly with the chapters on weight control and food and nutrition politics, policy, and legislation. Another big thank you to Kimberly Biango for her help with PowerPoint design.

Last, I would like to thank my loving and supportive parents, Neil and Gail Drucker, for cheerfully offering their babysitting services so that my work could get done; my sister, Jenny Drucker, for always believing in my abilities despite my own doubts; my husband, best friend, and role model, Itai Dinour, for keeping me grounded and safe through all the chaos; and my daughters, Orli, Talia, and Ilana Dinour, for making me laugh and providing me with a daily source of strength, perspective, and purpose.

Lauren M. Dinour

I am thankful indeed for the opportunity to collaborate with Arlene Spark, EdD, RD, FADA, FACN, and Lauren M. Dinour, DPH, RD; and more honored than I can possibly say to be considered a colleague.

Janel Obenchain

We cannot thank enough the contributors to this effort: Samantha (Sammi) Giertych, RD; Ellen Passov, MBA, RDN; Maggie Meehan, MA, MPH, RD, CDN; and Shakiba Muhammadi, MD, MPH; and families, colleagues, and friends who talked us through this project.

And of course, the talented CRC Press team: Randy Brehm, Iris Fahrer, and Adel Rosario, who so kindly guided us through to completion.

Arlene, Lauren, and Janel

1 Public Health and Nutrition

INTRODUCTION

The title of this book—*Nutrition in Public Health*—represents our view that nutrition is a component of the broad field of public health. Although the phrases *nutrition in public health*, *nutrition and public health*, and *public health nutrition* sound as if they are synonymous, subtle but important differences exist among these phrases.

- Public health nutrition refers to the population-focused branch of public health that monitors diet, nutrition status and health, and food and nutrition programs, and provides a leadership role in applying public health principles to activities that lead to health promotion and disease prevention through policy development and environmental changes. This definition of public health nutrition represents a distillation of the competencies for public health nutrition that were suggested by national and international leaders in the field (Hughes 2003; Johnson et al. 2001; Lawrence and Worsley 2007).
- Nutrition *and* public health suggests the coexistence of the fields of nutrition and public health, although not necessarily as equal partners.
- Nutrition *in* public health refers to a discipline of nutrition functioning as a branch of the vast field of public health.

All three phrases are used interchangeably in this book.

Public health nutritionists make up only a small fraction of the public health workforce engaged in nutrition. Our aim is to provide information that is useful to everyone who addresses food and nutrition issues as part of their public health duties—epidemiologists, grant writers, community health educators, public health nurses, public health physicians, and public health dentists, as well as nutritionists.

In the United States, credible training in public health is offered through master of public health (MPH) degree programs that have been accredited by the Council on Education in Public Health (CEPH 2011). Nevertheless, the study of nutrition is conspicuously absent from the fundamental areas of knowledge CEPH requires for accrediting public health programs and schools. These areas are biostatistics, epidemiology, environmental health, behavioral and social science, and health policy and management. In a sense, the tail wags the dog. As CEPH does not explicitly call for nutrition, schools and programs are not required to offer nutrition in their curricula. Therefore, one goal of this book is to provide an overview of nutrition in public health for public health professionals whose training lack sufficient preparation in this important area.

In particular, *Nutrition in Public Health* is designed to serve as a resource guide, reference book, textbook, roadmap, as well as a key to demystifying access to online information about nutrition in public health. *Nutrition in Public Health* may be used as the following:

- Resource guide for public health and community nutritionists.
- Reference book for nonnutritionist public health professionals who address food and nutrition issues as part of their duties.
- Textbook for traditional and online courses in community and public health and nutrition.
- Guide to accessing online information about topics related to nutrition in public health and government-financed food and nutrition programs, surveys, and research tools.

In this chapter, we introduce and describe a variety of processes, professionals, regulations, and regulatory agencies involved in the promotion of nutrition in public health, with an emphasis on the critical role of the federal government. As relevant, we make some references to the contents of the chapters, but this brief introduction is not meant to forecast the text in its entirety.

PUBLIC NUTRITION

"Public nutrition" has existed for a long time, although not by that name (Rogers and Schlossman 1997). The term first appeared in 1996 in a letter to the editor of the *American Journal of Clinical Nutrition* (Mason et al. 1996). The mission of public nutrition is to anticipate and address the nutritional outcomes of emergencies (malnutrition, mortality, and morbidity) by identifying the causes of malnutrition and mortality in emergency situations, and to identify the broad range of management skills needed in relation to humanitarian response initiatives, including nutrition assessment, policy development, and program design and implementation.

Nutritional problems exist at national, community, and individual levels, and include hunger, childhood malnutrition, famine, suboptimal growth, infection, dietary imbalance or deficiency, and chronic disease. Public nutrition is a broad-based, problem-solving approach to addressing nutritional problems of populations or communities.

Public nutrition recognizes that food insecurity is only one of the determinants of malnutrition in emergencies. Interventions need to address both the health and social environment to have an impact on malnutrition. To accomplish its mission, public nutrition uses a wide range of strategies that take into account public policies and programs in food-related fields, like economics, trade, and agriculture, as well as health (Harinarayan 1999). Some leaders in the field believe that putting public nutrition under the rubric of health would medicalize the field, whereas putting it under agriculture would marginalize it. Public nutrition has a distinct identity, incorporating the relevant aspects of the variety of disciplines that bear on the nutrition problem, as well as incorporating scientific advances in the understanding of nutritional problems (Rogers and Schlossman 1997).

PUBLIC HEALTH

According to The Future of Public Health, a landmark report released more than two decades ago by the Institute of Medicine (IOM), the mission of public health is to "assure conditions in which people can be healthy" (Institute of Medicine 1988). This mission is carried out through organized, interdisciplinary efforts that address the physical, mental, and environmental health concerns of communities and populations at risk for disease and injury, and through three core functions—*assessment*, *policy development*, and *assurance*. These core functions are addressed through the delivery of key services, nine of which are associated with specific core functions and are listed below. Research, the tenth essential public health service identified by the IOM, serves as an umbrella over all the other essential services.

ASSESSMENT

The purpose of assessment and monitoring of the health of communities and populations at risk is to identify health problems and priorities, and evaluate health services. Assessment and monitoring are carried out through the systematic collection, analysis, and dissemination of information about the health of the community in order to

1. Identify health problems in the community
2. Evaluate effectiveness, accessibility, and quality of personal and population-based health services

POLICY DEVELOPMENT

In collaboration with community and government leaders, public health policies are formulated in order to solve local and national health problems and priorities that have been identified. Comprehensive public health policies serve the public interest by their ability to

3. Support individual and community health efforts
4. Inform, educate, and empower people about health issues
5. Mobilize community partnerships to identify and solve health problems

ASSURANCE

Assurance sees to it that all populations have access to appropriate and cost-effective care, including health promotion and disease prevention services, and evaluation of the effectiveness of that care. This oversight assures that the public receives the services promised to them, which is designed to

6. Assure a competent public health and personal healthcare workforce
7. Ethically manage self, people, and resources
8. Enforce laws and regulations that protect health and ensure safety
9. Link people to needed personal health services and assure the provision of healthcare when otherwise unavailable

PUBLIC HEALTH NUTRITION

Public health nutrition is a professional discipline with its own body of knowledge and relevant skills. Imbedded in the practice of public health nutrition are services and activities to assure conditions in which people can achieve and maintain nutritional health. This array of services and activities includes

- Research and analysis; for example, surveillance and monitoring of nutrition-related health status and risk factors.
- Capacity building; for example, community- or population-based assessment, program planning, and evaluation.
- Leadership in community- and population-based interventions that collaborate across disciplines, programs, and agencies.
- Leadership in addressing the access and quality issues around direct nutrition services for populations (Hughes 2008).

We briefly introduce these activities below—surveillance and monitoring; assessment, program planning, and evaluation; and leadership. These activities are referenced throughout the text.

SURVEILLANCE AND MONITORING

Nutrition monitoring is a complex system of activities that provides information about the dietary, nutritional, and related health status of Americans, the relationships between diet and health, and the factors affecting dietary and nutritional status. The US Department of Health and Human Services (HHS) and the US Department of Agriculture (USDA) carry out national-level surveillance and monitoring through a wide array of surveys (Interagency Board for Nutrition Monitoring and Related Research and Bialostosky 2000). The data from these surveys are used in public health nutrition policymaking in the areas of food safety, food fortification, food labeling, dietary guidance, tracking progress toward nutrition and health objectives, and setting nutrition research priorities.

These surveillance and monitoring efforts are mentioned throughout the text when applicable; for example, as one might anticipate, there are numerous such efforts described in Chapter 13. Researchers at all levels of government have access to the USDA's food composition databases, described in more detail in Chapter 3. Several surveys of note are described in Appendix 1.1 to this chapter, and are worth reviewing for increased appreciation of their role in public health nutrition.

Coordinated Federal Nutrition Monitoring

The National Nutrition Monitoring and Related Research Act of 1990* (NNMRRA) was enacted to establish a comprehensive, coordinated program for nutrition monitoring and related research to improve the assessment of the health and nutritional status of the US population. The monitoring act called for the following: a program to achieve coordination of federal nutrition monitoring efforts within 10 years and assist states and local governments in participating in a nutrition monitoring network; an interagency board to develop and implement the program; and an advisory council to provide scientific and technical advice and evaluate program effectiveness.

To the dismay of many nutritional epidemiologists, NNMRRA expired in 2000, and very little of the infrastructure required to maintain a fully coordinated system remains in place today. Nevertheless, some of NNMRRA's major activities are maintained under other legislative authorities. For example, the *Dietary Guidelines* must be reviewed every 5 years, and full integration of Continuing Survey of Food Intake of Individuals (CSFII; USDA) and the National Health and Nutrition Examination Survey (NHANES; HHS) has been realized. Under this integrated framework, the HHS is responsible for sample design and data collection, whereas the USDA is responsible for dietary data collection methodology, maintaining the databases used to code and process the data, and data review and processing.

ASSESSMENT, PROGRAM PLANNING, AND EVALUATION

Assessment is the foundation for developing and implementing program planning. Assessment also serves as a baseline for program evaluation. In public health nutrition, assessment may be based on data obtained from national and statewide surveys as well as from information obtained from local community food and nutrition assessments. Chapter 10 describes community assessment.

LEADERSHIP: PUBLIC HEALTH AND COMMUNITY NUTRITIONISTS

Public health nutritionists are engaged in public health nutrition activities. They have data analysis skills and are proficient in community development, program planning, program management, program evaluation, budget development, and policy analysis and development (Solon 1997). Public health nutritionists include midlevel planners; researchers; and teachers, administrators, and directors of research and training programs. Public health nutritionists also function as macro planners, decision makers, and heads of governmental sectors. Public health nutrition professionals are employed by the public (that is, government or tax-supported) sector, as opposed to being employed by the private (for-profit) sector.

Public health nutritionists provide leadership in assessing the need for public health nutrition campaigns planning, and evaluating them. They are also responsible for assuring compliance with laws and regulations regarding the provision of community nutrition services and assuring competence of the nutrition workforce (Box 1.1).

Both public health nutrition and community nutrition focus on issues that affect the whole population rather than the specific dietary needs of individuals. The emphasis for each is on promoting health and preventing disease. The population included in community nutrition is

---

* P.L. 101–445.

BOX 1.1   NUTRITION IN COMMUNITY HEALTH

The phrase *nutrition in community health* refers to nutrition as a component of the community health branch of public health; *nutrition and community health* connotes the coexistence of nutrition and community health; and *community nutrition* refers to the branch of public health that focuses on promoting the health of individuals, families, and communities by providing quality services and community-based programs tailored to meet the unique nutritional needs of different communities and populations. Community nutrition comprises health promotion programs, policy and legislative initiatives, primary and secondary prevention, and healthcare across the life span. These three phrases are also used interchangeably in this book.

---

circumscribed to a local level. In contrast, the population under the aegis of public health nutrition is much broader.

Community nutrition focuses on the delivery of nutrition services in the areas where people live and work. Community nutritionists are engaged in the direct delivery of nutrition services in the community. The *community nutritionist* must have expertise in nutrition education and individual counseling for high-risk clients as well as experience in program planning, implementation, and evaluation. *Nutrition in the community* refers to tax-supported and private food and nutrition programs implemented for the purpose of decreasing the prevalence of undesirable nutrition-related conditions as well as increasing food security in the community.

Nutrition in the community also includes the local environment that affects food choices, such as the availability of and access to well-stocked supermarkets, and alternative foodways such as farmers markets, community-supported agriculture and farm shares, the food environment in schools, businesses that support breastfeeding mothers, as well as nutrition services provided by tax-supported, nonprofit, and for-profit entities. These include school meals; the Special Supplemental Nutrition Program for Women, Infants, and Children (WIC); local food stamp offices; congregate feeding programs for the elderly; and home-delivered meals for the frail, elderly, and others who are housebound.

Community nutritionists are largely employed by the public sector. Increasingly, however, nonprofit organizations (such as the United Way and Second Harvest) and for-profit healthcare organizations, such as health maintenance organizations and hospital outpatient departments, are employing community nutritionists to provide services to community groups. In addition, self-employed community nutritionists provide consultation services to the Special Supplemental Nutrition Program for WIC programs and senior centers that are required to have a credentialed professional (such as a registered dietitian or licensed nutritionist) provide nutrition education and approve menus.

Table 1.1 compares the scope of practice of community vs. public health nutritionists.

FEDERAL GOVERNMENT'S ROLE IN NUTRITION IN PUBLIC HEALTH

The field of public health nutrition is fueled by the public largesse. As a result, every discussion about nutrition in public health must include reference to its funding sources in the federal government. The federal government has enormous influence over public health nutrition.

To appreciate public health nutrition, it is therefore necessary to understand the organizational structure of the US government, including its various departments and agencies that oversee public health nutrition programs.

Federal, which also means *national*, refers to the government of the United States, as distinct from those of the individual states. A federal government is one in which power is divided between a central authority and a number of regional authorities. Federal systems are often evolved from

TABLE 1.1

Scope of Practice of the Community Nutritionist and the Public Health Nutritionist

	Community Nutritionist	Public Health Nutritionist
Focus	Focuses on issues that affect the whole population rather than the specific dietary needs of individuals	Focuses on issues that affect the whole population rather than the specific dietary needs of individuals
Emphasis	Emphasizes promoting health and preventing disease in populations and groups	Emphasizes promoting health and preventing disease in populations
Target population	The population is circumscribed to a local level that may consist of homogenous groups of people	The population includes a wide spectrum of people and needs
Practice	The practice of community nutrition may include the delivery of nutrition programs and services	The practice of public health nutrition may include the assessment for and design, management, and evaluation of nutrition programs and services
Supervision	Community nutrition programs and services may be delivered by professionals and also by paraprofessionals who are trained and supervised by professionals	Public health nutritionists may train and supervise community nutritionists
Rules	Community nutritionists adhere to laws and policies; suggest policy	Public health nutritionists enforce laws; create policy
Employment	Community nutritionists may be employed at the city or county levels, and by local nonprofit and for-profit agencies that deliver nutrition services; may also be self-employed.	Public health nutritionists may be employed at the federal, state, county, or city levels

confederations. The federal organization of the US government developed from an initial confederation of the 13 original colonies.

The structure and responsibilities of the federal government are outlined in the US Constitution (1787). Its first three articles establish the legislative branch (Article I), the executive (Article II), and the judiciary (Article III) (National Archives, http://www.archives.gov/exhibits/charters/constitution.html). Figure 1.1 is an organizational chart of the US government. A description of the three branches of government appears in Box 1.2.

BILL OF RIGHTS

Just as important as the governmental structure established by the Constitution are the personal freedoms guaranteed by the Bill of Rights and the Thirteenth, Fourteenth, and Fifteenth Amendments to the Constitution. Approved by the First Congress in 1789 and ratified by the states in 1791, the first 10 amendments to the Constitution, known collectively as the Bill of Rights, assure basic individual liberties essential to a free and democratic society. In the aftermath of the Civil War, the Thirteenth, Fourteenth, and Fifteenth Amendments (1865–1870) continued the mission of the Bill of Rights by abolishing slavery, by assuring citizens due process in actions taken under state governments, and by taking the first steps toward providing suffrage (the right to vote in political elections) or all adults. These constitutional guarantees stand as a bulwark against governmental abuses. The Constitution has been amended 17 additional times since the Bill of Rights, most recently in 1992 (National Archives, http://www.archives.gov/exhibits/charters/bill_of_rights.html). From time to time, amendments to the Constitution are cited in this book. For example, the First Amendment is examined during the discussion about advertising that appears in Chapter 5, and the Fourteenth Amendment is referred to in a discussion about healthcare for prison inmates, which is presented in Chapter 6.

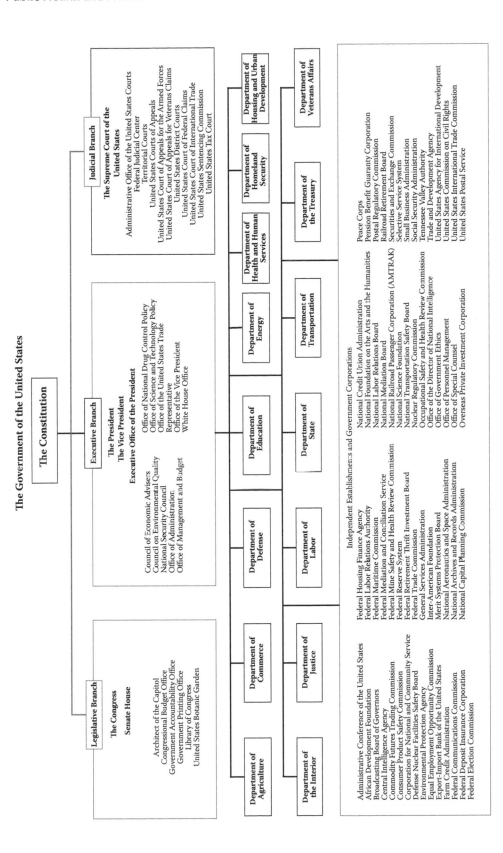

FIGURE 1.1 NetAge. US Gov Org Charts. US Government Organization Chart—Constitution Level. (From The Government of the United States. Available at: http://www.netage.com/economics/gov/Gov-chart-top.html, accessed June 28, 2015.)

LEGISLATIVE BRANCH OF THE FEDERAL GOVERNMENT

The US Congress is the legislative body of the federal government. It is bicameral (consisting of
two bodies), comprising the House of Representatives (the House) and the Senate. The House of
Representatives has 435 members, each representing a congressional district and serving a 2-year
term. House seats are apportioned among the states based on population, whereas each state has
two senators, regardless of population. There are 100 senators, serving staggered 6-year terms. Both
senators and representatives are chosen through direct election.

The US Constitution vests all legislative powers of the federal government in the Congress.
The powers of Congress are limited to those enumerated in the Constitution; all other powers are
reserved to the states and the people. Through acts of Congress, Congress may regulate interstate
and foreign commerce, levy taxes, organize the federal courts, maintain the military, declare war,
and exercise certain other "necessary and proper" powers.

Congress meets in the US Capitol in Washington, DC. Reckoned according to the terms of representatives, the 114th Congress was in session from 2015 through 2016, and so on (Box 1.3).

JUDICIAL BRANCH OF THE FEDERAL GOVERNMENT

The judicial branch hears cases that challenge or require interpretation of the legislation passed
by Congress and signed by the president. It consists of the Supreme Court and the lower federal
courts. Appointees to the federal bench serve for life or until they voluntarily resign or retire.
The Supreme Court is the most visible of all the federal courts. The number of justices is determined by Congress, and since 1869, the court has been composed of one chief justice and eight
associate justices. Justices are nominated by the president and confirmed by the Senate. In this
chapter, we introduce the judicial branch out of order, as we have quite a bit to say about the
executive branch.

EXECUTIVE BRANCH OF THE FEDERAL GOVERNMENT

The power of the executive branch is vested in the president, who also serves as commander in chief of the armed forces. In order for a person to become president, he or she must be a native-born citizen of the United States, be at least 35 years of age, and have resided in the United States for at least 14 years. Once elected, the president serves a term of 4 years and may be reelected only once.

The president appoints the cabinet and oversees the various agencies and departments of the federal government. The tradition of the cabinet dates back to the beginnings of the presidency itself. One of the principal purposes of the cabinet (drawn from Article II of the Constitution) is to advise the president on any subject relating to the duties of their respective offices. The cabinet includes the vice president and the heads (usually known as *secretaries*) of the 15 executive departments—Agriculture, Commerce, Defense, Education, Energy, Health and Human Services, Homeland Security, Housing and Urban Development, Interior, Justice (headed by the attorney general), Labor, State, Transportation, Treasury, and Veterans Affairs. Also included in the cabinet are the administrator of the Environmental Protection Agency, the director of the Office of Management and Budget, the director of the National Drug Control Policy, and the US trade representative.

In terms of nutrition in public health, the two most important cabinet departments—and the government agencies referred to most frequently in this book—are the USDA and the HHS, although allusions to other agencies occasionally appear.

DEPARTMENT OF AGRICULTURE

The USDA organizational chart appears in Figure 1.2. At least six USDA agencies have a profound effect on public health nutrition policy and practice. These six agencies are housed in three offices: Food, Nutrition, and Consumer Services (Food and Nutrition Service, Center for Nutrition Policy and Promotion); Food Safety (Food Safety and Inspection Service); and Research, Education, and Economics (Agricultural Research Service, Economic Research Service, National Agricultural Statistics Service).

The three offices (and their agencies) are briefly described below.

Food, Nutrition, and Consumer Services

Food and Nutrition Service

The Food and Nutrition Service (FNS) administers the USDA food assistance programs, which serve one in four Americans, and represent the nation's commitment to the principle that no one in the United States should fear hunger or experience want (US Department of Agriculture 2012). FNS works in partnership with the states and tribal governments in all its programs. State and local agencies determine most administrative details regarding distribution of food benefits and eligibility of participants, and FNS provides commodities and funding for additional food and to cover administrative costs. FNS administers a number of supplemental food assistance programs, including the Supplemental Nutrition Assistance Program (SNAP), the Child and Adult Care Food Program (CACFP), the School Breakfast Program (SBP), the National School Lunch Program (NSLP), and the Summer Food Service Program (SFSP). FNS food and nutrition assistance programs are discussed in Chapter 11.

Center for Nutrition Policy and Promotion

The Center for Nutrition Policy and Promotion (CNPP) coordinates nutrition policy in the USDA and provides overall leadership in nutrition education for the American public, by developing and promoting dietary guidance that links scientific research to the nutrition needs of consumers. It also coordinates with the HHS in the review, revision, and dissemination of the *Dietary Guidelines for Americans*, the federal government's statement of nutrition policy formed by a consensus of

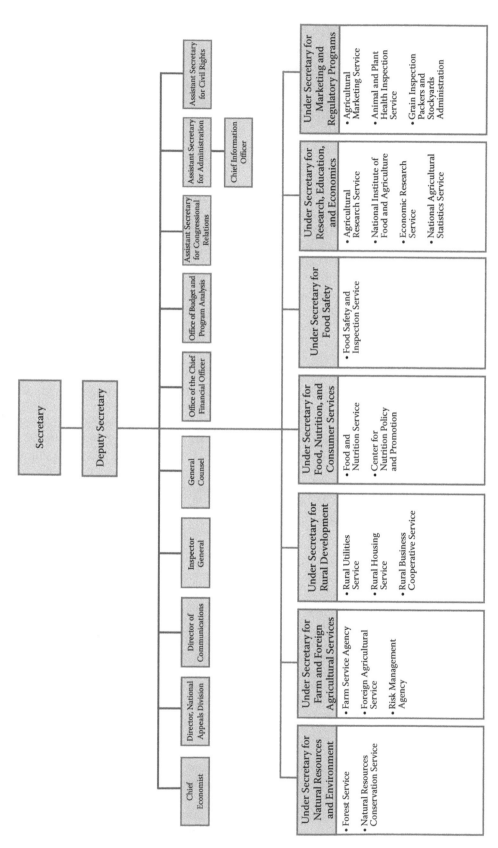

FIGURE 1.2 US Department of Agriculture organizational chart. (From http://www.usda.gov/img/content/agencyworkflow.jpg, last updated November 25, 2013, accessed January 20, 2015.)

scientific and medical professionals.* Chapter 9 examines the food guidance system and dietary guidelines developed and maintained by CNPP.

Food Safety

Food Safety and Inspection Service

The Food Safety and Inspection Service (FSIS) regulates the processing and distribution of meat and meat products, poultry and poultry products, and egg products, to ensure that those products moving in intrastate, interstate, and foreign commerce are wholesome, unadulterated, and properly labeled and packaged. Chapter 13 describes the role of FSIS in protecting the food supply from unintentional and intentional contamination.

Research, Education, and Economics

Agricultural Research Service

The Agricultural Research Service (ARS) serves as the USDA's principal in-house research agency, conducting research and providing information access and dissemination to ensure safe food and to assess the nutritional needs of Americans.

Economic Research Service

The Economic Research Service (ERS) functions as the USDA's principal social science research agency, and it provides decision makers with economic and policy-related social science information and analysis in support of the USDA's goals of enhancing the protection and safety of US agriculture and food, and improving US nutrition and health. Research from the ARS and ERS is cited throughout this book (Box 1.4).

National Agricultural Statistics Service

The National Agricultural Statistics Service (NASS) conducts surveys and prepares official USDA data and estimates of production, supply, prices, and other information necessary to maintain orderly agricultural operations (US Department of Agriculture, http://www.nass.usda.gov). NASS also conducts the census of agriculture, which is currently done every 5 years.

National Institute of Food and Agriculture

The National Institute of Food and Agriculture (NIFA) links the research and education resources and activities of the USDA (http://www.csrees.usda.gov/about/about.html) with academic and land-grant institutions throughout the nation as well as other public and private organizations to advance a global system of extramural research, extension, and higher education in the food and agricultural sciences. NIFA's partnership with the land-grant universities is critical to effective shared planning, delivery, and accountability for research, higher education, and extension programs. NIFA provides research, extension, and education leadership through economic and community systems; families, 4-H, and nutrition; and competitive research, education, and extension programs. NIFA, a major source of funds for demonstration projects and experiments in public health and nutrition, is discussed in Chapter 14 (Box 1.5).

DEPARTMENT OF HEALTH AND HUMAN SERVICES

The HHS organization chart can be viewed in Figure 1.3 or at http://www.hhs.gov/about/orgchart. All 11 agencies in this department interface with nutrition, but particularly noteworthy are the Centers for Disease Control and Prevention (CDC), the Food and Drug Administration (FDA), the

---

* PowerPoint slides regarding the 2015 edition of the *Dietary Guidelines for Americans* are available for textbook adopters. Current information is also available at the *Dietary Guidelines* home page: http://health.gov/dietaryguidelines/.

BOX 1.4   FOOD SUPPLY AND CONSUMPTION RESEARCH TIP

The USDA's ERS provides a number of food-related reports, including a food availability (per capita) data system, which includes data series on food availability, loss-adjusted food availability, and nutrient availability. The series provides continuous data beginning from 1909. It is typically used to measure changes in food consumption over time and to determine the approximate nutrient content of the food supply. Food supply data, also known as *food disappearance data*, reflect the amount of the major food commodities entering the market, regardless of their final use. The total amount available for domestic consumption is estimated by determining the residual after exports, industrial uses, seed and feed use, and year-end inventories are subtracted from the sum of production, beginning inventories, and imports. Consumption estimates derived from food disappearance data tend to overstate actual consumption because they include spoilage and waste accumulated through the marketing system and in the home. Conversion factors are needed to compensate for processing, trimming, spoilage, and shrinkage within the distribution system. Nevertheless, food disappearance data are useful as indicators of trends in consumption over time.

Source: US Department of Agriculture, Food Availability (Per Capita) Data System. Available at http://www.ers .usda.gov/data-products/food-availability-(per-capita)-data-system/faqs.aspx, accessed February 17, 2015.

BOX 1.5   NATIONAL AGRICULTURAL LIBRARY

Additionally, the USDA's National Agricultural Library (NAL) ensures and enhances access to agricultural information. The NAL administers the Food and Nutrition Information Center (FNIC), which serves as a source of food and nutrition information for nutrition and health professionals, educators, government personnel, and consumers.

Indian Health Service (IHS), the Administration for Community Living (ACL) and the National Institutes of Health (NIH).

Centers for Disease Control and Prevention

The CDC organization chart can be viewed in Figure 1.4 or at http://www.cdc.gov/maso/mab_Charts .htm. In terms of public health and nutrition, the most important units in the CDC are the Office of Public Health Scientific Services, within which are the National Center for Health Statistics (NCHS) and the Center for Surveillance, Epidemiology, and Laboratory Services; and the Office of Noncommunicable Diseases, Injury, and Environmental Health, within which are the National Center for Chronic Disease Prevention and Health Promotion (NCCDPHP) and the National Center on Birth Defects and Developmental Disabilities (NCBDDD). Many programs under the jurisdiction of the CDC are discussed throughout this book.

National Center for Health Statistics

CDC's NCHS is the nation's principal health statistics agency, providing data to identify and address health issues. NCHS compiles statistical information to help guide public health and health policy decisions. Collaborating with the USDA and other public partners, NCHS employs a variety of data collection mechanisms to obtain accurate information from multiple sources. This process provides a broad perspective to help understand the population's health, influences on health, and health outcomes, allowing researchers, policymakers, public health practitioners, journalists, academics, and students to identify health problems, risk factors, and disease patterns; plan and assess public health programs; and compare populations, providers, and geographic areas.

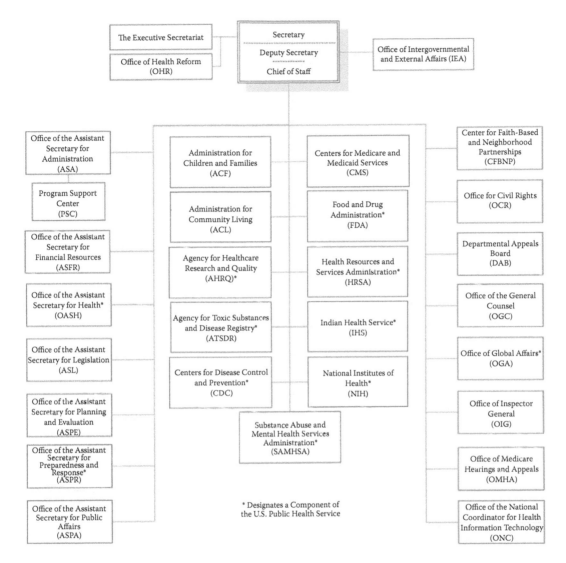

FIGURE 1.3 US Department of Health and Human Services organizational chart. (From http://www.hhs .gov/about/orgchart/index.html, accessed July 30, 2013.)

Food and Drug Administration

FDA is responsible for protecting the public health by assuring the safety, efficacy, and security of human and veterinary drugs, biological products, medical devices, our nation's food supply, cosmetics, and products that emit radiation (US Food and Drug Administration 2014). As discussed in Chapter 13, FDA safeguards the nation's food supply by making sure that all ingredients used in foods are safe; that food is free of contaminants such as disease-causing organisms, chemicals, or other harmful substances; that new food additives are safe; that the safety of dietary supplements is monitored as well as the content of infant formulas and medical foods; and that food labels are regulated.

Indian Health Service

IHS is responsible for providing federal health services to American Indians and Alaska Natives. The IHS is the principal federal healthcare provider and health advocate for Indian people. Its goal is to raise their physical, mental, social, and spiritual health status to the highest possible level. The IHS (http://www.ihs.gov/aboutihs/overview/) currently provides health services to approximately

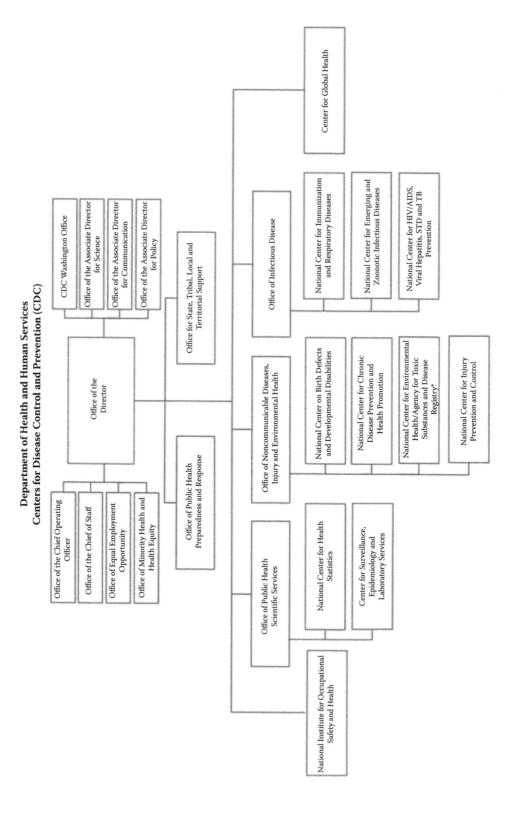

FIGURE 1.4 Centers for Disease Control and Prevention organizational chart. (From http://www.cdc.gov/maso/pdf/CDC_Official.pdf, accessed July 30, 2013.)

1.5 million American Indians and Alaska Natives who belong to 566 federally recognized tribes in 35 states. (Indian Health Service: Agency Overview) American Indian and Alaska Native communities suffer a disproportionately high rate of type 2 diabetes when compared with other populations in the United States.

Administration for Community Living

ACL's mission is to maximize the independence, well-being, and health of older adults, people with disabilities across the life span, and their families and caregivers. The agency is striving to ensure that all Americans—including people with disabilities and older adults—are able to live at home with the support they need, participating in communities that value their contributions (US Department of Health and Human Services, http://www.acl.gov/About_ACL/Index.aspx). ACL serves as one of the nation's largest providers of home- and community-based care for older persons and their caregivers.

National Institutes of Health

NIH, comprising 27 separate institutes and centers, is the federal focal point for medical research in the United States. The NIH National Library of Medicine (NLM) collects, organizes, and makes available biomedical science information to scientists, health professionals, and the public. The library's web-based databases, including PubMed/Medline and MedlinePlus, are used extensively around the world. Grants administered by NIH are discussed in Chapter 14. NIH-sponsored programs, such as *We Can!*, are referenced throughout the text (Box 1.6).

NUTRITION IN PUBLIC HEALTH: PROSPECTIVE

This text aims to provide insight about principles, policies, and practice. The principles of public health nutrition are presented in chapters examining nutritional epidemiology, programs to reduce disparities in the prevalence of diet-related chronic disease, weight control challenges and solutions, and an examination of special populations—breastfeeding mothers, people with HIV and AIDS, and prison inmates. The nutrition policy of the United States is addressed in the two chapters that deal with food and nutrition politics and dietary advice. Additional chapters support the practice of public health nutrition, by presenting the tools for conducting a food and nutrition assessment of a community, designing and carrying out a social marketing campaign, and writing a grant proposal.

As this chapter suffices as both introductory and conclusory, we end on a prospective note.

The vast array of books, social media, and discourse on food, nutrition, health concerns, and the food system is astounding. In this sense, nutrition has become truly public.

Chapter 2 of this text proposes a focus on health promotion rather than disease prevention. New advances in food technologies, such as nanotechnology applications that enhance micronutrient delivery, may end up as public health nutrition solutions. Will such solutions improve health or prevent disease? In Chapter 4 of this text, we highlight some of the demographic changes in society, and researchers have identified new challenges and opportunities stemming from both technological advances and changes in social dynamics, including the following (Pelletier 2013):

- Increased awareness, interest, and/or concern for food and nutrition on public and private agendas, as seen in the attention given to the global spreading of obesity and chronic diseases, continued and heightened focus on food insecurity and malnutrition, and the increased understanding of the impact multinational food corporations have on our diet and food systems.
- Recognition of the interconnected nature of nutrition and health problems with agriculture; food systems and environmental sustainability; poverty and social justice; and the social, organizational, and political processes that seek to maintain or change the trend.
- Increasing demand for evidence of the effectiveness of interventions when implemented at scale and growing interest in and funding of *action-oriented research* such as implementation or translational science and community-based participatory research (CBPR).

BOX 1.6   THE NATIONAL INSTITUTES OF HEALTH

The institutes and offices within the NIH that serve as the custodians of funds that support the preponderance of nutrition-related research in human health and disease are as follows.

- The *National Cancer Institute* (NCI), established in 1937, addresses suffering and deaths due to cancer. Through basic and clinical biomedical research and training, NCI conducts and supports research aimed at preventing cancer before it starts, identifying at the earliest stage cancers that do develop, eliminating cancers through innovative treatment interventions, and biologically controlling those cancers that cannot be eliminated so they become manageable chronic diseases.
- The *National Heart, Lung, and Blood Institute* (NHLBI), established in 1948, provides leadership for a national program in diseases of the heart, blood vessels, lung, and blood; blood resources; and sleep disorders. Since October 1997, the NHLBI has also had administrative responsibility for the NIH Women's Health Initiative. The institute plans, conducts, fosters, and supports an integrated and coordinated program of basic research, clinical investigations and trials, observational studies, and demonstration and education projects.
- The *National Institute on Aging* (NIA), established in 1974, leads a national program of research on the biomedical, social, and behavioral aspects of the aging process; the prevention of age-related diseases and disabilities; and the promotion of a better quality of life for all older Americans.
- The *National Institute of Allergy and Infectious Diseases* (NIAID), established in 1948, supports research aimed at understanding, treating, and ultimately preventing the myriad infectious, immunologic, and allergic diseases.
- The *National Institute of Diabetes and Digestive and Kidney Diseases* (NIDDK), established in 1950, conducts and supports basic and applied research and provides leadership for a national program in diabetes, endocrinology, and metabolic diseases; digestive diseases, nutrition, and obesity; and kidney, urologic, and hematologic diseases. Several of these diseases are among the leading causes of disability and death; all seriously affect the quality of life of those who have them.
- The *National Center for Complementary and Alternative Medicine* (NCCAM), established in 1998, explores complementary and alternative medical practices in the context of rigorous science.
- The *National Institute on Minority Health and Health Disparities* (NIMHD), established in 2000, promotes minority health and leads, coordinates, supports, and assesses the NIH effort to reduce and ultimately eliminate health disparities. In this effort, NIMHD conducts and supports basic, clinical, social, and behavioral research; promotes research infrastructure and training; fosters emerging programs; disseminates information; and reaches out to minority and other communities with a disparity of health needs.

The researchers argue that these evident new lines of inquiry reflect a shift in motivation toward creating actionable knowledge addressing real-world problems. They further note that the vast majority of papers in leading nutrition journals still compromise conventional nutritional research, which traditionally concerns descriptive measurements of *who and what* and the use of essentially individual-level analysis in order to discern problems and intervening solutions about population health. The researchers argue that nutritional research needs to continue to incorporate expanded and broader methods, as focusing on individuals as the unit of analysis in research does not fully serve the intellectual or practical goals of population-level nutrition research. The authors argue that in order to create real-world solutions (arguably, solutions that promote health), we must recognize the social construction of not only the problems but also the solutions and the actors that decide and implement such solutions. We must use approaches for nutritional research that tend to be more engaged, participatory, and holistic, such as CBPR and prospective policy research.

In other words, nutrition in public health.

CONCLUSION

Nutrition in public health—the practice of nutrition within the public health arena—is a complex undertaking. Fueled by taxpayer dollars, public health involves all levels of government, from numerous agencies at the federal level to small, community-based organizations. Public health nutritionists, while seeking to improve the health of populations through improved nutrition, must also be proficient in community development; program planning, management, and evaluation; budget development; and policy analysis and development.

ACRONYMS

ARS	Agricultural Research Service
CDC	Centers for Disease Control and Prevention
CNPP	Center for Nutrition Policy and Promotion
ERS	Economic Research Service
FDA	Food and Drug Administration
FNCS	Food, Nutrition and Consumer Services
FNIC	Food and Nutrition Information Center
FSIS	Food Safety and Inspection Service
HHS	Department of Health and Human Services
NHLBI	National Heart, Lung, and Blood Institute
NIDDK	National Institute of Diabetes and Digestive and Kidney Diseases
NIFA	National Institute of Food and Agriculture
NIH	National Institutes of Health
NLM	National Library of Medicine
USDA	US Department of Agriculture
We Can!	Ways to Enhance Children's Activity and Nutrition!
WIC	Special Supplemental Nutrition Program for Women, Infants, and Children
WISEWOMAN	Well-Integrated Screening and Evaluation for Women Across the Nation

APPENDIX 1.1

Surveys: National Health Interview Survey (NHIS), Behavioral Risk Factor Surveillance System (BRFSS), Youth Risk Behavior Surveillance System (YRBSS), National Health and Nutrition Examination Survey (NHANES).

NATIONAL HEALTH INTERVIEW SURVEY

The NHIS is the principal source of information on the health of the civilian, noninstitutionalized population of the United States and one of the major data collection programs of NCHS (Centers for Disease Control and Prevention, http://www.cdc.gov/nchs/nhis/about_nhis.htm). The NHIS is a cross-sectional household interview survey. Since 1957, its data have been used to monitor trends in illness and disability and to track progress toward achieving national health objectives, such as those of Healthy People 2020. Questionnaires, data sets, and documentation are available from 1963 to date at http://www.cdc.gov/nchs/nhis/nhis_questionnaires.htm. NHIS data are also used by the public health research community for epidemiologic and policy analysis of such timely issues as characterizing those having various health problems, determining barriers to accessing and using appropriate healthcare, and evaluating federal health programs. The main objective of the NHIS is to monitor the health of the US population through the collection and analysis of data on a broad range of health topics.

Although the NHIS has been conducted continuously, its content has been revised roughly every 10–15 years. Starting in 1997, the NHIS questionnaire has core questions and supplements. The core questions remain largely unchanged, which allows for trend analysis and data pooling over a number of years to increase the sample size for analysis. The supplements allow the survey to be responsive to emerging public health data needs. For example, in 2014, about 4000 additional households containing one or more Native Hawaiian and Pacific Islander were added to the NHIS, and a public-use data file will be available in the fall of 2015 (Centers for Disease Control and Prevention, http://www .cdc.gov/nchs/nhis/nhpi.html). The CDC (http://www.cdc.gov/nchs/nhis/supplements_cosponsors .htm) publishes a list of NHIS supplements and co-sponsors by year and topic that includes details about the sponsoring agency, questionnaires, and data file location. The Cancer Control Supplement is administered every 5 years, and covers a variety of topics, including diet and nutrition (National Cancer Institute, http://appliedresearch.cancer.gov/nhis/what.html).

The sampling plan is redesigned after each census. For example, in the previous sample design, all eligible adults in contacted families had an equal chance to be the sample adult; now adults over 65 who are black, Hispanic, or Asian have an increased chance of being selected as the sample adult. The NHIS sample is drawn from each state. Although the NHIS sample is too small to provide state-level data with acceptable precision, estimates may be drawn from combined data, and its design facilitates the use of NHIS data with state-level telephone health surveys.

Sampling and interviewing are continuous throughout the year. Households selected for interviewing are a probability sample representative of the target population. Beginning in 2011, the expected sample size (completed interviews) was collected from approximately 35,000 households containing about 87,500 persons. Survey participation is voluntary, and the confidentiality of responses is assured under Section 308(d) of the Public Health Service Act. The annual response rate of the NHIS is close to 90% of the eligible households in the sample.

Data are collected through a personal interview conducted in the participant's household by interviewers employed and trained by the US Bureau of the Census. The NHIS questionnaire is conducted using a computer-assisted personal interviewer (CAPI). The interviewer uses a laptop computer and enters responses directly into it during the interview. This computerized mode offers distinct advantages over the previous pencil-and-paper formats in terms of timeliness of the data and improved data quality. Since 2004, questionnaires have been available in Spanish as well as in English.

BEHAVIORAL RISK FACTOR SURVEILLANCE SYSTEM

The BRFSS is the world's largest ongoing telephone health survey system—over 500,000 interviews were conducted in 2011 (Centers for Disease Control and Prevention, http://www.cdc.gov/brfss /about/about_brfss.htm). By the early 1980s, there was universal agreement that personal health behaviors play a significant role in premature morbidity and mortality. Although national estimates of health-risk behaviors among the US adult population had been periodically obtained through surveys conducted by the NCHS, these data were not available on a state-specific basis. This deficiency was viewed as critical for state health agencies, which have the primary role of targeting resources to reduce behavioral risks and their consequent illnesses. Although national data may not be appropriate for any given state, state and local agency participation was critical to achieving national health goals. As a result, the CDC established the BRFSS to collect state-level data that would provide the basis for monitoring state-level prevalence of the major behavioral risks among adults associated with premature morbidity and mortality. The basic philosophy was to collect data on actual behaviors—rather than on attitudes or knowledge—that would be especially useful for planning, initiating, supporting, and evaluating health promotion and disease prevention programs.

Over the years, data from BRFSS have been used to monitor the prevalence of high-risk health behaviors, specific diseases, and use of preventive health services; dictate the design, focus, implementation, and evaluation of prevention health programs and strategies; and monitor progress toward achieving local, state, and national health objectives.

To provide data that could be compared across states, CDC developed a core of standard questions for states to incorporate into their own questionnaires, which are administered by telephone, including interviews of households that use only cell phones. As of 2011, all 50 US states, the District of Columbia, Puerto Rico, the US Virgin Islands, Guam, American Samoa, and Palau participated; more than 506,000 interviews were conducted in total. Starting in 2010, CDC (http://www.cdc.gov/brfss/about/brfss_today.htm) is piloting and testing other modes of data collection.

All health departments must ask the core questions without modification; however, the optional modules and additional questions are at the discretion of the state. The BRFSS questionnaire (Centers for Disease Control and Prevention, http://www.cdc.gov/brfss/questionnaires.htm) comprises three parts, described as follows:

- The *core component* consists of a *fixed*, a *rotating*, and an *emerging* core. The fixed core is a standard set of questions asked by all states and includes queries about current behaviors that affect health (for example, tobacco use and women's health) and questions on demographic characteristics. The *rotating core* consists of two distinct sets of questions, each asked in alternating years by all states, addressing different topics. In the years that a rotating topic is not used in the core, it is supported as an optional module. The *emerging core* is a set of up to five questions added to the fixed and rotating cores. Emerging core questions typically focus on issues of a late-breaking nature and are evaluated during the current year or soon thereafter to determine if inclusion in future surveys as a regular core component is warranted.
- The *optional modules* are sets of questions on specific topics that states may elect to use, but if they are used, they must not be modified. Module topics have included questions on smokeless tobacco, oral health, cardiovascular disease, and firearms.
- The *state-added questions* are questions on topics of particular interest to an individual state that it may choose to add. In the past, categories of interest to public health nutritionists have included cholesterol, folic acid, food consumption, food handling, lead poisoning, physical activity, and weight control.

YOUTH RISK BEHAVIOR SURVEILLANCE SYSTEM

CDC (http://www.cdc.gov/HealthyYouth/yrbs/index.htm) launched the YRBSS in 1990 to monitor health-risk behaviors that contribute markedly to the leading causes of death, disability, and social problems among youth in the United States, including behaviors contributing to accidental injury and violence, sexual behaviors contributing to sexually transmitted diseases and unintended pregnancy, alcohol and other drug use, tobacco use, unhealthy dietary behaviors, and inadequate physical activity. The stated purpose of the YRBSS is to determine the prevalence of health-risk behaviors, assess trends in these behaviors, and examine co-occurrence of these behaviors. There was a conscious decision to focus on behaviors rather than determinants. YRBSS also measures the prevalence of obesity and asthma (Centers for Disease Control and Prevention, http://www.cdc.gov/healthyyouth/data/surveillance.htm). (Note: the acronym for the survey itself is YRBS).

YRBSS data are used at the national, state, and local levels in a variety of policy and program applications, such as monitoring progress toward achieving Healthy People 2020 objectives. YRBSS data can be used to describe risk behaviors, create awareness, set program goals, develop programs and policies, support health-related legislation, and seek funding.

The questionnaire is anonymous and self-administered, with either a computer-scannable booklet or an answer sheet. The system includes national, state, and local school-based surveys of representative samples of 9th- through 12th-grade students. The national survey provides data representative of high school students in both public and private schools in the 50 states and the District of Columbia.

A voluntary component of the program is the provision of funding and technical support to states and major cities to conduct their own surveys. The national survey is conducted during February– May of each odd-numbered year, and most sites conduct their own surveys during this time as well. Sites can add or delete questions in the core questionnaire to meet the needs of their state and local departments of education and health.

Special-population surveys that are related to short-term federal initiatives are also included with the YRBSS. From 2007 to 2009 communities participating in the Steps to a HealthierUS program conducted surveys, and between 2010 and 2013, communities participating in the Communities Putting Prevention to Work program conducted surveys. CDC also provides assistance to conduct YRBS surveys of Native American youth (Brener et al. 2013).

Comprehensive information about the results of YRBSS can be found on CDC's website at http://www.cdc.gov/HealthyYouth/yrbs/index.htm. The site includes a copy of the most recent questionnaire and item rationale; links to the Morbidity and Mortality Weekly Report Surveillance Summaries that highlight YRBSS data; the data and codebooks for the national YRBSS; related publications, journal articles, and fact sheets; and Youth Online.

NATIONAL HEALTH AND NUTRITION EXAMINATION SURVEY

The major food and nutrition survey that shapes nutrition policy in the United States is known as What We Eat in America–NHANES, an integration of two prior surveys: the Continuing Survey of Food Intake of Individuals (CSFII) conducted by the USDA and NHANES conducted by HHS (Centers for Disease Control and Prevention, http://www.cdc.gov/nchs/nhanes.htm). The year 2002 was the first year of full integration of these two surveys.

NHANES serves as the data collection mechanism for the joint HHS/USDA effort to monitor the diet and nutritional status of Americans, providing information needed for food policy and dietary guidelines (US Department of Health and Human Services 2014). NHANES can link food intake data to anthropometric, clinical, and biochemical indices, allowing researchers to explore relationships between diet and health status.

NHANES Background

The NCHS National Health Examination Survey (NHES) was launched in the 1950s. By the late 1960s, with a burgeoning awareness of and concern about domestic hunger and other nutrition issues, it became apparent that the lack of a nutrition component in NHES was a serious flaw. A nutrition component was added in 1971, and NHES expanded into NHANES.

Initially, NHANES was conducted episodically, NHANES I from 1971 through 1974, NHANES II from 1976 through 1980, and NHANES III from 1988 through 1994. Since 1999, the survey has been conducted continuously, with results reported for 2-year cycles, such as NHANES 2009–2010 and NHANES 2011–2012.

NHANES Methodology

NHANES is a continuous, annual survey that collects data from a nationally representative sample of the civilian, noninstitutionalized US population aged 2 months or older through in-home personal interviews, physical examinations in mobile examination centers (MECs), and mail follow-up food frequency questionnaires (FFQs). The survey is conducted among a nationally representative sample of about 5000 people each year. Certain groups are oversampled, such as Hispanics, African Americans, persons 60 years or older, and most recently, Asian Americans, to allow for more precise estimates of their populations. (Centers for Disease Control and Prevention, http://www.cdc.gov/nchs/nhanes/about_nhanes.htm).

Diet-related conditions studied include cardiovascular disease, diabetes, kidney disease, obesity, oral health, and osteoporosis. Environmental exposures are also studied, some of which may be dietary-based exposures, such as phthalates. MEC data collection includes physical examinations, a standardized dental examination, physiological measurements, and laboratory tests on blood and urine. With each NHANES cycle, test components are dropped and added. For example, the National Cancer Institute (http://appliedresearch.cancer.gov/nhanes/) proposed and coordinated funding from multiple NIH institutes and the Department of Defense for a new electronic physical activity monitor to be worn on the wrist, which will provide the first objective measurement of sleep duration in a nationally representative sample (Box 1.7).

NHANES Dietary Measures

What We Eat in America is the dietary interview component of NHANES. It consists of dietary recalls, an FFQ, and interview questions about the use of vitamin and mineral supplements.

The NHANES participant is first interviewed at home. A follow-up physical examination is conducted at the mobile exam center (MEC). Dietary behavior information is collected during the home interview. A 24-hour dietary recall is obtained at the MEC, along with the physical exam. A second 24-hour dietary recall is collected by telephone about 3–10 days after the MEC exam (Centers for Disease Control and Prevention, http://www.cdc.gov/nchs/tutorials/dietary/SurveyOrientation/Dietary DataOverview/Info2.htm).

The automated multiple-pass method (AMPM) is used to collect the recalls. This computerized protocol, developed by the USDA, collects interviewer-administered 24-hour dietary recalls either in person or by telephone. The software program provides a series of questions or prompts to help skilled interviewers elicit precise information. Designed to enhance recall accuracy and reduce

---

BOX 1.7   NHANES HEALTH EXAMINATION COMPONENTS

Select health measurements by participant age and gender for 2013–2014

- Physician's exam—all ages.
- Blood pressure—ages 8 years or older.
- Body composition—ages 8–59 years.
- Bone density—ages 8 years or older.
- Oral health exam—ages 2 years or older.
- Fitness test—ages 12–49 years.
- Body measurements—all ages.

Select laboratory tests by participant age and gender for 2013–2014

- Albumin—6 years or over.
- Celiac disease—6 years or over.
- Estradiol—6 years or over (introduced in 2013–2014).
- Glucose—12 years or older.
- Herpes 1 and 2 antibody—14–49 years.
- Human papillomavirus (HPV) (males)—14–59 years.
- HPV (females, swab)—14–59 years.

Source: National Health and Nutrition Examination Survey, 1999–2014 Survey Content Brochure. Available at http://www.cdc.gov/nchs/data/nhanes/survey_content_99_14.pdf, accessed February 17, 2015.

respondent burden, it is the primary instrument used to collect dietary intake data from individuals sampled in national surveys (Bliss 2004). An FFQ was also mailed to participants several days after the in-person data collection in the 2003–2004 and 2005–2006 NHANES cycles.

The food intake data collected by NHANES can be linked to the health status data from other NHANES components, if such components are available, allowing researchers to explore relationships between dietary intakes and health status. For example, results from NHANES 1999–2000, conducted after the implementation of food fortification and educational efforts to increase folate consumption, indicate that these efforts have been effective in increasing folate status among US women of childbearing age (Centers for Disease Control and Prevention, 2000).

REFERENCES

Bliss RM. Researchers produce innovation in dietary recall. *Agric Res.* 2004;52(6):10–12.

Brener ND, Kann L, Shanklin S, Kinchen S, Eaton DK, Hawkins J, Flint KH. Methodology of the youth risk behavior surveillance system—2013. Recommendations and reports. *MMWR.* 2013;62(RR01):1–23. Available at http://www.cdc.gov/mmwr/preview/mmwrhtml/rr6201a1.htm?s_cid=rr6201a1_w, accessed February 17, 2015.

Centers for Disease Control and Prevention. Folate status in women of childbearing age—United States, 1999. *MMWR. Weekly.* 2000;49:962–965.

Council on Education in Public Health (CEPH). Accreditation Criteria Public Health Programs. Amended June 2011. Available at http://www.ceph.org/i4a/pages/index.cfm?pageid=3350, accessed January 20, 2015.

Harinarayan A. What is public nutrition? *ENN (Emergency Nutrition Network) Field Exchange.* No. 8, 13, 1999.

Hughes R. Definitions for public health nutrition: A developing consensus. *Public Health Nutr.* 2003;6:615–620.

Hughes R. Workforce development: Challenges for practice, professionalization and progress. *Public Health Nutr.* 2008;11:765–767.

Institute of Medicine. *The Future of Public Health.* Washington, DC: National Academy Press, 1988.

Interagency Board for Nutrition Monitoring and Related Research and Bialostosky K, ed. *Nutrition Monitoring in the United States: The Directory of Federal and State Nutrition Monitoring and Related Research Activities.* Hyattsville, MD: National Center for Health Statistics, 2000. Available at http://www.cdc.gov /nchs/data/misc/direc-99.pdf, accessed January 20, 2015.

Johnson DB, Eaton DL, Wahl PW, Gleason C. Public health nutrition practice in the United States. *Am Diet Assoc.* 2001;101:529–534.

Lawrence M, Worsley T. *Understanding Public Health Nutrition.* Allen & Unwin, Crow's Nest, Australia, 2007.

Mason J, Habicht J-P, Greaves JP, Jonsson U, Kevany J, Martorell R, Rogers B. Public nutrition. Letter to the editor. *Am J Clin Nutr.* 1996;63:399–400.

National Archives. Bill of Rights. Available at http://www.archives.gov/exhibits/charters/bill_of_rights.html, accessed January 20, 2015.

National Archives. Constitution of the United States. Available at http://www.archives.gov/exhibits/char ters/constitution.html, accessed January 20, 2015.

Pelletier DL, Porter CM, Aarons GA, Wuehler SE, Neufeld LM. Expanding the frontiers of population nutrition research: New questions, new methods, and new approaches. *Adv Nutr.* 2013;4(1):92–114.

Rogers B, Schlossman N. "Public nutrition": The need for cross-disciplinary breadth in the education of applied nutrition professionals. *Food Nutr Bull.* 1997;18(2) (June);120–133

Solon FS. Developing a national training pyramid. *Food Nutr Bull.* 1997;18(2) (June).

US Department of Agriculture. USDA Mission Areas. Food, Nutrition and Consumer Services, Food and Nutrition Service. Updated March 23, 2012. Available at http://www.usda.gov/wps/portal/usda /usdahome?contentid=missionarea_FNC.xml, accessed January 20, 2015.

US Department of Agriculture. National Agricultural Statistics Service. Available at http://www.nass.usda.gov/, accessed February 17, 2015.

U.S. Food and Drug Administration. About FDA. What We Do. Last updated August 5, 2014. Available at http://www.fda.gov/aboutfda/whatwedo/, accessed January 20, 2015.

2 Preventing Disease or Promoting Health?*

The most sophisticated and effective healthcare in the world cannot produce results as good as simply remaining healthy in the first place.

Robert G. Evans

INTRODUCTION

Over the last three centuries, changes in dietary patterns and physical activity have accelerated in varying degrees in different regions of the world (Popkin 2006). Modernization, urbanization, economic development, and the rise of income level lead to predictable shifts in diet and activity patterns, referred to as nutrition transitions (The Nutrition Transition, http://www.hsph.harvard.edu/obesity-prevention-source/nutrition-transition/#references). These nutrition transitions, which include structural and composition shifts in diet and activity patterns, are reflected in nutritional outcomes, such as changes in body composition, and health outcomes, such as increases in obesity and noncommunicable diseases (NCDs). In addition, the dietary and activity pattern changes parallel demographic and socioeconomic changes; various cultural and knowledge factors; disease patterns; and sociologic considerations (for example, the role of women and family structure) (Popkin 2006).

Findings from the World Health Organization's (WHO's) 2013 Global Burden of Disease Study, analyzing data from 188 countries between 1980 and 2013, conclude that over the past 33 years, overweight or obesity rates worldwide have risen 28% among adults and 47% among children. Obesity now afflicts people of all ages, incomes, and regions, with two-thirds of the world's obese population living in developing countries. Not a single country during this time span has successfully reduced its obesity rate, although during the last 8 years, obesity rates in wealthier nations have been slowing (Ng et al. 2014). Along with obesity arrive increases in hypertension, cardiovascular disease (CVD), type 2 diabetes, and a host of other ills. Given these chronic health issues now confronting both developed and developing nations, we can ask what role public health should play in the relationship between the individual and the environment, both natural and built.

During the past century, public health has become increasingly guided by epidemiology and by technological advances in medicine. Yet scientific knowledge is only one of several elements fundamental to effective public health practice. Scientific knowledge must be combined with engagement in civil society and social movements to result in effective action (Beaglehole et al. 2004).

This chapter suggests that we need a broader-based interpretation of effective public health in the United States, with health promotion as its overarching theme. Although public health has had great success in combating certain specific disease-causing pathogens, the modern diseases of cancer, heart disease, and obesity do not fit this paradigm. Accepting that the health of an individual arises from the health of the society and of the environment, if the practice of public health is to be effective, the ideology of health promotion must pervade all fields impacting the public good—from environmental protection to healthcare.

---

* Maggie Meehan, MA, MPH, RD, CDN, and Shakiba Muhammadi, MD, MPH, contributed primary research and prepared draft versions of portions of this chapter.

DEFINING HEALTH

Health is an amorphous concept. The word derives from the Greek word meaning "whole" and is defined as "wholeness, being whole, sound or well" (Online Etymology Dictionary, http://www .etymonline.com). This idea of *wholeness* is open to broad interpretation and may refer to the health of the individual, the community, or the nation.

Historically, the concept of health was often synonymous with the health needs of the nation-state, such as a steady supply of soldiers or laborers well enough to fight or work, control of over-population, protection of the elite, and environmental stability (Detels et al. 2009). Developments in public health have often historically arisen from the poor physical state of military recruits, but more recently, retired military leaders have worried that potential soldiers are too overweight to fight (Hemmerly-Brown 2010).

In 1948, the WHO defined health as "a state of complete physical, mental, and social well-being and not merely the absence of disease or infirmity." This definition has not been amended since 1948 (Preamble to the Constitution of the World Health Organization, New York, June 19–22, 1946, http://www.who.int/about/definition/en/print.html). Ambitious in breadth, critics suggest that if the definition of health is to be a useful guiding principle, it must refer to a less idealistic state, one that can be agreed upon as an achievable level of *well-being* (Seedhouse 2009).

It is also worth examining a more carefully parsed definition of health. Seedhouse's *foundations theory of health* (Seedhouse 2009), which ultimately results in individual achievement of human potential, describes people as being enabled by foundations to achieve chosen and biological potentials. A state of optimum health would be one in which the foundations are complete in context for the person. Although the number and content of foundations (imagined as building blocks) will vary by individual and circumstance, at least four basic building blocks generally can be thought of as necessary for all people:

1. Basic needs such as food, shelter, and clothing
2. Access to as much information as possible about all factors affecting one's life
3. The skill and confidence needed to assimilate this information
4. The understanding that one does not operate in isolation but as part of one's physical and societal surroundings

The fifth block (or additional blocks) differs for each individual, depending on what additional support may be needed in difficult circumstances. The additional foundation becomes necessary when a life problem, such as an adverse medical event or the loss of a job or home, diminishes or destroys the ability of the four primary building blocks to support a person's present way of life.

Seedhouse's foundations theory of health is particularly valuable in that it does not rely on biology alone, and thus not on the traditional sphere of medicine as health. Rather, it places the individual within a context and recognizes that information, skills, and socialization are needed by the individual in order to negotiate that context while attempting to fulfill his or her potential. Unfortunately, the foundations theory is limited in that although it recognizes the impact of an individual's environment on his or her health, it also tends to individualize environmental context and solutions. A health promotion model, conversely, is based on the ideal of providing a healthy environment within which an individual lives and makes choices, and by extension, for all individuals.

HISTORY OF PUBLIC HEALTH: A BRIEF REVIEW

The contemporary practice of public health in the United States has perhaps been sidetracked by a focus on medical intervention and technical solutions. It has been observed that while "public health has evolved into a subdivision of medicine with minimal and subordinate inclusion of the ancillary disciplines of engineering and the social sciences … *health has been improved by many non-medical factors*—economic prosperity, town planning, architecture, religious and humanitarian charity, the power of organized labor, and even broader political changes resulting in the greater availability of political or economic rights …" (emphasis added) (Detels et al. 2009).

One of the earliest roles of public health was in reaction to an epidemic crisis. Classically, the reaction to an epidemic had been abject resignation. Facing plague and leprosy, medieval Christian Latin countries took a more activist role, although the actions taken (quarantine and pogroms) by no means benefited everyone. A populace acting precipitously and independently (such as by burning groups of its citizens to death) threatened civil and ecclesiastical institutions. It is in institutional responses to such actions threatening the security of the nation-state that public health emerges as a form of public authority (Detels et al. 2009).

Historically, public health in Western societies also regulated community social goods, such as enforcing rules for sanitation and construction, caring for the poor, regulating work hours, conducting markets and the quality of the goods sold, maintaining population statistics, and regulating medical practice—activities still within the purview of public health today. When regulation of medical practice served the interests of established practitioners, it was done under the guise of maintaining the quality of public medical care (Detels et al. 2009).

During the course of the nineteenth century, public health developed an association with a right of citizenship. Public health grew less reactive and regulatory and more oriented toward the goal of reducing rates of morbidity and mortality (Detels et al. 2009). This new focus on prevention paralleled and stimulated the growth in scientific knowledge and preventative acts. However, whereas some countries embraced sanitation—comprehensive systems of water and sewerage—as a means not only to improved health but also, in Britain's case, for a "prettier," happier, and better world, the United States remained alone among Western nations in adhering to a policy that an individual's health was solely a private matter (Detels et al. 2009).

By the 1880s, germ theory was well known, and, as described by Hamlin, the "Golden Age of Public Health" was well underway. Public health regulation of an individual's life—home, work, family relations, recreation activities, and sex—expanded beyond that of the previous century's medical police. Although public health regulation began infringing to a greater extent on personal individual liberties, such infringement proved eminently successful in reducing morbidity and mortality, and was generally seen by citizens as an appropriate and desirable role of the state. By providing support for the health of the public, a reciprocal social contract was induced, one in which the state can then, in turn, expect its citizens to strive to be healthy, i.e., productive members of society.

With the emergence of cancers and other chronic illnesses, such as type 2 diabetes, that lacked single preventive strategies, the question arose as to the extent of this social contract. How far reaching now were the health obligations of the liberal state to its citizens? Because many of these newly prominent diseases are not infectious, they do not disrupt the social and economic functions of the community or state in the same obvious manner as plague, or impure drinking water, decreasing the value of the established reactive and policing approaches to public health. Yet, these diseases do interfere with fulfillment of human potential—and citizens can justly demand attention by the state (Detels et al. 2009).

Presently, the "problem of the relationship between the institutions of public health and the citizenry on whose behalf they claim to act is the greatest challenge currently facing public health in the developed world" (Detels et al. 2009). It is from this perspective that we suggest the role of public health demands a paradigm shift. A strictly reactive, policing, or preventive approach to public health ignores the current health conditions confronting individuals, if not worldwide, certainly in the United States and other developed countries. A holistic or systems approach accepts that health does not exist in a vacuum and that the health of a society's physical environment, culture, and economics manifests in the individual health status of its citizens.

DISEASE PREVENTION

Why does disease prevention not suffice as a model for public health? What is the relationship between public health, the health of the individual, and disease prevention? A focus on disease prevention assumes exposure to causative factors of disease; in order to prevent disease, a known state of disease already exists, and attention is paid to the specifically known causative factors of that disease. By the time the disease prevention model is implemented, it is already too late to promote health. Health promotion preempts disease; it shifts the concentration of effort, positing a state of health (or wholeness) as the norm, as something to be supported and encouraged, rather than a state of disease, of something that must be battled. Thus, although disease prevention and health promotion are often conjoined, we argue that the two are distinct activities with distinct motivations and goals.

Incontrovertibly, disease prevention remains the overriding approach to health in the United States as evinced by a search of articles available on PubMed and Medline in 2014, listed in Table 2.1, retrieved using a limited set of search strings.

More than twice as many articles deal with disease prevention as with health promotion. Although 870 articles describe *some form of research on* promoting a healthy weight, over 30,000 deal with obesity prevention. Promoting nonsmoking got only 34 hits, whereas smoking cessation, over 50,000. Increasing physical activity and physical activity appeared in 51,272 and 371,622 articles, respectively, whereas the chronic condition diseases that are fostered through lack of physical activity appeared in 3,445,673 articles.

Clearly, the disease prevention paradigm is not working as effectively as desired to enhance the health of our populace. According to the Centers for Disease Control and Prevention (CDC), the top three causes of death in the United States in 2013 were heart disease, cancer, and at a distance, chronic lower respiratory disease (Centers for Disease Control and Prevention 2013). None of these diseases cause widespread panic in the community in the manner of a raging epidemic. These diseases do not require policing as an unsafe water supply would require, and to date, none are preventable by a vaccine. Yet, all would benefit from a health promotion model.

Because the nature of the predominant health issues confronting our society has changed, so must public health change the way in which it confronts these issues. Cancer may often be attributed to environmental causes, although many remain unidentified or speculative. Although diseases such as heart disease and diabetes can be attributed in part to lifestyle choices, even individual lifestyle

TABLE 2.1
Articles Retrieved Using Various Prevention/Promotion Search Strings

String	Number of Articles Retrieved
Health *promotion*	156,114
Disease *prevention*	344,345
Promoting healthy weight	870
Obesity *prevention*	33,216
Promoting nonsmoking	34
Smoking *cessation*	54,594
Increase fruit and vegetable consumption	1361
Reduce fat intake	2496
Increase physical activity	51,272
Physical activity	371,622
Diabetes mellitus	657,606
Cardiovascular disease	2,022,620
Hypertension	765,447

choices are driven by economic conditions such as poverty or environmental conditions such as a lack of sidewalks in suburban neighborhoods. Furthermore, some of the lifestyle choice risks, such as trans-fat consumption and heart disease, became, through ubiquity in our food supply, hardly choices at all.

The public health workforce and infrastructure are unprepared to meet these challenges. "In most developed countries, public health has narrowed in focus and to a large extent, is driven by the research agenda of academic epidemiologists and biomedical scientists. Its focus has often been on what can be measured easily, such as cholesterol or blood pressure, rather than on the immensely more complex issues of the broader social forces that also affect health, directly or indirectly, such as economic transitions" (Hamlin 2009). A strictly quantitative approach to health neglects critical examination of many of the causes of lack of health. In short, the public health activities induced by a disease prevention model are inadequate.

CURRENT HEALTH BEHAVIORS OF THE US ADULT POPULATION

Only a small portion of the US population adheres to a healthy lifestyle. Four healthy lifestyle characteristics (HLCs)—nonsmoking, healthy weight, fruit and vegetable consumption, and regular physical activity—taken together can serve as a single healthy lifestyle indicator. Using data from the 2000 Behavioral Risk Factor Surveillance System, which surveyed more than 153,000 adults aged 18–74 by phone, researchers determined that only 3% of US adults practiced all four healthy lifestyle behaviors (Reeves and Rafferty 2005).

A subsequent study, using the same four HLCs, examined data from the third National Health and Nutrition Examination Survey (1988–1994) (NHANES III), with a pool of 16,176 adults 21 or older. They found that 6.8% of the population engaged in all four healthy lifestyle factors and concluded that "there is a long road to travel" before a preponderance of Americans adopt a healthy lifestyle (Ford et al. 2001).

Berrigan and colleagues, using five HLCs—they added low alcohol consumption—found that only 6% of US adults adhere to a healthy lifestyle, while at the other end of the spectrum, 5% follow none of the recommendations at all (Berrigan et al. 2003). These findings were further corroborated by a study of people with and without coronary heart disease (CHD), using three HLCs: nonsmoking, fruit and vegetable consumption, and physical activity. Among those without heart disease, 5% adhered to all three behaviors; among those with heart disease, 7% adhered to all three behaviors (adopting a healthier lifestyle subsequent to a heart incident) (Miller et al. 2005).

These studies make abundantly clear that the vast majority of the American public does not engage in healthy lifestyle practices. Yet, as discussed in Chapter 9, *Dietary Guidelines for Americans*—developed jointly by the Department of Health and Human Services (HHS) and the US Department of Agriculture (USDA)—have been available in one form or another since 1980 (*Nutrition and Your Health* 1995). Of note, these guidelines were intended for healthy Americans—and thus adhere to a health promotion model. Yet there are very few healthy Americans according to any of the definitions offered thus far. The guidelines, although exemplary in many ways, may be an instance of *too little, too late*.

The original impetus for the guidelines was the 1977 Dietary Goals for the United States, also known as the McGovern report, issued by the Senate Select Committee on Nutrition and Human Needs. This report was particularly distressing to certain special-interest groups because of its recommendation for Americans to reduce their consumption of meat, soft drinks, and total calories (Dietary Guidelines Advisory Committee 2010). In addition, the involvement of the USDA in developing dietary guidelines is considered by many to be in direct conflict with its goal of promoting agriculture, which can be interpreted as a goal to increase consumption (Nestle 2002). Awareness of both these issues—the negative impact of lobbying by private industry and potential conflicts of interest of government agencies—must be maintained when developing a health-promoting ideology.

Furthermore, the questionable efficacy of these guidelines and the accompanying MyPlate (though a significant improvement over the preceding MyPyramid) in producing a healthy population—regardless of their scientific/quantitative accuracy—indicates that simply tossing such guidance out into the public arena without simultaneously providing a supportive environment in which to follow them is basically futile.

DISEASE PROMOTION

Compounding the inadequacies of disease prevention in our society are activities that are directly disease promoting. As Freudenberg notes, "Inadequate housing is associated with a variety of physical and mental problems" (Freudenberg 2000). Homelessness or overcrowding results from a number of disease-promoting policies including reduced federal support for low-income housing, conversion of low-income housing to middle- or upper-income housing, increases in the number of people living in poverty or having low-wage jobs, and deinstitutionalization of the mentally ill without compensating community mental health services (Freudenberg 2000).

Further, whereas the last 25 years have seen environmental conditions in the United States generally improve, air, lead, particulate matter, and other forms of pollution in urban communities continue to be associated with increased rates of illness and death.

The activities of the tobacco industry, gun manufacturers, the alcohol industry, illicit drug dealers, and producers of high-fat, low-nutrient-value foods all encourage disease promotion (Freudenberg 2000).

Urban dwellers often feel unsafe in their own neighborhoods because of real or perceived potential for crime, whereas suburbanites, deprived of sidewalks, also feel unsafe, deterred from physical activity by fear of speeding traffic. Although urban planners have been rethinking designs to integrate physical activity within the natural flow of daily routines, such as encouraging children to walk to school and play in playgrounds, and adults to jog and cycle, these efforts must continue to increase, particularly in suburban and rural communities.

HISTORY OF HEALTH PROMOTION

Generally, a broader-based interpretation of health promotion has international origins, stemming from the work of WHO to define health and to make explicit the role of governments in the health of their citizens. In 1978, a combined conference of WHO and the United Nations International Children's Emergency Fund (UNICEF) in Alma Ata, Soviet Union, with 134 nations present, confirmed WHO's original definition of health and noted that people are affected by their social, economic, and natural environments. This declaration led to the development in 1981 of the Global Strategy for Health for All by the Year 2000. Although the Global Strategy failed to meet this deadline for health for all, the tenets of the Global Strategy are illustrative. The major components of this strategy include equity in health; health promotion; preventive activity in primary healthcare settings; cooperation between government, communities, and the private sector; and increased community participation (*Global Strategy for Health* 1981).

However, the Alma Ata Declaration failed to provide an identifiable framework for action, spurring a series of international conferences on health promotion. The first of these conferences, held in Ottawa in 1986, resulted in the Ottawa Charter for Health Promotion. The Ottawa Charter stressed that health promotion is "the process of enabling people to increase control over, and to improve their health" (World Health Organization, http://www.who.int/healthpromotion/Milestones_Health _Promotion_05022010.pdf) and that "health promotion is not just the responsibility of the health sector" (*Ottawa Charter for Health Promotion* 1986). WHO has continued pushing and developing a health promotion agenda, holding Global Conferences on Health Promotion in Adelaide, Australia (1988); Sundsvall, Sweden (1991); Jakarta, Indonesia (1997); Mexico City, Mexico (2000); Bangkok, Thailand (2005); Nairobi, Kenya (2009); and Helsinki, Finland (2013).

The main theme of the 2013 conference was "Health in All Policies" (HiAP), and its focus was on implementation, the *how-to*, which is structured around the following six themes (World Health Organization, http://www.who.int/entity/healthpromotion/conferences/8gchp/background/en/index .html):

1. Facilitate the exchange of experiences and lessons learned and give guidance on effective mechanisms for promoting intersectoral action.
2. Review approaches to address barriers and build capacity for implementing HiAP.
3. Identify opportunities to implement the recommendations of the Commission on Social Determinants of Health through HiAP.
4. Establish and review the economic, developmental, and social case for investing in HiAP.
5. Address the contribution of health promotion in the renewal and reform of primary healthcare.
6. Review progress, impact, and achievements of health promotion since the Ottawa Conference.

The documents arising from these conferences contain sensitive analyses, impressive goals, and sweeping calls to action. But has this work fallen on deaf ears? Are individual nations acting upon the ideas and philosophies espoused by these conference findings?

For instance, in the United States, the CDC's Healthy Communities Program (formerly Steps to a HealthierUS, discussed in Chapter 4) "aims to prevent chronic diseases by working to reduce health-risk factors. It also supports efforts to attain health equity—that means making sure all people can reach their full health potential," (Centers for Disease Control and Prevention 2014), an idea in agreement with a health promotion perspective. Yet, the USDA's online description of the initiative is this: "The programs focus on reducing the burden of diabetes, obesity and asthma and address three related risk behaviors—physical inactivity, poor nutrition, and tobacco use" (US Department of Agriculture 2012). In other words, the primary targets of this initiative remain personal choices made by individuals, without including or acknowledging the impact of the physical, social, political, or commercial environments on individual health.

ROLES OF HEALTH PROMOTION

How does an emphasis on health promotion change our perception of the appropriate activities of public health? How do we go about promoting health promotion? How do we make it fundamental to various fields outside of, but connected to, public health—for example, town planning, where children can no longer walk safely to school, or architecture, where inadequately thought-through designs result in sick-building syndrome.

Public health cannot be seen as isolated within its own self-contained bubble. Rather, public health must become a component of urban planning, architecture, engineering, legislation, and so on. The concept of environment refers to more than just the physical arena in which people live, work, and play, and also includes social, economic, and cultural dimensions (Tones 2002).

Grounding public health in health promotion recognizes and appreciates that numerous professions—law, engineering, human relations, public service, and so on—are currently, though perhaps unwittingly, engaged in public health. That "many disciplines are needed to understand the links between the underlying and proximal determinants of health" (Beaglehole et al. 2004) is as much a potential strength of public health as it is a weakness. The goal would then be to make explicit the ideal of health promotion in fields of study as disparate as law, engineering, architecture, and city planning. Exposing students of these fields to the concepts of public health and health promotion is fundamental to achieving a true paradigm shift. Expanding the definition of who is a public health worker increases the ability of the public health workforce to meet current challenges.

TOWARD IMPROVED HEALTH PROMOTION

Different individuals and organizations have developed their own definitions of health promotion, interpreting the term to match their agendas and philosophies, often equating health promotion with health education. Yet, the traditional preventive approach of relying on health education has limited effectiveness (Tones 2002). Within traditional healthcare settings, health promotion gasps for life as an almost irrelevant subset of disease prevention. Health promotion is a phenomenon that takes place almost entirely outside the 10–20 minutes available for a clinical encounter (longest for babies and for the elderly) and targets specific health risks or behaviors. Health promotion is considered to include nutrition counseling and advice; smoking cessation education; weight loss and weight management education; prenatal education; health-risk assessment; sexually transmitted disease (STD) prevention; stress management education; and substance abuse counseling (McMenamin et al. 2004). This pale attempt at health promotion in which physicians might play only a very small role is the wrong mindset, and many of the programs listed arise from a disease prevention perspective, not one of health promotion. A smoking cessation or substance abuse program, for example, is not health promoting in the same manner as a nutrition education program, nor is nutrition education through a program at a local clinic health promoting in the same manner as it would be if provided within the flow of elementary school education.

Moving beyond the healthcare setting, an ecological approach to health promotion consisting of integrating environmental and individual targets of intervention across a variety of settings (Richard et al. 1996) risks being not broad based enough in application. Without national and supranational support, grassroots efforts are attempting to slay giants. Confronting asthma among children in the South Bronx will always pit David against Goliath—with David's slingshot sometimes hitting its mark after prodigious effort—until Goliath agrees that situating a preponderance of bus stations, transfer stations, and waste incinerators and their ilk in low-income neighborhoods is not a health-promoting policy. This is in no way meant to denigrate grassroots programs, without which the health status of our nation would be further diminished. Nor does it predict their demise. We intend to suggest a shift in perspective whereby the goals of grassroots programs would be supported by the system at large.

Freudenberg, a distinguished professor of Urban Health at Hunter College, City University of New York, suggests 10 ways, some overlapping, to promote health. Although the suggestions are specifically aimed at urban environments, they are applicable as well to suburban, ex-urban, and rural environments.

1. Give access to quality primary care.
2. Increase health knowledge (*this, presumably, would contribute to the next point*).
3. Reduce risky behaviors.
4. Increase social support (*not clear how this differs from item 9 and possibly item 5*).
5. Reduce stigma and marginalization.
6. Advocate health-promoting policies.
7. Improve urban physical environments (*a direct result of item 6 in the right environment*).
8. Meet basic needs (*not clear how this differs from item 10*).
9. Create supportive social environments (*essentially the same as 4*).
10. Reduce income inequality.

Although Freudenberg does not prioritize these strategies, a health promotion model embracing these goals would do so, placing advocacy of health-promoting policies at the top of the list and access to quality primary healthcare toward the bottom as the first would reduce the need for the second. Interestingly, two of these strategies directly coincide with two of the four primary building blocks for health discussed at the beginning of this chapter, namely, basic needs (item #8 here), and access to information (item #2 here). These include building the first block, basic needs (item #8 here), and the second block, access to information (item #2 here), as well.

EXAMPLES OF HEALTH PROMOTION ACTIVITIES

CARDIOVASCULAR DISEASE

A comprehensive community program for health promotion was initiated in Finland in 1972 after a *petition by the local population* was submitted to the government, asking that something be done to reduce high CVD rates in the area (McAlister et al. 1982). The government had failed the population in helping to provide a health-promoting environment. Although the aims of the program were to improve detection and control of hypertension, reduce smoking, and improve dietary habits, an intriguing by-product of the intervention, in addition to improved health in neighboring townships due to "leakage," was the creation of new food products such as a sausage that substituted mushrooms for some meat and fat and low-fat milk (at no increase in cost), as well as increased consumer demand for these products. As the authors note, "The environment is often a determining influence on behavior and may be a direct influence on health" (McAlister et al. 1982).

Even though this appears to have been initiated at a grassroots level, it must be noted that the population, knowing their health was at risk, asked the government to intervene to help create a health-promoting environment rather than a disease-promoting environment (or even a disease-preventing one). Thus, health promotion requires a coordinated systems approach and cannot be relegated only to the piecemeal efforts of community-based organizations.

TOBACCO AND SUGAR CONTROL MEASURES

Although cigarette smoking remains the leading cause of preventable death in the United States, a disease prevention rather than a health promotion perspective on public health gives rise to escalating wars of advertising by tobacco companies and counterintelligence by community organizations, national organizations such as the American Heart Association (AHA), and private foundations. As long as health-promoting policies such as limitations on advertising for known causes of cancer are denigrated as contrary to the First Amendment and freedom of speech, defensive disease prevention actions such as increases in taxes on cigarettes, the Smoke-Free Air Act passed in 2002, and nicotine-dependence treatment guidelines for physicians are imperative.

Of these actions described above, the cigarette tax was most effective in reducing smoking. The tax inherently disproportionately affected low-income users yet nonetheless exposed 67,000 fewer nonsmokers to the negative health impact of exposure to cigarette smoke (Frieden et al. 2005). Yet, even though tobacco taxation has shown efficacy, efforts to encourage similar taxation solutions that reduce the consumption of junk food or sugar have been much harder to implement.

Sugar-sweetened beverages in particular have been linked to obesity and other health concerns (Olsen and Heitmann 2009). Most states in the United States already have small taxes on sugared beverages and snack items (Brownell and Frieden 2009). However, unlike localities that have introduced tobacco taxation with an eye toward guiding behavior, these small taxes on junk food items are usually in line with tax rates on other food items and do not provide a clear message or incentive as to the desired behavior. For example, as of 2011, 40 states tax soda at an average rate of 5.2%, but only in 5 states is the tax 7.0% or higher (Wang et al. 2012).

Following Kelley Brownell's 1994 proposal of a tax on junk food, derided as a "Twinkie tax" or a "fat tax," attempts have been made across the United States to introduce such taxes, and 20 years later, we are finally seeing progress. As of September 2014, nine states had sugar-sweetened beverage tax proposals filed in the current legislative session, some as sales tax, some as excise tax, and many with the idea of earmarking the proceeds to support health-related foods or activities, or obesity prevention (Yale Rudd Center for Food Policy and Obesity, http://www.yaleruddcenter.org/legislation/legislation_trends.aspx).

Taxation strategy is also being pursued at a local municipality level. In November of 2014, Berkeley, California, passed a tax on sugar-sweetened beverages that included café-served coffee beverages (Aliferis 2014). The Berkeley tax is based on the amount of sugar added, instead of the size of the beverages. A June 2014 study funded by the Robert Wood Johnson Foundation found that a calorie-based tax on sugar-sweetened beverages was more effective than a volume-based tax as it would achieve a greater reduction in calories with a smaller effect on the amount that consumers would be willing to pay for a product, and generally, people were more inclined to purchase the cheaper drink (Zhen et al. 2014).

LIFESTYLE COMPARED TO MEDICATION INTERVENTIONS

Herman and colleagues' study of the cost-effectiveness of lifestyle modification compared with the use of the drug metformin in preventing type 2 diabetes perfectly exemplifies the fundamental difference between health promotion and disease prevention (Herman et al. 2005). Whereas both interventions were effective in comparison to a placebo, the lifestyle intervention (health promoting) outclassed the drug (disease preventing) in terms of delaying onset, reducing absolute incidence, and cost per quality of life-year.

Lifestyle intervention increased life expectancy by 0.5 year whereas metformin increased life expectancy by 0.2 year. Associated morbidities such as blindness, end-stage renal disease, amputation, stroke, and CHD were decreased by greater percentages with lifestyle rather than metformin intervention. Overall, the lifestyle intervention provided greater health benefits at lower cost than the metformin intervention (Herman et al. 2005).

WOULD A HEALTH PROMOTION MODEL NEGLECT THE REALITY OF DISEASE?

Health promotion cannot, ultimately, be naive. It would be irresponsible for a health promotion perspective to neglect the reality of disease and the need for clinical and social interventions. However, the need for such interventions would be reduced by a truly health-promoting model.

Paul Farmer, a medical anthropologist and physician, is a founding director of Partners in Health, an international nonprofit organization that, since 1987, has provided direct healthcare services and undertaken research and advocacy activities on behalf of those who are sick and living in poverty. Farmer and his colleagues have pioneered strategies in community-based treatment.

In "The Consumption of the Poor: Tuberculosis in the 21st Century," Farmer details the occurrence of tuberculosis (TB) in three separate individuals. Of the first, Jean Dubuisson, Farmer writes, "… Jean is a member of [Haiti's] only truly productive class: the rural peasantry. But membership in that class brought certain 'birthrights.'" As a subsistence farmer, Jean belongs to the poorest class in the hemisphere and is thus ensured the "right" not to attend school, to lack electricity or safe drinking water, and to have little access to medical care. He also has no role whatsoever in running the country he and those like him support (Farmer 2000).

A health promotion model would not permit lack of education, lack of safe water, denial of medical care, and political disenfranchisement. These are fundamental to the concept of health promotion.

The second individual, Corina Bayona, a Peruvian woman who migrated from an unforgiving countryside to a sprawling slum, typifies Latin Americans living with multidrug-resistant TB. Although Peru has been praised for its improved TB control program, Corina was sick and infectious for at least 6 years, during which she worked, taking crowded buses across Lima twice a day (Farmer 2000). Throughout the course of her illness, Corina was frequently upbraided for noncompliance rather than receiving help (or, at the very least, sympathy), because she did not have the time to travel to distant clinics, could not afford the medicines prescribed, or remained untreated because of a health workers' strike (Farmer 2000).

The story of the third individual reveals perhaps the most egregious failure of the disease prevention model. Calvin Loach—a United States citizen, a Vietnam vet, an African American, and an injection-drug user—received inappropriate care and was eventually "lost to follow-up." Farmer cites a 1991 study conducted at Harlem Hospital that found that nearly 90% of patients did not complete their drug therapy for TB. The New York City Department of Health's overview for 1992 observed that the TB case rate in central Harlem of 222 per 100,000 exceeded that of many Third World countries (Farmer 2000).

Farmer wisely contends that even if we lack the means to reduce poverty and social inequalities, "few data ... support the hypothesis that there are insufficient means to cure all tuberculosis cases, everywhere" (Farmer 2000). As we move toward a health promotion model, it is imperative to persist in disease treatment and prevention and avoid a blame-the-victim mentality. Yet the causes of Jean's, Corina's, and Calvin's illnesses are rooted not in disease but in social displacement and economic deprivation. In 1923, Allen Krause had observed, "More or less poverty in a community will mean more or less tuberculosis, so will more or less crowding and improper housing, more or less unhygienic occupations and industry" (Farmer 2000).

Without a health promotion model, other diseases or TB itself will recur with continued displacement of populations, with devaluation of agricultural workers, and with overcrowding.

Although Haiti and Peru are poorer countries than the United States (Haiti significantly more so than Peru), the poor face similar problems in all three countries. Thus, it is not a matter simply of money but of political will.

HEALTH PROMOTION: POLITICS AND PUBLIC POLICY

Health promotion is inherently political (Seedhouse 2009). Seedhouse's observation that there are facts, there are opinions masquerading as facts, and many health promotion strategies are value driven is well taken. Seedhouse writes: "In all cases [whether consciousness-raising about social injustice or non-smoking strategies] it is political philosophy (however implicit) which fires health promotion" (Seedhouse 2009). This understanding of the political nature of health promotion is also evident in Freudenberg's sixth strategy—advocating health-promoting policies. Freudenberg notes that public health strategies for policy change encompass legislative and electoral advocacy, media campaigns, and lawsuits (Freudenberg 2000).

The Jakarta Declaration of 1997 (http://www.ldb.org/iuhpe/jakdec.htm) noted that trends such as urbanization threaten "the health and well-being of millions of people." Urbanization is far more than a trend. Urbanization is a direct result of governmental policies that support agribusiness, monocropping, and crop exportation rather than small, local food systems and farmers. Such policies deprive subsistence farmers of their land, driving them into overcrowded cities where the spread of disease is rampant. Thus, public health practitioners need to acknowledge the political nature of the urbanization process and developing health policy and act accordingly (Beaglehole et al. 2004).

This is not to suggest, however, that our current policies are completely devoid of a health-promoting ideology. In fact, a number of policies codified as federal, state, or local law have been instituted throughout the course of our history. The following provide examples of positive health-promoting policies:

- Theodore Roosevelt's creation of national parks, 1900–1901.
- Poultry Products Inspection Act, 1957.
- Federal Meat Inspection Act, 1967.
- Egg Products Inspection Act, 1970.
- Clean Water Act, 1987 (a reauthorization of a 1972 act).
- Clean Air Act, 1990.
- American with Disabilities Act, 1990.
- Senate Appropriations Committee's $2 million expansion of the USDA Fruit and Vegetable Snack Program, 2005.

- Healthy People 2020 and predecessors.
- Affordable Care Act, 2010.
- US surgeon general's national prevention and health promotion strategy, 2011.

There is, however, no unified approach with a consistent philosophical base. These policies are enforced under the aegis of many different agencies, are often not perceived as public health initiatives *per se*, and are frequently undermined by monetary interests of private industry.

Health Promotion and Universal Healthcare

Healthcare is an important component of health promotion. Farmer asks, "As a global economy is 'restructured', is there no room for alternative strategies of development—alternative visions of providing healthcare to the poor?" He notes that the pharmaceutical, insurance, and healthcare industries as well as international agencies (particularly financial institutions) increasingly determine who has access to effective medical care. Refreshingly, he contends that the power of technological advancement stems not merely from the wonders of science but from the power of moral persuasion. We can insist on certain measures not because they are cost-effective but because they are the best we can do for the sick (Farmer 2000).

However, healthcare should not receive undue focus as a solution. Universal healthcare, although imperative, is not a substitute for a health promotion paradigm. In fact, one could argue that the weaker the health promotion ethos within a society, the greater the need for healthcare—poor health being a logical outcome of poor health promotion.

On a more detailed level, evaluation of health education programs and responsibility for their implementation and effectiveness are key aspects of health promotion. McMenamin and colleagues' study of *health promotion* in physician practice groups found that with each additional reporting requirement, there was a 37% increase in the odds of offering some type of health promotion program (McMenamin et al. 2004).

Role of the Individual in Public Health

The role of personal responsibility in achieving health cannot be overlooked or overemphasized. Traditionally, public health in the United States has taken a market-based approach that limits government responsibility for public health and places the burden of health improvement on the individual (Beaglehole et al. 2004).

But the United States is nowhere near an ideal, health-promoting society where the healthier choice would be the easier choice, and health cannot be left solely to personal responsibility. Most of us are outsiders some of the time, not compelled by the need to behave according to the "rules," whether by being overly lazy or daring, or by consuming less than the recommended five to nine fruits and vegetables every day or more than the recommended shot (or two, for men) of alcohol (Seedhouse 2009). Low-income people, for example, eating a less-than-optimal diet, may be perfectly aware of what they *should* be eating but nonetheless unable to access or afford the recommended healthy diet. In a society with health promotion as its overriding agenda, access to fresh, good-quality produce would be comparable to access to saturated fats and added sugars that are easily and cheaply available today.

Many people, regardless of socioeconomic status, may make less-than-optimal choices in order to fill psychological needs. In our present society, "even those diseases most closely linked to lifestyle choice could be attributed to the broader social environment ... To expect disciplined personal behavior from alienated people living in a stressful world would be unrealistic, and the institutions of public health should recognize this ... How absurd, for example, for a state to subsidize the production of tobacco and the addiction to it of people in other nations, whilst blaming its own citizens for smoking" (Detels et al. 2009). How absurd it would be to blame Jean Dubuisson, Corina Bayona, or Calvin Loach for contracting TB.

NEW DEFINITION OF PUBLIC HEALTH'S ROLE

The goal of health promotion should be fundamental to, and pervasive across, disciplines, with the ultimate goal being a healthy and enabling environment. Collective action is justified because health is both an end in itself—a human right—as well as a prerequisite for achieving human potential (Beaglehole et al. 2004; Seedhouse 2009). Public health must acknowledge the direct impact of environmental and socioeconomic circumstances on decisions individuals make about health (Beaglehole et al. 2004; Tones 2002). A health-promoting environment enables the individual to make choices, even if the choices an individual makes may not always be what a public health practitioner or another informed citizen might define as healthy.

A health-promoting society is one with coherent public policy initiatives, constant evaluation of policy, universal healthcare, the ability to see beyond market-driven imperatives, and a clearly articulated definition of health. It also requires full engagement of the community in decision making, planning, and implementation.

Health Promotion Is Three-Dimensional

In their book *Just and Lasting Change*, Daniel Taylor-Ide and Carl E. Taylor (2002) describe how health-focused change has been implemented, successfully or otherwise, in communities around the world and the lessons learned over the last 100 years. Collaboration amongst three dimensions are fundamental and *of equal importance* to community change (in other words, creation of a health-promoting environment):

1. Bottom-up actions by people (the community)
2. Top-down policies from government (support through policy initiatives)
3. Outside-in contributions of ideas and skills (expertise)

In addition, these actions must be based on locally specific *and gathered* data. And, finally, a simple annual community work plan—no logic models, no situational analyses, just an assignment of who will do what for the coming year—can support a change in collective behavior.

The authors' model for inclusive change is termed Self-Evaluation for Effective Decision Making and Systems for Communities to Adapt Learning and Expand (SEED-SCALE). SEED promotes the idea that "decisions not grounded in local data often are isolated from the people" through the use of generating a local database that allows the yearly work plan to self-correct. It is not full-scale research about a community.

SCALE defines the growth of program implementation along the three dimensions—beginning with the community, through contributions from outside experts such as community and public health nutritionists, to an enabling environment of policies and financing. Programs that initially succeed but are co-opted by one dimension or another, such as government oversight replacing community volunteers, ultimately fail. As Kim Travers notes, experts often determine barriers to nutritional health and make recommendations without consulting the "victims," resulting in health promotion that disempowers people by denying them knowledge of root causes of nutrition problems and the opportunity to act for change on their own behalf (Travers 1997).

CONCLUSION

The need to shift the focus of public health in the United States from disease prevention to health promotion—as described both here and in documents produced by bodies such as the WHO and international conferences on health promotion—is a vital and fascinating topic, which deserves further exploration. The observations in this chapter are but the tip of the iceberg, raising more questions than they answer.

Medicine and public health are two complementary and interacting approaches for promoting and protecting health. Epidemic events and humanitarian emergencies have created new relationships among medicine, public health, ethics, and human rights. Each domain has seeped into the others, making allies of public health, pressing the need for an ethics of public health, and revealing the rights-related responsibilities of physicians and other healthcare workers (Mann 1997). In the United States, the American Board of Preventive Medicine combines public health and general preventive medicine to prevent disease and manage the health of communities. These practitioners gain public health skills and tailor them in primary, secondary, and tertiary prevention-oriented clinical practice in a wide range of settings (Board of Certification, American Board of Preventive Medicine, https://www.theabpm.org/certification.cfm).

The change in the nature of the diseases most affecting society—from germ based to environmental based—must be reflected in the practice of public health. The current health behaviors of the US adult population indicate that the disease prevention model of public health is ineffective at best and destructive at worst. Public health in the United States must develop a unified approach with a consistent philosophical base, coordinated among the numerous government agencies whose efforts impact the public health.

As a call for action, two changes affecting public policy and professional education in the United States are suggested. First, just as an environmental impact statement must be prepared prior to construction of bridges, dams, and tunnels, a health impact statement should be written for housing projects, employment and unemployment policies, healthcare plans, the building of roadways, agricultural policies, and so on. Second, awareness of public health issues must influence the practice of professions from politics to transportation. Therefore, public health and health promotion must become a part of the core curriculum of numerous professional programs throughout the country.

ACRONYMS

AHA	American Heart Association
CHD	Coronary heart disease
CVD	Cardiovascular disease
HHS	United States Department of Health and Human Services
HLC	Health lifestyle characteristic
NCD	Noncommunicable disease
NHANES III	Third National Health and Nutrition Examination Survey
SCALE	Systems for Communities to Adapt Learning and Expand
SEED	Self-Evaluation for Effective Decision Making
STD	Sexually transmitted disease
TB	Tuberculosis
UNICEF	United Nations International Children's Emergency Fund
USDA	United States Department of Agriculture
WHO	World Health Organization

STUDENT ASSIGNMENTS AND ACTIVITIES DESIGNED TO ENHANCE LEARNING AND STIMULATE CRITICAL THINKING

1. Describe how the role of public health changed over the twentieth century and how it has developed to the present. What do you think will be the role of public health in the future?

2. What is the present role of government, schools, communities, parents, children, and role models in public health? What do you think would be the best way to increase public health awareness? What are some of the challenges to improving the population's lifestyle to be a healthier one?

3. Fashion models are often considered to be underweight. Search the Internet for policies that set a minimum weight for models. Use the following key words to help guide your search: models, rules/policies/laws, underweight, minimum weight. Where did you find this website? What is your opinion of this policy?

4. List three nutrition-related diseases. Describe how each of these diseases can be prevented through strong public health policy initiatives.

5. Research the social–ecological model as a framework for health promotion. How can this model be used to promote the four healthy lifestyle characteristics (HLCs): nonsmoking, healthy weight, fruit and vegetable consumption, and regular physical activity? Give an example of an intervention at each level for each HLC.

	Nonsmoking	Healthy Weight	Fruit and Vegetable Consumption	Regular Physical Activity
Individual				
Interpersonal				
Organizational				
Community				
Society/Policy/Systems				

6. The National Environmental Policy Act (NEPA) requires all federal agencies to consider the potential environmental impact of their proposed actions. To meet this requirement, federal agencies prepare a detailed statement—known as an environmental impact statement (EIS)—to help ensure that all environmental effects are thought of in the policy and decision-making process. Unfortunately, similar efforts are not required to assess potential health impacts; many public policies and federal programs, such as transportation, education, housing, and welfare, do not have health impact as their primary goal and do not consider health when making decisions. A potentially useful tool for policy makers, then, is a health impact statement (HIS), which would take into account the health impact of proposed policies or programs.

Part 1. Search the Internet for some examples of HISs.
   a. How has the HIS been applied?
   b. What were the findings?
   c. Did the proposed policy or program change as a result of the HIS?

Part 2. Using http://www.congress.gov (formerly THOMAS), choose a piece of legislation related to education or housing that has been introduced to the current Congress.
   a. What questions would you ask if you were performing an HIS on this piece of legislation?
   b. With what other health and/or nonhealth professionals and stakeholders would you need to collaborate?
   c. What organizations and/or agencies would be able to provide you with the additional information you need?
   d. How do you think the results of your efforts would affect the final legislation?

REFERENCES

Aliferis L. Here's what would be taxed—Or not—In SF, Berkeley soda tax measures, *KQED*, October 29, 2014. Available at http://blogs.kqed.org/stateofhealth/2014/10/29/heres-what-would-be-taxed-or-not-in-sf -berkeley-soda-tax-measures/, accessed February 2, 2015.

Beaglehole R, Bonita R, Horton R, Adams O, McKee M. Public health in the new era: Improving health through collective action. *Lancet*. 2004;363(9426):2084–2086.

Berrigan D, Dodd K, Troiana RP, Krebs-Smith SM, Barbash RB. Patterns of health behavior in U.S. adults. *Prev Med*. 2003;36:615–623.

Board of Certification. American Board of Preventive Medicine. Available at https://www.theabpm.org/certification .cfm, accessed February 2, 2015.

Brownell KD, Frieden TR. Ounces of prevention—The public policy case for taxes on sugared beverages. *N Engl J Med*. 2009;360:1805–1808.

Centers for Disease Control and Prevention. Deaths and Mortality. 2013. Available at http://www.cdc.gov/nchs /fastats/deaths, accessed June 29, 2015.

Centers for Disease Control and Prevention. CDC's Healthy Communities Program, Program Overview. Last updated October 31, 2014. Available at http://www.cdc.gov/nccdphp/dch/programs/healthycommunitiesprogram /overview/index.htm, accessed February 2, 2015.

Detels R, Beaglehole R, Lansang MA, Gulliford M, eds. *Oxford Textbook of Public Health*, 5th ed. Oxford, UK: Oxford University Press, 2009.

Dietary Guidelines Advisory Committee. Report of the Dietary Guidelines Advisory Committee on the Dietary Guidelines for Americans, Appendix E-4, History of the Dietary Guidelines for Americans, 2010. Available at http://origin.www.cnpp.usda.gov/Publications/DietaryGuidelines/2010/DGAC/Report/E-Appendix-E -4-History.pdf, accessed February 2, 2015.

Farmer PE. The consumption of the poor: Tuberculosis in the 21st century. *Ethnography*. 2000;1(2):183–216.

Ford ES, De Proost Ford MA, Will JC, Galuska DA, Ballew C. Achieving a healthy lifestyle among United States adults: A long way to go. *Ethn Dis*. 2001;11:224–231.

Freudenberg N. Health promotion in the city: A review of current practice and future prospects in the United States. *Ann Rev Public Health*. 2000;21:473–503.

Frieden TR, Mostashari F, Kerker BD, Miller N, Hajat A, Frankel M. Adult tobacco use levels after intensive tobacco control measures: New York City, 2002–2003. *Am J Public Health*. 2005;95:1016–1023.

Global Strategy for Health for All by the Year 2000. Geneva: World Health Organization, 1981, reprinted 1989. Available at http://whqlibdoc.who.int/publications/9241800038.pdf, accessed December 4, 2014.

Hamlin C. The history and development of public health in developed countries. In *Oxford Textbook of Public Health*. Detels R. et al. 2009 (eds.) Oxford, UK: Oxford University Press, 2009, pp. 20–38. Available at http://oxfordmedicine.com/view/10.1093/med/9780199218707.001.0001/med-9780199218707-chapter -0102, accessed February 2, 2015.

Hemmerly-Brown A. Retired military leaders worry recruit population is 'Too Fat to Fight'. U.S. Army, August 24, 2010. Available at http://www.army.mil/article/44173, accessed February 2, 2015.

Herman WH, Hoerger TJ, Brandle M et al. The cost-effectiveness of lifestyle modification or metformin in preventing type 2 diabetes in adults with impaired glucose tolerance. *Ann Intern Med*. 2005;142:323–332.

The Jakarta Declaration on Health Promotion into the 21st Century. Available at http://www.ldb.org/iuhpe /jakdec.htm, accessed February 2, 2015.

Mann JM. Medicine and public health, ethics and human rights. *Hastings Cent Rep*. 1997;27(3):6–13.

McAlister A, Puska P, Salonen J, Tuomilehto J, Koskela K. Theory and action for health promotion: Illustrations from the North Karelia project. *AJPH*. 1982;72:43–49.

McMenamin SB, Schmittdiel J, Halpin HA, Gillies R, Rundall TG, Shortell SM. Health promotion in physician organizations: Results from a national study. *Am J Prev Med*. 2004;26:259–264.

Miller RR, Sales AE, Kopjar B, Fihn SD, Bryson CL. Adherence to heart-healthy behaviors in a sample of the U.S. population. *Prev Chron Dis*. 2005;2(2):A18.

Nestle M. *Food Politics*. Berkeley, CA: University of California Press, 2002.

Ng M, Fleming T, Robison M et al. Global, regional, and national prevalence of overweight and obesity in children and adults during 1980–2013: A systematic analysis for the Global Burden of Disease Study 2013. *Lancet*. 2014;384(9945):766–781.

Nutrition and Your Health: Dietary Guidelines for Americans, 4th ed., 1995. Appendix I: History of dietary guidelines for Americans. Available at http://www.health.gov/dietaryguidelines/dga95/12DIETAP.HTM, accessed February 2, 2015.

The Nutrition Transition. Obesity Prevention Source. School of Public Health. Harvard. Available at http:// www.hsph.harvard.edu/obesity-prevention-source/nutrition-transition/#references, accessed February 2, 2015.

Olsen N, Heitmann BL. Intake of calorically sweetened beverages and obesity. *Obesity Rev.* 2009;10(1):68–75.

Online Etymology Dictionary, Health. Available at http://www.etymonline.com, accessed February 2, 2015.

Ottawa Charter for Health Promotion, 1986. Available at http://www.euro.who.int/en/publications/policy -documents/ottawa-charter-for-health-promotion,-1986, accessed February 2, 2015.

Popkin BM. Global nutrition dynamics: The world is shifting rapidly toward a diet linked with noncommunicable diseases. *Am J Clin Nutr.* 2006;84(2):289–298.

Preamble to the Constitution of the World Health Organization as adopted by the International Health Conference, New York, June 19–22, 1946; signed on July 22, 1946 by the representatives of 61 States (Official Records of the World Health Organization, no. 2, p. 100) and entered into force on April 7, 1948. Available at http://www.who.int/about/definition/en/print.html, accessed December 23, 2014.

Reeves MJ, Rafferty AP. Healthy lifestyle characteristics among adults in the United States. *Arch Intern Med.* 2005;165:854–857.

Richard L, Potvin L, Kishchuk N, Prlic H, Green LW. Assessment of the integration of the ecological approach in health promotion programs. *Am J Health Promot.* 1996;10:318–328.

Seedhouse D. *Health Promotion: Philosophy, Prejudice, and Practice*, 2nd ed. Wiley, Chicester, 2009.

Taylor-Ide D, Taylor CE. *Just and Lasting Change: When Communities Own Their Futures.* Johns Hopkins University Press, Baltimore, 2002.

Tones K. Health promotion, health education, and the public health. In Detels R, McEwen J, Beaglehole R, Tanaka H, eds. *The Oxford Textbook of Public Health*, 4th ed. The Scope of Public Health. Oxford, UK: Oxford University Press, 2002, pp. 829–863.

Travers KD. Nutrition education for social change: Critical perspective. *JNEB.* 1997;29(2):57–62.

United States Department of Agriculture. National Institute of Food and Agriculture. Steps to a Healthier US. Last updated February 2, 2012. Available at http://www.nifa.usda.gov/nea/food/part/health_part_steps .html, accessed February 2, 2015.

Wang YC, Coxson P, Shen YM, Goldman L, Bibbins-Domingo K. Tax policy measure: A penny-per-ounce tax on sugar-sweetened beverages would cut health and cost burdens of diabetes. *Health Affairs.* 2012;31:1199–1207. doi:10.1377/hlthaff.2011.0410.

World Health Organization. Health Promotion. Milestones in Health Promotion. Statements from Global Conferences. Available at http://www.who.int/healthpromotion/Milestones_Health_Promotion_05022010 .pdf, accessed December 23, 2014.

World Health Organization. The Eighth Global Conference on Health Promotion. Available at http://www.who .int/entity/healthpromotion/conferences/8gchp/background/en/index.html, accessed February 2, 2015.

Yale Rudd Center for Food Policy and Obesity, Legislation Database. Available at http://www.yaleruddcenter .org/legislation/legislation_trends.aspx, accessed September 4, 2014.

Zhen C, Brissette IF, Ruff RR. By ounce or by calorie: The differential effects of alternative sugar-sweetened beverage tax strategies. *Am J Agr Econ.* 2014;96(4):1070–1083.

3 Nutritional Epidemiology

Statistics are no substitute for judgment.

Henry Clay (1777–1852)

INTRODUCTION

Nutritional epidemiology is defined as the study of the nutritional determinants of disease in human populations (Langseth 1996). The function of nutritional epidemiology is to identify and study associations between diet and disease in defined populations. Although it originally focused on nutrient deficiency diseases, contemporary nutritional epidemiology greatly concerns the study of heart disease, cancer, diabetes, osteoporosis, and neural tube defects (NTDs). These irreversible chronic conditions have multiple causes and long latency periods, occur with relatively low frequency (despite a substantial cumulative lifetime risk), and are associated with excessive as well as insufficient intake of nutrients and other food factors (Willett 1998a). A major enterprise of nutritional epidemiology is to assess the efficacy of nutrition interventions—including nutrition education, policies, and programs—and to develop diet assessment methods that enable public health officials and researchers to monitor dietary intake and other health-related behaviors of defined populations. Epidemiological methods are widely applied in public health nutrition, and even practitioners who do not carry out surveys themselves will find that their public health practice is influenced by epidemiological observations.

In this chapter, we first look at some of the dietary assessment tools used to determine what people eat, including food frequency questionnaires (FFQs) and diet histories, and biochemical markers that indicate dietary intake. We then examine the types of studies used in nutritional epidemiology, including the use of controlled clinical trials. Two landmark experimental studies in nutritional deficiencies are included in this review: Lind's (1747) experiment that demonstrated that limes cure scurvy and Goldberger's (1914) experiments demonstrating that a diet containing animal products prevents and cures pellagra. We then review how controlled clinical trials are used to research diet-related chronic disease conditions. We conclude with a brief look at the US Department of Agriculture's (USDA's) role in providing data and tools of key importance to nutritional epidemiology, such as information on the food supply and composition.

DIETARY ASSESSMENT

The dietary assessment component of nutritional epidemiology focuses on the various approaches to collecting and analyzing dietary data. There are two functions of the dietary assessment component of nutritional epidemiology. One is to determine the appropriateness of different assessment methods for specific applications, nutrients, and populations. The other is to determine what people eat.

How do we know what people eat? We can watch them, ask them, perform biochemical assays that indicate nutrient intake, or use a combination of these methods. As indicated in Table 3.1, each methodology for determining food intake has its strengths and weaknesses.

OBSERVATION

There are two methods used to determine what people eat by watching them. In the first method, a trained observer is assigned the task of estimating and recording everything eaten by one or several

TABLE 3.1

Strengths and Weaknesses of the Various Methodologies for Determining Food Intake

	Observation	Food/Diet Record	Dietary Recall	Food Frequency Questionnaire	Biomarkers
Strengths	Does not rely on memory or self-report Low respondent burden	Does not rely on memory Can provide data about eating habits and food preparation Can provide detailed intake data Allows for an unlimited level of specificity	Quick and easy to administer Inexpensive Low respondent burden Does not alter usual diet Allows for an unlimited level of specificity	Quick and easy to administer Can be self-administered Inexpensive for large samples Machine-readable: low burden on researcher for analysis and data entry Moderate respondent burden	Does not rely on memory or self-report Can validate other methods of determining dietary intake
Weaknesses	Not appropriate for large studies High researcher burden Requires labor-intensive data collection	Requires high degree of cooperation Not appropriate for large studies Requires labor-intensive analysis and data entry Act of recording may alter diet High respondent burden Respondent must be literate	Relies on memory Requires labor-intensive analysis/data entry Frequent overreporting and underreporting Omissions of dressings and sauces can lead to low estimates of high-fat, sodium-rich foods	Expensive and time-consuming to develop When self-administered, respondent must be literate Depends on ability of respondent to describe diet May not represent usual foods or portion sizes consumed	Expensive Invasive Not all biochemical indicators can be used as markers of nutrient intake

Source: Lee, R.D. and Nieman, D.C., *Nutritional Assessment*, 6th ed., McGraw-Hill, Boston, 2013. Willett, W., *Nutritional Epidemiology*, 2nd ed., Oxford University Press, New York, 1998.

people during a given meal. The second method is known as a plate-waste study. The two most common types of plate-waste studies are weighed and visual. In the weighed study, the amount of food consumed is calculated by subtracting the amount of food waste left after a meal from the amount of food served. Alternatively, the amount of waste can be visually estimated by subtracting the estimated plate waste from the weighed food served (Kirks and Wolff 1985). Using direct observation to determine what people eat is a laborious process that makes it impractical for working with large populations.

SELF-REPORT

Examples of surveys that provide information about an individual's dietary intake include 3- and 7-day diet records, 24-hour dietary recalls, and FFQs.

Diet Records

The diet record is a prospective tool that asks the individual to record everything he or she eats for a specified number of days. Diet records have been found to be superior to FFQs when estimating the amount of nitrogen (a marker for protein), potassium, and sodium consumed (Daya et al. 2001), but the burden on the individual is high, making diet records impractical for large-scale studies. Additionally, diet records require that subjects are literate and motivated. Nevertheless, the American Academy of Family Physicians has posted a sample food diary with instructions at http://familydoctor.org/familydoctor/en/prevention-wellness/food-nutrition/healthy-food-choices/nutrition-keeping-a-food-diary.html.

24-Hour Dietary Recall

The 24-hour dietary recall is a retrospective method that asks the individual to provide detailed information about all foods and beverages consumed over the past 24 hours. Dietary recalls are open-ended and therefore allow for an unlimited level of specificity, which is especially useful when studying culturally diverse groups (Buzzard 1998). Although dietary recalls do not necessitate that respondents be literate, the method does rely on memory and requires a highly trained interviewer. The USDA uses a computerized method—called the automated multiple-pass method (AMPM)—for collecting interviewer-administered 24-hour dietary recalls in What We Eat in America (WWEIA), the dietary interview component of the National Health and Nutrition Examination Survey (NHANES). Information obtained by the AMPM includes a description of the food, additions to the food (such as milk added to cereal), amount of food consumed, time eaten, where the food was obtained, and whether the food was eaten at home. The WWEIA nutrient intake tables are available at http://www.ars.usda.gov/Services/docs.htm?docid=18349.

Food Frequency Questionnaires and Checklists

An FFQ is a common method used to assess individual long-term dietary intake of foods and nutrients. FFQs are retrospective tools used to determine estimates of usual dietary intakes over time (typically 6 months to 1 year) of individuals belonging to groups. The questionnaires elicit a subjectively reported "usual frequency" of consuming an item from a list of foods. The FFQ lists specific foods and asks the subjects if they eat them and, if so, how often and how much. FFQs must be culture specific, with different lists of foods appropriate for assessing diverse diets. Both short (60 food items) and long (100 food items) FFQs have been developed, but none assess current energy intake. Modified FFQs were designed for identification of people with a high intake of dietary fat and/or low intakes of fiber, fruits, and vegetables. Some of these questionnaires were developed to identify potential candidates for enrollment into intervention research studies (Johnson 2002). FFQs are often used in large cohort studies to place individuals into broad categories along a distribution of nutrient intake.

As developing an FFQ is laborious, time-consuming, and costly, the development of FFQs usually requires a major national effort or coordinated task force. Subsequently, FFQs are validated using serial 24-hour recalls, food records, or biomarkers as the gold standard. One well-known and validated FFQ was developed by Dr. Gladys Block at the National Cancer Institute (NCI) for research into the role of diet in health and disease. (NutritionQuest, http://nutritionquest.com/company/our-research-questionnaires). Variations of the Block questionnaire include an FFQ specifically for dialysis patients, FFQs for children of various age groups, and an FFQ focusing on meat. (NutritionQuest, http://nutritionquest.com/assessment/list-of-questionnaires-and-screeners). A list of published studies related to the development and validation of Block assessment tools can be found at http://nutritionquest.com/company/our-research-questionnaires/.

BIOMARKERS

Asking people about their food intake results in self-reports that may be less than accurate. One way to verify self-reports is by the use of biomarkers. Biomarkers are external indicators that reflect food intake by measuring metabolites in urine and serum. Biomarkers have been identified to verify self-reported intake of protein, fatty acids, fruits and vegetables, and energy (Johnson and Hankin 2003). Doubly labeled water (DLW) is currently the most widely used and well-accepted biomarker. It provides an accurate measure in free-living subjects of their total energy expenditure and, hence, energy intake, which is frequently underreported. The use of DLW is based on the principle of energy balance, i.e., if a person is weight stable, then his or her energy expenditure, as measured by DLW, must be equal to his or her energy intake. Because of the high cost and sophisticated technology associated with DLW, it does not lend itself to routine use in clinical settings, but it is used for validating energy intakes obtained from other dietary intake methods (Schoeller 1988).

IMPROVING DIET AND PHYSICAL ACTIVITY ASSESSMENT MODALITIES

Diet and physical activity are lifestyle and behavioral factors that play a role in the etiology and prevention of many chronic diseases, such as cancer and coronary heart disease. Both also play roles in preventing overweight/obesity and in maintaining weight loss. Therefore, diet and physical activity are assessed for both surveillance and epidemiologic/clinical research purposes. The measurement of usual dietary intake or physical activity over varying time periods or in the past, by necessity, has relied on self-report instruments. Such subjective reporting instruments are cognitively difficult for respondents, and they are prone to considerable measurement errors that may vary among population subgroups and depend on the time frame considered and the characteristics of the respondents. As such, the NCI; the National Institute of Diabetes and Digestive and Kidney Diseases (NIDDK); the National Heart, Lung, and Blood Institute (NHLBI); the National Institute on Alcohol Abuse and Alcoholism (NIAAA); the National Institute of Child Health and Human Development (NICHD); the National Institute of Nursing Research (NINR); and the National Institutes of Health (NIH) are interested in promoting innovative research to enhance the quality of measurements of dietary intake and physical activity.

Therefore, through at least 2015, the NIH (2012) will accept proposals for the development of (1) novel assessment approaches; (2) better methods to evaluate instruments; (3) assessment tools for culturally diverse populations or various age groups, including older adults; (4) improved technology or applications of existing technology; (5) statistical methods to assess or correct for measurement errors or biases; (6) methods to investigate the multidimensionality of diet and physical activity behavior through pattern analysis; and (7) integrated measurement of diet and physical activity along with the environmental context of such behaviors.

STUDY DESIGNS IN NUTRITIONAL EPIDEMIOLOGY

Several types of research study designs are used in epidemiology. Their purposes are to (1) describe relevant risk factors (common factors or characteristics that contribute to a disease) and health outcomes, (2) generate hypotheses, or (3) study causal linkages between risk factors and diseases. The types of studies used in nutritional epidemiology include case studies and case series (what clinicians see), ecological studies (geographical comparisons), cross-sectional studies (a "snapshot" in time), case–control studies (compare people with and without a disease), cohort studies (follow people over time to see who gets the disease), and randomized controlled trials (RCTs; human experiments).

Study designs that provide descriptions and help to generate hypotheses include case studies, case series, ecological studies, and cross-sectional studies. These four types of studies are used to

---

BOX 3.1 A WORD ABOUT PROSPECTIVE VS. RETROSPECTIVE STUDIES

A prospective study watches for outcomes, such as the development of a disease, during the study period and relates this to other factors such as suspected risk or protection factor(s). The study usually involves taking a group (or *cohort*) of subjects and watching them over a long period. The outcome of interest should be common; otherwise, the number of outcomes observed will be too small to be statistically meaningful (indistinguishable from those that may have arisen by chance). All efforts should be made to avoid sources of bias such as the loss of individuals to follow-up during the study. Prospective studies usually have fewer potential sources of bias and confounding than retrospective studies. A retrospective study looks backward and examines exposures to suspected risks or protective factors in relation to an outcome that is established at the start of the study. Most sources of error due to confounding and bias are more common in retrospective studies than in prospective studies.

Source: Food and Drug Administration. Office of Food Additive Safety. *Redbook 2000. Toxicological Principles for the Safety Assessment of Food Ingredients.* July 2000. Updated July 2007. Chapter VI.B: Epidemiology (October 2001). Available at http://www.fda.gov/Food/GuidanceRegulation/GuidanceDocumentsRegulatoryInformation/IngredientsAdditivesGRASPackaging/ucm078401.htm, accessed January 20, 2015.

- Provide data regarding the magnitude of disease load and types of disease problems in the community in terms of morbidity and mortality rates and ratios.
- Provide clues to disease etiology, and help in the formulation of an etiological hypothesis.
- Provide background data for planning, organizing, and evaluating preventive and curative services.
- Contribute to research by describing variations in disease occurrence by time, place, and person.

From the perspective of causal linkages, a weakness of these four types of studies is their lack of comparison groups. Although case studies and case series provide information about possible linkages, they cannot control for the effects of alternative explanations or confounding variables. Cross-sectional studies provide limited information about comparison groups at the time of data analysis. Rather, two common observational epidemiologic study designs used to examine causal linkages between risk factors and diseases are case–control studies and cohort studies (Kelsey et al. 1996). Likewise, the RCT is an experimental epidemiologic study design used to determine causation. Each of these study designs is explained in detail in the sections that follow, and the strongest evidence comes from studies that are presented last (Box 3.1).

CASE REPORTS AND CASE SERIES

Case studies are descriptions of individual cases of disease, whereas a case series describes a group of similar cases of disease. They are useful because they may generate ideas for future epidemiologic investigations. Strongly suggestive anecdotal or clinical observations may indicate a possible causal relationship. Analytic epidemiologic studies can then be designed to verify and quantify the risks, and to determine the role of confounding factors. Case reports or case series may be used to track toxicity reports of new foods or to document the beginning of an epidemic. A case series is of greater value than a case report because the series provides more documentation of evidence for the suggested hypothesis (Sherry et al. 2003).

Case reports are a type of descriptive epidemiology study frequently evaluated by the Food and Drug Administration's (FDA's) Center for Food Safety and Applied Nutrition (CFSAN). There are two principal avenues through which case reports come to CFSAN's attention—reports published in the

BOX 3.2   MEDWATCH SAFETY ALERTS

The MedWatch website is used by consumers and healthcare professionals to voluntarily report a serious adverse event, product quality problem, product use error, or therapeutic inequivalence/failure suspected to be associated with the use of an FDA-regulated drug, biologic, medical device, dietary supplement or cosmetic. The FDA also publishes safety alerts on the MedWatch site; safety alerts for food, infant formula, and medical nutrition therapy may be found under "Safety Alerts for Human Medical Products."

For example, in late 2014/early 2015, the FDA posted a warning notifying healthcare professionals and their medical care organizations of the ongoing investigation of an outbreak of listeriosis linked to commercially produced, prepackaged caramel apples.[1] In 2009, the FDA published a safety alert warning consumers not to eat any varieties of a certain brand of prepackaged, refrigerated cookie dough due to the risk of contamination with *E. coli* 0157:H7, a bacterium that causes abdominal cramping, vomiting, and diarrhea (often with bloody stools).[2] In 2003, the FDA issued a public health advisory on the basis of several reports of toxicity, including death, associated with the use of FD&C Blue No. 1 (Blue 1) in enteral feeding solutions. Blue 1 was administered in order to help in the detection and/or monitoring of pulmonary aspiration in patients being fed by an enteral feeding tube. Reported cases indicated that seriously ill patients, particularly those with a likely increase in gut permeability (e.g., patients with sepsis), were manifesting blue discoloration of the skin, urine, feces, or serum, and some developed serious complications such as refractory hypotension and metabolic acidosis and death.[3]

Source:
[1]Data from Food and Drug Administration. MedWatch The FDA Safety Information and Adverse Event Reporting Program. Caramel Apples: Warning—Illnesses, Including Deaths, Linked to *Listeria Monocytogenes* Contamination. Available at http://www.fda.gov/Safety/MedWatch/SafetyInformation/SafetyAlertsforHumanMedicalProducts /ucm428113.htm, accessed January 20, 2015.
[2]Data from Food and Drug Administration. MedWatch The FDA Safety Information and Adverse Event Reporting Program. Nestle Toll House Prepackaged, Refrigerated Cookie Dough. June 19, 2009. Available at http://www .fda.gov/Safety/MedWatch/SafetyInformation/SafetyAlertsforHumanMedicalProducts/ucm168005.htm, accessed January 20, 2015.
[3]Data from Food and Drug Administration. MedWatch The FDA Safety Information and Adverse Event Reporting Program. FD&C Blue No. 1 (Blue 1) in enteral feeding solutions. Available at http://www.fda.gov/Safety/MedWatch /SafetyInformation/SafetyAlertsforHumanMedicalProducts/ucm169530.htm, accessed January 20, 2015.

peer-reviewed medical literature and reports captured in one or more of CFSAN's ongoing voluntary (also called *passive*) adverse event monitoring systems, such as the Adverse Reaction Monitoring System (ARMS). ARMS collects spontaneous reports from consumers and health professionals regarding alleged adverse effects from food products. In addition, CFSAN receives adverse event reports through the FDA's (http://www.fda.gov/Safety/MedWatch/default.htm) MedWatch program. The FDA uses the MedWatch reporting system to issue public health advisories regarding unsafe nutritional products, such as dietary supplements, infant formulas, and medical foods (Box 3.2).

ECOLOGICAL OR CORRELATIONAL STUDIES

Ecological studies examine disease rates of a population in a given geographical area based on average measures of exposure. In an ecological or correlational study, the unit of analysis is an aggregate of individuals, and information is collected on this group rather than on individual members. In other words, ecological or correlational studies do not examine the relationship between exposure and disease among individuals. Rather, the association between an aggregate measure of disease and an aggregate measure of exposure is studied.

Ecological studies are relatively quick and inexpensive. Because they often rely on data that have been routinely collected by government agencies for standard surveillance initiatives, ecological studies can provide a useful first look at relationships. As such, they are useful for generating, rather than definitively testing, a scientific hypothesis. They may also be used for a preliminary evaluation of a new hypothesis to determine whether more extensive and expensive investigations are warranted (Langseth 1996). Thus, the results of ecological studies would be insufficient to demonstrate a relationship without other types of data to support them.

Examples of Ecological Studies

As discussed by Willett in his book, *Nutritional Epidemiology* (1998) (Willett 1998b), ecological studies of migrant and other special populations have been widely used to differentiate between genetic and environmental determinants of NTDs, whereas other ecological studies relate the intake of dietary factors to the incidence of coronary heart disease (CHD).

A genetic component in the etiology of NTDs had long been suspected because previously affected pregnancy and family history of an affected pregnancy are risk factors for subsequent NTDs. However, ecological studies demonstrated that rates of NTDs vary by geographic area, in populations that migrate from areas of high to low incidence, among populations that are malnourished, and among populations that consume fortified cereals. Migration studies have shown that groups that migrated from high-risk areas in Ireland to low-risk areas in the United States and the south of Britain manifest lower risks of a pregnancy with an NTD. An additional retrospective ecological study revealed that an epidemic of NTDs appears to have occurred in Boston during the Great Depression. And finally, it was an ecological study that demonstrated the decline in the prevalence of NTDs after breakfast cereals in Dublin were fortified with folic acid and vitamin B_{12}.

Ancel Keys, MD, was known worldwide for his landmark epidemiological seven-country study of Finland, Greece, Italy, Japan, the Netherlands, the United States, and Yugoslavia, which demonstrated that the intake of saturated fat as a percentage of calories was strongly correlated with coronary death rates. His studies provided evidence that a diet rich in vegetables, fruits, and pasta and low in meat, eggs, and dairy products is associated with a reduced occurrence of CHD. In Keys' sample, the less industrialized countries manifested low saturated fat intake and low incidence of CHD. In addition to differences in intake of saturated fat, the less and more industrialized countries also differed in terms of physical activity, obesity, and smoking. The percentage of energy from total fat had little relationship with CHD incidence or mortality, which led Willet as well as Keys to recommend a Mediterranean-style diet (Willett 2001).

Among men of Japanese ancestry, there is a gradient in CHD mortality increasing from Japan to Hawaii to California. A study of 11,900 Japanese men in Hiroshima and Nagasaki, Honolulu, and the San Francisco Bay Area of California was conducted to investigate this disease difference (Syme et al. 1975). According to Willett (1998c), when the investigators compared the saturated fat intake of Japanese men living in Japan, Hawaii, and California, the three populations were found to have saturated fat intakes as a percentage of calories of 7%, 23%, and 26%, respectively. With transition to the United States, the men in the study manifested increases in mean serum cholesterol and weight (but not height) parallel to the observed changes in dietary saturated fat. Distributions of serum cholesterol, glucose, uric acid, and triglycerides were also examined. In every age group, the mean for each of the biochemical variables was lower for men in Japan than in Hawaii and California (Nichaman et al. 1975). Examination of public health records indicated that age-adjusted CHD rates were consistently and significantly lower in Japan than in American Japanese (Worth et al. 1975). This ecological study supports the hypothesis that an increased intake of saturated fat is associated with an increased risk of CHD.

Ecological Fallacy

A fallacy is an error in reasoning, usually based on mistaken assumptions. Researchers should be familiar with the fallacies they are susceptible to. Errors based on ecological studies occur when conclusions are drawn about individuals from data that are associated with groups. This is because relationships observed for groups do not necessarily hold for individuals. The ecological fallacy occurs when one makes conclusions about individuals based only on analyses of group data. For example, we know from ecological studies that a positive correlation exists between consumption of saturated fat and CHD across many nations. However, it is not possible to infer that the specific people with CHD actually had a high saturated fat intake. Thus, while we can conclude that saturated fat consumption is a risk factor for CHD, it would be an error of reasoning (an ecological fallacy) to further conclude that people with CHD actually had high saturated fat consumption. Because ecological studies are not based on the actual exposure of individuals, they are less sophisticated than case–control and cohort studies, and results should be treated with caution.

Cross-Sectional or Prevalence Studies

Cross-sectional studies are snapshots of risk factors, health outcomes, and other relevant factors in a population at a single point in time. Such information can be very useful in assessing the health status and needs of a population. Some cross-sectional studies are surveys. Cabinet-level departments of the US government conduct many important surveys, many of which are administered regularly over time. For example, the USDA and the Department of Health and Human Services (HHS) oversee national food and nutrition surveys. Whereas many of the surveys offer a representative overview of the health of the population, they cannot shed light on disease etiology (Sherry et al. 2003). Another cross-sectional survey that has a major impact on nutrition in public health is the decennial census, conducted by the Commerce Department's Census Bureau.

Other cross-sectional studies include a biologic measurement of disease or of nutrient exposure. These studies provide information about disease prevalence and factors associated with that prevalence. Information is collected about dietary exposures for individuals so that in cross-sectional studies, unlike ecologic studies, it is known whether the individuals with the disease are those with the exposure. In other words, the presence or absence of disease and the presence or absence of suspected etiologic factors are determined in each member of the study population or in a representative sample at a particular time. An example is a study that linked calcium intake with blood pressure measurements in healthy populations. The calcium and blood pressure data indicated whether the individuals with higher blood pressure were those with lower intakes of calcium (Hamet 1995).

The advantages of cross-sectional studies are that the people are contacted only once, so these studies are relatively inexpensive to conduct and can be completed relatively quickly. But this also limits their usefulness. Cross-sectional studies reveal nothing about the temporal sequence of exposure and disease. It is not known whether the dietary exposure as measured is a consequence of the disease or a causal factor. In the calcium and blood pressure example, it is not known from cross-sectional data if individuals with higher blood pressure had altered their diets and their intake of calcium in response to a previous diagnosis of high blood pressure (Freidenheim 1999). Another limitation of cross-sectional studies is that they can only measure disease prevalence, not incidence (Food and Drug Administration 2001).

Case–Control Studies

In case–control studies, individuals who already have a certain health outcome (cases) are compared to similar individuals who do not have the health outcome (controls). In these retrospective studies, effect sizes are calculated as ratios of likelihood (known as *odds ratios* [*ORs*]) of exposure to the risk factors. Such studies frequently include a biologic measurement of disease or of nutrient exposure. Case–control studies are designed to answer such questions as "Do persons with osteoporosis (cases) consume diets that differ from those consumed by individuals without this disease (controls)?"

Whereas case–control studies can be done quickly and relatively inexpensively, they are less than ideal for studying diet because information is gathered from the past. People with illnesses often recall past behaviors differently from those without illness (known as *recall bias*), which exposes these studies to potential inaccuracies and bias. In addition, choosing appropriate controls is always biased unless they are a random sample of the population. Despite these challenges, carefully designed case–control studies can provide useful results.

The FDA, for example, often looks carefully at the results of case–control studies in the setting of outbreaks of foodborne disease to identify the food vehicle that was most likely responsible for transmitting the infectious agent. The results then can be used to help target specific food vehicles for microbiologic testing as a means of recovering the pathogen from the implicated food. In addition, results of case–control studies have been frequently used in safety evaluations at the FDA, primarily to add further information to the overall assessment of safety (Sherry et al. 2003).

Examples of Case–Control Studies

A case–control study was carried out in Northern Ireland to compare dietary intake and biochemical indices of nutritional status in women following the birth of a baby/termination of a pregnancy affected by NTDs and women with a normal baby. Dietary records and blood samples were obtained from 15 women who had been referred to the study following an affected pregnancy (cases) and the same number of women whose pregnancy outcome was normal (controls). Although there were no statistically significant differences in nutrient intake between the two groups, the cases demonstrated a tendency for lower fruit and vegetable consumption compared to the controls. Blood tests revealed that levels of serum vitamin B_{12} were significantly lower in cases compared to controls, and activities of two of the nucleotide salvage pathway enzymes were significantly higher, findings that are consistent with other research on NTDs and the metabolism of folate and vitamin B_{12}. This early study suggested the need for a focus on vitamin status to prevent NTDs (Wright 1995).

Researchers conducted a case–control study of 462 confirmed pancreatic cancer cases and 4721 population-based controls to assess associations between specific and total carotenoid intakes and the risk of pancreatic cancer. Dietary intake was assessed by a self-administered FFQ. After adjustment for age, body mass index (BMI), smoking, educational attainment, dietary folate, and total energy intake, lycopene consumption—provided mainly by tomatoes—was associated with a 31% reduction in pancreatic cancer risk among men when comparing the highest and lowest quartiles of intake. Both beta-carotene and total carotenoids were associated with a significantly reduced risk among those who never smoked, suggesting that a diet rich in tomatoes and tomato-based products with high lycopene content may help reduce pancreatic cancer risk (Nkondjock et al. 2005).

Next to tobacco, saccharin may be the substance that has been most studied epidemiologically. Literally thousands of patients with bladder cancer have participated in case–control studies (Morgan and Wong 1985). In 1972, the FDA removed saccharin from the list of generally recognized as safe (GRAS) substances and issued an interim food additive regulation limiting the use of saccharin in foods. On the basis of subsequent studies demonstrating that saccharin caused bladder cancer in rats, Congress instituted product-labeling requirements for saccharin-sweetened foods and beverages.

In 1977, the NCI and the FDA conducted a case–control study to reveal the possible roles of the artificial sweeteners saccharin and cyclamate in human urinary bladder cancer. More than 500 patients with confirmed bladder cancer and an equal number of matching controls participated. Questionnaires revealed no significant differences between subjects' and controls' previous intake of artificial sweeteners. Because these findings persisted after simultaneous adjustment for the effects of smoking, occupation, age, diabetes mellitus, and a number of other potentially confounding factors, the researchers concluded that neither saccharin nor cyclamate is likely to be carcinogenic, at least at the moderate dietary ingestion levels reported by the patient sample (Kessler and Clark 1978). The results of this study, together with findings of additional research with laboratory

---

BOX 3.3   FORMER WARNING LABEL ON SACCHARIN-SWEETENED FOODS AND BEVERAGES

"Use of this product may be hazardous to your health. This product contains saccharin, which has been determined to cause cancer in laboratory animals."

Source: National Institutes of Environmental Health Sciences, Panel Recommends that Saccharin Remain on U.S. List of Carcinogens, October 31, 1997. Available at http://www.nih.gov/news/pr/oct97/niehs-31.htm, accessed January 20, 2015.

---

animals, convinced the FDA in December 2000 to remove the warning label that had been used on saccharin-sweetened foods since 1977 (Box 3.3).

COHORT STUDIES

Cohort or follow-up studies follow large groups of people over a long period of time. In these studies, the investigator begins with two groups that are initially free of the health outcome. One of the groups is exposed to the risk factor of interest, whereas the other group is not. Researchers regularly gather information from the people in the study on a wide variety of variables, such as meat intake, physical activity level, and weight. The incidences of health outcomes among the exposed and nonexposed individuals are then followed prospectively. The effect size is expressed as the ratio (relative risk [RR]) of the incidence of disease among exposed compared to nonexposed individuals. Once a specified amount of time has elapsed, the characteristics of people in the group are compared to test specific hypotheses, such as the link between carotenoids and glaucoma, or meat intake and prostate cancer. Figure 3.1 depicts the temporal differences between cross-sectional, case–control, and cohort study designs.

Cohort studies generally provide more reliable information than case–control studies because cohort studies do not rely on information from the past and can account for temporal sequence. Cohort studies gather the information over a long duration of time, from before anyone develops the disease being studied. As a group, these types of studies have provided valuable information about the link between lifestyle factors and disease. Two of the largest and longest-running cohort studies of diet are the Harvard-based Nurses' Health Study (NHS; http://www.channing.harvard.edu/nhs/) and the Health Professionals Follow-Up Study (HPFS) (http://www.hsph.harvard.edu/hpfs/).

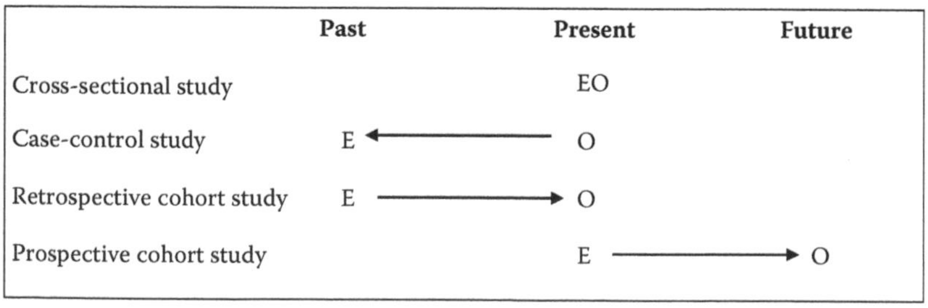

E: exposure, O: outcome, →: direction of investigation

FIGURE 3.1   Temporal differences in various observational study designs. (Adapted from Friis RH and Sellers TA, *Epidemiology for Public Health Practice*, 3rd ed., Sudbury, MA: Jones and Bartlett, p. 270, 2004.)

TABLE 3.2
Strengths and Weaknesses of Case–Control and Prospective Cohort Studies

	Case–Control Study	Prospective Cohort Study
Strengths	Less expensive	More efficient for studying rare exposures
	Smaller number of people	Less bias in risk factor data
	Time to carry out study is shorter	May find associations with other diseases
	Suitable for rare diseases	Yields incidence rates as well as relative risk
Weaknesses	Incomplete information about past events	Large numbers of subjects required
	Biased recall of exposures may occur	Lengthy follow-up period
	Problems of selecting controls and matching variables	Attrition
		Changes in criteria and methods over time
	May yield only relative risk (odds ratio)	More expensive

Conversely, although a powerful design, a cohort study is more time-consuming and expensive than a case–control study because a cohort study requires both large study populations and long periods of observations to achieve definite results. Cohort studies are also open to problems of loss of study participants to follow-up, and bias may be introduced if not every member of the cohort is followed. A cohort study is not suitable for studying rare diseases or those that take a long time to develop, since the length of the study may be less than the latency period of the disease. For example, if the study is stopped before the participants reach old age, many important diseases such as cancer may be missed.

However, given a set of exposures, multiple outcomes can be studied using a cohort study design. In nested case–control study designs, a case–control study is embedded (nested) within a longitudinal prospective cohort study. Presented in Table 3.2 are the major strengths and weaknesses of case–control and prospective cohort studies.

Retrospective Cohort Studies

Cohort studies can be retrospective or prospective (or both). In a retrospective cohort study, historical data—such as those found in medical records—are used to determine exposure level at some baseline in the past. Investigators then perform a follow-up to determine subsequent occurrences of disease between baseline and the present. Because retrospective cohort studies utilize measurements of exposure that occurred in the past, they require less time and money to perform than prospective cohort studies (Friis and Sellers 2004).

The first recommendations about increasing intake of folic acid were made in 1992. In order to help reduce the incidence of NTDs in the United States, in 1996, the FDA mandated that all enriched breads and grains sold in the country be fortified with folic acid by January 1998. However, other developed countries (such as Norway, Finland, the Northern Netherlands, England and Wales, Ireland, France, Hungary, Italy, Portugal, and Israel) responded to the mounting mass education campaigns without fortifying the food supply. To evaluate the effectiveness of policies and recommendations on folic acid aimed at reducing the occurrence of NTDs, a retrospective cohort study was conducted of births monitored by birth defect registries in these countries. Researchers examined the incidences and trends in rates of NTDs before and after 1992 and before and after the year of local recommendations (when applicable). No detectable improvement in the incidence of NTDs was found. As recommendations alone did not seem to influence trends in NTDs up to 6 years after the confirmation of the effectiveness of folic acid in clinical trials, the researchers concluded that a reasonable strategy would be to quickly integrate food fortification with fuller implementation of recommendations on supplements, similar to the policy in the United States (Botto et al. 2005).

Prospective Cohort Studies

In prospective cohort studies, a population is assembled and then followed to see if those with the highest exposure to a particular factor develop certain conditions at a higher rate than those with lower exposure. Examples of this kind of study are the Framingham study of cardiovascular disease (CVD), which began in 1948; the NHS I, which has examined the effect of lifestyle factors on disease since 1976; the HPFS; the NHS II and NHS III; and the Growing Up Today Study I and II (GUTS I and GUTS II), started in 1996 and 2004, respectively, to follow children 9–14 years of age whose mothers participated in the NHS II.

Nutritional epidemiologic research at Harvard University primarily involves the investigation of dietary factors in the cause and prevention of CVD, cancer, and other conditions. The development of methods to measure dietary intake in large populations has been fundamental to this work. A substantial effort has been devoted to the development, evaluation, and refinement of methods to measure various aspects of diet in the context of large epidemiologic studies. This has resulted in the development and validation of separate FFQs for women, men, and children. Although the FFQs developed for the NHS II, HPFS, and GUTS have been demonstrated to provide reasonably accurate assessments of a wide spectrum of dietary factors, their validity has been questioned, as discussed in the Biomarkers section earlier in this chapter that deals with biochemical indicators of dietary intake. Researchers at Harvard and elsewhere have been developing and evaluating biological markers of dietary intake, particularly using plasma and toenail samples, indicators that are primarily utilized in nested case–control studies using the large specimen banks collected prospectively as part of such ongoing studies as the NHS II.

Framingham Heart Study (1948–)

In 1948, the National Heart Institute (now the NHLBI) established the longitudinal Framingham Heart Study to identify CVD risk factors by following its development in a large cohort who had not yet developed overt symptoms of CVD or suffered a heart attack or stroke. Since 1971, the study has been conducted under the aegis of Boston University. The original cohort consisted of 5209 respondents of a random sample of two-thirds of the adult population, 30–62 years of age, residing in Framingham, MA. Researchers began the first round of extensive physical examinations and lifestyle interviews that they would later analyze for common patterns related to CVD development. Since 1948, participants have continued to return to the study every 2 years for a detailed medical history, physical examination, and laboratory tests. Exam 30 for this original cohort ended in February 2010.

In 1971, the study enrolled a second-generation cohort of 5124 of the original cohort's adult children and their spouses to participate in similar examinations. The Offspring Study was initiated when the need for establishing a prospective epidemiologic study of young adults was recognized. Offspring exam 9 began in 2011. A third generation (the children of the Offspring cohort) of 4095 participants was initiated in July 2005 to further understand how genetic factors relate to CVD. These participants are given an extensive cardiovascular examination similar to that of their parents and grandparents. The forms from the most recent examinations of each of these cohorts are available at: http://www.framinghamheartstudy.org/researchers/exam-forms.php.

Since its inception in 1948, more than 2800 research articles have been published using Framingham Heart Study data. A bibliography (1950–2014) of these studies can be found at http://www.framinghamheartstudy.org/fhs-bibliography/index.php. Highlights of some of the most significant diet-related research milestones of the Framingham Heart Study are listed in Table 3.3.

Health Professionals Follow-Up Study (1986–)

The HPFS began in 1986 to evaluate a series of hypotheses about men's health relating nutritional factors to the incidence of serious illnesses, such as cancer, heart disease, and other vascular diseases. This all-male national longitudinal study was designed to complement the all-female NHS I, which examines similar hypotheses. In the beginning, a cohort of 51,529 men in health professions

TABLE 3.3
Selection of Research Milestones in the Framingham Heart Study

1960	Cigarette smoking found to increase the risk of heart disease.
1961	Cholesterol level and blood pressure found to increase the risk of heart disease.
1967	Risk of heart disease found to be decreased by physical activity and increased by obesity.
1970	High blood pressure found to increase the risk of stroke.
1976	Menopause found to increase the risk of heart disease.
1978	Psychosocial factors found to affect heart disease.
1988	High levels of HDL-C found to reduce risk of death.
1994	Enlarged left ventricle chamber of the heart shown to increase the risk of stroke.
1996	Progression from hypertension to heart failure described.
1999	Lifetime risk of developing coronary heart disease at 40 years of age is one in two for men and one in three for women.
2001	High-normal blood pressure associated with an increased risk of cardiovascular disease.
2002	Obesity is a risk factor for heart failure.
2005	Lifetime risk of becoming overweight exceeds 70%, obese about 50%.
2008	Social networks exert key influences on decision to quit smoking.
2009	High leptin levels may protect against Alzheimer's disease and dementia.
2009–2010	Discovery of hundreds of new genes underlying major heart disease risk factors: body mass index, blood cholesterol, cigarette smoking, blood pressure, and glucose/diabetes.
2010	Fat around the abdomen is associated with smaller, older brains in middle-aged adults.
2010	Stroke by age 65 years in a parent increased risk of stroke in offspring threefold.

Source: Framingham Heart Study Research Milestones. Available at http://www.framinghamheartstudy.org/about/mile
stones.html, accessed January 20, 2015.

enlisted to participate in the study (58% dentists, 20% veterinarians, 8% pharmacists, 7% optometrists, 4% osteopathic physicians, and 3% podiatrists), of whom 1.7% are Asian American and 1% are African American. (In research where ethnic background is a focus, the researchers oversample ethnic groups in order to draw valid results.) The researchers selected health professionals in the belief that men who chose these types of careers would be motivated and committed to participating in a long-term project and would appreciate the necessity of answering the survey questions accurately. Every 2 years, study participants receive questionnaires asking about diseases and health-related topics like smoking, physical activity, and medications taken. The questionnaires that contain FFQs are administered in 4-year intervals. Approximately 93% of the original cohort still participates. Since its inception, more than 100 research articles have been published using data from the study (Harvard School of Public Health, http://www.hsph.harvard.edu/hpfs/). Based on analysis of HPFS data to date, the following were observed:

- For every kilogram of weight gained, the risk of developing type 2 diabetes increased by 7.3%. Researchers prospectively examined the relations between changes in body weight and body fat distribution (1986–1996) and the subsequent risk of diabetes (1996–2000) among 22,171 men in the HPFS. A gain in abdominal fat was positively associated with risk of diabetes, independent of the risk associated with weight change. Compared with men who had a stable waist, men who increased waist circumference by 14.6 cm or more had 1.7 times the risk of diabetes after controlling for weight gain. In addition, men who lost more than 4.1 cm in hip girth had 1.5 times the risk of diabetes compared with men with stable hip circumference. In this cohort, 56% of the cases of diabetes could be attributed to weight gain greater than 7 kg, and 20% of the cases could be attributed to a gain in waist measurement exceeding 2.5 cm. The findings of this study highlight the importance of maintaining body weight and waist circumference to reduce the risk of diabetes (Koh-Banerjee et al. 2004).

- Abdominal adiposity is associated with the incidence of symptomatic gallstone disease, and measures of abdominal adiposity, abdominal circumference, and waist-to-hip ratio predict the risk of developing gallstones independently of BMI. As part of the HPFS, men reported newly diagnosed symptomatic gallstone disease on questionnaires mailed to them every 2 years. The researchers prospectively studied measures of abdominal obesity in relation to the incidence of symptomatic gallstone disease in a cohort of 29,847 men who were free of prior gallstone disease and who provided complete data on waist and hip circumferences. Data on weight and height, and waist and hip circumferences, were collected in 1986 and in 1987 through self-administered questionnaires. The researchers documented 1117 new cases of symptomatic gallstone disease. After adjustment for BMI and other risk factors for gallstones, men with a height-adjusted waist circumference 102.6 cm (40.4 in.) had an RR of 2.29 compared with men with a height-adjusted waist circumference <86.4 cm (34 in.). Men with a waist-to-hip ratio 0.99 had an RR of 1.78 compared with men with a waist-to-hip ratio <0.89 (Tsai et al. 2004).

- Low birth weight (LBW) is associated with an increased risk of hypertension and diabetes, and high birth weight (HBW) is associated with an increased risk of obesity, findings that support the hypothesis that early life exposures, for which birth weight (BW) is a marker, are associated with several chronic diseases in adulthood. The researchers examined the relation between BW and cumulative incidence of adult hypertension, incidence of non–insulin-dependent diabetes mellitus, and prevalence of obesity in a cohort of 22,846 men in the HPFS. BWs, medical histories, family histories, and other factors were collected by biennial mailed questionnaires. Compared with men in the referent BW category (7.0–8.4 lb.), men who weighed <5.5 lb. had an age-adjusted OR of 1.26 for hypertension and 1.75 for diabetes mellitus. Compared with men in the referent group, the age-adjusted OR of being in the highest vs. the lowest quintile of adult BMI for men with BW >10.0 lb. was 2.08 (Curhan et al. 1996).

- Data from the HPFS and NHS support an association between the Overall Nutritional Quality Index (ONQI) and lower risks of chronic disease and all-cause mortality. Created by a multidisciplinary panel of nutrition and public health experts, the ONQI is a nutrient-profiling algorithm that incorporates over 30 dietary components and aims to rank foods by relative healthfulness. The raw scores are converted to a 1-to-100 scale; the higher the score, the higher the nutritional quality of the food or beverage item. Dietary data were collected using FFQs administered at baseline (1986), and the ONQI algorithm was applied to each item on the FFQ (ONQI-f), resulting in an average ONQI-f score for the diet consumed by each participant. Information on lifestyle habits, medical history, and newly diagnosed disease was also collected at baseline and updated biennially. Individuals with a previously diagnosed chronic disease (CVD, diabetes, and cancer) and those with invalid dietary data at baseline were excluded from analyses, resulting in 42,382 men and 62,284 women included in analysis. During the 20 years of follow-up, there were 13,520 cases of major chronic disease in men and 20,004 cases of major chronic disease in women. The ONQI-f score was inversely associated with risk of total chronic disease, CVD, diabetes, and all-cause mortality (p-trend ≤ 0.01), but not cancer, in both cohorts. For example, compared to the lowest-quintile ONQI-f score, the risk of CVD in the highest quintile was 25% lower in men and 21% lower in women. Likewise, the risk of diabetes in the highest quintile was 30% lower in men and 22% lower in women in the lowest quintile. The results suggest that, in these two cohorts, consumption of foods with higher ONQI scores is associated with lower risk of chronic disease and total mortality (Chiuve et al. 2011).

Nurses' Health Studies (1976–)

The Nurses' Health Studies are among the largest prospective investigations into the risk factors for major chronic diseases in women. Relations between diet, physical activity, weight gain, and risk of chronic diseases are studied. Dr. Frank Speizer established the NHS I in 1976 with funding from the NIH. The original goal for the NHS I was to investigate the potential long-term consequences of the use of oral contraceptives in normal women. Registered nurses (RNs) were selected to be followed prospectively as it was anticipated that because of their nursing education, they would be able to respond with a high degree of accuracy to brief, technically worded questionnaires and would be motivated to participate in a long-term study. Married RNs who were aged 30–55 in 1976, who lived in the 11 most populous states (California, Connecticut, Florida, Maryland, Massachusetts, Michigan, New Jersey, New York, Ohio, Pennsylvania, and Texas), and whose state nursing boards agreed to supply the study with their members' names and addresses were enrolled in the cohort if they responded to the baseline questionnaire. Approximately 122,000 RNs responded out of the 170,000 queried. Every 2 years, cohort members receive a follow-up questionnaire with questions about diseases and health-related topics including smoking, hormone use, and menopausal status. Because it was recognized that diet and nutrition would play important roles in the development of chronic diseases, dietary intake was measured by an FFQ (developed and validated by Willett and his colleagues at Harvard). The first FFQ was collected in 1980, a second in 1984, a third in 1986, and every 4 years thereafter. Physical activity has been repeatedly assessed, and ongoing validation studies show it to be a valid measure. Quality-of-life (QOL) questions were added in 1992 and repeated every 4 years. Because certain aspects of diet cannot be measured by questionnaire—particularly minerals that become incorporated in food from the soil in which it is grown—RNs submitted 68,000 sets of toenail samples between the 1982 and 1984 questionnaires. Similarly, to identify potential biomarkers, such as hormone levels and genetic markers, 33,000 blood samples were collected in 1989–1990 followed by second samples from 18,700 of these participants in 2000–2001. These samples are stored and used in case–control analyses. The response rates to NHS I questionnaires are at approximately 90% for each 2-year cycle (The Nurses' Health Study, http://www.channing.harvard.edu/nhs/?page_id=70).

In 1989, with funding from the NIH, Willett and his colleagues established the NHS II to study oral contraceptives, diet, and lifestyle risk factors in a population younger than the NHS I cohort. The initial target population was women between the ages of 25 and 42 years in 1989; the upper age was to correspond with the lowest age group in the NHS I. A total of 116,686 women remained in the NHS II. Every 2 years, cohort members receive a follow-up questionnaire asking about diseases and health-related topics including smoking, hormone use, pregnancy history, and menopausal status. In 1991, the first FFQ was collected, and subsequent FFQs are administered at 4-year intervals. A two-page QOL supplement was included in the first mailing of the 1993 and 1997 questionnaires. Blood and urine samples from approximately 30,000 RNs were collected in the late 1990s. The response rates to NHS II questionnaires are at approximately 90% for each 2-year cycle (Nurses' Health Study 3, http://www.nhs3.org/). A newsletter detailing the progress of the NHS I and II is sent to each participant annually, and past newsletters can be found at http://www.channing.harvard.edu/nhs/?page_id=351.

In 2010, Willett and his colleagues started the NHS III to study health issues related to lifestyle, fertility/pregnancy, environment, and nursing exposures in a more representative sample of nurses ages 20–46 years living in the United States or Canada. For the first time, the study will be entirely web based, and NHS III participants will commit to completing a 30-minute online survey every 6 months. Each survey has a different focus, such as demographic data and medical history, reproductive history and current diet, and lifetime physical activity. Participants will also have the opportunity to participate in optional substudies on specific topics like fertility. Similar to the previous studies, the NHS III (http://www.nhs3.org/) continues throughout the lifespan of the participants.

Table 3.4 summarizes some diet-related research findings of the Nurses' Health Studies.

TABLE 3.4

Selection of Diet-Related Research Findings from the Nurses' Health Studies

	Breast Cancer	Coronary Heart Disease (CHD)/ Stroke	Colon Cancer	Hip Fracture	Cognitive Functioning	Eye Disease
Obesity	Increases risk among postmenopausal women. Weight loss after menopause is associated with reduced risk.	Strong positive relationship between weight (BMI) and risk of CHD and stroke. Weight gain after age 18 increases risk of stroke and CHD.	Increases risk.	Strong protection against hip fracture, in large part due to extra padding around the hips.	Not examined.	Increases risk of cataracts and age-related macular degeneration (AMD).
Alcohol	Having one or more drinks per day increases risk.	Moderate alcohol intake reduces the risk of CHD.	Having two or more drinks per day increases risk.	High consumption increases risk. However, low or moderate consumption is associated with greater bone density.	Moderate intake (0.5–1 serving per day) reduces risk of cognitive impairment.	No relation.
Diet	Higher intake of red meat increases risk of premenopausal breast cancer.	A Mediterranean-type diet reduces risk of incident CHD and stroke. Fish intake reduces risk of stroke. Nut and whole-grain consumption reduces risk of CHD. Refined carbohydrates and trans fats increase risk.	Higher intakes of folate, vitamin B_6, calcium, and vitamin D reduce risk. High intake of red and processed meats increases risk.	Reduction of risk with calcium supplement use among women with low calcium diets; higher dietary calcium intake has no effect. Vitamin D intake reduces risk, and retinol intake increases risk.	Higher vegetable intake, especially green leafy vegetables, reduces risk of cognitive impairment.	Some antioxidants reduce risk of cataracts and AMD. Higher intake of fish may reduce risk of cataracts and AMD.

Source: The Nurses' Health Study. Findings: Some Highlights. Available at http://www.channing.harvard.edu/nhs/?page_id=197, accessed January 20, 2015.

The Growing Up Today Study (1996–)

GUTS I was established in 1996 to assess the predictors of dietary intake, physical activity, and weight changes in youth. Invitations to participate and baseline sex-specific questionnaires were initially mailed in the fall of 1996 to 13,261 girls and 13,504 boys, ages 9–14, whose mothers participate in the NHS II. At baseline, 9039 girls and 7843 boys returned completed questionnaires and thus enrolled in the cohort (Gillman et al. 2001). The cohort is 93.3% white, 1.5% Asian, 0.9% African American, 1.5% Hispanic, 0.8% Native American, and 2.2% other ethnicity (Berlan et al. 2010). At baseline, each child provided his or her current height and weight and a detailed assessment of typical past-year dietary intakes; physical activities; recreational "inactivities" (television, videos, and video/computer games); and other behaviors and lifestyle patterns. Included was a validated FFQ designed specifically for children and adolescents. GUTS I participants have completed questionnaires annually from 1996 to 2001 and every 2 years after 2001. The questionnaires are revised over time to support the instrument's alignment with the developmental stage of cohort participants and to optimize the information collected. Questions typically address weight and height, health-risk behaviors across a range of domains, and psychosocial experiences (Skinner et al. 2012).

In 2004, 10,923 children ages 10–17 years with mothers participating in the NHS II were enrolled in the second GUTS cohort (GUTS II) (Growing Up Today Study, http://www.gutsweb.org/index.php/the-study/guts-then-and-now). Because of the age differences between the participants in the GUTS I cohort and the GUTS II cohort, each cohort originally received different questionnaires on different schedules that asked age-appropriate questions. As of 2013, however, both GUTS cohorts will receive the same annual questionnaire, since all participants are now adults. Questionnaires can be completed on paper or online (Growing Up Today Study 2012). A newsletter detailing updates and findings from GUTS is sent to each participant, and previous newsletters can be found at the study website at http://www.gutsweb.org/index.php/news/newsletters. Nearly 100 papers have been published between 1999 and 2013 by researchers working with GUTS data (Growing Up Today Study 2012). Of note:

- Infants who were fed breast milk more than infant formula, or who were breastfed for longer periods, had a lower risk of being overweight during older childhood and adolescence. In order to examine the extent to which overweight status among adolescents is associated with the type of infant feeding (breast milk vs. infant formula) and duration of breastfeeding, mothers of the children in the GUTS cohort were mailed a supplemental questionnaire in 1997. In the first 6 months of life, 9553 subjects (62%) were only or mostly fed breast milk, and 4744 (31%) were only or mostly fed infant formula. A total of 7186 subjects (48%) were breastfed for at least 7 months, while 4613 (31%) were breastfed for 3 months or less. At ages 9–14 years, 404 girls (5%) and 635 boys (9%) were overweight (Gillman et al. 2001).
- Weight-related issues of parents are transmitted to their children, suggesting that peers, parents, and the media must be targeted for intervention to prevent children and adolescents from developing extreme concern with weight and unhealthy weight control behaviors (Field et al. 2001).
- For many adolescents, dieting to control weight not only is ineffective but may actually promote weight gain. Dieting to control weight, binge eating, and dietary intake were assessed annually from 1996 through 1998. In 1996, 25.0% of the girls and 13.8% of the boys were infrequent dieters, and 4.5% of the girls and 2.2% of the boys were frequent dieters. Among the girls, the percentage of dieters increased over the following 2 years. During 3 years of follow-up, dieters gained more weight than nondieters. Among the girls, frequency of dieting was positively associated with increases in age; among the boys, both frequent and infrequent dieters gained 0.07 z-score of BMI more than nondieters. In addition, boys who engaged in binge eating gained significantly more weight than nondieters (Field et al. 2003).

- A bidirectional relationship has been found between depressive symptoms and both over-eating and binge eating among adolescent and young adult females. Females who reported depressive symptoms at baseline were twice as likely than their peers to start overeating and binge eating during 2 years of follow-up. Likewise, females who engaged in overeating or binge eating at baseline were twice as likely as their peers to develop high levels of depressive symptoms during 2 years of follow-up (Skinner et al. 2012).
- Although snack foods may have low nutritional value, they do not appear to be an important independent determinant of weight gain among children and adolescents (Field et al. 2004).
- Children who drank more than three servings a day of milk gained more in BMI than those who drank smaller amounts, but the added calories appeared responsible. Dietary calcium and skim and 1% milk were associated with weight gain, but dairy fat was not. The authors concluded that drinking large amounts of milk might provide excess energy to some children (Berkey et al. 2005).

META-ANALYSES

Meta-analyses are increasingly used to address the problem of the explosion of information in the scientific literature coupled with the pressure for timely, informed decisions in public health. A meta-analysis combines and analyzes the results of a (preferably) large number of previous reports to yield overall conclusions about a hypothesis. Unlike narrative scientific reviews of the literature, meta-analyses provide a quantitative synthesis of the available data. The technique is best used when examining studies addressing the same question and employing similar methods to measure relevant variables. Meta-analysis can be a valuable tool to aggregate relevant findings across studies and help to explain differences among studies. However, the strength of conclusions from meta-analyses can vary according to such factors as criteria for inclusion of studies, statistical methods used, and the type of studies being analyzed, i.e., observational vs. RCTs. Although meta-analyses restricted to RCTs is usually preferred to meta-analyses of observational studies, the number of published meta-analyses concerning observational studies in health has increased substantially (Box 3.4) (Stroup et al. 2000).

The use of meta-analyses systematically combining the results of RCTs to determine best practices in clinical nutrition support has become routine (Brown and Dattilo 2003; Tolley and Headley 2005; Willett 1998d). However, meta-analyses are also conducted to study issues of community-based nutrition practice, such as examining the efficacy of school-based nutrition education (McArthur 1998), determining the most effective means to promote breastfeeding (Guise et al. 2003) and weight management (Mullen et al. 1997), determining nutrition recommendations concerning fish consumption to decrease CHD mortality (He et al. 2004), and so on.

Because of the inherent limitations of meta-analysis, it often serves not as primary evidence for a hypothesis but, rather, as a source of supporting evidence that can confirm the validity of data concerning a hypothesis, or it may suggest avenues for new investigations. The results of a well-done meta-analysis may be accepted as a way to present the conclusions of disparate studies by using a common scale (Food and Drug Administration 2001). In order to conduct a meta-analysis, one must develop a research protocol that explains how the researcher will (1) identify criteria for the inclusion and exclusion of studies and avoid biases in this process; (2) decide whether the characteristics of study subjects, their interventions, and outcomes in each study are comparable; (3) use well-defined methods to extract data from the studies; (4) express the results of multiple studies in a consistent fashion; and (5) use statistical methods to assess the data (Food and Drug Administration 2001).

CONTROLLED TRIALS

A controlled clinical trial is a human experiment in which people are assigned to receive one out of two or more treatments. This treatment is often a drug, since clinical trials of drugs are required

BOX 3.4   META-ANALYSIS OF THE ASSOCIATION OF ALL-CAUSE MORTALITY WITH OVERWEIGHT AND OBESITY

In January 2013, much discussion surrounded a meta-analysis[1] published in the *Journal of the American Medical Association*, which systematically reviewed the association of all-cause mortality with overweight and obesity using standard BMI categories. Data were extracted from 97 prospective, observational cohort studies, providing a combined sample size of more than 2.88 million individuals and over 270,000 deaths. Results show that, compared to those in the "normal" weight category (BMI of 18.5 to <25), both overall obesity (BMI of ≥30) and grades 2 and 3 obesity (BMI of ≥35) are associated with significantly higher all-cause mortality (hazard ratio [HR] 1.18, 95% confidence interval [CI] 1.12–1.25, and HR 1.29, 95% CI 1.18–1.41, respectively). However, grade 1 obesity (BMI of 30 to <35) is not associated with increased mortality relative to normal weight (HR 0.95, 95% CI 0.88–1.01), suggesting that the excess mortality in obesity may be due to elevated mortality at higher BMI levels. Conversely, overweight status (BMI of 25 to <30) is associated with significantly lower mortality compared to normal weight status (HR 0.94, 95% CI 0.91–0.96). Similar patterns emerged when analysis considered only those studies (*N* = 53) defined as "adequately adjusted," meaning that results were adjusted for age, sex, and smoking and not adjusted for factors in the causal pathway between obesity and mortality.[1]

These findings led many to question whether concerns about overweight are valid, and the study's authors and others acknowledge several limitations to the study, including the following:

- The study only addresses all-cause mortality and not morbidity or cause-specific mortality.[1]
- The study only addresses findings related to BMI (an imperfect predictor of adiposity and metabolic risk) and not other aspects of body composition, such as visceral fat or fat distribution.[1,2]
- Persons with a BMI between 18.5 and 22 have higher mortality than those with a BMI between 22 and 25. Placing these persons in a single group raises the mortality rate for the normal weight group, which may then affect comparisons with overweight and obese groups.[2]
- Publication bias and/or selective reporting may have limited the number of published studies showing null or negative results.[1]

Source:
[1]Data from Flegal KM et al., *JAMA*. 2013;309(1):71–82.
[2]Data from Heymsfield SB, Cefalu WT, *JAMA*. 2013;309(1):87–8.

before being licensed for prescription. The treatment may also be a health intervention, such as a weight loss or smoking cessation program. In clinical trials, the aim is to replicate the *real-life* situation so that the results obtained are as close as possible to what would happen if the treatment were used in the natural setting (real life). Clinical trials tend to be extremely expensive and are unsuitable for use in some situations. For instance, it is not ethical to ask people to drink heavily in order to investigate the effects of alcohol.

The gold standard of epidemiological studies is the double-blind RCT, where participants are randomly assigned to a treatment group, and neither the participant nor the researcher knows which treatment the participant is receiving (in other words, they are *blind* to the treatment assigned). The superiority of the double-blind RCT over other designs is based on the fact that randomization controls for unknown confounders, and blinding reduces potential sources of bias. For example, knowing which treatment a participant receives may alter the participant's behavior and/or the researcher's assessment of the participant.

Nonblind, Nonrandomized Controlled Trials

We start our examination of controlled clinical trials by examining the nonblind, nonrandomized experiments of Lind (1716–1794) and Goldberger (1874–1929), whose studies represent seminal nutritional epidemiologic research.

Lind and Scurvy

The reputation of James Lind rests mainly on his conducting the first clinical trial in nutrition (1747), in which the potencies of a number of supposed antiscorbutic remedies were compared (Hughes 1975), as described in Lind's own words. Lind took six pairs ($n = 12$) of scorbutic sailors and provided each pair with one of six different standard treatments. The experiment demonstrated that citrus fruit was a more effective treatment for scurvy than the other therapies he administered (Brown 2003). As the sailors receiving two of his six chosen interventions had such a dramatic recovery, he felt ethically obligated to end his trial and administer these treatments to all the remaining sailors (Box 3.5) (Doig 1998).

**BOX 3.5   IN JAMES LIND'S OWN WORDS,
FROM HIS *TREATISE ON THE SCURVY* (1753)**

CLINICAL DESCRIPTION OF SCURVY

"The first indication ... of this disease, is generally a change of colour in the face ... to a pale and bloated look ... Their ... aversion to motion degenerates soon into an universal lassitude, with a stiffness and feebleness of the knees upon using exercise with which they are apt to be much fatigued, and upon occasion subject to a breathlessness or panting. Their gums soon after become itchy, swell, and are apt to bleed upon the gentlest friction. Their breath is then offensive; and upon looking into their mouths, the gums appear of an unusual redness, are soft and spongy and ... putrid. They ... are prone to fall into haemorrhages from other parts of the body. Their skin at this time feels dry ... and when examined, it is found covered with several reddish, bluish, or rather black and livid spots ... as it were a bruise ... Many have a swelling of their legs; which is first observed on their ancles [sic] towards the evening, and hardly to be seen next morning; but ... it gradually advances up the leg, and the whole member becomes oedematous ..."

DESCRIPTION OF CONTROLLED TRIAL ON THE TREATMENT OF SCURVY

"On the 20th of May 1747, I selected twelve patients in the scurvy, on board the *Salisbury* at sea. Their cases were as similar as I could have them. They all in general had putrid gums, the spots and lassitude, with weakness of the knees. They lay together in one place, being a proper apartment for the sick in the fore-hold; and had one diet common to all, viz. water gruel sweetened with sugar in the morning; fresh mutton-broth often times for dinner; at other times light puddings, boiled biscuit with sugar, etc., and for supper, barley and raisins, rice and currants, sago and wine or the like. Two were ordered each a quart of cyder a day. Two others took twenty-five drops of elixir vitriol three times a day ... Two others took two spoonfuls of vinegar three times a day ... Two of the worst patients were put on a course of sea-water ... Two others had each two oranges and one lemon given them every day ... The two remaining patients, took ... an electary recommended by a hospital surgeon ... The consequence was, that the most sudden and visible good effects were perceived from the use of oranges and lemons; one of those who had taken them, being at the end of six days fit for duty ... The other was the best recovered of any in his condition; and ... was appointed to attend the rest of the sick. Next to the oranges, I thought the cyder had the best effects ..."

Source: Dunn PM, *Arch Dis Child Fetal Neonatal Ed.* 1997;76(1):F64–5.

Contemporary historians (Bartholomew 2002) claim that by the time Lind conducted his experiment, Woodall (1612) and Strother (1725), among others, had already established that fresh fruit prevented scurvy, but Lind's contribution was in recording the natural history of the disease and demonstrating through the use of controlled conditions of experimentation how scurvy might best be treated (and, indeed, prevented). The commendable features of Lind's experiment included his selecting participants who were similar at the beginning of the experiment (they were all scorbutic) and maintaining them throughout the experiment under the same general environmental and dietary conditions. The groups differed from each other only in respect to the type of treatment used. It remained for the antiscorbutic factor (found in adrenal glands and plants) to be isolated and synthesized almost 200 years after Lind's experiments, described in the next section.

Vitamin C

In 1928, Hungarian-American biochemist Szent-Györgyi (1893–1986) isolated from the adrenal cortex orange juice and paprika (which was widely available in his native Hungary), a substance he named hexuronic acid. He subsequently sent large supplies of it to Paul Karrer (1889–1971) and Walter N. Haworth (1883–1950, the first British organic chemist) and his colleagues, who determined the structure of hexuronic acid and synthesized it in 1932. It was the first vitamin to be synthesized. Similarly, American biochemist Charles Glen King isolated vitamin C in 1931–1932 by studying the antiscorbutic activities of guinea pigs with preparations from lemon juice. The chemical identity of King's active substance was almost identical to Szent-Györgyi's hexuronic acid. In the spring of 1932, first King and then, two weeks later, Szent-Györgyi published articles declaring that vitamin C and hexuronic acid were indeed the same compound. In 1937, Haworth shared the Nobel Prize in Chemistry and Szent-Györgyi received the Nobel Prize in Physiology or Medicine in part for their work on vitamin C. Controversy remains over whether King as well as Szent-Györgyi deserve equal credit for their work on the vitamin. King is not mentioned in the speech used to present Szent-Györgyi to the king of Sweden for the 1937 Nobel Prize in Physiology or Medicine (Hammarsten 1937). King's research is referred to in Szent-Györgyi's Nobel Lecture, but he then goes on to intimate that King was not interested in collaborating (Box 3.6).

BOX 3.6   EXCERPT FROM SZENT-GYÖRGYI'S NOBEL LECTURE

"... At the same time King and Waugh also reported crystals obtained from lemon juice, which were active antiscorbutically and resembled our hexuronic acid ... Suddenly the long-ignored hexuronic acid moved into the limelight, and there was an urgent need for larger amounts of the substance, so that on the one hand its structural analysis could be continued and on the other its vitamin nature confirmed. However, in the course of our vitamin experiments we had used up the last remnants of our substance, and we had no chance of preparing the substance from adrenals, every other material was unsuitable for large-scale work ... My town, Szeged, is the centre of the Hungarian paprika industry. Since this fruit travels badly, I had not had the chance of trying it earlier. The sight of this healthy fruit inspired me one evening with a last hope, and that same night investigation revealed that this fruit represented an unbelievably rich source of hexuronic acid, which, with Haworth, I re-baptized ascorbic acid ... It was still possible by making use of the paprika season, which was then drawing to a close, to produce more than half a kilogram, and the following year more than three kilograms of crystalline ascorbic acid. *I shared out this substance among all the investigators who wanted to work on it* [emphasis added]. I also had the privilege of providing my two prize-winning colleagues P. Karrer and W. N. Haworth with abundant material, and making its structural analysis possible for them."

Source: Szent-Györgyi, A. Oxidation, energy transfer, and vitamins. *Nobel Lecture*, December 11, 1937. Available at http://www.nobelprize.org/medicine/laureates/1937/szent-gyorgyi-lecture.pdf, accessed January 20, 2015.

Goldberger and Pellagra

Rarely encountered in the US today, pellagra is defined by its classic triad of symptoms: dermatitis, diarrhea, and dementia (referred to as the three Ds of pellagra—a fourth D is death). In the beginning of the twentieth century, pellagra was a leading cause of death in the southern United States. Between 1900 and 1940, at least 100,000 individuals died of the disease. Women between the ages of 22 and 44 years, children between the ages of 2 and 10 years, and the elderly were the most frequent casualties. Most pellagrous patients were rural and poor, and lived in cotton mill villages; half of them were African American, and more than two-thirds were women. Also affected were thousands of institutional inmates. Pellagra was uncommon among children younger than 2 years of age, postpubertal adolescents, and active men (Marks 2003). The central figure in the US government's efforts to combat this malady was Joseph Goldberger, MD, a physician educated in New York City who specialized in infectious diseases. In 1914, the US surgeon general appointed Goldberger to direct investigations into pellagra, which was widely considered to be an infectious disease and one that was becoming epidemic in orphanages, asylums, and mill towns. It seems reasonable to assume that he was selected for the project because of his expertise in infectious disease (Klevay 1997).

Like the first cases of AIDS, pellagra was limited to populations toward whom there was public apathy, if not hostility. As the epidemic grew, concluding that pellagra was from malnutrition and poverty, rather than infection, would have forced acknowledging the existence of an underclass and taking steps to ameliorate their condition. Consequently, the investigation of the disease and introduction of preventive measures were impeded for years.

Following community observation that many of the afflicted people subsisted on a limited diet of pork fat, corn bread, and molasses, Goldberger challenged previous theories that pellagra was infectious, noting that it was more consistent with a dietary deficiency. To validate his hypothesis, Goldberger intervened in the diets of orphanages, asylums, and prisons both to cure and induce pellagra. Goldberger demonstrated that changing the diet—by including meat, dairy products, and legumes—decreased the incidence of pellagra. He also demonstrated that healthy volunteers could not be inoculated with the disease.

Goldberger conducted pellagra prevention experiments in two orphanages in Mississippi and a Georgia state sanitarium. Pellagra had been endemic in these institutions for several years. The diets at the three institutions were modified with a liberal intake of fresh animal foods and legumes beginning in the fall of 1914. By the following spring, there was only one case of recurrence among the 172 pellagrins from both the orphanages, and no new cases of pellagra occurred. In the Georgia sanitarium, after dietary modification, there was no recurrence of pellagra among the 72 pellagrins, though the recurrence rate was 50% among controls. During the study period, the sanitary conditions of the orphanages and the asylum remained unchanged. With these studies, Goldberger was convinced that pellagra was a preventable dietary disease (Rajakumar 2000).

In an experiment conducted at a state prison farm, he produced pellagra in convicts by feeding them a traditional, monotonous Southern diet. Goldberger persuaded authorities in Mississippi to allow 12 prisoners to volunteer to eat for 6 months an experimental diet that might induce pellagra. In return, the prisoners would be released at the end of the experiment. The diet had abundant corn and other cereals but no meat or dairy products. (With hindsight, we know that meat and dairy products can protect against pellagra because they supply the amino acid tryptophan, which is converted to niacin in the body.) After 5 months, six of the men had developed dermatitis on the scrotum and, in a few cases, on the backs of their hands. Goldberger was satisfied that this was pellagra, but the volunteers immediately fled after obtaining their release, and he could not demonstrate their condition to physicians who doubted whether he truly had produced the disease (Cooper 2003).

Upon observing that pellagra was contracted by prisoners (but not guards) and by patients (but not nurses), Goldberger hypothesized that the disease is not contagious. His null hypothesis was that germs cause pellagra. To prove that pellagra was not infectious, Goldberger, his wife, and 14 associates ingested or were injected with urine, blood, skin scrapings, and feces from patients with

TABLE 3.5

Goldberger's Use of the Scientific Method to Determine the Cause of Pellagra

Scientific Method	Pellagra Is Caused by Diet	Pellagra Is Not Infectious
Observation	Observed that people who contracted pellagra subsisted on a limited diet of pork fat, corn bread, and molasses, whereas those who did not contract the disease had more varied diets.	Observed that prisoners contracted pellagra but not guards.
Hypothesis	Hypothesized that pellagra is caused by limited diets. His null hypothesis was that a restricted diet will not produce pellagra.	Hypothesized that the disease is not contagious. His null hypothesis was that germs cause pellagra.
Test	Tested his hypothesis by feeding convicts the traditional, monotonous Southern diet, which produced pellagra.	Tested his hypothesis by inoculating healthy volunteers with substances from pellagrins, which did not produce pellagra.
Conclusion	Concluded that pellagra is caused by eating a limited diet.	Concluded that pellagra is not contagious.

pellagra. Pellagra did not develop in any of them, thus leading Goldberger to conclude that *pellagra is not a contagious disease* (Kraut 2003).

Next, Goldberger established the socioeconomic epidemiology of pellagra. Seven cotton mill villages in South Carolina were chosen. The entire population was screened for pellagra, and meticulous dietary data for all households were collected. Pellagrous households had restricted intake of animal protein. There was no association of development of pellagra with consumption of corn or sanitary conditions. Pellagrous households were all poor. The poverty and diet of those affected could be linked to cotton. Cotton was king among the cash crops: sharecroppers and tenant farmers cultivated cotton at the expense of other crops. Lack of diversification and the speculative nature of cotton prices during the Depression made the tenant farmer and the sharecropper vulnerable to poverty, poor diet, and pellagra. By now, Goldberger concluded that pellagra was a socioeconomic malady, its occurrence in epidemic proportions in the South reflecting the extent of Southern poverty. If poor diet resulting from poverty among Southern tenant farmers and mill workers was the root cause of pellagra, then the only real cure was social reform, especially changes in the land tenure system (Rajakumar 2000).

Using the scientific method (making observations, posing a question, formulating a hypothesis, testing the hypothesis, and drawing conclusions), Goldberger proved that pellagra is a noncommunicable disease caused by a faulty diet linked to the prevailing economic conditions in the South. Table 3.5 summarizes Goldberger's use of the scientific method in determining the cause of pellagra.

Next, we turn to controlled trials that are randomized (RCTs). Like cohort studies, RCTs follow a group of people over time. However, with RCTs, the researchers actually intervene to see how a specific behavior change or treatment, for example, affects a health outcome. They are called *randomized trials* because people in the study are randomly assigned to either receive or not receive the intervention. This randomization helps researchers hone in on the true effect the intervention has on the health outcome. However, randomized trials also have drawbacks, especially when it comes to diet. For example, although RCTs are good at looking at the effects of vitamin supplementation and health outcomes, when the change in diet is more involved than taking a vitamin pill, participants begin to have trouble keeping to their prescribed diets. Such involved interventions can also become very expensive.

Nonblind, Randomized Clinical Trial

The Multiple Risk Factor Intervention Trial (MRFIT) was a nonblind, randomized primary prevention trial conducted at 22 US clinical centers from 1973 to 1982 to test whether lowering elevated serum cholesterol and diastolic blood pressure, and ceasing cigarette smoking would reduce CHD mortality. From the 361,662 men 35–57 years of age who were screened, 12,866 volunteers were selected for the trial. All of the volunteers had one or more of three risk factors for CHD (elevated cholesterol, hypertension, cigarette smoking). Half of the participants were assigned to the special intervention group (SI) and half to the usual care (UC) group, and followed for 6–8 years. The SI group was advised to follow an eating pattern designed to result in a nutrient intake of 30–35% of calories from fat, with 10% (later 8%) from saturated and 10% from polyunsaturated fat, approximately 300 mg (later 250 mg) of cholesterol, and modification of carbohydrates as needed for individual requirements. This group was also encouraged to cease cigarette smoking by a combination of techniques, including counseling and audiovisual aids. Hypertension management was based on a stepped-care program of weight reduction and medications. SI men had risk factor assessments every 4 months. Those in the UC group were referred to their personal physician or another source of care for such risk factor management as considered appropriate by these providers. Men in both groups returned annually for a medical history and physical examination. The primary end point was death due to CHD. An electrocardiogram was also obtained to identify nonfatal myocardial infarction as an additional end point (Kjelsberg et al. 1997).

The three risk factors declined in both groups, but the reductions were larger throughout the trial in the SI group, being significant at $P < .01$ at each annual visit. For example, after 6 years, 50% of SI men who were smokers had quit compared with 29% of the UC men. Diastolic blood pressure fell in the two groups by 10.5 and 7.3 mm Hg, respectively. Plasma cholesterol fell in the two groups by 12.1 and 7.5 mg/dL, respectively, which primarily represented changes in low-density lipoprotein cholesterol (LDL-C) and not high-density lipoprotein cholesterol (HDL-C). The unexpected decline in cholesterol in the UC group and a smaller-than-predicted decline in the SI group meant that the SI–UC difference was about half of that expected. At the end of the follow-up period, the CHD death rates were 17.9 per 1000 in the SI group and 19.3 per 1000 in the UC group. Total mortality rates were 41.2 per 1000 in the SI group and 40.4 per 1000 in the UC group. Neither death rates from CHD nor any other cause was reported as significantly different in the two groups. The researchers concluded that it is possible to apply an intensive long-term intervention program against the three coronary risk factors with considerable success in terms of risk factor changes, but the overall results do not show a beneficial effect on CHD or total mortality from this multifactor intervention (The Multiple Risk Factor Intervention Trial Research Group 1982).

Posttrial mortality surveillance of the 12,300 participants still living at the end of active intervention in 1982 continued through 1998. After 16 years, 370 SI and 417 UC men had died from CHD, which represents an 11.4% lower mortality rate for SI vs. UC men. Results for total mortality followed a similar pattern—991 SI and 1050 UC men had died by the end of follow-up. Differences between SI and UC men in mortality rates from acute myocardial infarction, CHD, and all causes were greater during the posttrial follow-up period than during the trial. The researchers conclude that these results demonstrate a long-term, continuing mortality benefit from the program (The Multiple Risk Factor Intervention Trial Research Group 1996). Using the National Death Index, a mortality follow-up of the 361,662 men screened for the MRFIT was continued thorough 1998.

Double-Blind, Randomized Controlled Clinical Trials

Physicians' Health Studies

In 1980, investigators from Harvard Medical School and Brigham and Women's Hospital, with funding from the NCI and NHLBI, launched the first Physicians' Health Study (PHS I) to study the effects of aspirin and beta-carotene in the primary prevention of CVD and cancer. PHS I was the first large, double-blind RCT conducted entirely by mail. At baseline in 1982, invitation letters, consent forms, and enrollment questionnaires were sent to 261,248 male physicians between 40 and 84 years of age residing in the United States and registered with the American Medical Association (AMA). Physicians were chosen for this study because of their ability to give true informed consent, their knowledge of possible side effects, and their ability to provide complete and accurate information. Of the 59,285 physicians who were willing to participate, 33,223 were eligible. Following an initial trial phase where participants received active aspirin and placebo (an inactive, or inert, treatment) beta-carotene, an additional 11,152 participants were excluded from the study, because they changed their minds, reported a reason for study exclusion, or did not reliably take the study pills. The remaining 22,071 physicians were then randomly assigned to receive active aspirin and active beta-carotene (n = 5517), active aspirin and beta-carotene placebo (n = 5520), aspirin placebo and active beta-carotene (n = 5519), or aspirin placebo and beta-carotene placebo (n = 5515). Follow-up questionnaires were sent at 6 and 12 months of treatment, and then annually afterward. Questions asked about compliance with taking the pills, use of nonstudy medications, occurrence of major illnesses or adverse effects, and other risk factor information. The primary end points of the study were total cancer, prostate cancer, CVD, and eye disease (i.e., cataracts and macular degeneration). The aspirin arm of the study was terminated early in 1988 because it was found that low-dose aspirin reduced the risk of first myocardial infarction by 44% ($P < .00001$). The beta-carotene arm of the study continued until 1995, and researchers found that after 13 years of supplementation, beta-carotene produced neither benefit nor harm, suggesting that beta-carotene alone is not responsible for the health benefits seen among people who eat large amounts of fruits and vegetables. Although PHS I ended in 1995, participants continue to complete annual questionnaires. Between 1984 and 2012, over 400 publications have been published on data from PHS I (Physicians' Health Study I, http://phs.bwh.harvard.edu/phs1.htm).

A second double-blind RCT, PHS II, was started in 1997 to test whether vitamin C, vitamin E, beta-carotene, and a multivitamin were beneficial in the primary prevention of CVD, total cancer, and prostate cancer, as well as colon cancer, age-related eye disease, and early cognitive decline. Recruitment for PHS II began in 1997, when PHS I participants were invited to join. A total of 7641 PHS I participants agreed to participate in PHS II. Invitation packets were also mailed to 254,597 US male physicians aged 50 years or older who were registered with the AMA and had not taken part in PHS I. Of the 16,743 who were willing to participate, 11,128 were eligible, and 7001 remained in the study following an initial trial period. A final total of 14,642 participants were randomized into 1 of 16 possible combinations of vitamin C, vitamin E, beta-carotene, and a multivitamin, or their placebos. Each year, PHS II participants receive a 12-month supply of study pills in foil-backed calendar packs, along with an annual follow-up questionnaire that asks about treatment compliance, use of nonstudy medications, occurrence of major illnesses or adverse effects, and other risk factor information. The beta-carotene arm ended as planned in 2003, and researchers found that beta-carotene did not reduce the risk of total CVD, total cancer, or total mortality. The vitamin C and vitamin E arms ended as planned in 2007 and found that these supplements do not prevent major cardiovascular events, cancer, or eye disease (Physicians' Health Study II, http://phs.bwh.harvard.edu/phs2.htm). In 2011, the multivitamin arm ended as planned, and results show that, among the PHS II population, taking a multivitamin does not reduce major CVD events, myocardial infarction, stroke, CVD mortality, prostate cancer, colorectal cancer, other site-specific cancers, or cancer mortality after more than 10 years of treatment and follow-up (Gaziano et al. 2012; Sesso et al. 2012). Daily multivitamin supplementation was found to modestly, yet significantly, reduce the risk of total cancer incidence (Sesso et al. 2012). Although the trial is over, researchers have submitted a grant proposal to continue collecting annual data from PHS participants in an observational follow-up study (Physicians' Health Study, http://phs.bwh.harvard.edu/faqs.htm).

USDA'S AGRICULTURAL RESEARCH SERVICE

The research of the Agricultural Research Service (ARS) is organized into National Programs to best coordinate the over 800 research projects of the ARS. Human Nutrition is National Program #107. The mission of the Human Nutrition Program is to define the role of food and its components in optimizing health throughout the life cycle for all Americans by conducting high-national-priority research. The program's vision is that of well-nourished Americans making health-promoting dietary choices based on scientific evidence. The program components consist of (1) linking agricultural practices and beneficial health outcomes, (2) monitoring food composition and nutrient intake of the nation, (3) scientific basis for dietary guidance, (4) prevention of obesity and obesity-related diseases, and (5) life stage nutrition and metabolism (US Department of Agriculture, http://www .ars.usda.gov/research/programs/programs.htm?NP_CODE=107). Work is carried out in Beltsville, Maryland; Boston, Massachusetts; Davis, California; Grand Forks, North Dakota; Houston, Texas; Ithaca, New York; and Little Rock, Arkansas.

BELTSVILLE HUMAN NUTRITION RESEARCH CENTER

The mission of the Beltsville Human Nutrition Research Center (BHNRC) is to define, through research, the role of foods and their components in optimizing human health and reducing the risk of nutritionally related disorders. As of 2014, the center consists of five laboratories (US Department of Agriculture, http://www.ars.usda.gov/main/site_main.htm?modecode=80-40-05-00).

- Food Composition and Methods Development Laboratory.
- Food Components and Health Laboratory.
- Diet, Genomics, and Immunology Laboratory.
- Nutrient Data Laboratory (NDL).
- Food Surveys Research Group (FSRG).

Nutrient Data Laboratory

The NDL (US Department of Agriculture, http://www.ars.usda.gov/main/site_main.htm?modecode =80-40-05-25) is one of the BHNRC laboratories. The NDL and its predecessor organizations have been compiling and developing food composition databases for over a century. (The USDA has borne primary responsibility for characterizing the nutrient content of the US food supply for over 115 years. The first food composition tables were published in 1891 by Atwater and Woods, who assayed the refuse, water, fat, protein, ash, and carbohydrate content of approximately 200 foods.) The mission of the NDL's interdisciplinary team of nutritionists, dietitians, food technologists, and computer specialists is to develop authoritative food composition databases and state-of-the-art methods to acquire, evaluate, compile, and disseminate composition data on foods available in the US. USDA food composition data, developed by the NDL, are used in many government databases and provide core data for commercial and foreign databases, as well as serve as tools for epidemiological research, national nutrition policy planning, and dietetics and food service planning. Among these are the following:

- USDA ARS, FSRG.
- Food and Nutrient Database for Dietary Studies (FNDDS) surveys and search tool.
- Foodlink.
- USDA FNS, Child Nutrition Database.
- USDA AMS Food & Commodity Connection.
- USDA Center for Nutrition Policy and Promotion.

The principle database is the USDA National Nutrient Database for Standard Reference (NDSR). The NDSR is maintained by the NDL and BHNRC, and online access is provided to the public via a website jointly developed by the USDA NDL, and the Food and Nutrition Information Center and Information Systems Division of the National Agricultural Library.

Nutrient Database for Standard Reference

The USDA NDSR was designed specifically to collect and disseminate food composition data (Syme et al. 1975). The current version of the NDSR as of September 2014 is release 27, with over 8000 foods (US Department of Agriculture, http://ndb.nal.usda.gov/ndb/). The NDL's databases need constant revision as the food supply constantly changes. The completeness of analytical data varies from nutrient to nutrient (Willett 1998c). As of early 2015, the database is available here: http://ndb.nal.usda.gov/. A search tool enables the user to search by food item, group, or list to retrieve the nutrient content of foods. The NDSR files can also be downloaded onto a personal computer. This database is the successor to the *Agriculture Handbook No. 8, Composition of Food*, published in hard copy until 1992 but no longer available in print form. This database (release 13) was also used to create the most recent edition (2002) of *Nutritive Value of Foods, Home and Garden Bulletin 72* (HG-72). Since its first publication in 1960, this reference has been an important source of food composition data for consumers, as well as a useful educational tool for dietitians and other professionals. The current version contains data on almost 1300 foods typically consumed in the US, expressed in common household units. The nutrients and other food factors in the table are water; calories; protein; total fat; fatty acids (saturated, monounsaturated, and polyunsaturated); cholesterol; total dietary fiber; calcium; iron; potassium; sodium; vitamin A (in IU and RE units); thiamin; riboflavin; niacin; and ascorbic acid (US Department of Agriculture, http://www.ars.usda.gov/is/np/NutritiveValueofFoods/Nutritive ValueofFoodsIntro.htm).

Food Surveys Research Group

The FSRG (US Department of Agriculture, http://www.ars.usda.gov/main/site_main.htm?mode code=80-40-05-30), housed at the BHNRC, is responsible for NHANES's dietary data collection methodology, maintenance of the databases used to code and process the data, and data review and processing. The FRSG provides a view of dietary survey data about food consumption patterns in the US, articles regarding USDA dietary intake research methods, and previous dietary intake surveys. Uses of FSRG survey data include assessment of dietary intakes, dietary trends, and food consumption economics; development of policies for food assistance, food labeling, and food safety programs; and implementation of dietary guidance and nutrition education programs.

The mission of the FSRG is to monitor and assess food consumption and related behavior of the US population by conducting surveys and providing the resulting information for food- and nutrition-related programs and public policy decisions (Ahuja et al. 2013). The FSRG is responsible for implementing food consumption surveys, dietary method research, as well as a number of databases and tools: WWEIA (dietary intake from NHANES), the search tool What's In the Foods You Eat (a database of commonly consumed foods), FNDDS (used to analyze dietary intake data, see Box 3.7), a prototype version of FNDDS containing branded foods, the AMPM, the Food Patterns Equivalents Database (used to compare intake data to US dietary guidance), and Food Intakes Converted to Retail Commodities. Information for all of these (as well as access to many of the tools) can be found at http://www.ars.usda.gov/Services/docs .htm?docid=23887.

BOX 3.7   FOOD AND NUTRIENT DATABASE FOR DIETARY STUDIES (FNDDS)

FNDDS is designed for the analysis of dietary intake and contains no missing nutrient values. It includes comprehensive information that can be used to code individual foods and portion sizes and contains nutrient values for calculating nutrient intakes. FNDDS data are for foods and beverages reported in WWEIA, NHANES. Many of the foods in FNDDS are mixtures not available in the NDSR. The NDSR is the source of the nutrient values for foods in FNDDS, including the mixed foods whose nutrient values are calculated by combining the NDSR data for separate ingredients. The FNDDS portion weights are for the portion sizes survey respondents report. Therefore, FNNDS includes additional weights for common food portion sizes not available in the NDSR.

Various government agencies provide technical support for nutritional epidemiological research.

- The Clinical and Epidemiological Nutrition Research program at the NIDDK supports clinical research focused on observational/interventional studies in nutrition, as well as nutritional epidemiology studies, but does not support research regarding obesity, energy balance, or weight control. (US Department of Health and Human Services, http://www.niddk.nih.gov/research-funding/research-programs/Pages/clinical-epidemiological-nutrition-research-program.aspx).
- The Nutritional Epidemiology Branch of the NCI (NEB) studies the causal relations between nutrition, nutrition-related factors, and human cancer. Its research encompasses diet, energy balance and obesity, physical activity, specific nutrients and supplements, diet-related additives, contaminants, metabolites, and intermediate biologic markers. NEB also trains researchers and develops software tools and other resources (US Department of Health and Human Services, http://dceg.cancer.gov/about).
- The University of North Carolina's Nutrition Obesity Research Center (UNC NORC) is one of 12 centers in the country funded by the NIDDK that is specifically designed to provide support and expertise to scientists studying the role of nutrition and obesity in public health. UNC NORC aims to support investigators, enhance nutrition and obesity research at the university, strengthen clinical nutrition training programs, and translate findings from obesity and nutrition research to the general public to use to improve their overall health and well being (University of North Carolina, http://www.sph.unc.edu/norc/).

CONCLUSION

Nutritional epidemiology is fundamental to the practice of nutrition in public health. Through the keen observational skills of its practitioners, numerous advances in public health have been made—from an appreciation of a clean water supply to an understanding of the relationship between food and nutrition, as in Lind's and Goldberger's studies. The history and development of epidemiology as a science is an engaging narrative and a continually evolving story, moving from an initial focus on deficiency diseases to our current spotlight on chronic diseases, such as heart disease, diabetes, and obesity.

Although the gold standard of research is often considered to be the RCT, other study designs are both possible and desirable. Longitudinal prospective studies, for example, though costly and cumbersome, are a powerful tool in the study of the effects of diet on health as these effects take years to manifest themselves. Epidemiologic research is supported by data analysis efforts and nutritional databases that allow interpretation of findings and trends. As technology continues to evolve and expand, it will prove a useful adjunct to the pursuit of nutritional epidemiology and our understanding of nutrition and health.

ACRONYMS

AMA	American Medical Association
AMPM	Automated multipass method
ARMS	Adverse Reaction Monitoring System
ARS	Agricultural Research Service
BHNRC	Beltsville Human Nutrition Research Center
BMI	Body mass index

BW	Birth weight
CFSAN	Center for Food Safety and Applied Nutrition
CHD	Coronary heart disease
CI	Confidence interval
CVD	Cardiovascular disease
DLW	Doubly labeled water
FDA	Food and Drug Administration
FFQ	Food frequency questionnaire
FNDDS	Food and Nutrient Database for Dietary Studies
FSRG	Food Surveys Research Group
GRAS	Generally recognized as safe
GUTS I and II	Growing Up Today Study I and II
HBW	High birth weight
HDL-C	High-density lipoprotein cholesterol
HHS	United States Department of Health and Human Services
HPFS	Health Professionals Follow-Up Study
HR	Hazard ratio
LBW	Low birth weight
LDL-C	Low-density lipoprotein cholesterol
MRFIT	Multiple Risk Factor Intervention Trial
NCI	National Cancer Institute
NDL	Nutrient Data Laboratory
NDSR	National Nutrient Database for Standard Reference
NEB	Nutritional Epidemiology Branch of the NCI
NHANES	National Health and Nutrition Examination Study
NHLBI	National Heart, Lung, and Blood Institute
NHS I, II, and III	Nurses' Health Study I, II, and III
NIAAA	National Institute on Alcohol Abuse and Alcoholism
NICHD	National Institute of Child Health and Human Development
NIDDK	National Institute for Diabetes and Digestive and Kidney Diseases
NIH	National Institutes of Health
NINR	National Institute of Nursing Research
NTDs	Neural tube defects
ONQI	Overall Nutritional Quality Index
OR	Odds ratio
PHS I and II	Physicians' Health Study I and II
QOL	Quality of life
RCT	Randomized controlled trial
RN	Registered nurse
RR	Relative risk
SI	Special intervention
UC	Usual care
UNC NORC	University of North Carolina Nutrition Obesity Research Center
USDA	United States Department of Agriculture

STUDENT ASSIGNMENTS AND ACTIVITIES DESIGNED TO ENHANCE LEARNING AND STIMULATE CRITICAL THINKING

1. Search the Internet for job descriptions of a nutritional epidemiologist. What skills are necessary to work in this field? In what types of settings are nutritional epidemiologists employed? Describe at least three topics of current interest in nutritional epidemiology.

2. Discuss the costs and benefits of the various dietary assessment methods.
3. Keep a 3-day dietary record (2 weekdays and 1 weekend day). Refer to the sample record and instructions provided by the American Academy of Family Physicians at the FamilyDoctor website: http://familydoctor.org/familydoctor/en/prevention-wellness/food -nutrition/healthy-food-choices/nutrition-keeping-a-food-diary.html. Enter and analyze your 3-day dietary record using the online SuperTracker (food tracker) available from the US Department of Agriculture at https://www.supertracker.usda.gov/default.aspx. Print a copy of the following reports: meal summary report, nutrients report, and food groups and calories report.

   The following week, complete the National Cancer Institute's automated, self-administered 24-hour dietary recall available at http://appliedresearch.cancer.gov/asa24/ (instructors will need to register for free access). Enter and analyze your 3-day dietary record using the online SuperTracker (food tracker) available from the US Department of Agriculture at https://www.supertracker.usda.gov/default.aspx. Print a copy of the following reports: meal summary report, nutrients report, and food groups and calories report.

   In addition to submitting your dietary records, 24-hour recall, and food tracker print-outs, write a reaction paper discussing your results from each method and any findings that surprise you, including answers to the following questions:
   a. Describe the results of your 3-day dietary record and 24-hour dietary recall regarding your energy intake; carbohydrate; protein; total fat; saturated fat; polyunsaturated fat; cholesterol; vitamins A, C, and E; calcium; iron; and sodium. Conduct a self-assessment of your diet. What food group(s)/nutrient(s) need improvements for you to obtain optimal health?
   b. Do you believe that the 3-day dietary record and 24-hour dietary recall are accurate and valid representations of your dietary intake? Why or why not? How did the results from your 3-day dietary record compare with those from your 24-hour dietary recall? What implications might this have for large surveys attempting to test relationships between diet and disease? If you had to conduct a study to collect dietary intake data from a large cohort, say 300 participants, what would be your preferred method and why?
   c. Can you think of a new, innovative method (or an improved modification to an existing method) for collecting accurate dietary data?
4. Download the sample of the National Cancer Institute's Diet History Questionnaire II at http://appliedresearch.cancer.gov/dhq2/. After completing the questionnaire, describe your experience. Include in your discussion answers to the following:
   a. How long did it take you to complete this questionnaire? Did you find the questionnaire easy to understand and complete? Why or why not?
   b. What, if any, attempts were made to reflect cultural differences in dietary intake? Why is this important?
   c. What, if any, attempts were made to reflect seasonal changes in dietary habits? Why is this important?
   d. Are any of the foods listed in the questionnaire uncommon or unknown to you? Which ones? Why do you think these foods were included?
   e. Were there any foods that you feel are missing from the questionnaire? What are they, and why do you think they were not included?
   f. How accurate do you think your recall was? How does this affect the results of the questionnaire?
5. Describe how the complexity of our food supply poses challenges in studying the relationship between diet and disease.
6. Does the daily variation in an individual's dietary intake have important implications for population-based nutritional epidemiologic studies? Explain your answer.

7. A nurse practitioner wants to know whether her patient can safely consume caffeine during pregnancy. Using PubMed (http://www.ncbi.nlm.nih.gov/pubmed/), find three epidemiological studies in humans that will help you answer her question. Then, answer the following for each study:
   a. What were the objectives of the study?
   b. What type of study design was conducted? Discuss the strengths and weaknesses of this type of study design.
   c. Describe the source of the study population, process of sample selection, and sample size.
   d. What type(s) of dietary assessment method was used in this study? Was this method the most appropriate choice? Why or why not?
   e. What were the major results of the study?
   f. What study limitations were addressed in the discussion section? What other limitations of the study were not mentioned?
   g. What were the authors' main conclusions?
   h. What do you conclude?
   Based on your review of these three studies, what will you tell the nurse practitioner?
8. Using PubMed (http://www.ncbi.nlm.nih.gov/pubmed/), find a nutrition-related example of three of the following epidemiological study designs, at least one from each column. Articles must have been published within the past 5 years.

Ecological study	Prospective cohort study
Cross-sectional study	Meta-analysis
Case–control study	Nonrandomized controlled trial
Retrospective cohort study	Randomized controlled trial

   For each study, answer the following questions:
   a. What were the objectives of the study?
   b. What type of study design was conducted? Discuss the strengths and weaknesses of this type of study design.
   c. Describe the source of the study population, process of sample selection, and sample size.
   d. What type(s) of dietary assessment method was used in this study? Was this method the most appropriate choice? Why or why not?
   e. What were the major results of the study?
   f. What study limitations were addressed in the discussion section? What other limitations of the study were not mentioned?
   g. What were the authors' main conclusions?
   h. What do you conclude?
9. Review the publications and newsletters detailing the progress of the *Health Professionals Follow-Up Study* at http://www.hsph.harvard.edu/hpfs/hpfs_publications.htm. Describe five of the most recent findings from these studies. Discuss the strengths and weaknesses of these studies.
10. Your supervisor has asked you to conduct a 12-month cohort study of infant feeding among first-time Chinese-American mothers. The purpose of this study is to determine how long mothers breastfeed their infants, at what age infants are first given solid foods, and the food preparation techniques mothers use to prepare food for their infants.
   a. Develop 10 interview questions you would ask each study participant. State your reasons for asking each question. Consult the questionnaires used in the *Nurses' Health Studies* (http://www.channing.harvard.edu/nhs/?page_id=246) and *Growing Up Today Studies* (http://www.gutsweb.org/index.php/the-survey/guts-questionnaires) as guides.

    b. Discuss how you would conduct your study. Include the following:
        i. What criteria would you use to include/exclude potential participants? How many participants would you recruit?
       ii. Describe where, when, and how the interviews would take place.
      iii. Develop a time frame for the study.
      iv. List the advantages and disadvantages of using a cohort study design.
    c. Explain how another study design could be used to answer the same research questions and discuss the advantages and disadvantages of using this design.
    d. Discuss the strengths and weaknesses of collaborating with universities, hospitals, health clinics, nonprofit organizations, and/or a health department to conduct this study.
    e. Sometimes, additional funding is needed to complete a study, so researchers will apply for grant money. Search the federal government grants at http://www.grants.gov and the *Foundation Center* at http://fdncenter.org/funders/. List potential grant sources for your research study. Explain why you chose these grants.

11. Write a research paper discussing both sides of a controversial issue in nutritional epidemiology. (Alternatively, have two students or teams each present one side of the issue in a debate-like format.) What types of studies have been performed to assess a relationship? Which side of the debate does the research support most (consider both the quantity and quality of the research available on both sides)? Possible topics may include the following:

- Does portion size influence body weight?
- Should the US supply of infant formula be fortified with long-chain omega-3 polyunsaturated fatty acids?
- Should soft drinks be taxed to prevent diabetes and cancer?
- Does a diet high in fructose increase body fat?
- Are all calories created equal?
- Should Americans be encouraged to consume soy?
- Should body mass index (BMI) be used to assess obesity?
- Are organically grown foods healthier than conventionally grown foods?

12. The following epidemiologic case studies on foodborne disease are available from the Centers for Disease Control and Prevention for classroom discussions (come with instructor's guide):

- Botulism in Argentina: http://www.cdc.gov/epicasestudies/classroom_botulism.html.
- Gastroenteritis at a University in Texas: http://www.cdc.gov/epicasestudies/classroom_gast.html.
- Multistate Outbreak of Cyclosporiasis: http://www.cdc.gov/epicasestudies/classroom_cyclo.html.
- Multistate Outbreak of *E. coli* O157:H7 Infection: http://www.cdc.gov/epicasestudies/classroom_ecoli.html.
- *Salmonella* in the Caribbean: http://www.cdc.gov/epicasestudies/classroom_salmonella.html.

REFERENCES

Ahuja JKC, Juan W, Egan K, Buzby J, Trumbo P, Moshfegh A, Holden J. Federal monitoring activities related to food and nutrition: How do they compare? *Procedia Food Sci.* 2013;2:165–171. Available at http://www.sciencedirect.com/science/article/pii/S2211601X13000254, accessed February 17, 2015.

Bartholomew M. James Lind and scurvy: A revaluation. *J Marit Res.* 2002;4(1):1–4.

Berkey CS, Rockett HRH, Willett WC, Colditz GA. Milk, dairy fat, dietary calcium, and weight gain: A longitudinal study of adolescents. *Arch Pediatr Adolesc Med.* 2005;159(6):543–550.

Berlan ED, Corliss HL, Field AE, Goodman E, Austin SB. Sexual orientation and bullying among adolescents in the Growing Up Today Study. *J Adolesc Health.* 2010;46(4):366–371.

Botto LD, Lisi A, Robert-Gnansia E et al. International retrospective cohort study of neural tube defects in relation to folic acid recommendations: Are the recommendations working? *BMJ.* 2005;330(7491):571.

Brown L, Dattilo A. Meta-analysis in nutrition research. In Monsen E, ed. *Research: Successful Approaches.* Chicago: American Dietetic Association, 2003, chap. 11.

Brown SR. *Scurvy: How a Surgeon, a Mariner, and a Gentleman Solved the Greatest Medical Mystery of the Age of Sail.* New York: Thomas Dunne Books (St. Martin's Press), 2003.

Buzzard M. 24-hour recall and food record methods. In Willett W, ed. *Nutritional Epidemiology,* 2nd ed. New York: Oxford University Press, 1998, chap. 4.

Chiuve ST, Sampson L, Willett WC. Adherence to the Overall Nutritional Quality Index and risk of total chronic disease. *Am J Prev Med.* 2011;40(5):505–513.

Cooper KJ. A short history of nutritional science: Part 3 (1912–1944). Pellagra in the United States. *J Nutr.* 2003;133(10):3023–3032.

Curhan GC, Willett WC, Rimm EB, Spiegelman D, Ascherio AL, Stampfer MJ. Birth weight and adult hypertension, diabetes mellitus, and obesity in U.S. men. *Circulation.* 1996;94(12):3246–3250.

Daya NE, McKeown N, Wong MY, Welch A, Bingham S. Epidemiological assessment of diet: A comparison of a 7-day diary with a food frequency questionnaire using urinary markers of nitrogen, potassium and sodium. *Int J Epidemiol.* 2001;30(2):309–317.

Doig GS. Interpreting and using clinical trials. *Crit Care Clin.* 1998;14(3):513–524.

Field AE, Camargo CA Jr., Taylor CB, Berkey CS, Roberts SB, Colditz GA. Peer, parent, and media influences on the development of weight concerns and frequent dieting among preadolescent and adolescent girls and boys. *Pediatrics.* 2001;107(1):54–60.

Field AE, Austin SB, Taylor CB et al. Relation between dieting and weight change among preadolescents and adolescents. *Pediatrics.* 2003;112(4):900–906.

Field AE, Austin SB, Gillman MW, Rosner B, Rockett HR, Colditz GA. Snack food intake does not predict weight change among children and adolescents. *Int J Obes Relat Metab Disord.* 2004;28(10):1210–1216.

Food and Drug Administration. Office of Food Additive Safety. *Redbook 2000. Toxicological Principles for the Safety Assessment of Food Ingredients, July 2000.* Updated July 2007. Chapter VI.B: Epidemiology, October 2001. Available at http://www.fda.gov/Food/GuidanceRegulation/GuidanceDocumentsRegulatoryInforma tion/IngredientsAdditivesGRASPackaging/ucm078401.htm, accessed January 20, 2015.

Freidenheim JL. Study design and hypothesis testing: Issues in the evaluation of evidence from research in nutritional epidemiology. *Am J Clin Nutr.* 1999;69(6):1315S–1321S.

Friis RH, Sellers TA. Study designs: Cohort studies. In Friis RH, Sellers TA, eds. *Epidemiology for Public Health Practice,* 3rd ed. Sudbury, MA: Jones and Bartlett, 2004, chap. 7.

Gaziano JM, Sesso HD, Christen WG et al. Multivitamins in the prevention of cancer in men: The Physicians' Health Study II randomized controlled trial. *JAMA.* 2012;308(18):1871–1880.

Gillman MW, Rifas-Shiman SL, Camargo CA Jr. et al. Risk of overweight among adolescents who were breastfed as infants. *JAMA.* 2001;285(19):2461–2467.

Guise JM, Palda V, Westhoff C, Chan BK, Helfand M, Lieu TA; U.S. Preventive Services Task Force. The effectiveness of primary care-based interventions to promote breastfeeding: Systematic evidence review and meta-analysis for the U.S. Preventive Services Task Force. *Ann Fam Med.* 2003;1(2):70–78.

Growing Up Today Study. Then and Now. Available at http://www.gutsweb.org/index.php/the-study/guts-then -and-now, accessed January 20, 2015.

Growing Up Today Study. Summer 2012 Newsletter. Available at http://www.gutsweb.org/images/PDFs /newsletters/2012newsletter.pdf, accessed January 20, 2015.

Hamet P. The evaluation of the scientific evidence for a relationship between calcium and hypertension. *J Nutr.* 1995;125(2 Suppl):311S–400S.

Hammarsten E. The 1937 Nobel Prize in Physiology or Medicine Presentation Speech, December 10, 1937. Available at http://www.nobelprize.org/nobel_prizes/medicine/laureates/1937/press.html, accessed January 20, 2015.

Harvard School of Public Health. President and Fellows of Harvard College. Health Professionals Follow-Up Study. About the Study. Available at http://www.hsph.harvard.edu/hpfs/, accessed January 20, 2015.

He K, Song Y, Daviglus ML, Liu K, Van Horn L, Dyer AR, Greenland P. Accumulated evidence on fish consumption and coronary heart disease mortality: A meta-analysis of cohort studies. *Circulation.* 2004;109(22):2705–2711.

Hughes RE. James Lind and the cure of scurvy: An experimental approach. *Med Hist.* 1975;19(4):342–351.

Johnson RK. Dietary intake—How do we measure what people are *really* eating? *Obes Res.* 2002;10(Suppl 1):63S–68S.

Johnson RK, Hankin JH. Dietary assessment and validation. In Monsen E, ed. *Research: Successful Approaches,* 2nd ed. Chicago: American Dietetic Association, 2003, chap. 15.

Kelsey JL, Whittemore AS, Evans AS, Thompson WD. *Methods in Observational Epidemiology*, 2nd ed. New York: Oxford University Press, 1996.

Kessler II, Clark JP. Saccharin, cyclamate, and human bladder cancer: No evidence of an association. *JAMA*. 1978;240(4):349–355.

Kirks BA, Wolff HK. A comparison of methods for plate waste determinations. *J Am Diet Assoc.* 1985;85(3):328–331.

Kjelsberg MO, Butler JA, Dolecek TA. Brief description of the Multiple Risk Factor Intervention Trial. *Am J Clin Nutr.* 1997;65(1 Suppl):191S–195S.

Klevay LM. And so spake Goldberger in 1916: Pellagra is not infectious! *J Am Coll Nutr.* 1997;16(3):290–292.

Koh-Banerjee P, Wang Y, Hu FB, Spiegelman D, Willett WC, Rimm EB. Changes in body weight and body fat distribution as risk factors for clinical diabetes in U.S. men. *Am J Epidemiol.* 2004;159(12):1150–1159.

Kraut AM. *Goldberger's War: The Life and Work of a Public Health Crusader.* New York: Hill and Wang, 2003.

Langseth L. *Nutritional Epidemiology: Possibilities and Limitations.* Brussels, Belgium: International Life Sciences Institute, 1996.

Marks HM. Epidemiologists explain pellagra: Gender, race, and political economy in the work of Edgar Sydenstricker. *J Hist Med Allied Sci.* 2003;58(1):34–55.

McArthur DB. Heart healthy eating behaviors of children following a school-based intervention: A meta-analysis. *Issues Compr Pediatr Nurs.* 1998;21(1):35–48.

Morgan RW, Wong O. A review of epidemiological studies on artificial sweeteners and bladder cancer. *Food Chem Toxicol.* 1985;23(4–5):529–533.

Mullen PD, Simons-Morton DG, Ramirez G, Frankowski RF, Green LW, Mains DA. A meta-analysis of trials evaluating patient education and counseling for three groups of preventive health behaviors. *Patient Educ Couns.* 1997;32(3):157–173.

National Institutes of Health (NIH). Improving Diet and Physical Activity Assessment (R01). Funding Opportunity Announcement (FOA) Number: PAR-12-198. Release date: June 6, 2012. Available at http://grants.nih.gov/grants/guide/pa-files/PAR-12-198.html, accessed January 15, 2015.

Nichaman MZ, Hamilton HB, Kagan A, Grier T, Sacks T, Syme SL. Epidemiologic studies of coronary heart disease and stroke in Japanese men living in Japan, Hawaii and California: Distribution of biochemical risk factors. *Am J Epidemiol.* 1975;102(6):491–501.

Nkondjock A, Ghadirian P, Johnson KC, Krewski D. Canadian cancer registries epidemiology research group: Dietary intake of lycopene is associated with reduced pancreatic cancer risk. *J Nutr.* 2005;135(3):592–597.

The Nurses' Health Study. History. Available at http://www.channing.harvard.edu/nhs/?page_id=70, accessed January 20, 2015.

Nurses' Health Study 3. Available at http://www.nhs3.org/, accessed January 20, 2015.

NutritionQuest. Assessment & Analysis Services. Questionnaires and Screeners. Available at http://nutritionquest.com/assessment/list-of-questionnaires-and-screeners, accessed January 20, 2015.

NutritionQuest. Our Research: Questionnaires. Available at http://nutritionquest.com/company/our-research-questionnaires, accessed January 20, 2015.

Physicians' Health Study I. Available at http://phs.bwh.harvard.edu/phs1.htm, accessed January 20, 2015.

Physicians' Health Study II. Available at http://phs.bwh.harvard.edu/phs2.htm, accessed January 20, 2015.

Physicians' Health Study. FAQs. Available at http://phs.bwh.harvard.edu/faqs.htm, accessed January 20, 2015.

Rajakumar K. Pellagra in the United States: A historical perspective. *Southern Med J.* 2000;93(3):272–277.

Schoeller DA. Measurement of energy expenditure in free living humans by using doubly labeled water. *J Nutr.* 1988;118(11):1278–1289.

Sesso HD, Christen WG, Bubes F et al. Multivitamins in the prevention of cardiovascular disease in men: The Physicians' Health Study II randomized controlled trial. *JAMA*. 2012;308(17):1751–1760.

Sherry B, Archer S, VanHorn L. Descriptive epidemiologic research. In Monsen ER, ed. *Research: Successful Approaches*, 2nd ed. Chicago: American Dietetic Association, 2003, chap. 8.

Skinner HH, Haines J, Austin SB, Field AE. A prospective study of overeating, binge eating, and depressive symptoms among adolescent and young adult women. *J Adolesc Health.* 2012;50(5):478–483.

Stroup DF, Berlin JA, Morton SC et al. Meta-analysis of observational studies in epidemiology: A proposal for reporting. Meta-analysis of Observational Studies in Epidemiology (MOOSE) group. *JAMA*. 2000;283(15):2008–2012.

Syme SL, Marmot MG, Kagan A, Kato H, Rhoads G. Epidemiologic studies of coronary heart disease and stroke in Japanese men living in Japan, Hawaii and California: Introduction. *Am J Epidemiol.* 1975;102(6):477–480.

The Multiple Risk Factor Intervention Trial Research Group. Multiple Risk Factor Intervention Trial: Risk factor changes and mortality results. *JAMA*. 1982;248(12):1465–1477.

The Multiple Risk Factor Intervention Trial Research Group. Mortality after 16 years for participants random-ized to the Multiple Risk Factor Intervention Trial. *Circulation.* 1996;94(5):946–951.

Tolley EA, Headley AS. Meta-analyses: What they can and cannot tell us about clinical research. *Curr Opin Clin Nutr Metab Care.* 2005;8(2):177–181.

Tsai CJ, Leitzmann MF, Willett WC, Giovannucci EL. Prospective study of abdominal adiposity and gallstone disease in U.S. men. *Am J Clin Nutr.* 2004;80(1):38–44.

US Department of Agriculture. Agriculture Research Service. Food Surveys. Available at http://www.ars.usda.gov/main/site_main.htm?modecode=80-40-05-30, accessed February 17, 2015.

US Department of Agriculture. Agricultural Research Service. Human Nutrition. Available at http://www.ars.usda.gov/main/site_main.htm?modecode=80-40-05-00, accessed February 17, 2015.

US Department of Health and Human Services. National Institutes of Health. National Cancer Institute. Nutritional Epidemiology Branch. Available at http://dceg.cancer.gov/about, accessed January 20, 2015.

US Department of Health and Human Services. National Institutes of Health. National Institute of Diabetes and Digestive and Kidney Diseases. Clinical and Epidemiological Nutrition Research. Available at http://www.niddk.nih.gov/research-funding/research-programs/Pages/clinical-epidemiological-nutrition-research-program.aspx, accessed January 20, 2015.

US Department of Agriculture. Agricultural Research Service. National Nutrient Database for Standard Reference Release 27. Available at http://ndb.nal.usda.gov/ndb/, accessed February 17, 2015.

US Department of Agriculture. Agriculture Research Service. National Program 107: Human Nutrition. Available at http://www.ars.usda.gov/research/programs/programs.htm?NP_CODE=107, accessed February 17, 2015.

US Department of Agriculture. Agricultural Research Service. Nutrient Data. Available at http://www.ars.usda.gov/main/site_main.htm?modecode=80-40-05-25, accessed February 17, 2015.

US Department of Agriculture. Agricultural Research Service. Nutritive Value of Foods. Available at http://www.ars.usda.gov/is/np/NutritiveValueofFoods/NutritiveValueofFoodsIntro.htm, accessed February 17, 2015.

US Food and Drug Administration. MedWatch: The FDA Safety Information and Adverse Event Reporting Program. Available at http://www.fda.gov/Safety/MedWatch/default.htm, accessed January 20, 2015.

University of North Carolina. Gillings School of Global Public Health. Nutrition Obesity Research Center. Available at http://www.sph.unc.edu/norc/, accessed January 20, 2015.

Willett W. Overview of nutritional epidemiology. In Willett W, ed. *Nutritional Epidemiology*, 2nd ed. New York: Oxford University Press, 1998a, chap. 1.

Willett W. Folic acid and neural tube defects. In Willett W, ed. *Nutritional Epidemiology*, 2nd ed. New York: Oxford University Press, 1998b, chap. 18.

Willett W. Diet and coronary heart disease. In Willett W, ed. *Nutritional Epidemiology*, 2nd ed. New York: Oxford University Press, 1998c, chap. 17.

Willett W. Issues in analysis and presentation of dietary data. In Willett W, ed. *Nutritional Epidemiology*, 2nd ed. New York: Oxford University Press, 1998d, chap. 13.

Willett WC. *Eat, Drink, and Be Healthy.* New York: Simon and Schuster Source, 2001.

Worth RM, Kato H, Rhoads GG, Kagan K, Syme SL. Epidemiologic studies of coronary heart disease and stroke in Japanese men living in Japan, Hawaii and California: Mortality. *Am J Epidemiol.* 1975;102(6):481–490.

Wright ME. A case-control study of maternal nutrition and neural tube defects in Northern Ireland. *Midwifery.* 1995;11(3):146–152.

4 Diet-Related Chronic Disease
*Disparities and Programs to Reduce Them**

Injustice anywhere is a threat to justice everywhere.

Martin Luther King, Jr. (1929–1968)

INTRODUCTION

The term *health disparities* generally refers to a higher burden of incidence, prevalence, morbidity, and mortality of diseases and other adverse health conditions experienced by one population group relative to another group. In the United States, a health disparity is commonly viewed as affecting racial and ethnic populations; however, health disparity burdens may manifest in groups characterized by socioeconomic status (SES), age, location, gender, disability status, immigration status, and sexual identity and orientation; the medically underserved; and rural populations. The term *health-care disparity* refers to differences between groups in health insurance coverage, access to and use of care, and quality of care (The Henry R. Kaiser Family Foundation 2012). Healthcare disparities may contribute to health outcome disparities.

Public health nutrition programs and policies must address health disparities, as diet-related conditions such as infant mortality, heart disease, stroke, cancer, and type 2 diabetes affect racial and ethnic minority populations and other subpopulations to a greater extent than the general population:

- *Infant mortality*: The infant mortality rate is twice as high among African Americans compared to whites, and nearly 60% higher in Native Americans/Alaska Natives compared to whites (MacDorman and Mathews 2013).
- *Heart disease*: Heart disease is the leading cause of death in the United States, for both men and women. There exists a disproportionate burden of death and disability from cardiovascular disease (CVD) in minority and low-income populations. African Americans are 30% more likely to die from heart disease, and African American women are 1.6 times as likely to have high blood pressure as whites (US Department of Health and Human Services 2012). African American women in particular carry a high burden of risk; the age-adjusted rate of heart disease for African American women is 72% higher than for white women (Women's Heart Foundation, http://www.womensheart.org/content/HeartDisease/heart_disease_facts.asp).
- *Stroke*: Stroke is the fourth leading cause of death in the United States, killing approximately 130,000 Americans every year (Hoyert and Xu 2012). African Americans are 1.8 times more likely to die of stroke than whites (Go et al. 2013).
- *Cancer*: Cancer is the second most common cause of mortality in the United States. Many minority groups suffer disproportionately from cancer. African Americans have the highest overall risk of cancer at any site, as well as, specifically, pancreas, prostate, lung cancer, and myeloma, while rates of stomach and liver cancers (and associated mortality) are highest among Asian Americans and Pacific Islanders (US Cancer Statistics Working Group 2013).

---

* Samantha (Sammi) Giertych, RD, contributed primary research and prepared draft versions of portions of this chapter.

- *Type 2 diabetes*: Diabetes affects nearly 26 million Americans and leads to more than 70,000 deaths annually. It is also the leading cause of end-stage renal disease (ESRD), adult blindness, and amputation. The prevalence of diabetes is nearly 70% higher in African Americans than in whites. Some Native American, Hispanic, and Asian and Pacific Islander subpopulations are also at particularly high risk for this disease (Centers for Disease Control and Prevention 2011a).

This chapter selects three chronic conditions for examination—diabetes, CVD, and cancer—because collectively, these three conditions account for over half of all deaths in the United States (Kochanek et al. 2014). First, we briefly highlight the common general prevention guidelines and the common risk factors shared by these chronic conditions—overweight and obesity, which is addressed in more detail in Chapter 5. We also review metabolic syndrome, which is a common risk factor for both diabetes and CVD. Finally, we then identify federal agencies significantly involved with addressing health disparities. We examine the selected conditions of diabetes, CVD, and cancer; related health disparities; and associated public health initiatives.

COMMON RISK FACTORS AND PREVENTION

LEADING DIET-RELATED CHRONIC DISEASES

The profile of diseases contributing most heavily to illness, disability, and death among Americans changed dramatically during the last century. Today, chronic diseases—such as diabetes, CVD (primarily heart disease and stroke), and cancer—are among the most prevalent, costly, and preventable of all health problems. Over the 3-year period of 2003–2006, the combined cost of health inequalities and premature death was estimated to be $1.24 trillion (LaVeist et al. 2009). The common causes of these chronic illnesses—physical inactivity, poor diet, and obesity—are not unique to any one of these conditions but are shared by each of them. These shared risk factors provide opportunities for prevention. Focusing research, outreach, and education efforts on particular risk factor areas in populations who disproportionately experience these diseases holds the potential to achieve greater progress in health promotion and disease prevention. Easily understood recommendations designed to reduce individual risk for CVD, cancer, and diabetes can foster advocacy and action for communities, organizations, individuals, families, and clinicians (US Department of Health and Human Services 2011a).

GENERAL PREVENTION GUIDELINES

In 2004, the American Diabetes Association (ADA), the American Heart Association (AHA), and the American Cancer Society (ACS) reviewed strategies for the prevention and early detection of diabetes, CVD, and cancer. The organizations launched a collaborative initiative to (1) create national commitment to prevention and improvement in primary prevention and early detection, (2) promote greater public awareness about healthy lifestyles, (3) support and initiate legislative action that results in more funding for and access to primary prevention programs and research, and (4) reconsider the concept of the periodic medical checkup as an effective platform for prevention, early detection, and treatment (Eyre et al. 2004).

As a component of these efforts, the three organizations developed general prevention guidelines for all average-risk adults that focus on primary prevention through diet and exercise, monitoring body mass index (BMI) and blood pressure, and screening for diabetes and CVD by periodically checking plasma glucose and serum lipid levels. The general prevention guidelines include a schedule of these screening tests, which should be performed on individuals beginning at age 20, as shown in Table 4.1.

At each regular healthcare visit, BMI should be calculated and blood pressure measured (unless blood pressure is <120/80 mm Hg, then measurement is only recommended once every 2 years). A test for blood glucose should be performed every 3 years starting at age 40, and a lipid profile is

TABLE 4.1

Screening Test Schedules Recommended by the ACS, ADA, and AHA

Screening Test	Frequency
BMI	Each regular healthcare visit.
Blood pressure	Each regular healthcare visit. Reduce to at least once every 2 years if BP is <120/80 mm Hg.
Lipid profile	Every 5 years.
Blood glucose test	Every 3 years after age 40.
Clinical breast exam (CBE) and mammography	CBE every 3 years until age 40; annually thereafter. Mammography annually starting at age 40.
Pap test[a]	Age 21–30, every 1–3 years; every 1–5 years thereafter until age 65 with simultaneous HPV type; depending on type of test and past results.
Colorectal screening	Screening frequency depends on test preferred, starting at age 50.
Prostate-specific antigen test and digital rectal exam	Offer test and exam yearly, and assist informed decisions starting at age 50.

Source: Eyre, H. et al., *CA Cancer J. Clin.*, 54, 2004.

[a] In 2012, the US Preventive Services Task Force released new recommendations to reduce the frequency of cervical screening. A summary can be accessed here: http://www.uspreventiveservicestaskforce.org/uspstf11/cervcancer/cervcancerrs .htm#clinical, accessed September 26, 2014.

recommended every 5 years. The statement also contains recommendations for colorectal screening, as well as prostate-specific antigen (PSA) testing and digital rectal exams for men over age 50.

ADA, AHA, and ACS also encourage primary care practitioners to review these general preventive guidelines with all average-risk adults (Eyre et al. 2004):

- Achieve and maintain a healthy weight.
- Exercise for at least 30 minutes on 5 or more days a week.
- Eat at least 5 servings of vegetables and fruits daily.
- Encourage tobacco cessation.

Although drafted prior to the 2010 *Dietary Guidelines for Americans*, these are essentially the recommendations in the 2010 edition of the *Dietary Guidelines for Americans*. The preventive impact of adhering to these four guidelines has been shown in subsequent studies (Ford et al. 2009). (ACS has updated specific cancer prevention guidelines, which changed the reference from servings to cups for fruit and vegetable consumption and includes other dietary factors. The updated ACS guidelines are discussed later in this chapter).

OVERWEIGHT AND OBESITY: THE COMMON RISK FACTOR

Obesity is a major risk factor for CVD, diabetes, and cancer. For example, according to data from the third National Health and Nutrition Examination Survey (NHANES III, 1988–1994) and NHANES (1999–2002), half of the adults in the United States who are diagnosed with diabetes are obese. Specifically, the prevalence of obesity among adults with diabetes was 45.7% (1988–1994) and 54.8% (1999–2002) (Centers for Disease Control and Prevention 2004). Avoidance of weight gain has also been determined to have a cancer-preventive effect with regard to cancers of the pancreas, gallbladder, colon, rectum, breast (postmenopausal), endometrium, kidney (renal cell), and esophagus (adenocarcinoma) (World Cancer Research Fund 2007).

Understanding population health disparities in overweight and obesity rates is crucial for effective preventative public health initiatives. Although overweight and obesity statistics are discussed in Chapter 5, some highlights regarding obesity-related health disparities are worth noting for the purposes of this chapter.

Age

The prevalence of overweight and obesity varies somewhat by age. The prevalence of obesity is higher among older women compared with younger women, but this trend is not found in men. In children, obesity rates are highest among adolescents (Ogden et al. 2012a).

Previously, the term *obesity* was not used to define child and adolescent BMI. In 2010, the National Center for Health Statistics (NCHS) formally changed the terms for BMI cutoffs in children—at or above the 85th percentile of BMI for age from "at risk for overweight" to "overweight," and at or above the 95th percentile from "overweight" to "obese." The variation in terminology over time and by organization demonstrates the complexity of assessing body fatness in child and adolescent populations (Ogden and Flegal 2010). Although BMI is mostly highly correlated with body fatness levels, NHANES has observed that non-Hispanic black children have significantly lower levels of body fat than other children at the same BMI level. Body fatness may or may not be a stronger predictor of health-related outcomes than BMI (Ogden et al. 2012b).

Gender, Race, and Ethnicity

The prevalence of obesity varies by gender, race, and ethnicity. In 2009–2010, overweight and obesity were more prevalent among minority women than among non-Hispanic white women. Non-Hispanic black women had the highest prevalence of obesity (58.5%), followed by Mexican American women (41.4%) and non-Hispanic white women (32.2%). Black men were more likely to be obese than their non-Hispanic white and Hispanic counterparts, although the prevalence of obesity among men differed little by race and ethnicity (36.2–38.8%) (Ford et al. 2009).

Socioeconomic Status

An overall inverse relationship between poverty and obesity in adults and children exists (National Center for Health Statistics 2013a), illustrated in Table 4.2. Socioeconomic status (SES) affects the prevalence of overweight and obesity in the population as a whole; however, most obese adults are not of low SES, and the effect varies by gender. Women of lower SES are more likely to be obese than women with higher incomes. However, the likelihood that men will be overweight or obese

TABLE 4.2
Percentage of Overweight and Obese Adults (20–74, Age Adjusted) and Obese Children According to Poverty Status, 2007–2010

Poverty Level	Overweight Adults	Obese Adults	Obese Children Aged 2–5	Obese Children Aged 6–11	Obese Children Aged 12–19
Below 100%	69.5	37.9	13.2	22.2	24.3
100–199%	70.9	38.2	11.8	20.7	20.1
200–399%	68.8	37.6	13.9	18.9	16.3
400% or more	66.7	31.4	5.8[a]	12.5[a]	14.0

Source: National Center for Health Statistics, Health, United States, 2012: With Special Feature on Emergency Care, 2013. Available at http://www.cdc.gov/nchs/data/hus/hus12.pdf, accessed January 7, 2015.

Note: Includes persons of all races and Hispanic origins. Data based on measured height and weight. Poverty status is based on family income and family size.

[a] Estimates considered unreliable.

was reported as approximately equal as of 2001 regardless of SES group (Office of the Surgeon General et al. 2001). This variance in effect of SES by gender has continued to be reported in the scientific literature (Food Research and Action Center, http://frac.org/initiatives/hunger-and-obesity /are-low-income-people-at-greater-risk-for-overweight-or-obesity/). Additionally, the impact of family income on prevalence of overweight may vary by ethnicity at the lower thresholds of income. Analysis of NHANES 1999–2004 showed that overweight in non-Hispanic white and Mexican American children decreased with family income, though previous studies have found mixed results. In black children, higher family income was associated with reduced prevalence of overweight (Freedman et al. 2007).

METABOLIC SYNDROME

The term *metabolic syndrome* references a cluster of five risk factors in an individual. These factors are abdominal obesity (thought to be a better indicator of diabetes risk than BMI), hypertriglyceridemia, reduced high-density lipoprotein (HDL), hyperglycemia, and hypertension. Individuals who exhibit at least three of these five medical conditions are considered to have metabolic syndrome (US Department of Health and Human Services et al. 2002).

Table 4.3 presents the clinical diagnostic criteria for metabolic syndrome conditions. Of interest to those working with minority populations are the ethnic-group–specific waist circumference guidelines, suggested by the International Diabetes Federation for people from Europe, Central and Latin America, the Middle East, Asia, India, and Japan, regardless of their current residence.

People with metabolic syndrome are at increased risk for developing diabetes and CVD as well as for increased mortality both from CVD and from all causes (Ford et al. 2002).

NHANES III data indicate that consumption of fruits and vegetables is low among people with metabolic syndrome. At the same time, adults with the syndrome have suboptimal concentrations of several antioxidants, which may partially explain their increased risk for diabetes and CVD (Ford et al. 2003).

Prevalence of Metabolic Syndrome

A study of NHANES 2003–2006 data reported that about one-third of US residents have metabolic syndrome. Among metabolic syndrome criteria, abdominal obesity (52.8%), high blood pressure (39.5%), and elevated blood glucose (38.6%) were most prevalent (Ervin 2009). A noticeable change observed in NHANES 2003–2006 data as compared to NHANES III (1998–2002) data was a higher prevalence of the syndrome among non-Hispanic white males (37.2%) than Mexican American males (33.2%), though the syndrome remains most prevalent among Mexican American females (Ford et al. 2002).

In a comparison of NHANES III (1988–1994) data to NHANES 2003–2004 data, the average unadjusted waist circumference in adults increased from 95.3 to 100.4 cm among men (age adjusted, 96.0 to 100.4 cm) and from 88.7 to 94.2 cm, among women (age adjusted, 89.0 to 94.0 cm). These results demonstrate the rapid increase in obesity, particularly abdominal obesity, among US adults in the time period (Li et al. 2007).

Increasing prevalence of abdominal obesity remains a current issue. A 2013 study that used NHANES data from 1999 to 2010 found that over the period of 1999–2010, the age-adjusted prevalence of metabolic syndrome decreased from 25.5% to 22.9%. Some of the risk factors decreased in prevalence, such as hypertriglyceridemia (from 33.5% to 24.3%) and elevated blood pressure (from 32.3% to 24.0%), but others increased in prevalence, such as hyperglycemia (from 12.9% to 19.9%) and elevated waist circumference (from 45.4% to 56.1%). Furthermore, these trends varied considerably by sex and race/ethnicity. White male adults were more likely to have abdominal obesity than their counterparts of other race/ethnicity, but the opposite was true for white female adults. Black male adults and black female adults consistently had a higher prevalence of elevated blood pressure than other groups. Mexican Americans, both overall and by sex, consistently had a higher

TABLE 4.3

Clinical Identification of Metabolic Syndrome

Indicator	United States Adult Treatment Panel III[a]	International Diabetes Federation[b]
Abdominal obesity, as measured by waist circumference A high-risk waist line exceeds these measures	Women, 88 cm (35 in.); men, 102 cm (40 in.)	Europe: women, 80 cm (31.5 in.); men, 94 cm (37 in.) Central and Latin America, Middle East, Asia, India: women, 80 cm (31.5 in.); men, 90 cm (35.4 in.) Japan: women, 90 cm (35.4 in.); men, 85 cm (33.5 in.) Other countries (excluding North America): women, 80 cm (31.5 in.); men, 94 cm (37 in.)
Triglycerides	≥150 mg/dL (1.69 mmol/L)	≥150 mg/dL (1.70 mmol/L), or specific treatment for this lipid abnormality
HDL cholesterol	Men <40 mg/dL (1.03 mmol/L) Women <50 mg/dL (1.29 mmol/L)	<40 mg/dL (1.03 mmol/L) <50 mg/dL (1.29 mmol/L), or specific treatment for this lipid abnormality
Blood pressure	≥130/85 mm Hg	≥130/85 mm Hg, or treatment of previously diagnosed hypertension
Fasting glucose[c]	≥100 mg/dL (6.1 mmol/L)	≥100 mg/dL (6.1 mmol/L), or previously diagnosed type 2 diabetes

Source: National Heart, Lung, and Blood Institute, Table 3: Classification of Blood, Evaluation, and Treatment of High Blood Pressure, US Department of Health and Human Services, National Institutes of Health, August 2004. Available at http://www.nhlbi.nih.gov/guidelines/hypertension/jnc7full.pdf, accessed February 4, 2015.

[a] National Cholesterol Education Program, National Heart, Lung, and Blood Institute, Third Report of the National Cholesterol Education Program (NCEP) Expert Panel on Detection, Evaluation, and Treatment of High Blood Cholesterol in Adults (Adult Treatment Panel III) Final Report, NIH Publication No. 02-5215, National Institutes of Health, September 2002, Table II.6-1: Clinical Identification of the Metabolic Syndrome, p. II-27, http://www.nhlbi.nih.gov /health-pro/guidelines/current/cholesterol-guidelines/final-report.htm, accessed February 4, 2015.

[b] International Diabetes Federation (IDF), The IDF Consensus Worldwide Definition of the Metabolic Syndrome, http:// www.idf.org/webdata/docs/MetSyndrome_FINAL.pdf, accessed February 4, 2015.

[c] In 2003, the American Diabetes Association changed the definition of impaired fasting glucose from 110 to 100 mg/dL. Genuth, S. et al., Diabetes Care, 26, 2003.

prevalence of low HDL cholesterol (HDL-C), high triglycerides, and high blood glucose than other subgroups. Overall, the metabolic syndrome remains most prevalent among Mexican American female adults (Beltrán-Sánchez et al. 2013).

Metabolic Syndrome in Youth

In a sample of adolescents included in NHANES 2001–2006, the overall prevalence of the metabolic syndrome was 8.6% or roughly 2.5 million individuals. Prevalence of the metabolic syndrome was higher in Hispanics (11.2%) and lower in non-Hispanic blacks (4.0%) than non-Hispanic whites (8.9%). Prevalence was higher in non-Hispanic white and Hispanic males than females of the same ethnicity, while prevalence was similar between non-Hispanic black males and females (Johnson et al. 2009).

Of the constellation of risk factors that make up the metabolic syndrome, elevated triglycerides were the most prevalent factor (25.6%). Waist circumference, triglycerides, and HDL levels were found to be the most influential risk factors. Hispanic adolescents were most likely to experience central adiposity, while non-Hispanic black adolescents were disproportionately affected by elevated blood pressure (≥90th percentile) (Johnson et al. 2009).

When the effect of different degrees of overweight on the prevalence of the metabolic syndrome was studied in 430 overweight children and adolescents, the prevalence of metabolic syndrome not only was found to be high but also increased with increasing BMI. The prevalence of the syndrome reached 50% in the most overweight children and adolescents, a finding that has significant implications both for public health and clinical interventions (Weiss et al. 2004).

Small studies suggest hypotheses for larger investigations, such as secondary analyses of NHANES data. For example, a study of metabolic syndrome in 163 predominantly white, ostensibly low-risk college students unexpectedly found that 27% were overweight, 10% were dyslipidemic, and 6% were prediabetic (Huang et al. 2004). Similar studies have noted a significant prevalence of the metabolic syndrome and its risk factors among this "low-risk" cohort (Dalleck and Kjelland 2012; Fernandes and Lofgren 2011). However, these results need to be confirmed in studies with larger sample sizes in order to confidently recommend aggressive education among low-risk as well as high-risk groups, even in the absence of disease.

Because the implications of the metabolic syndrome for healthcare are substantial from a public health standpoint, identification of individuals with metabolic syndrome may provide opportunities to intervene earlier in the development of shared disease pathways that predispose individuals to both diabetes and CVD.

FEDERAL EFFORTS ADDRESSING HEALTH DISPARITIES

Racial and ethnic minority groups will comprise an increasingly larger portion of the US population in coming years. While continuing the progress achieved in improving the overall health of the American people, the federal government supports programs and projects specifically aimed at reducing health disparities. Significantly, the Department of Health and Human Services (HHS), leveraging opportunities in the Affordable Care Act (ACA) of 2010, has developed a broad federal plan addressing health disparities (Koh et al. 2011), the 2011 *HHS Action Plan to Reduce Racial And Ethnic Disparities: A Nation Free of Disparities in Health and Health Care* (Disparities Action Plan) (US Department of Health and Human Services 2011b).

The ACA addresses health disparities through provisions increasing access to and affordability of care, expanding community-level care, and increasing prevention efforts for underserved groups. Community-based strategies are encouraged, along with improving the diversity and cultural competency of our healthcare workforce (Koh et al. 2011).

Department of Health and Human Services

According to the Government Accountability Office (GAO), the HHS is the primary federal entity involved in projects and research aimed at understanding and addressing disparities in healthcare, including the areas of diabetes, heart disease, and cancer (Box 4.1). The HHS also plays a major role in financing healthcare for minority groups (US Government Accountability Office 2003).

Eliminating health disparities is one of the HHS secretary's Strategic Initiatives (US Department of Health and Human Services, http://www.hhs.gov/strategic-plan/priorities.html). In 2011, leveraging the opportunities provided by ACA, the HHS published the Disparities Action Plan (US Department of Health and Human Services 2011b). The Disparities Action Plan, a broad plan aimed at providing national direction, is the first federal strategic disparities plan (Koh et al. 2011).

The Disparities Action Plan identifies the following four major health issues disproportionately affecting minority populations: (1) lack of medical insurance and access to primary and quality care,

BOX 4.1   GOVERNMENT ACCOUNTABILITY OFFICE

The US Government Accountability Office (GAO) is an independent, nonpartisan agency that works for Congress. Often called the *congressional watchdog*, GAO investigates how the federal government spends taxpayer dollars. The head of the GAO is the comptroller general of the United States, who is appointed to a 15-year term by the president from a slate of candidates proposed by Congress.

The GAO's mission is to support Congress in meeting its constitutional responsibilities and to help improve the federal government's performance and accountability.

The work of the GAO is done at the request of the comptroller general or congressional committees or subcommittees, or is mandated by public laws or committee reports. The GAO audits agency operations, investigates allegations of illegal and improper activities, evaluates how well federal programs and policies are meeting their objectives, performs policy analyses and outlines options for congressional consideration, and issues legal decisions and opinions (such as reports on agency rules).

GAO documents are available through the GAO's website (http://www.gao.gov), which contains abstracts and full-text files of current reports and testimony, and an archive of older products. Each day, a list of newly released GAO materials is posted under "Reports and Testimonies," which contains links to the full-text document files. E-mail subscription is available.

Source: US Government Accountability Office, About GAO. Available at http://www.gao.gov/about/, accessed January 12, 2015.

(2) lack of diversity in the healthcare workforce, (3) reduced access to healthy lifestyle options and subsequent high mortality rates, and (4) lack of useful data on the ethnicity and language makeup of the patient population.

The five goals set for 2010–2015 to address these issues are to (1) transform healthcare, (2) strengthen the nation's HHS infrastructure, (3) advance the health and well-being of all Americans, (4) advance scientific knowledge and innovation, and (5) increase the transparency and accountability of HHS programs. Multiple interdisciplinary agencies have been recruited to aid in attaining these goals (US Department of Health and Human Services 2011c). Appendix 4.1 of this chapter describes HHS' Strategic Plan and the Disparities Action Plan.

In general, several branches of the HHS have significant health disparity responsibilities—the Office of the Secretary, which oversees the Office of Disease Prevention and Health Promotion (ODPHP) and the Office of Minority Health (OMH); the National Institutes of Health (NIH); and the Centers for Disease Control and Prevention (CDC). The organization chart of the HSS (http://www.hhs.gov/about/orgchart/index.html) can be found at the agency's website.

Furthermore, as mandated by ACA, HHS has created offices of minority health within certain agencies, including within the Agency for Healthcare Research and Quality (AHRQ), the Food and Drug Administration (FDA), the Health Resources and Services Administration (HRSA), the Centers for Medicare & Medicaid Services (CMS), and the Substance Abuse and Mental Health Services Administration (SAMHSA). Although the existence of the new offices within these agencies will further promote efforts addressing health disparities, work has already been done by these agencies in this area. For example, since 2002, AHRQ has produced annual national health disparities reports documenting the status of healthcare disparities and quality of care received by racial, ethnic, and socioeconomic groups in the United States (US Department of Health and Human Services 2011b). Some of the work done by HHS offices and operating divisions is described below.

Office of Disease Prevention and Health Promotion

The mission of ODPHP is to work to strengthen the disease prevention and health promotion priorities of HHS within the collaborative framework of the HHS agencies. Health promotion programs under the aegis of the ODPHP include the following:

- *Dietary Guidelines for Americans*: Published jointly with the USDA every 5 years since 1980, this publication is the statutorily mandated basis for many federal food assistance programs and for nutrition education activities. The 2010 edition is the most recent published as of the writing of this chapter.*
- Healthy People 2020: Released in 2010, Healthy People 2020 presents a comprehensive set of disease prevention and health promotion objectives developed to improve the health of all people in the United States during the next decade. An overarching goal of Healthy People 2020 is to achieve health equity, eliminate disparities, and improve the health of all groups.

ODPHP programs have recently directed their focus to health communication as an area for initiative and improvement. A number of Healthy People 2020 objectives address health communication goals, including health literacy (HC-1), access to online health information (HC-9), and social marketing in health promotion and disease prevention (HC-13) (Office of Disease Prevention and Health Promotion, http://www.healthypeople.gov/2020/topics-objectives/topic/health-communication-and-health-information-technology).

As of 2014, ODPHP manages three independent websites to disseminate news and health information: http://www.health.gov, as ODPHP's home, provides disease prevention and health promotion information; http://www.healthypeople.gov provides up-to-date information on Healthy People 2020 objectives; and http://www.healthfinder.gov provides consumer resources to make informed health choices. These are all available as tabs at http://www.health.gov. In an ever-increasingly technology-driven society, current and future public health strategies should utilize appropriate tech-based tools to increase coverage and capture audiences' attention.

Office of Minority Health

The OMH was established in 1986 to improve and protect the health of racial and ethnic minority populations through the development of health policies and programs that will eliminate health disparities. The OMH advises the secretary of HHS and the Office of Public Health and Science (OPHS) on public health program activities affecting the racial and ethnic minority groups identified by the federal government. The OMH convened numerous stakeholders from around the country at a National Leadership Summit for Eliminating Racial and Ethnic Disparities in Health in 2008. The resulting National Partnership for Action to End Health Disparities, a partnership of widely diverse organizations, made recommendations that resulted in the 2011 National Stakeholder Strategy for Achieving Health Equity. The main principles of the Stakeholder Strategy include improving local awareness of health disparities, enhancing local data collection efforts, and emphasizing public–private partnerships to improve access to care; the strategies can be tailored for specific community use (Koh et al. 2011).

National Institutes of Health

As the primary federal agency for conducting and supporting medical research, the NIH's mission is to "enhance healthy life, lengthen life, and reduce illness and disability" (US Department of Health and Human Services, http://www.nih.gov/about/mission.htm). NIH provides leadership and direction to programs designed to improve the health of the nation by conducting and supporting research in the causes, diagnosis, prevention, and cure of human diseases. Composed of

---

* PowerPoint slides regarding the 2015 edition of the *Dietary Guidelines for Americans* are available for textbook adopters. Current information is also available at the *Dietary Guidelines* home page: http://health.gov/dietaryguidelines/.

27 institutes and centers, listed in Appendix 4.2 of this chapter, NIH provides leadership and financial support to researchers nationally and internationally. Each institute and center has its own specific research agenda, and all but three receive their funding directly from Congress and administer their own budgets. The Office of the Director is the central office, responsible for setting policy for NIH (http://www.nih.gov/about/organization.htm) and for planning, managing, and coordinating the programs and activities of all the NIH components. Two offices are highlighted below.

Office of Disease Prevention

The Office of Disease Prevention (ODP) is located within the Office of the Director of NIH. Its function is to coordinate research on disease prevention and health promotion across the institutes and centers that comprise NIH. In particular, the ODP fosters, coordinates, and assesses research in prevention by collaborating with other federal agencies, academic institutions, the private sector, nongovernmental organizations, and international organizations in the formulation of research initiatives and policies that promote public health. The ODP advises the NIH on research related to disease prevention and health promotion and works with the NIH research institutes to initiate and develop requests for proposals (RFPs), requests for applications (RFAs), and program announcements (PAs) to enhance program development. Refer to Chapter 14 for more information on grant writing.

National Institute on Minority Health and Health Disparities

The National Institute on Minority Health and Health Disparities (NIMHD) was first established as the Center on Minority Health and Health Disparities under the Minority Health and Health Disparities Research and Education Act of 2000, P.L. 106-525, and transitioned to full institute in 2010. The mission of NIMHD is "to lead scientific research to improve minority health and eliminate health disparities" (US Department of Health and Human Services, http://www.nimhd .nih.gov/about/visionMission.html). The general purpose of the institute is to conduct and support minority health disparities research, training, dissemination of information, and other programs with respect to minority health conditions and other populations with health disparities.

Centers for Disease Control and Prevention

The CDC has a number of initiatives that address health and a number of units that have a specialized disease prevention or health promotion focus on (1) cancer prevention and control; (2) heart disease and stroke; (3) diabetes; and (4) nutrition, physical activity, and obesity.

Several CDC initiatives that address health disparities are described below; other initiatives are included in Section 3 to illustrate prevention efforts for diabetes, CVD, and cancer.

Racial and Ethnic Approaches to Community Health

Racial and Ethnic Approaches to Community Health (REACH) is a cornerstone of the CDC's initiative to eliminate the disparities in health status experienced by ethnic minority populations. The program was initially funded from 2000 to 2006 as REACH 2010, supporting community coalitions in designing, implementing, and evaluating community-driven strategies to eliminate health disparities. This approach is also described as community-based participatory research or programming (CBPR). Successes included improvements in cholesterol screening rates among Hispanics and African Americans and an increase in the percentage of women receiving pap smears. After these initial successes, Congress allocated $39.6 million for continuation of the program as REACH US in fiscal year 2010. REACH US currently funds 40 communities to implement changes in key health disparities areas (US Department of Health and Human Services 2010). The latest REACH projects include efforts in obesity and hypertension prevention (Centers for Disease Control and Prevention 2013a).

Healthy Communities

Through the National Center for Chronic Disease Prevention and Health Promotion (NCCDPHP), the CDC's Healthy Communities Program (formerly ODPHP's Steps to a HealthierUS) connects communities with national prevention resources to provide a springboard for action in health-related behavioral and environmental areas. Healthy Communities recruits and trains leaders in funded communities to implement education and policy efforts to improve individual and population health (CDC, http://www.cdc.gov/nccdphp/dch/programs/healthycommunitiesprogram/index.htm).

VERB: It's What You Do

VERB (CDC, http://www.cdc.gov/youthcampaign/index.htm) was a national, multicultural social marketing campaign that ran from 2002 to 2006 encouraging young people ages 9–13 years to be physically active. Utilizing ethnic-specific advertisements and promotion through schools and other community organizations, the VERB campaign influenced tweens to engage in more physical activity, as well as have more positive attitudes toward the benefits of being physically active. For current campaign efforts geared toward children and adolescents, see *Let's Move!* in this chapter and in Chapter 5.

Division of Cancer Prevention and Control

Through the Division of Cancer Prevention and Control (DCPC), the CDC (http://www.cdc.gov /DHDSP/index.htm) works with national cancer organizations, state health agencies, and other key groups to develop, implement, and promote effective strategies for preventing and controlling cancer.

Division of Heart Disease and Stroke Prevention

The Division of Heart Disease and Stroke Prevention (DHDSP) of the CDC (http://www.cdc.gov /DHDSP/index.htm), formed in 2006, aims to provide public health leadership to improve cardiovascular health for all, reduce the burden of heart disease and stroke, and eliminate disparities associated with heart disease and stroke. The CDC released the *Public Health Action Plan to Prevent Heart Disease and Stroke* (Action Plan) to prevent heart disease and stroke in 2003; it was updated in 2008 and again in 2014 (US Department of Health and Human Services 2008). The Action Plan is described in more detail in Section 3 of this chapter.

Division of Diabetes Translation

The CDC has had a diabetes division since 1977. In 1989, the name of the division was updated with the addition of "Translation," reflecting the division's mission to translate science into daily practice. Now known as the Division of Diabetes Translation (DDT), the division is active in strengthening the public health surveillance systems for diabetes by working with those states using the diabetes-specific modules of the Behavioral Risk Factor Surveillance System (BRFSS) to develop a nationwide, state-based surveillance system. It also conducts applied research that focuses on translating research findings into clinical and public health practice, such as the effectiveness of health practices to address risk factors for diabetes and demonstration of primary prevention of type 2 diabetes. The division provides funding for state-based Diabetes Prevention and Control Programs (DPCPs) throughout the United States. Analysis of these funded programs produced Effective Public Health Strategies to Prevent and Control Diabetes: A Compendium, detailing effective intervention strategies for preventing development of type 2 diabetes and complications from diabetes (US Department of Health and Human Services 2013).

In 2004, CDC published Diabetes: A National Plan for Action (US Department of Health and Human Services 2004). The plan provides detailed strategies for preventing diabetes, as well as obesity and heart disease. Specific strategies are proposed for school personnel, healthcare providers, employers, community leaders, media spokespeople, researchers and professional educators, and government officials.

Division of Nutrition, Physical Activity, and Obesity

The Division of Nutrition, Physical Activity, and Obesity (DNPAO) takes a public health approach to addressing the role of nutrition and physical activity in improving the public's health and preventing and controlling obesity and other chronic diseases. The scope of the DNPAO activities includes epidemiological and behavioral research, surveillance, training and education, intervention development, health promotion and leadership, policy and environmental change, communication and social marketing, and partnership development. The DNPAO website includes a "Policy Resources" section for professionals working in areas of obesity prevention (CDC, http://www.cdc.gov/nccdphp /dnpao/index.html).

A CLOSE-UP ON DIABETES, CARDIOVASCULAR DISEASE, AND CANCER

DIABETES

Diabetes is the seventh leading cause of death in the United States (Centers for Disease Control and Prevention 2014a). Diabetes also contributes to higher rates of morbidity through serious complications, such as heart disease and stroke, blindness, kidney failure, and lower-limb amputation (Centers for Disease Control and Prevention 2014b). The prevalence of diabetes increases with age and is higher among certain racial and ethnic minority populations. The growth, aging, and increasing racial and ethnic diversity of the US population portends a substantial increase in the segment of the population with diabetes. Additionally, researchers have begun to collect data on both diagnosed and undiagnosed estimates of diabetes prevalence, revealing statistics that suggest that a much larger proportion of the US population is afflicted with the disease than previously estimated.

Prevalence of Diabetes

In 2014, 29.1 million people were estimated to have diabetes, with an estimated 8.1 million undiagnosed cases, and 86 million Americans over the age of 20 were estimated to be pre-diabetic. Asian Americans, Hispanics, non-Hispanic blacks, and Native Americans/Alaska Natives were all at increased risk for diabetes diagnosis compared with non-Hispanic whites (Centers for Disease Control and Prevention 2014c). The percentage of diagnosed diabetes was twice as high in Native American/Alaska Native populations as in the non-Hispanic white population. Rates also vary significantly among subgroups within these populations, and understanding these variations is significant for public health planning. For example, the rate among Alaska Natives is 6.0%, whereas the rate among Native Americans in southern Arizona is 24.1% (Centers for Disease Control and Prevention 2014c).

If diabetes prevalence rates were to remain constant over time, controlling for age, sex, race, and ethnicity, then based on Census Bureau population projections, the number of people with diabetes, diagnosed and undiagnosed, could increase to anywhere between 84 million and 132 million by 2050 (variations due to use of conservative versus liberal estimates). The main reasons for this rapid predicted increase include aging of the US population, increase in high-risk minority populations, and reduced mortality among people with diabetes due to improved treatment. The ability to predict rates of undiagnosed cases has vastly expanded on the magnitude of this epidemic (Boyle et al. 2010).

Direct and Indirect Cost of Diabetes

In 2012, per-capita medical expenditures totaled $13,700 for people with diabetes, with $7900 of that total attributed to diabetes treatment. When adjusted for differences in age, sex, and race/ethnicity, people with diabetes had medical expenditures that were almost 2.3 times higher than expenditures that would be incurred by the same group in the absence of diabetes (American Diabetes Association 2012). End-stage renal disease is an example of such a cost (Box 4.2).

The direct and indirect costs of diabetes in 2012 were estimated at $176 billion and $69 billion, respectively, totaling $245 billion. This estimate likely underestimates the true burden of diabetes because it omits intangibles such as pain and suffering, care provided by nonpaid (usually family) caregivers, and several areas of healthcare spending where people with diabetes most likely use services at higher rates than people without diabetes (i.e., dental care, optometry care, and the services

---

BOX 4.2   END-STAGE RENAL DISEASE (ESRD)

ESRD is a complete or near-complete failure of the kidneys to excrete wastes, concentrate urine, and regulate electrolytes. The most common cause of ESRD in the United States is diabetes. African Americans are four times as likely and Native Americans are twice as likely to have ESRD than non-Hispanic whites. ESRD occurs when the kidneys are no longer able to function at a level necessary for day-to-day life. It usually occurs as chronic renal failure progresses to the point where kidney function is less than 10% of baseline. At this point, kidney function is so diminished that without dialysis or kidney transplantation, complications are multiple and severe, and death will occur from accumulation of fluids and waste products in the body. Dialysis and kidney transplantation are the only treatments for ESRD. In the United States, more than 400,000 people are on long-term dialysis, and nearly 200,000 have a functioning transplanted kidney (US Renal Data System 2012).

---

of registered dietitians). In addition, this cost estimate excludes undiagnosed cases of diabetes, as well as costs due to prediabetes (American Diabetes Association 2012).

Diagnostic Criteria

Over the past decade, measurement of diabetes diagnoses by the CDC, NHANES, and the National Health Interview Survey (NHIS) has gradually transitioned from reliance on fasting plasma glucose to the addition of hemoglobin A1c as a diagnostic tool, paralleling the increased use of this measure as the preferred method for clinical diagnosis. Table 4.4 compares the diagnostic thresholds for diabetes using the methods of fasting plasma glucose (FPG), oral glucose tolerance test (OGTT), and hemoglobin A1c (Boxes 4.3 and 4.4).

Screening

The ADA also publishes an annual Standards of Medical Care in Diabetes (Standards of Care), providing components of diabetes care, general treatment goals, and tools to evaluate the quality of care, including screening, diagnostic, and therapeutic actions (American Diabetes Association 2015a). In the 2015 Standards of Care, the ADA suggests that screening for type 2 diabetes, independent of risk factors, beginning at age 30 or 45 years is highly cost-effective. If the results of

---

TABLE 4.4

Diagnostic Thresholds for Diabetes and Lesser Degrees of Impaired Glucose Regulation

Category	Fasting Plasma Glucose	2-Hour 75 g Oral Glucose Tolerance Test	Hemoglobin A1c
Normal	100 mg/dL (5.6 mmol/L)	<140 mg/dL (7.8 mmol/L)	<5.7%
Prediabetes	100–125 mg/dL (5.6–6.9 mmol/L)	140–199 mg/dL (7.8–11.0 mmol/L)	5.7–6.4%
Diabetes	≥126 mg/dL (7.0 mmol/L)	200 mg/dL (11.1 mmol/L)	≥6.5%

Source: American Diabetes Association, *Diabetes Care*, 37, 2014.

Note: When both tests are performed, impaired fasting glucose (IFG) or impaired glucose tolerance (IGT) should be diagnosed only if diabetes is not diagnosed by the other test. A diagnosis of diabetes needs to be confirmed on a separate day. A diagnosis of diabetes may also be made with the presence of severe hyperglycemic symptoms and a random plasma glucose >200 mg/dL (11.1 mmol/L).

BOX 4.3   DIAGNOSTIC TESTS FOR DIABETES

Fasting plasma glucose: The FPG test checks blood glucose levels after fasting for at least 8 hours. Diabetes is diagnosed at fasting blood glucose of greater than or equal to 126 mg/dL.

Oral glucose tolerance: The OGTT checks blood glucose levels before consumption of a sweet drink and then again in 2 hours to determine how well glucose is being processed. Diabetes is diagnosed at 2-hour blood glucose of greater than or equal to 200 mg/dL.

A1c: Diabetes is diagnosed at an A1c of greater than or equal to 6.5%.

BOX 4.4   HEMOGLOBIN A1c

A1c is formed by the nonenzymatic attachment of glucose to the N-terminal valine of the β-chain of hemoglobin. Because the life span of erythrocytes is about 120 days, the measurement of A1c reflects long-term glycemic exposure, representing the average glucose concentration over the preceding 8–12 weeks. A1c measurements are strongly correlated with microvascular complications, such as retinopathy; factors such as acute illness, short-term lifestyle changes (e.g., exercise), recent food ingestion, and sample handling do not significantly alter A1c values.

The significant reduction in microvascular complications with lower A1c combined with other advantages (such as the convenient lack of fasting requirement and better sample stability/reproducibility) has led to the recommendation that A1c be used for screening and diagnosis of diabetes. However, the interpretation of A1c depends on the erythrocytes having a normal life span; hemoglobin variants can affect some A1c measurements, and some conditions prevent A1c from being measured. The hemoglobin variants problem affects people of African, Mediterranean, and Southeast Asian heritage. Additionally, the A1c test is less sensitive than the glucose tests, meaning that the test identifies fewer cases of diabetes.

Source: Sacks DB. A1c versus glucose testing: A comparison. Diabetes Care February 2011 vol. 34 no. 2, 518–523. Available at http://care.diabetesjournals.org/content/34/2/518.full, accessed December 23, 2014; Comparing tests for diabetes and prediabetes: A quick reference guide. Updated June 18, 2014. Available at http://diabetes.niddk.nih.gov/dm/pubs/comparingtests/, accessed December 23, 2014.

---

screening are normal, testing should be repeated in at least 3-year intervals; if the results reflect a prediabetes status, testing should be repeated more frequently. The ADA also recommends that testing be considered for an adult of any age who is overweight (BMI ≥ 25 kg/m^2 or ≥ 23 kg/m^2 for Asian Americans) and who has any additional risk factors (Box 4.5) (American Diabetes Association 2015a).

As of October 2014, the US Preventive Services Task Force has issued a draft recommendation for screening type 2 diabetes in adults to include multiple-risk-factor-based type 2 diabetes screening for asymptomatic patients. Screening those with high blood pressure was previously the only screening guideline under the existing recommendation from 2008.

Risk-factor-based screening for type 2 diabetes will identify more individuals with the disease. The recommendation is currently drafted with a B rating (a suggestion for practitioners to provide this service), and under the ACA, preventive services that receive A or B ratings are covered through private insurance without cost sharing. Thus, if the draft recommendation stands, individuals at risk will have greater access to diabetes screening (American Diabetes Association 2014a).

BOX 4.5   ADA STANDARDS OF CARE: ADDITIONAL RISK FACTORS TO PROMPT SCREENING OF OVERWEIGHT ADULTS FOR DIABETES

- Physical inactivity.
- First-degree relative with diabetes.
- High-risk race/ethnicity (e.g., African American, Latino, Native American, Asian American, Pacific Islander).
- Women who delivered a baby weighing more than 9 lb. or were diagnosed with gestational diabetes mellitus.
- Hypertension or on therapy for hypertension.
- HDL cholesterol level <35 mg/dL (0.90 mmol/L) and/or a triglyceride level >250 mg/dL (2.82 mmol/L).
- Women with polycystic ovarian syndrome.
- A1c ≥ 5.7%, IGT, or IFG on previous testing.
- Other clinical conditions associated with insulin resistance (e.g., severe obesity, acanthosis nigricans).
- History of CVD.

Source: American Diabetes Association. Diabetes Care. Standards of Medical Care in Diabetes—2015. Diabetes Care January 2015 38 (Supplement 1). Available at http://care.diabetesjournals.org/content /suppl/2014/12/23/38.Supplement_1.DC1/January_Supplement_Combined_Final.6-99.pdf, accessed February 4, 2015.

Prediabetes

Type 2 diabetes develops over a long period of time in adults. The CDC (2014) uses data from NHANES to predict the prevalence of prediabetes but has noted that fasting glucose and A1c have limitations in identifying populations with prediabetes, and the implications of the age and race differences between groups in the prediabetes estimates are not known, with research ongoing to determine the best blood tests for prediabetes (American Diabetes Association 2014b). In 2009–2012, 37% of US adults aged over 20 years had prediabetes, and this increased to 51% in those aged over 65 years. Prediabetes has similar prevalence among non-Hispanic whites, non-Hispanic blacks, and Hispanics (Centers for Disease Control and Prevention 2014).

Because strong evidence exists that appropriate changes in lifestyle can delay or prevent the progression from prediabetes to type 2 diabetes, emphasis has been placed on implementation of programs and policies for diabetes prevention. The ADA (http://www.diabetes.org/are-you-at-risk /lower-your-risk/cua.html) has implemented a national prevention initiative, Check Up America, aimed at assisting the general public in lowering their risk for type 2 diabetes and heart disease by addressing a constellation of risk factors.

Diabetes Prevention and Treatment

Lifestyle intervention in high-risk individuals provides greater health benefits at a lower cost than drug therapy and is thus the most fiscally responsible intervention choice for addressing the US diabetes epidemic. The Diabetes Prevention Program (DPP, 2013), a large-scale, multisite randomized clinical trial designed to evaluate the safety and efficacy of interventions that may delay or prevent development of diabetes in people at increased risk for type 2 diabetes, demonstrated that lifestyle modification is a cost-effective strategy to prevent type 2 diabetes in adults having impaired glucose tolerance (Box 4.6).

The Joslin Diabetes Center periodically releases clinical guidelines, including nutrition guidelines for overweight and obese adults with type 2 diabetes or prediabetes, or at high risk for developing type 2 diabetes. The 2011 Joslin nutrition and physical activity guidelines recommend that

BOX 4.6   THE DIABETES PREVENTION PROGRAM (DPP)

DPP[1] was a large-scale, multisite randomized clinical trial designed to evaluate the safety and efficacy of interventions that may delay or prevent development of diabetes in people at increased risk for type 2 diabetes. Randomization of participants into the DPP over 2.7 years ended in June 1999. Nondiabetic persons ($n = 3234$) with elevated fasting and postload plasma glucose concentrations were randomly assigned to placebo, metformin (850 mg twice daily), or a lifestyle modification program. The medication group received standard lifestyle recommendations in the form of written information and in an annual 20- to 30-minute individual session that emphasized the importance of a healthy lifestyle. Participants were encouraged to follow the then-current US dietary recommendations (the Food Guide Pyramid) and the equivalent of a National Cholesterol Education Program step 1 diet,[2] to reduce their weight, and to increase their physical activity. The goals for the participants assigned to the intensive lifestyle intervention were to achieve and maintain a weight reduction of at least 7% of initial body weight through a healthy, low-calorie, low-fat diet and to engage in physical activity of moderate intensity, such as brisk walking, for at least 150 minutes per week. A 16-lesson curriculum covering diet, exercise, and behavior modification was designed to help the participants achieve these goals. The curriculum, taught by case managers on a one-to-one basis during the first 24 weeks after enrollment, was flexible, culturally sensitive, and individualized. Subsequent individual monthly sessions and group sessions with the case managers were designed to reinforce the behavioral changes.

The mean age of the participants was 51 years, and the mean body mass index was 34.0. The population was 68% female, and 45% were members of minority groups. The average follow-up was 2.8 years. The program was able to demonstrate that the most effective treatment was lifestyle intervention, followed by medication and placebo. The incidence of diabetes was 4.8, 7.8, and 11.0 cases per 100 persons in the lifestyle, drug, and placebo groups, respectively. The lifestyle intervention reduced the incidence of diabetes by 58% (95% confidence interval, 48–66%) and the drug by 31% (95% confidence interval, 17–43%), as compared with placebo.

For more information on the study and the lifestyle intervention manuals developed by the DPP study group, see the DPP home page at http://www.bsc.gwu.edu/dpp/index.htmlvdoc.

Source:
[1]Data from Knowler, WC et al., *N. Engl. J. Med.* 2002 Feb 7;346(6):393–403.
[2]Data from Step by step: Eating to lower your high blood cholesterol. Bethesda, MD. National Heart, Lung, and Blood Institute Information Center, 1987.

approximately 45% of a person's daily calories come from carbohydrates, 20–30% from protein (unless the person has kidney disease), and less than 35% from fat (mostly monounsaturated and polyunsaturated fats), and consumption of at least 20–35 g of fiber (Joslin Diabetes Center & Joslin Clinic 2011).

To initiate and continue weight reduction, a modest goal of 1 lb. every 1–2 weeks is advised by reducing daily caloric intake by 250–500 calories. Total daily calories should not be less than 1000–1200 for women and 1200–1600 for men. A target of 60–90 minutes of moderately intensive physical activity most days of the week is encouraged and should include cardiovascular, flexibility, and resistance activities to maintain or increase lean body mass. Joslin's 2011 guidelines complement the 2010 *Dietary Guidelines for Americans.*

HHS programs addressing diabetes include CDC's National Diabetes Prevention Program (NDPP) and the National Diabetes Education Program (NDEP). The CDC awarded NDPP $6.75 million in 2012 for the funding of six organizations to support program development. Individuals participating in the program develop lifestyle skills and strategies to incorporate physical activity and healthy eating habits in daily life through year-long group coaching sessions. NDPP also recognizes local organizations that have developed their own lifestyle intervention programs for the prevention of type 2 diabetes (CDC, http://www.cdc.gov/diabetes/prevention/index.htm).

National Diabetes Education Program

HHS's NDEP was launched in 1997 to improve diabetes management and thus reduce the morbidity and mortality from diabetes and its complications among Americans with diabetes. NDEP is sponsored by the National Institute of Diabetes and Digestive and Kidney Diseases (NIDDK) of the NIH and the CDC's DDT unit described above. The results of the DPP clinical trial noted above added a dramatic message to NDEP's outreach: among high-risk individuals, the onset of diabetes can be prevented or delayed. Modest weight loss through regular physical activity and healthy eating could cut the risk of developing type 2 diabetes by more than half in people with prediabetes (Knowler et al. 2002). Beginning in 2002, NDEP released messages and materials to translate the science of diabetes prevention into clinical practice and to raise awareness among high-risk individuals. *Small Steps. Big Rewards. Prevent Type 2 Diabetes*, the first national diabetes prevention campaign, targets Americans with prediabetes with tailored materials and messages for each high-risk audience (US Department of Health and Human Services, http://www.ndep.nih.gov/campaigns/SmallSteps /SmallSteps_index.htm).

In 2009, NDEP also launched a diabetes management campaign—*Control Your Diabetes. For Life* (US Department of Health and Human Services, http://ndep.nih.gov/partners-community -organization/campaigns/ControlYourDiabetesForLife.aspx). The campaign emphasizes tight regulation of blood glucose for people with diabetes through healthy eating, physical activity, effective use of medication, and frequent blood glucose testing. Materials and messages highlight the importance of knowing the *ABC*s of diabetes:

A: A1c < 7%
B: Blood pressure < 140/80 mm Hg
C: Cholesterol levels appropriate to the individual

NDEP strategies for diabetes education include culturally and linguistically appropriate diabetes awareness education campaigns. Campaign materials are available in over 20 languages.

DIABETES IN CHILDREN

The occurrence of type 2 diabetes in youth has emerged to the forefront of public health over the past two decades, reflecting the increasing rates of childhood obesity discussed in Chapter 5. In 1992, type 2 diabetes was a rare occurrence in most pediatric centers; however, by 1994, it represented up to 16% of new cases of diabetes diagnosed in urban areas, and by 1999, the incidence of new type 2 diagnoses in children ranged between 8% and 45%, depending on geographic location (Kaufman 2002).

In response to the growing public health concern about type 2 diabetes in children, CDC and the NIDDK funded a 5-year multicenter study—SEARCH for Diabetes in Youth (2000–2005)— to examine the current status of diabetes among children and adolescents in the United States. The main objectives of the project were to assess the magnitude and burden of diagnosed diabetes through a multicenter registry system that covers more than 6% of the children and adolescents in the United States, and to develop criteria to differentiate between the types of diabetes among young people in the United States (The SEARCH Writing Group 2004). SEARCH is currently in its third phase (2010–2015) (The SEARCH for Diabetes in Youth Study Group 2010). Data gathered from SEARCH are reported throughout this section. Environmental factors studied in SEARCH include SES, education level of parents, as well as unhealthy behaviors such as smoking and dietary intake. Prevalence data were collected based on physician diagnosis or self-reports of the presence of diabetes and do not include estimates of undiagnosed cases.

Prevalence of Diabetes in Youth and Children

In 2012, an estimated 208,000 youth, or 0.25% of this population, had diagnosed type 1 or type 2 diabetes (Centers for Disease Control and Prevention 2014c). Prevalence of diabetes in youth varies by age, race/ethnicity, and gender. The average age at diagnosis is 8.4 years. Type 2 diabetes is rare in children younger than 10, and though prevalence of type 2 diabetes increases with age, more than 80% of cases remain type 1 in youth 10–19 years of age. Prevalence of total diabetes was found to be slightly higher in females (The SEARCH for Diabetes in Youth Study Group 2006).

Race and ethnicity are significant risk factors but vary between type 1 and type 2 diabetes. Type 1 diabetes incidence is highest among non-Hispanic white youth and lowest among American Indian and Asian/Pacific Islander youth, while the converse is partially true for type 2 diabetes; rates of type 2 diabetes are highest among American Indian and African American youth and lowest among non-Hispanic white youth (The Writing Group 2007). Asian/Pacific Islander and American Indian youth are disproportionately affected by type 2 diabetes. African American and Hispanic youth experience similar rates of type 1 and type 2 diabetes. Finally, the number of newly diagnosed cases each year occurs disproportionately in non-Hispanic white youth, mainly due to the high occurrence of type 1 in this population (Mayer-Davis 2009). Both type 1 and type 2 diabetes are increasing in prevalence in youth. From 2001 to 2009, analysis of SEARCH data reports that the prevalence of type 1 in US youth increased 21.1% and type 2 in youth increased 30.5% (Dabelea et al. 2014).

Rising Incidence of Type 1 Diabetes in Children

A pediatrics registry study of Philadelphia children spanning 20 years (1985–2005) has found that the incidence of type 1 diabetes among Philadelphian children has increased at an average yearly rate of 1.5%, or an average 5-year cohort rate of 7.3% over 20 years; however, the sharpest rise occurred since 1995–1999. The most significant increase was a doubling of incidence in white children aged 10–14 since the 1995–1999 cohort (Lipman et al. 2013).

Furthermore, the data for the youngest children (ages 4 and under) showed an increase in type 1 of 70% over the 20-year period of the study. Similar rises have been reported in Finland and Sweden (Lipman et al. 2013). Theories of the recent rise in type 1 diagnoses include reduced exposure of young children to immune-strengthening environments (the hygiene hypothesis), an increase of vitamin D deficiency, and an increase in early exposure to cow's milk (Lipman et al. 2013), as well as the possibility of exposure to enterovirus (Harjutsala et al. 2013).

The Philadelphia study also reported an extreme rise in the incidence of type 1 diabetes among black children 0–4 years of age in the 2000–2004 cohort, noting an increase of 140% since the 1995–1999 cohort and an increase of more than 200% over 20 years (Lipman et al. 2013).

Complications in Diabetes Diagnoses in Children

The increasing co-occurrence of obesity with type 1 diabetes, as well as the increasing appearance of diabetic ketoacidosis (DKA) with type 2 cases (now nearly 10%) (Rewers et al. 2008), has made distinguishing between type 1 and type 2 cases in children increasingly difficult. DKA is a life-threatening condition caused by the body burning fat for energy when glucose is lacking. Ketones are acids produced in this process, and at high levels, they can poison the body (American Diabetes Association, http://www.diabetes.org/living-with-diabetes/complications/ketoacidosis-dka.html).

Other types of diabetes diagnoses in youth include maturity-onset diabetes in youth (early onset of type 2 diabetes) and hybrid diabetes (presence of both insulin resistance and autoimmune dysfunction). Though the proportion of type 2 diagnoses in youth increases with age, incidences of type 2 diabetes are occurring more frequently in youth under the age of 10 (The SEARCH for Diabetes in Youth Study Group 2006).

As in adults, type 2 diabetes in youth is associated with obesity. In addition, these youth show early signs of insulin resistance and cardiovascular risk. A study of diabetic youth over the period 2001–2004, reported that for youth with type 2 diabetes, 10.4% were overweight, while 79.4% were obese (Liu et al. 2010).

In addition to obesity, other risk factors for the development of diabetes in youth include insulin resistance, ethnicity, and onset of puberty. The constellation of these risk factors may be problematic during the critical period of adolescent development, especially in individuals who may have compromised β-cell function and an inability to compensate for severe insulin resistance (Goran et al. 2003). Exposure to diabetes or obesity *in utero* coupled with being large for gestational age (birth weight > 90th percentile) has shown an increased risk for the development of metabolic syndrome and obesity later in life (Boney et al. 2005).

Screening Recommendations for Children

The ADA screening recommendation for type 2 diabetes and prediabetes in children (persons aged 18 years or younger) recognizes the risk factors of race and ethnicity. The recommendation is to consider clinical testing starting at age 10 or at onset of puberty (if prior to age 10) for any child who is overweight (BMI > 85th percentile for age and gender, weight for height > 85th percentile, or weight > 120% of ideal weight for height) and who also has any two of the following risk factors (American Diabetes Association 2015b):

- Family history of type 2 diabetes in first- or second-degree relative.
- Race/ethnicity of Native American, African American, Hispanic/Latino, Asian American, or Pacific Islander.
- Signs of insulin resistance or conditions associated with insulin resistance, such as acanthosis nigricans (the skin around the neck or in the armpits appears dark and thick, and feels velvety), hypertension, dyslipidemia, polycystic ovarian syndrome, or small-for-gestational-age birth weight.
- Maternal history of diabetes or gestational diabetes while pregnant with the child.

However, recent data have suggested that BMI may not be an accurate indicator of body fat or disease risk in minority youth populations. Analysis of SEARCH data showed that adjustment of BMI cutoffs in Asian (overweight = 23 kg/m^2, obese = 25 kg/m^2) and Pacific Islander (overweight = 26 kg/m^2, obese = 32 kg/m^2) youth yielded a 60% higher risk of diabetes in Asians than non-Hispanic whites and suggests that Asians and Pacific Islanders should be considered distinct ethnic groups (Liu et al. 2009).

Prevention of Type 2 Diabetes in Children

Primary prevention of type 2 diabetes in children should ideally include a public health approach with community-level strategies. Collaboration with health organizations, healthcare providers, and private businesses can increase the resources and reach of government and school-centered efforts. Programs that provide children and their families with the knowledge, attitudes, behavioral skills, and encouragement to consume a healthy diet and engage in regular physical activity can be effective in attenuating the expanding problem.

Primary prevention strategies focused on children include increasing physical activity and improving nutrition. More specifically, this includes reducing the amount of "screen time" spent playing video games, watching television, and using the internet, and reducing the amount of sweetened beverages consumed. Successful programs have targeted interventions to reduce these behaviors—improving school menus, installing water coolers, and implementing exercise-based curricula have all led to reductions in obesity rates of study populations. Governmental efforts should be focused on improving access to community-level health resources, such as increasing open spaces in urban areas and supporting healthier food vendors in schools (Kaufman 2007).

For children who are obese and who have impaired glucose tolerance, intensive efforts to reduce obesity in children through increased physical activity and better eating habits are likely to help to prevent the development of type 2 diabetes. Women of childbearing age are also being targeted because exposure to obesity with or without diabetes *in utero* may be a major contributor to the increase in type 2 diabetes during childhood and adolescence (Adamo et al. 2012).

Ongoing efforts to prevent and treat type 2 diabetes will require community and government involvement to reduce obesity in both pediatric and adult populations. A number of government initiatives are underway to address obesity in the youth population, such as We Can! and Let's Move!, which are discussed in Chapter 5. We will not highlight these again here, except to add that both programs suggest encouraging children to drink more water in place of sweetened beverages. Following up on this suggestion, the first lady launched the Drink Up campaign in 2013 to encourage kids to drink more water (*Let's Move!*, http://www.letsmove.gov). Although the message does not directly assert anything about drinking less soda, the adoption of the positive behavior may squeeze out less desired behaviors.

CARDIOVASCULAR DISEASE

One-third of the US population has some form of CVD. Nationally, heart disease and stroke are the first and fourth leading causes of mortality, accounting for nearly 30% of all deaths. More than 800,000 Americans—men and women, old and young—die of CVD each year, and 150,000 of these deaths occur in individuals aged less than 65 years. Six out of 10 stroke deaths occur in women. However, looking at mortality alone understates the health effects of these two conditions. The economic effects of CVD on the US healthcare system are increasing as the population ages, with an estimated $312.6 billion in healthcare costs and lost productivity annually (Million Hearts, http://millionhearts.hhs.gov/abouthds/cost-consequences.html).

Heart Disease

Heart disease, which killed nearly 600,000 Americans in 2010, accounted for 24% of all deaths in the United States (Murphy et al. 2013). Nonetheless, during the last two decades, the age-adjusted rate of deaths from coronary heart disease (CHD) has declined sharply, falling from 186.8 per 100,000 in 2000 to 113.6 in 2010, but the decrease still falls short of reaching the Healthy People 2020 target of 103.4 per 100,000 (objective HDS-2) (HealthyPeople.gov, http://www.healthypeople.gov/2020/topics-objectives/topic/heart-disease-and-stroke/objectives).

Furthermore, the improvements in the rate of death are not equally shared among the population. In 2008, the rate of death from heart disease ranged from 22% to 84% higher among blacks than whites, varying with age, and was 54% higher among men than women (National Institutes of Health, National Heart Lung, and Blood Institute 2012). Among racial/ethnic groups, blacks consistently show the greatest disparity from the average. Both black men and women have higher death rates from CHD and stroke before the age of 75 than other groups. Geographically, during 2008–2010, CHD death rates were highest in the South (Centers for Disease Control and Prevention, http://www.cdc.gov/heartdisease/facts.htm).

Prevention of Heart Disease

In 2010, heart disease cost the nation $108.9 billion (Heidenreich et al. 2011). About 28% of heart attacks each year occur in those who have previously had a heart attack (Go et al. 2014).

The major risk factors of heart disease are high blood pressure, high blood cholesterol, tobacco use, diabetes, physical inactivity, and poor nutrition. Modest reductions in the rates of one or more of these risk factors can have a large public health impact. For individuals, comparing tobacco usage and diet shows that the greatest gains of risk reduction, both for individuals and the population as a group, can be achieved through improving nutrition.

Based on 2009–2010 NHANES data, 76% of adults have ideal smoking behavior (never having smoked or having quit more than 12 months ago). Less than 1% of adults have ideal dietary behaviors, specifically meeting four out of five dietary components of a healthy dietary plan consistent with a Dietary Approaches to Stop Hypertension (DASH)-type eating pattern. The five components of ideal DASH eating patterns are to consume at least 4.5 cups per day of fruits and vegetables, at least 2 servings per week of fish, and at least 3 servings per day of whole grains, as well as consuming no more than 36 oz. per week of sugar-sweetened beverages and 1500 mg of sodium per day. In children, the prevalence of ideal diet is nearly 0% (Roger et al. 2012). In other words, almost everyone can make some dietary improvements.

Prevention Initiatives

Life's Simple 7

The AHA released Life's Simple 7 in 2010 as part of the plan to achieve its 2020 Impact Goal of improving the cardiovascular health of all Americans by 20% while reducing deaths from CVDs and stroke by 2% (Go et al. 2013). Table 4.5 charts the Life's Simple 7 key cardiovascular health and behavior factors on a spectrum of poor, intermediate, and ideal. Along with this list of health and behavior factors that impact health and quality of life, the AHA (http://mylifecheck.heart.org) designed My Life Check, an assessment that individuals can request via a form on the AHA website. The assessment produces personalized steps to improve health behaviors.

Million Hearts

Another national initiative is the Million Hearts initiative, launched by HHS in September 2011. The goal of Million Hearts is to prevent 1 million heart attacks and strokes by 2017, and it uses four approaches: enhanced surveillance, environmental approaches, health systems interventions, and community–clinical links. One innovative part of this program was the comparison of telephonic nurse disease management with a home monitoring program for controlling blood pressure among African Americans enrolled in a national health plan.

Public Health Action Plan to Prevent Heart Disease and Stroke

The Action Plan was initially released in 2003 as the work of the CDC and more than 80 people representing 66 national and international organizations. The collaboration led to the formal organization of the National Forum for Heart Disease and Stroke Prevention (National Forum), an independent nonprofit 501(c)(3) voluntary health organization that implements the Action Plan. Members of the National Forum include more than 80 US and international organizations representing public, private, healthcare, advocacy, academic, policy, and community sectors (Labarthe et al. 2014). The 2003 Action Plan outlined public health strategies to prevent heart disease and stroke (Box 4.7).

The Action Plan was first updated in 2008. The update highlighted the following specific actions for addressing health disparities (US Department of Health and Human Services 2008):

- Develop communication strategies to effectively communicate with those populations most at risk and address inequities in access to healthcare.
- Understand the changing dynamics of communication and the increasingly interactive nature of communications. Incorporate electronic (web-based) forms of communication in strategies. In outreach, identify and use communication devices that are accessible in a particular community.
- Educate key decision makers to support heart disease and stroke prevention policies and programs.
- Foster effective systems for healthcare delivery (e.g., utilizing care models with emphasis on patient self-management and community resources).

The National Forum updated the Action Plan again in 2014 (Ten-Year Update), noting that persisting health disparities resulting from CVD reflect unequal exposure to the causes and that unequal access to prevention and treatment for minority and other vulnerable populations remains a need for action. Citing the final report of Healthy People 2010, the Ten-Year Update states that disparities

TABLE 4.5

American Heart Association's *Life's Simple 7*: Key Health Factors and Behaviors for Cardiovascular Health

Health Factor/Behavior	Poor	Intermediate	Ideal
Blood Pressure			
Adults >20 years of age	SBP ≥ 140 or DBP ≥ 90 mm Hg	SBP 120–139 or DBP 80–89 mm Hg or treated to goal	<120/<80 mm Hg
Children 8–19 years of age	>95th percentile	90th–95th percentile or SBP ≥ 120 or DBP ≥ 80 mm Hg	<90th percentile
Physical Activity			
Adults >20 years of age	None	1–149 minutes/week mod, 1–74 minutes/week vig, or 1–149 minutes/week mod + vig	150+ minutes/week mod, 75+ minutes/week vig, or 150+ minutes/week mod + vig
Children 12–19 years of age	None	0–59 minutes of mod or vig every day	60+ minutes of mod or vig every day
Cholesterol			
Adults >20 years of age	≥240 mg/dL	200–239 mg/dL or treated to goal	<170 mg/dL
Children 6–19 years of age	≥200 mg/dL	170–199 mg/dL	
Healthy Diet			
Adults >20 years of age	0–1 components	2–3 components	4–5 components
Children 5–19 years of age	0–1 components	2–3 components	4–5 components
Healthy Weight			
Adults >20 years of age	≥30 kg/m^2	25–29.9 kg/m^2	<25 kg/m^2
Children 2–19 years of age	>95th percentile	85th–95th percentile	<85th percentile
Smoking Status			
Adults >20 years of age	Current smoker	Former ≤2 months	Never/quit ≥12 months
Children 12–19 years of age	Tried in the prior 30 days		Never tried; never smoked whole cigarette
Blood Glucose			
Adults >20 years of age	≥126 mg/dL	100–125 mg/dL or treated to goal	<100 mg/dL
Children 12–19 years of age	≥126 mg/dL	100–125 mg/dL	<100 mg/dL

Source: Go, A.S. et al., *Circulation*, 127, 2013.
Note: DBP, is diastolic blood pressure; SBP, is systolic blood pressure.

by race/ethnicity and education attainment persist, often with a 50% or greater gap, and in many instances widened even while overall improvements have taken place (Labarthe et al. 2014).

Overall, the National Forum's goal is that heart disease and stroke will no longer be the leading cause of death for all Americans by 2020. The work to achieve this goal is informed by three priorities: cardiovascular surveillance, health equity, and sodium reduction (National Forum for Heart

BOX 4.7   CDC'S PUBLIC HEALTH STRATEGIES
TO PREVENT HEART DISEASE AND STROKE

1. Develop policies for preventing heart disease and stroke at national, state, and local levels to assure effective public health action, including new knowledge on the efficacy and safety of therapies to reduce risk factors. Implement intervention programs in a timely manner and on a sufficient scale to permit rigorous evaluation and the rapid replication and dissemination of those most effective. Active intervention is needed continually to develop and support policies (both in and beyond the health sector) that are favorable to health, change those that are unfavorable, and foster policy innovations when gaps are identified. Policies that adversely affect health should be identified because they can be major barriers to the social, environmental, and behavioral changes needed to improve population-wide health.

2. Promote *cardiovascular health* and prevent heart disease and stroke through interventions in multiple settings, for all age groups, and for the whole population, especially high-risk groups. This recommendation defines the scope of a comprehensive public health strategy to prevent heart disease and stroke. Such a strategy must emphasize promotion of desirable social and environmental conditions and favorable population-wide and individual behavioral patterns to prevent major risk factors and assure full accessibility and timely use of quality health services among people with risk factors or disease.

3. Strengthen public health agencies to assure that they develop and maintain sufficient capacities and competencies. Public health agencies at state and local levels should establish specific programs designed to promote cardiovascular health and prevent heart disease and stroke. Skills are required in the new priority areas of policy and environmental change, population-wide health promotion through behavioral change, and risk factor prevention. Public health agencies must also be able to manage and use health data systems to effectively monitor and evaluate interventions and prevention programs.

4. Define criteria and standards for population-wide health data sources. Expand these sources as needed to assure adequate long-term monitoring of population measures related to heart disease and stroke. Such measures include mortality, incidence, and prevalence rates; selected biomarkers of CVD risk; risk factors and behaviors; economic conditions; community and environmental characteristics; sociodemographic factors (e.g., age, race/ethnicity, sex, place of residence); and leading health indicators.

5. Upgrade and expand health data sources to allow systematic monitoring and evaluation of policy and program interventions. To learn what works best, all programs funded by public health agencies should allocate resources for evaluation up-front, and staff must be trained to develop and apply evaluation methods. The resulting data must be communicated effectively to other agencies and to policy makers.

6. Emphasize the critical roles of atherosclerosis and high blood pressure, which are the dominant conditions underlying heart disease and stroke, within a broad prevention research agenda. Prevention research on policy, environmental, and sociocultural determinants of risk factors is critical, as is rapid translation of this information into healthcare practice. Such research should focus especially on children and adolescents because atherosclerosis and high blood pressure can begin early in life. The

prevention research agenda should be developed and updated collaboratively among interested parties, taking current and planned research programs into account.

7. Develop innovative ways to monitor and evaluate policies and programs, especially for policy and environmental change and population-wide health promotion. Public health agencies and their partners should conduct and promote research to improve surveillance methods in multiple areas, settings, and populations. Marketing research can be used to evaluate public knowledge and awareness of key health messages and to update these messages over time. Methodological research can help assess the impact of new technologies and regulations on surveillance systems.

Source: US Department of Health and Human Services. *A Public Health Action Plan to Prevent Heart Disease and Stroke.* Centers for Disease Control and Prevention. 2003. Available at http://www.cdc .gov/dhdsp/action_plan/pdfs/action_plan_full.pdf, accessed February 4, 2015.

Disease and Stroke Prevention, http://www.nationalforum.org/organization). The Ten-Year Update calls for seven action priorities, which are summarized in Table 4.6.

Community-Based Prevention for Heart Disease

Research conducted during the 1970s demonstrates that community interventions that change the environment are particularly effective in reducing heart disease throughout the entire community. For example, when a workplace adopts a no-smoking policy, all employees will benefit, whether they smoke or not.

North Karelia Project

The first major community-based heart disease control program was conducted in North Karelia, Finland, which had a high CVD mortality rate. The North Karelia Project was launched in 1972 as a community-based program to influence diet and other lifestyles crucial in the prevention of CVD. The intervention employed comprehensive strategies. Broad community organization and the strong participation of community members were key elements. Evaluation of the project has studied how diet (particularly fat consumption) has changed and how these changes have led to a major reduction in population serum cholesterol and blood pressure levels. From 1971 to 1995, ischemic heart disease mortality in the working-age population declined by 73% in North Karelia and by 65% throughout Finland.

North Karelia is an example of a health disparity population within industrialized Finland. North Karelia was rural, with a lower socioeconomic stratum, and with many social problems. The project was based on low-cost intervention activities, where individual participation and community organizations played a key role. Comprehensive interventions in the community were eventually supported by national activities—from expert guidelines and media activities to industry collaboration and policy (Pekka et al. 2002).

Similar changes have been implemented in the United States and other countries. In the United States, NIH financed three major community-based intervention projects: the Stanford Five-City Project (Farquhar et al. 1990), the Minnesota Heart Health Program (Luepker et al. 1994), and the Pawtucket Heart Health Program (Carleton et al. 1995). Other projects have been carried out in Israel (Abrahamson et al. 1981), Germany (GCP Study Group 1988), and Sweden (Brännström et al. 1993).

WISEWOMAN

The WISEWOMAN program is administered through CDC's DHDSP but operated on the local level in states and tribal organizations. The program provides low-income, underinsured, and uninsured women aged 40–64 with chronic disease risk factor screening, lifestyle intervention, and

TABLE 4.6

The Public Health Action Plan to Prevent Heart Disease and Stroke: Ten-Year Update's Seven Immediate Action Priorities for 2014 and Beyond

Priority	Focus	Action Needed
Effective communication	Prevention and public health	Communicate to legislators, policy makers, and the public at large the nation's vital stake in sustaining and building upon the prevention and public health provisions in the Affordable Care Act, e.g., the National Prevention Council, Prevention and Public Health Fund, and others.
Strategic leadership, partnerships, and organization	Public health–healthcare collaboration and integration	Integrate public health and healthcare into a public health system effective in supporting community-level prevention policies and programs, e.g., the Million Hearts Initiative.
Taking action	Cardiovascular health and health equity	Develop, advocate, and implement policies, programs, and practices aimed to improve the nation's cardiovascular health in terms of the Healthy People 2020 objectives and AHA metrics—addressing tobacco use, overweight/obesity, physical activity, healthy diet (including reduction in sodium and artificial trans fat intake), blood pressure, cholesterol, and fasting plasma glucose); ensure that all such actions reach everyone, especially those most vulnerable due to unfavorable social and environmental conditions.
Building capacity	Prevention workforce	Make full use of resources for education and training of the prevention workforce at local, state, national, and global levels.
Evaluating impact	Monitoring cardiovascular health	Advocate for a comprehensive, robust, and timely system of monitoring cardiovascular events (heart attacks, stroke, heart failure) and cardiovascular health metrics for the US population, including full adoption of the "developmental" heart disease and stroke objectives of Healthy People 2020.
Advancing policy	Research on critical questions to advance policy and practice	Pursue needed implementation and dissemination of science and health economics research, including needed education and training for this research, in support of health policy development, implementation, and dissemination.
Engaging in regional and global collaboration	Initiatives linking CVD and noncommunicable disease (NCD) prevention	Undertake collaborations in major regional and global cardiovascular health and NCD initiatives, in the interest of improving cardiovascular health and reducing the burden of NCDs in the United States and globally.

Source: Labarthe, D. et al., *The Public Health Action Plan to Prevent Heart Disease and Stroke: Ten-Year Update,* Washington, DC, National Forum for Heart Disease and Stroke Prevention, 2014. Available at http://nationalforum.org/sites /default/files/Action%20Plan%20-%20Ten%20Year%20Update%20April%202014.pdf, accessed February 4, 2015.

referral services in an effort to prevent CVD. Projects provide standard preventive services including blood pressure and cholesterol testing, and programs to help women develop a healthier diet, increase physical activity, and stop using tobacco (CDC, http://www.cdc.gov/wisewoman/).

HYPERTENSION

The World Health Organization estimates that high blood pressure causes one out of every six deaths worldwide, making hypertension the third leading cause of death in the world (World Health Organization 2013). Blood pressure diagnostic categories for normal blood pressure, prehypertension, and stages 1 and 2 hypertension in adults are presented in Table 4.7.

TABLE 4.7
Blood Pressure Diagnostic Categories in Adults

Category	Systolic Blood Pressure, mm Hg	Diastolic Blood Pressure, mm Hg
Normal	<120	<80
Prehypertension	120–139	80–89
Hypertension stage 1	140–159	90–99
Hypertension stage 2	160–179	100–109

Source: Table 3, Classification of Blood Pressure for Adults, National Heart, Lung, and Blood Institute, *Seventh Report of the Joint National Committee on Prevention, Detection, Evaluation, and Treatment of High Blood Pressure*, US Department of Health and Human Services, National Institutes of Health, August 2004. Available at http://www.nhlbi.nih.gov/files/docs/guidelines/jnc 7full.pdf, accessed January 12, 2015.

Uncontrolled high blood pressure can lead to stroke, heart attack, or heart or kidney failure by placing stress on a number of target organs. Elevated blood pressure is also associated with pregnancy complications and compromised sexual functioning, and may result in organ damage if it occurs in children. Hypertension affects the heart, brain, kidneys, eyes, bones, sexual function, and pregnancy outcome (Box 4.8).

Prevalence of Hypertension

In 2012, the CDC reported that the estimated prevalence of hypertension among US adults aged greater than 18 years in 2003–2010 was 30.4%, or almost 67 million people. Hypertension was uncontrolled in at least half of this population (Centers for Disease Control and Prevention 2012). The percentage of individuals with hypertension receiving treatment has improved, and the percentage of patients with blood pressure controlled to <140/90 mm Hg has improved from 10% to 45.9%. These changes have been associated with highly favorable trends in the morbidity and mortality attributed to hypertension. The prevalence of hypertension has shown an increasing trend over time from 24.7% (NHANES 1988–1994) to 29.9% (NHANES 2005–2008) but has remained stable through 2009–2012 (HealthyPeople.gov, http://www.healthypeople.gov/2020/topics-objectives/topic/heart-disease-and-stroke/national-snapshot).

Furthermore, disparities in the prevalence of hypertension still exist in multiple populations, as described in Table 4.8. Hypertension prevalence increases with age and decreases with education and income level. Rates of hypertension are significantly higher in blacks than in whites and are lowest in Mexican Americans (Centers for Disease Control and Prevention 2011b).

Managing high blood pressure is the most important thing an individual can do to reduce the risk of stroke. Although stroke is the fourth leading cause of death for Americans, the risk of having a stroke varies with race and ethnicity. The risk of having a first stroke is nearly twice as high for blacks than for whites, and blacks are more likely to die following a stroke. The highest death rates from stroke are in the southeastern United States (Go et al. 2014).

Prevention of Hypertension

The prevention of high blood pressure is a major public health challenge in the United States. Clinicians should target people with prehypertension. On the other hand, decreasing individuals' blood pressure levels by even modest amounts could lead to a substantial reduction in morbidity and mortality in the general population. The National High Blood Pressure Education Program (NHBPEP) estimates that a 5 mm Hg reduction of systolic blood pressure in the population would result in a 14% overall reduction in mortality due to stroke, a 9% reduction in mortality due to CHD, and a 7% decrease in all-cause mortality (Whelton et al. 2002).

BOX 4.8   HYPERTENSION AND ITS SEQUELAE

Heart: High blood pressure places stress on a number of organs, including the kidneys, eyes, and heart. More than two-thirds of people who suffer a first heart attack have hypertension. Depending on severity, high blood pressure increases the risk of a heart attack by up to five times and precedes the development of congestive heart failure (CHF) in more than 70% of cases.[1]

Brain: High blood pressure contributes to 75% of all strokes and heart attacks, and is particularly deadly in African Americans. Malignant hypertension, an emergency condition resulting from untreated primary hypertension, can be lethal. About three-quarters of people who suffer a first stroke have moderately elevated blood pressure (≥140/90 mm Hg). Hypertensive people have up to 10 times the normal risk of stroke, depending on the severity of the blood pressure. Dementia and cognitive impairment occur more commonly in patients with hypertension. Hypertension is associated with vascular dementia and mixed dementia (the coexistence of Alzheimer's disease with vascular dementia).[2–4]

Kidney: In patients with diabetes, both hyperglycemia and hypertension are independent risk factors for renal disease. High blood pressure is strongly associated with diabetic nephropathy. Blood pressure control is paramount in reducing CVD risk and the development of diabetic nephropathy: the target blood pressure is <140/80 mm Hg in patients with type 2 diabetes.[5] Men with high blood pressure may also have a higher risk of kidney cancer.[6]

Eyes: High blood pressure can lead to retinopathy.[7]

Bone loss: Hypertension increases the excretion of calcium in urine, which may lead to loss of bone mineral density, a significant risk factor for fractures.[8,9]

Sexual dysfunction: Sexual dysfunction is more common and more severe in men with hypertension, particularly in smokers, than it is in the general population.[10]

Pregnancy and eclampsia: Severe, sudden high blood pressure in pregnant women is one component of preeclampsia (commonly called *toxemia*), which can be serious for both mother and child. Preeclampsia occurs in up to 10% of pregnancies, usually in the third trimester of a first pregnancy, and resolves immediately after delivery. The condition may be caused by a failure of the placenta to embed properly in the uterus, which causes it to misconnect with the mother's blood vessels. As a result, the fetus does not receive a sufficient blood supply, and the mother's own blood pressure increases to replace it. The reduced supply of blood to the placenta can cause low birth weight and eye or brain damage in the fetus. Severe cases of preeclampsia can cause kidney damage, convulsion, and coma in the mother and can be lethal to both mother and child. Women with existing hypertension are at risk for preeclampsia.[11]

Hypertension in children: Early abnormalities, including an enlarged heart and abnormalities in the kidney and eyes, may occur even in those children with mild hypertension. Children and adolescents with hypertension should be monitored and evaluated for possible early organ damage.[12,13]

Source:
[1]Data from Go, AS et al., *Circulation*. 127, e6–e245, 2013.
[2]Data from Di Bari, M et al., *Am. J. Epidemiol*. 153, 72–78, 2001.
[3]Data from Feigin, V et al., *J. Neurol. Sci*. 229–230, 151–155, 2005. Epub 2005 January 7.
[4]Data from Sacco, RL et al., *Stroke*. 28, 1507–1517, 1997.
[5]Data from American Diabetes Association. Diabetes Care. Standards of Medical Care in Diabetes—2014. Diabetes Care January 2014 37(Supplement 1): S14–S80. Available at http://care .diabetesjournals.org/content/37/Supplement_1/S14/T5.expansion.html, accessed December 23, 2014.

[6]Data from Choi, MY et al., *Kidney Int.* 67(2), 647–52, February 2005.
[7]Data from Wong, TY and Mitchell, P, *N. Engl. J. Med.* 351, 2310–2317, 2004.
[8]Data from Cappuccio, FP et al., *J. Nephrol.* 13, 169–77, 2000.
[9]Data from Blackwood, AM et al., *J. Hum. Hypertension.* 15, 229–237, 2001.
[10]Data from Giuliano, FA et al., *Urology.* 64, 1196–1201, 2004.
[11]Data from August, P et al., *Am. J. Obstet. Gynecol.* 191, 1666–1672, 2004.
[12]Data from Sorof, J and Daniels, S *Hypertension.* 40, 441–447, 2002.
[13]Data from US Department of Health and Human Services. National Institutes of Health. National Heart, Lung, and Blood Institute. The Fourth Report on the Diagnosis, Evaluation, and Treatment of High Blood Pressure in Children and Adolescents. NIH Publication No. 05-5267. Originally printed September 1996 (96-3790). Revised May 2005.

A public health intervention should be aimed at modifying these causal factors of hypertension:

- *Overweight*: More than 200 million Americans are overweight or obese. Maintain normal body weight (BMI 18.5–24.9 kg/m^2) (Flegal et al. 2012).
- *Low physical activity*: Engage in regular physical activity, at least 30 minutes per day, most days of the week. Fewer than half of American adults achieve this recommended amount of weekly exercise (National Center for Health Statistics 2013b).
- *High sodium intake*: The average sodium consumption for adult Americans aged 20 or over is 3592 mg per day, mostly from processed and restaurant foods (US Department of Agriculture 2011–2012). The Institute of Medicine recommends limiting dietary sodium intake to 1500 mg per day, while the 2010 Dietary Guidelines recommend a limit of 2300 mg per day in addition to consuming potassium-rich fruits and vegetables.
- *Low intake of fruits and vegetables*: Less than 20% of Americans consume at least 5 servings of fruits and vegetables per day (Kruger et al. 2007). Consuming a diet rich in fruits, vegetables, and low-fat dairy products and with a reduced content of saturated and total fat (i.e., DASH eating plan) can lower blood pressure by as much as 11.5 mm Hg (Sacks et al. 2001) and help maintain an adequate intake of dietary potassium (3500 mg per day).
- *High alcohol consumption*: Limit alcohol consumption to no more than one drink per day for women and two drinks per day for men.

Population-Based Strategies for Hypertension Prevention

A population-based approach aimed at achieving a downward shift in the distribution of blood pressure in the general population is an important component for any comprehensive plan to prevent hypertension. A small decrement in the distribution of systolic blood pressure is likely to result in a substantial reduction in the burden of blood pressure-related illness. Environmental approaches, such as lowering sodium content or caloric density in the food supply, and providing attractive, safe, and convenient opportunities for exercise are ideal population-based approaches for reduction of average blood pressure in the community. Community-wide education campaigns, school-based physical education, and enhanced access to appropriate facilities (parks, walking trails, bike paths) have been proven to be effective strategies for increasing physical activity in the general population (Task Force on Community Preventive Services 2002).

Sodium Reduction in Communities Program

The CDC launched the Sodium Reduction in Communities Program (SRCP) in 2010 as a 3-year program to promote local and state sodium reduction strategies in six communities across the United States. These communities have implemented low-sodium guidelines in local government offices and school districts; worked with food suppliers, independent restaurants, and grocery stores to provide lower-sodium options; and improved availability of lower-sodium options in hospitals and senior meal

TABLE 4.8

Disparities in Adult Hypertension by Selected Demographic Characteristics

Characteristic	Hypertension[b]		Controlled Hypertension[c]	
	%	(95% CI)	%	(95% CI)
Sex				
Male	30.6	(29.0–32.3)[e]	38.6	(34.6–42.6)[e]
Female (referent)	28.7	(27.5–30.0)	52.0	(48.7–55.3)
Age Group (Years), Unadjusted[a]				
18–44 (referent)	10.5	(9.0–11.9)	37.5	(31.2–43.7)
45–64	40.6	(38.1–43.2)[e]	48.9	(45.4–52.3)[e]
≥65	70.3	(67.5–73.2)[e]	45.6	(42.9–48.4)
Race/Ethnicity				
Mexican American	25.5	(23.4–27.7)[e]	31.8	(26.1–37.6)[e]
Black, non-Hispanic	42.0	(39.6–44.3)[e]	41.2	(37.4–44.9)
White, non-Hispanic (referent)	28.8	(27.1–30.4)	46.5	(42.9–50.1)
Education (Persons Aged ≥25 Years)[a]				
<High school	37.3	(34.6–40.0)[e]	36.5	(27.8–45.1)
High school graduate	35.9	(33.8–38.0)[e]	47.2	(41.7–52.7)
Some college	33.6	(31.5–35.8)[e]	44.6	(39.4–49.9)
College graduate or above (referent)	29.6	(27.5–31.6)	50.2	(43.5–56.9)
Family Income, US Poverty Level, %[d]				
<100	32.6	(30.4–34.8)[e]	42.4	(33.2–51.5)
100–199	32.7	(30.3–35.0)[e]	37.3	(30.0–44.6)
200–399	30.8	(28.6–33.1)	45.2	(39.8–50.6)
400–499	28.6	(25.0–32.2)	44.5	(34.0–55.0)
≥500 (referent)	27.4	(24.9–29.8)	47.9	(41.9–53.8)

Source: Age-Adjusted Percentage of Hypertension and Controlled Hypertension Among Adults Aged ≥18 Years, by Selected Demographic and Health Characteristics—National Health and Nutrition Examination Survey, United States, 2005–2008, CDC Health Disparities and Inequalities Report—United States, 2011. Available at http://www.cdc.gov/mmwr/pdf/other/su6001.pdf, accessed January 5, 2015.

[a] $P < 0.05$, test of trend for hypertension prevalence; not significant for controlled hypertension.

[b] Systolic blood pressure (SBP) ≥ 140 mm Hg, diastolic blood pressure (DBP) ≥ 90 mm Hg, or taking high blood pressure medicine.

[c] SBP < 140 mm Hg and DBP < 90 mm Hg among persons with hypertension.

[d] Family income: income of all persons within a household who are related to each other by blood, marriage, or adoption. Poverty level: family income relative to family size and age of the members adjusted for inflations by using the poverty thresholds developed by the US Bureau of the Census.

[e] $P < 0.05$ compared with the referent group, with Bonferroni adjustment for variables with more than two categories.

services. Each SRCP coordinates with local nutrition and disease prevention efforts to maximize the impact of these changes (CDC, http://www.cdc.gov/dhdsp/programs/sodium_reduction.htm). In 2013, the CDC funded another 3-year program cycle for 10 communities. The program seeks to increase accessibility, availability, purchase, and/or selection of lower-sodium products. The primary strategies are developing and implementing food service guidelines and nutrition standards, implementing menu changes, working with food distributors to increase availability and identify lower-sodium products, instituting strategies that may enhance selection of lower-sodium foods, and providing consumer information (CDC 2014).

CANCER

Unlike heart disease, there has been no appreciable decline in deaths from cancer. Cancer is the leading cause of death among women ages 35–79 and among men ages 50–79 (CDC 2010). In 2007, 475,211 Americans younger than 85 died of cancer; 380,791 died of heart disease (Jemal et al. 2010). As cardiac deaths (the previous leading cause of death) fell sharply, cancer (the second leading cause) replaced heart disease in the hierarchy of mortality.

Cancer incidence and death rates vary by gender, race, and ethnicity. The National Cancer Institute's (NCI's) Surveillance, Epidemiology, and End Results Program (SEER) collects and publishes cancer incidence and survival data from population-based cancer registries covering approximately 28% of the US population (National Cancer Institute, http://seer.cancer.gov/about/overview .html). The NCI and the CDC produce a comprehensive federal report, *United States Cancer Statistics (USCS): Cancer Incidence and Mortality Data*. Table 4.9 correlates cancer incidence by type of cancer and race/ethnicity as of 2011. The leading cause of cancer death in the United States overall for both men and women is lung cancer. The sites of the leading causes of cancer diagnosed in men and women are cancers of the prostate and breast, respectively (Box 4.9) (US Cancer Statistics Working Group 2013).

Cancer Prevention

Lifestyle factors can increase the risk of developing cancer. It is estimated that at least half of the cancer deaths that occurred in the United States in 2014 were related to preventable causes, namely, tobacco use, obesity, lack of physical activity, exposure to ultraviolet light, and failures in using known protocols for treating or preventing infection by cancer-associated pathogens (American Association for Cancer Research 2014).

The ACS publishes Guidelines on Nutrition and Physical Activity for Cancer Prevention (Guidelines), which provides recommendations about dietary and lifestyle factors that can reduce cancer risk. Last published in 2006, the Guidelines were updated in 2012. The Guidelines make recommendations about individual choices but also comment on what communities can do to facilitate healthy behaviors (Kushi et al. 2012). The 2012 Guidelines are presented below.

- ACS recommendations for individual choices:
    - Achieve and maintain a healthy weight throughout life.
    - Be as lean as possible throughout life without being underweight.
    - Avoid excess weight gain at all ages. For those who are currently overweight or obese, losing even a small amount of weight has health benefits and is a good place to start.
    - Engage in regular physical activity and limit consumption of high-calorie foods and beverages as key strategies for maintaining a healthy weight.
    - Adopt a physically active lifestyle.
    - Adults should engage in at least 150 minutes of moderate-intensity or 75 minutes of vigorous-intensity activity each week, or an equivalent combination, preferably spread throughout the week.
    - Children and adolescents should engage in at least 1 hour of moderate or vigorous intensity activity each day, with vigorous-intensity activity occurring at least 3 days each week.
    - Limit sedentary behavior such as sitting, lying down, watching television, or other forms of screen-based entertainment.
    - Doing some physical activity above usual activities, no matter what one's level of activity, can have many health benefits.
    - Consume a healthy diet, with an emphasis on plant foods.
    - Choose foods and beverages in amounts that help achieve and maintain a healthy weight.
    - Limit consumption of processed meat and red meat.

TABLE 4.9

Year 2011 Age-Adjusted Invasive Cancer Incidence Rates and 95% Confidence Intervals by Primary Site and Race and Ethnicity, United States

Cancer Sites	All Races	White	Black	Asian/ Pacific Islander[a]	American Indian/Alaska Native[a]	Hispanic[a,b]
All cancer sites combined	507.5	499.7	554.5	310.1	293.5	393.5
All cancer sites combined[c]	498.9	490.9	548.5	304.1	288.8	386.7
Oral cavity and pharynx	17.0	17.4	14.8	10.8	10.9	11.4
Lip	1.0	1.1	0.1	e	e	0.5
Tongue	5.1	5.4	3.5	2.6	2.7	3.1
Salivary gland	1.6	1.7	1.3	1.0	e	1.1
Floor of mouth	0.8	0.8	0.9	e	e	0.6
Gum and other mouth	1.9	1.8	1.7	1.9	1.7	1.4
Nasopharynx	0.8	0.6	1.0	3.4	e	0.5
Tonsil	3.4	3.7	2.6	0.7	1.6	2.1
Oropharynx	0.8	0.8	1.2	0.3	e	0.6
Hypopharynx	1.1	1.1	1.8	0.6	e	1.0
Other oral cavity and pharynx	0.5	0.5	0.6	e	e	0.5
Digestive system	96.5	93.0	119.3	93.2	73.9	100.1
Esophagus	8.0	8.2	7.3	3.6	4.3	4.8
Stomach	9.2	8.4	13.9	14.1	7.8	13.2
Small intestine	2.6	2.5	4.2	1.2	1.5	1.9
Colon and rectum	46.1	44.9	55.0	38.3	33.5	43.1
Colon excluding rectum	32.0	31.0	41.0	23.8	22.3	29.4
Rectum and rectosigmoid junction	14.2	14.0	14.0	14.5	11.2	13.7
Anus, anal canal, and anorectum	1.4	1.4	1.9	0.5	e	1.0
Liver and intrahepatic bile duct	11.4	10.1	16.3	20.0	12.9	18.8
Gallbladder	0.8	0.7	1.5	1.0	e	1.3
Other biliary	2.1	2.1	1.9	3.2	e	2.6
Pancreas	13.8	13.7	16.2	10.2	9.9	12.3
Retroperitoneum	0.4	0.4	0.4	0.4	e	0.4
Peritoneum, omentum, and mesentery	0.1	0.1	e	e	e	e
Other digestive organs	0.5	0.5	0.7	0.6	e	0.7
Respiratory system	80.2	79.6	96.8	48.6	52.0	48.4
Nose, nasal cavity, and middle ear	0.8	0.8	0.7	0.6	e	0.8
Larynx	6.1	5.9	8.5	2.5	3.1	4.8
Lung and bronchus	73.0	72.5	87.3	45.3	47.8	42.5
Pleura	0.0	0.0	e	e	e	e
Trachea, mediastinum, and other respiratory organs	0.2	0.3	0.2	0.3	e	0.3
Bones and joints	1.0	1.1	0.8	0.7	1.2	1.0
Soft tissue including heart	3.8	3.8	3.5	2.7	1.4	3.4
Skin excluding basal and squamous	27.5	30.2	2.0	2.1	7.1	5.4
Melanomas of the skin	25.3	28.0	1.1	1.4	6.2	4.3
Other nonepithelial skin	2.2	2.3	0.9	0.7	e	1.1
Male breast	1.4	1.3	1.9	0.5	e	0.8
Male genital system	134.8	124.5	197.3	69.6	65.8	110.2
Prostate	128.3	117.2	194.7	67.1	62.2	104.4

(Continued)

TABLE 4.9 (CONTINUED)

Year 2011 Age-Adjusted Invasive Cancer Incidence Rates and 95% Confidence Intervals by Primary Site and Race and Ethnicity, United States

Cancer Sites	All Races	White	Black	Asian/ Pacific Islander[a]	American Indian/Alaska Native[a]	Hispanic[a,b]
Testis	5.3	6.2	1.5	1.9	2.8	4.3
Penis	0.9	0.9	0.9	0.4	e	1.3
Other male genital organs	0.2	0.2	0.2	e	e	0.2
Urinary system	57.4	59.5	43.0	26.1	32.7	40.2
Urinary bladder[d]	35.1	37.1	19.1	14.4	13.9	19.5
Kidney and renal pelvis	21.0	21.1	23.2	10.7	18.2	20.0
Ureter	0.8	0.9	0.3	0.7	e	0.4
Other urinary organs	0.5	0.5	0.4	e	e	0.3
Eye and orbit	0.9	1.0	0.2	0.4	e	0.6
Brain and other nervous system	7.6	8.1	4.7	4.0	3.6	5.9
Brain	7.2	7.7	4.3	3.8	3.4	5.6
Cranial nerves and other nervous system	0.4	0.4	0.3	0.3	e	0.3
Endocrine system	7.7	8.0	4.4	7.7	3.2	5.8
Thyroid	6.9	7.3	3.4	6.9	2.9	5.1
Other endocrine including thymus	0.8	0.7	0.9	0.9	e	0.6
Lymphomas	25.7	26.3	19.4	16.7	12.7	22.0
Hodgkin's lymphoma	3.1	3.2	3.2	1.4	1.1	2.8
Non-Hodgkin's lymphoma	22.6	23.1	16.2	15.3	11.6	19.3
Myeloma	7.5	6.9	13.6	4.3	4.2	7.3
Leukemias	16.5	16.8	12.1	9.7	8.2	12.5
Acute lymphocytic	1.8	1.9	1.1	1.4	1.0	2.4
Chronic lymphocytic	5.6	5.7	3.5	1.7	2.0	2.5
Acute myeloid	4.8	4.9	3.7	4.1	2.6	3.9
Chronic myeloid	2.1	2.1	1.7	1.2	1.4	2.1
Other leukemias	2.2	2.2	2.0	1.1	e	1.6
Mesothelioma	1.7	1.8	0.8	0.7	e	1.2
Kaposi sarcoma	0.7	0.5	1.7	0.2	e	1.0
Miscellaneous	19.6	19.8	18.2	11.9	14.7	16.2

Source: US Cancer Statistics Working Group, *United States Cancer Statistics: 1999–2011 Incidence and Mortality Web-Based Report*, Atlanta, US Department of Health and Human Services, Centers for Disease Control and Prevention and National Cancer Institute, 2014. Available at http://www.cdc.gov/uscs, accessed February 4, 2015.

Note: Rates are per 100,000 persons and are age-adjusted to the 2000 US standard population (19 age groups—Census P25-1130). Data are from selected statewide and metropolitan-area cancer registries that meet the data quality criteria for all invasive cancer sites combined. See registry-specific data quality information. Rates cover approximately 99% of the US population. Excludes basal and squamous cell carcinomas of the skin, except when these occur on the skin of the genital organs, and *in situ* cancers except the urinary bladder.

[a] Data for specified racial or ethnic populations other than white and black should be interpreted with caution. See Technical Notes.

[b] Hispanic origin is not mutually exclusive from race categories (white, black, Asian/Pacific Islander, American Indian/ Alaska Native).

[c] Excludes some endometrial cancers, papillary ependymomas and papillary meningiomas, chronic myeloproliferative diseases, and myelodysplastic syndromes. These cancers are classified and reported as malignant cancers according to ICD-O-3, beginning with 2001 diagnoses. See Technical Notes.

[d] Includes invasive and *in situ*.

[e] Rates are suppressed if fewer than 16 cases were reported in a specific category (site, race, ethnicity).

BOX 4.9 GENDER, RACIAL, AND ETHNIC VARIATIONS IN CANCER INCIDENCE AND DEATH RATES

The numbers in parentheses are the rates per 100,000 persons as of 2011. Incidence counts cover approximately 98% of the US population. Death counts cover 100% of the US population.

ALL CANCERS COMBINED, MEN

Incidence rates are highest among blacks (554.5), followed by whites (499.7), Hispanics (393.5), Asians/Pacific Islanders (310.1), and American Indians/Alaska Natives (293.5).

Death rates are highest among blacks (253.9), followed by whites (203.2), Hispanics (146.4), American Indians/Alaska Natives (136.0), and Asians/Pacific Islanders (126.2).

Black men have both the highest cancer incidence rate and the highest cancer death rate. American Indian/Alaska Native men have the lowest cancer incidence rates; however, Asian/Pacific Islander men have the lowest cancer death rates.

ALL CANCERS COMBINED, WOMEN

Incidence rates are highest among whites (414.8), followed by blacks (393.8), Hispanics (324.2), Asians/Pacific Islanders (279.8), and American Indians/Alaska Natives (261.0).

Death rates are highest among blacks (166.2), followed by whites (143.4), Hispanics (98.0), American Indians/Alaska Natives (93.9), and Asians/Pacific Islanders (90.1). White women have the highest cancer incidence rates; however, black women have the highest cancer death rates. American Indian/Alaska Native women have the lowest cancer incidence rates and the second lowest cancer death rates.

Source: US Cancer Statistics Working Group. *United States Cancer Statistics: 1999–2011 Incidence and Mortality Web-Based Report.* Atlanta: US Department of Health and Human Services, Centers for Disease Control and Prevention and National Cancer Institute, 2014. Available at http://www.cdc.gov /uscs, accessed February 4, 2015.

- Eat at least 2.5 cups of vegetables and fruits each day.
- Choose whole grains instead of refined grain products.
- If you drink alcoholic beverages, limit consumption.
- Drink no more than one drink per day for women or two per day for men.
- ACS recommendations for community actions:
  - Public, private, and community organizations should work collaboratively at national, state, and local levels to implement policy and environmental changes that achieve the following:
    - Increase access to affordable, healthy foods in communities, work sites, and schools, and decrease access to and marketing of foods and beverages of low nutritional value, particularly to youth.
    - Provide safe, enjoyable, and accessible environments for physical activity in schools and work sites, and for transportation and recreation in communities.

Tobacco Use

In addition to lung cancer, tobacco use also increases the risk of cancers of the mouth, lips, and nose, as well as pharyngeal, laryngeal, esophageal, stomach, pancreatic, renal, bladder, uterine, cervical, colorectal, and ovarian cancers. Although cigarette use has declined dramatically over the past half century, an estimated 42.1 million people or 18.1% of all adults smoke cigarettes

(Centers for Disease Control and Prevention 2014d). Cigarette smoking is the leading cause of preventable death in the United States, accounting for more than 480,000 deaths (1 in 5) each year (US Department of Health and Human Services 2014). Multiple government and medical organizations offer smoking cessation programs as part of an ongoing movement in lung cancer prevention (Centers for Disease Control and Prevention 2013b) (American Cancer Society, http://www.cancer.org/healthy/stayawayfromtobacco/index).

Obesity

A 2014 review article focusing on epidemiologic studies reports that the evidence base for a link between obesity and cancer is growing (Basen-Engquist and Chang 2011); a meta-analysis of 221 data sets from prospective observational studies reported strong relationships between excess BMI and esophageal adenocarcinoma, gallbladder cancer, kidney cancer, and esophageal cancer (Renehan et al. 2008). Another analysis of prospective studies that covered 900,000 adults and approximately 6.5 million person-years of follow-up reported that mortality was lowest for those in the normal BMI range (22.5–25 kg/m^2), and with each increase of 5 kg/m^2 came a 10% increase in cancer mortality (Prospective Studies Collaboration 2009).

Sedentary Behavior/Lack of Physical Activity

A 2011 literature review examining health outcomes and sedentary behaviors (defined as activities that do not increase energy expenditure substantially above the resting level, such as sleeping, sitting, lying down, watching TV, and other forms of screen-based entertainment, reports that based on three high-quality studies, there was no evidence for a relationship between sedentary behavior and mortality from cancer (Proper et al. 2011). The 2007 World Cancer Research Fund report, a systematic review of available evidence conducted by an expert panel, reported that evidence is convincing that physical activity protects against colon cancer and is probably protective against postmenopausal breast cancer and cancer of the endometrium. Although evidence for other cancers is limited, generally, the evidence is consistent with the message that people are better off when more physically active (World Cancer Research Fund 2007).

Exposure to Ultraviolet Light

Skin cancer is the most common type of cancer in the United States, accounting for nearly half of all cancer cases. Excessive exposure of skin to ultraviolet radiation is a major risk factor for this type of cancer (American Cancer Society 2013). The CDC's Division of Cancer and Control recommends avoiding direct sun exposure between the hours of 10 a.m. and 4 p.m., wearing protective clothing outdoors, applying sunscreen when exposing skin to the sun, and avoiding other sources of ultraviolet light, including tanning beds (CDC, http://www.cdc.gov/cancer/skin/basic_info/prevention.htm).

Cancer-Associated Pathogens

Globally, pathogens (bacteria, parasites, and viruses) are estimated to cause about 15–20% of cancer cases each year. The vast majority of these (more than 90%) are attributable to four pathogens—*Helicobacter pylori*, which can cause stomach cancer; hepatitis B virus (HBV) and hepatitis C virus (HCV), which can cause liver cancer; and human papilloma virus (HPV), which can cause cervical, anal, and oral cancers (American Association for Cancer Research 2014). Although the pathway from infection to cancer is not understood, it is clear that infection can cause cancer to develop in some people.

Cancer Prevention and Fruit and Vegetable Consumption

The possible relationship between the consumption of fruits and vegetables and reduced risk of cancer was a hot topic of research in the 1980s and 1990s, leading to an expert-panel report convened by the World Cancer Research Fund/American Institute for Cancer Research (World Cancer

Research Fund 1997) concluding that there was convincing evidence that high intakes of fruit and/ or vegetables decrease the risk for cancers of the mouth and pharynx, esophagus, stomach, colorectum, and lung. However, the same organization published an updated report in 2007 downgrading *convincing* to either *probable* or *limited-suggestive* (World Cancer Research Fund 2007), as newer results from large prospective studies did not confirm the earlier, mostly case–control study, results (Key 2011).

Nonetheless, the earlier enthusiasm regarding increasing fruit and vegetable consumption has been widely adopted into dietary guidance, such as the 2010 *Dietary Guidelines for Americans*. In 2011, USDA (http://www.choosemyplate.gov/food-groups/; http://www.choosemyplate.gov/print-materials -ordering/selected-messages.html) released MyPlate as its primary food guide, in place of previous pyramid-shaped tools, and MyPlate features recommendations to "focus on fruits" and "vary your veggies," and emphasizes messages to consumers to "make half your plate fruits and vegetables."

Although the advice to consume this amount of fruits and vegetables is generally nutritionally sound advice, some researchers argue that current available data suggest that emphasizing general increases in fruit and vegetable consumption is not likely to influence cancer rates in already well-nourished populations but that nonetheless, research focused on relevant biological pathways of specific types of cancer may be fruitful (Key 2011).

Cancer Prevention Programs

National Comprehensive Cancer Control Program

In 1998, the CDC established the National Comprehensive Cancer Control Program (NCCCP), a program to fund and support the development and implementation of comprehensive cancer control (CCC) plans. CCC is a process through which communities and organizations can utilize resources to reduce cancer risk, detect cases earlier, improve treatment methods, and increase the rate of cancer survival. These programs are focused on individual lifestyle behavior change, promotion of cancer screening, and improving access to quality cancer care. Success stories include tobacco education in Cherokee schools, increased cancer screening in women of the Midwest, and improving quality of life for cancer survivors in multiple communities (CDC, http://www.cdc.gov/cancer/ncccp).

Strengthening Families Program

The Strengthening Families Program (SFP), which focuses on high-risk families, is an evidence-based family skills training program found to significantly reduce problem behaviors, delinquency, and alcohol and drug abuse in children and to improve social competencies and school performance.

A National Institute on Drug Abuse (NIDA) research grant in the early 1980s found the effectiveness of the SFP program to be corroborated by more than 15 subsequent independent replications. Both culturally adapted versions and the core version of SFP have been found effective with African American, Hispanic, Asian, Pacific Islander, and American Indian families. The SFP (http://www.strengtheningfamiliesprogram.org/index.html) has continued to be updated and evaluated with similar results.

Body & Soul

Developed for African American churches, Body & Soul encourages church members to eat a healthy diet rich in fruits and vegetables every day for better health. Body & Soul was developed in partnership with NCI, ACS, and CDC. The four pillars of the program are (1) pastoral leadership, (2) educational activities, (3) a church environment that supports healthy eating, and (4) peer counseling (US Department of Agriculture, http://snap.nal.usda.gov/foodstamp/resource_finder_details .php?id=409).

Addressing Health Disparities in Cancer

The CDC monitors trends in cancer incidence and mortality in order to identify disparities in the burden of the disease. SES, access to healthcare, unhealthy behaviors, social and built environments, exposure to carcinogens, and quality of treatment have all been identified as contributing factors to the burden of cancer risk and disease.

The CDC supports data collection efforts on screening, risk factor, and incidence rates, and funds organizations that strengthen cancer control and prevention efforts in vulnerable communities. For example, the African American Women and Mass Media Campaign used radio and print media to increase awareness of mammogram screening for the early detection of breast cancer among African American women in several areas of Georgia (CDC 2013).

CONCLUSION

Reducing health disparities—such as the incidence rates of diabetes, CVD, and cancer—is one of the four overarching goals of Healthy People 2020. Although SES is often the most significant determinant of health status, disparities reveal themselves in comparing population subgroups of many different kinds to the general population.

Numerous programs at the federal, state, and local levels exist to assess health disparities and try to effect change. For programs focusing on health behaviors, it is important that these programs target the correct audiences with effective materials sensitive to cultural differences among groups. Reducing health disparities has potentially enormous economic and societal ramifications in light of our rapidly changing demographics and escalating healthcare costs.

ACRONYMS

A1c	Glycosylated hemoglobin
ACA	Affordable Care Act
ACS	American Cancer Society
ADA	American Diabetes Association
AHA	American Heart Association
AHRQ	Agency for Healthcare Research and Quality
BMI	Body mass index
BRFSS	Behavioral Risk Factor Surveillance System
CCC	Comprehensive cancer control
CDC	Centers for Disease Control and Prevention
CHD	Coronary heart disease
CMS	Centers for Medicare & Medicaid Services
CVD	Cardiovascular disease
DASH	Dietary Approaches to Stop Hypertension
DCPC	Division of Cancer Prevention and Control
DDT	Division of Diabetes Translation
DHDSP	Division of Heart Disease and Stroke Prevention
DKA	Diabetic ketoacidosis
DNPAO	Division of Nutrition, Physical Activity, and Obesity
DPCP	Diabetes Prevention and Control Program
DPP	Diabetes Prevention Program
ESRD	End-stage renal disease
FDA	Food and Drug Administration
FPG	Fasting plasma glucose
GAO	Government Accountability Office
HBV	Hepatitis B virus
HCV	Hepatitis C virus
HDL	High-density lipoprotein
HHS	Department of Health and Human Services

HPV	Human papilloma virus
HRSA	Health Resources and Services Administration
IFG	Impaired fasting glucose
IGT	Impaired glucose tolerance
NCCCP	National Comprehensive Cancer Control Program
NCCDPHP	National Center for Chronic Disease Prevention and Health Promotion
NCI	National Cancer Institute
NDEP	National Diabetes Education Program
NDPP	National Diabetes Prevention Program
NHANES	National Health and Nutrition Examination Survey (1999–2002)
NHANES III	Third National Health and Nutrition Examination Survey (1988–1994)
NHBPEP	National High Blood Pressure Education Program
NHIS	National Health Interview Survey
NHLBI	National Heart, Lung, and Blood Institute
NIDA	National Institute on Drug Abuse
NIDDK	National Institute of Diabetes and Digestive and Kidney Diseases
NIH	National Institutes of Health
NIMHD	National Institute on Minority Health and Health Disparities
ODP	Office of Disease Prevention
ODPHP	Office of Disease Prevention and Health Promotion
OGTT	Oral glucose tolerance test
OMH	Office of Minority Health
OPHS	Office of Public Health and Science
PA	Program announcement
PSA	Prostate-specific antigen
REACH	Racial and Ethnic Approaches to Community Health
RFA	Request for applications
RFP	Request for proposal
SEER	Surveillance Epidemiology and End Results Program
SES	Socioeconomic status
SFP	Strengthening Families Program
SRCP	Sodium Reduction in Communities Program

STUDENT ASSIGNMENTS AND ACTIVITIES DESIGNED TO ENHANCE LEARNING AND STIMULATE CRITICAL THINKING

1. Based on your age and gender, what are the recommended screening tests you should have according to the American Cancer Society, American Diabetes Association, and American Heart Association? Think back to your last few regular healthcare visits. Which of these screening tests were performed during your visit? Which were not performed? If any of these recommended screening tests were skipped, what are some reasons why? Discuss how individuals can ensure that their physicians perform all recommended screening tests.

2. Research community-based participatory research (CBPR) as mentioned in the discussion on REACH 2010. Briefly summarize the main concepts of CBPR, and discuss how this approach can be used to improve nutrition and physical activity within a community.

3. Using the Chronic Disease State Policy Tracking System, http://nccd.cdc.gov/CDPHP PolicySearch//Default.aspx, find three recent bills related to nutrition and physical activity in your state. Briefly summarize these bills and describe who will likely benefit the most from each of them.

4. Track your diet for a week. How well do you meet the ideal healthy eating pattern of meeting four out of five DASH recommendations? The five ideal DASH eating patterns

are to consume ≥4.5 cups per day of fruits and vegetables, ≥2 servings per week of fish, and ≥3 servings per day of whole grains and to consume no more than 36 oz. per week of sugar-sweetened beverages and 1500 mg per day of sodium. Discuss which categories (if any) you do not meet and how you can modify your eating patterns to meet these ideals.

5. Discuss the health and economic consequences of the increasing rates of type 2 diabetes in children. Based on the risk factors for type 2 diabetes in youth, describe the areas where prevention efforts should be focused.

6. Research and describe current sodium recommendations. What are the recommendations of the US Dietary Guidelines? Are they the same or different from the sodium recommendation of the DASH diet? (See http://www.nhlbi.nih.gov/health/health-topics/topics/dash/.) Are they different from the Institute of Medicine (IOM)? How is sodium information provided on labels regulated by the FDA? Track your own dietary sodium intake over several days. How can you estimate intake for restaurant food? Select a health disparity population, evaluate likely sources of dietary sodium, and tailor a recommendation for the population.

7. Review the approaches of the 2013–2016 CDC sodium reduction communities at http://www.cdc.gov/dhdsp/programs/sodium_reduction.htm. For each, describe the targeted population. Is it a health disparity population? In what way? Can you think of other approaches?

8. CDC's WISEWOMAN is implemented in 21 sites. Find reports from two sites and compare the details of each site's approach and results. Can information from one community-based initiative be useful for another? Why or why not? In what manner?

9. The State Department of Health has just been awarded a $10 million grant to reduce health disparities in your state. As the nutritionist, you have input into how this money should be spent.

   a. Your first step is to determine the health disparities in your state. Using the vital statistics from your State Department of Health (see http://www.cdc.gov/nchs/nvss .htm for links to State Health Departments), list the top three causes of death in your state.

   b. Then, for each of these causes of death, determine the rates based on race/ethnicity, age, and gender. Describe any disparities that exist.

   c. Based on your findings, how will you recommend allocating the grant money? Include a discussion of the local, state, and/or federal programs that currently exist to help reduce the health disparities in your state. What other programs could be created by the grant to address the risk factors for these diseases?

APPENDIX 4.1: HHS STRATEGIC PLAN FOR FISCAL YEARS 2014–2018, SECRETARY'S STRATEGIC INITIATIVES, AND THE DISPARITIES ACTION PLAN

HHS STRATEGIC PLAN, FISCAL YEARS 2014–2018

Every 4 years, HHS updates its Strategic Plan. An agency strategic plan is one of three main elements required by the Government Performance and Results Act (GPRA) of 1993 (P.L. 103-62) and the GPRA Modernization Act of 2010 (P.L. 111-352). An agency strategic plan defines the mission and goals of the agency, and the means by which it will measure its progress in addressing specific national problems over a 4-year period.

For the period of fiscal years (FY) 2014–2018, HHS is publishing its Strategic Plan as a web document at http://www.hhs.gov/strategic-plan/priorities.html, which will be updated periodically to reflect the department's strategies, actions, and progress toward its goals. Appendix C of the Strategic Plan documents provides updates.

The Overview to the Strategic Plan highlights that HHS, through programs and partnerships, "eliminates disparities in health, as well as healthcare access and quality, and protects vulnerable individuals and communities from poor health, public health, and human services outcomes" (http://www.hhs.gov/about/strategic-plan/introduction/index.html/#overview).

The strategic goals for FY 2014–2018 are as follows:

1. Strengthen healthcare
2. Advance scientific knowledge and innovation
3. Advance the health, safety, and well-being of the American people
4. Ensure efficiency, transparency, accountability, and effectiveness of HHS programs

Although health disparities are acknowledged or addressed in various strategies throughout the document, the *HHS Action Plan to Reduce Racial and Ethnic Health Disparities* is specifically associated with strategic goal 1: strengthen healthcare, objective E: ensure access to quality, culturally competent care, including long-term services and supports for vulnerable populations.

The objective E strategies are as follows:

- Monitor access to and quality of care across population groups and work with federal, state, local, tribal, urban Indian, and nongovernmental actors to address observed disparities and to encourage and facilitate consultation and collaboration among them.
- Evaluate the impact of Affordable Care Act provisions on access to and quality of care for vulnerable populations, as well as on disparities in access and quality.
- Leverage the nonprofit hospital community health needs assessment process, required by the Affordable Care Act, to improve community environments and related community health status.
- Promote expanded access to high-quality, culturally competent healthcare services to improve health equity, and address health disparities among populations including racial and ethnic minorities; individuals with disabilities; refugees; lesbian, gay, bisexual, and transgender (LGBT) individuals; and people with limited English proficiency and limited health literacy skills.
- Support programs that build the health literacy skills of children, youth, and their families, and promote proven methods of checking patient understanding to ensure that patients understand health information, recommendations, and risk and benefit trade-offs.
- Help eliminate disparities in healthcare by educating and training physicians, nurses, and allied healthcare professionals on disparities and cultural competency while increasing workforce diversity in medical and allied healthcare professions.
- Implement activities of the HHS Language Access Plan, including training staff; consulting with stakeholders; conducting self-assessments; adopting effective methods for providing language assistance services; improving practices for reaching and serving populations with limited English proficiency; and notifying external stakeholders about the availability of language assistance services through the web, social media, or other outreach initiatives.
- Improve access to care through implementation of health insurance market reforms, and prevention and correction of discriminatory actions and practices.
- Conduct outreach and education activities to promote the Health Insurance Marketplace and expanded Medicaid coverage to minority, underserved, and vulnerable populations.
- Deliver the most appropriate range of services at federally funded health centers, school-based health centers, patient-centered medical homes, health homes, and Indian Health Service (IHS)-funded health programs to enhance access to comprehensive primary and preventive services for historically underserved areas.
- Improve access to mental health and substance abuse treatment services at parity with medical and surgical services.

- Promote access to primary oral healthcare services and oral disease preventive services in settings including federally funded health centers, school-based health centers, and IHS-funded health programs that have comprehensive primary oral healthcare services, and state- and community-based programs that improve oral health, especially for children, pregnant women, older adults, and people with disabilities.
- Improve access to comprehensive primary and preventive medical services to historically underserved areas and support federally funded health centers, the range of services offered by these centers, and increased coordination with partners at the community level including the Aging Services Network.
- Assist states in strengthening and further developing high-performing long-term services and support systems that focus on the person, provide streamlined access, and empower individuals to participate in community living.
- Implement the HHS Strategic Plan in a manner that involves consulting with tribes; renewing and strengthening the department's partnership with tribes; conferring with urban Indian organizations; and ensuring that plan processes are accountable, transparent, fair, and inclusive.
- Consult with communities experiencing health disparities such as low-income groups and groups promoting environmental justice.
- Support efforts to ensure access to healthcare services by participating in coordinated transportation planning, particularly in rural areas, with a special emphasis placed on coordinated transportation funding efforts at all levels.
- Promote and test integrated care models that integrate primary care, acute care, behavioral healthcare, and long-term services and supports to provide comprehensive, coordinated, and quality care for older adults and people with disabilities.

The objective E performance goals are as follows:

- Increase the likelihood that the most vulnerable people receiving Older Americans Act home and community-based and caregiver support services will continue to live in their homes and communities.
- Increase the percentage of children receiving System of Care mental health services who report positive functioning at six-month follow-up.
- Increase the number of people receiving direct services through the office of Rural Health Policy outreach grants.
- Increase the number of patients served by health centers.
- Maintain the proportion of persons served by the Ryan White HIV/AIDS Program who are racial/ethnic minorities.
- Increase the number of adult volunteer potential donors of blood stem cells from minority race or ethnic groups.
- Reduce infertility among women attending Title X family planning clinics by identifying chlamydia infection through screening of females ages 15–24.
- Increase the number of American Indian and Alaska Native patients with diagnosed diabetes who achieve good glycemic control (A1c less than 8.0%).
- Increase the proportion of adults ages 18 and over who are screened for depression.
- Increase the number of program participants exposed to substance abuse prevention education services.
- Implement recommendations from tribes annually to improve the tribal consultation process.
- Increase the field strength of the National Health Service Corps through scholarship and loan repayment agreements.
- Increase the percentage of individuals supported by Bureau of Health Professions programs who completed a primary care training program and are currently employed in underserved areas.

HHS DISPARITIES ACTION PLAN

The vision: "A nation free of disparities in health and health care."

The framework for the 2011 HHS Disparities Action Plan is based on five goals from the HHS Strategic Plan for FY 2010–2015

1. Transform healthcare
2. Strengthen the nation's Health and Human Services infrastructure and workforce
3. Advance the health, safety, and well-being of the American people
4. Advance scientific knowledge and innovation
5. Increase the efficiency, transparency, and accountability of HHS programs

Some nutrition and related chronic disease objectives of the goals are listed below:

Goal I: Transform Healthcare
- *Develop, implement, and evaluate interventions to prevent cardiovascular diseases and their risk factors.* Heart attacks and strokes are the leading causes of premature death for racial and ethnic minorities. This initiative will focus multiple efforts on the prevention of cardiovascular diseases and their risk factors. HHS will implement interventions that will range from quality-of-care improvement opportunities to potential reimbursement incentives for policy and health system changes. This initiative will involve working with both minority providers and providers serving minority populations.

Lead/participating agencies: CDC, AHRQ, CMS, HRSA, NIH, Office of the Assistant Secretary for Health (OASH), Office of the National Coordinator for Health Information Technology (ONC)

Timeline: Starting in 2011

Goal II: Strengthen the Nation's Health and Human Services Infrastructure and Workforce
- *Promote the use of community health workers by Medicare beneficiaries.* This initiative will promote the use of community health workers as members of interdisciplinary teams and multisector teams. Enabling payment of community health workers as members of diabetes self-management training teams, for example, improves the provision of healthcare, health education, and disease prevention services, and connection to health homes will be enhanced. These workers will improve patients' diabetes self-management skills in many ways, including the provision of plain-language health-related information in nonclinical community settings.

Lead/participating agencies: CMS, CDC, HRSA, IHS, OASH

Timeline: Starting in FY 2011

Goal III: Advance the Health, Safety, and Well-Being of the American People
- *Build community capacity to implement evidence-based policies and environmental, programmatic, and infrastructure change strategies.* Through the Affordable Care Act, the CDC Community Transformation Grants Program will implement, evaluate, and disseminate evidence-based community preventive health activities. The goal is to reduce chronic disease rates, prevent the development of secondary conditions, address health disparities, and develop a stronger evidence base for effective prevention programming. Funded communities will work across multiple sectors to reduce heart attacks, cancer, and strokes by addressing a broad range of risk factors and conditions including poor nutrition and physical inactivity, tobacco use, and others. While the program is designed to reach the entire population, special emphasis is placed on reducing health disparities and reaching rural and frontier areas.

Lead/participating agencies: CDC
Timeline: Starting in FY 2011

*   *Implement an education and outreach campaign regarding preventive benefits.* The campaign will be a national public–private partnership to raise public awareness of health improvement across the life span supported by the Affordable Care Act. The campaign will reach racial and ethnic minority populations with messages on the importance of accessing preventive services relevant to nutrition, physical activity, and tobacco use.

Lead/participating agencies: CDC, CMS, HRSA, IHS, SAMHSA
Timeline: Starting in FY 2012

*   *Develop, implement, and evaluate culturally and linguistically appropriate evidence-based initiatives to prevent and reduce obesity in racial and ethnic minorities.* HRSA will sponsor a Healthy Weight Learning Collaborative to disseminate evidence-based and promising clinical and community practices to promote healthy weight in communities across the nation. The Childhood Obesity Research Demonstration Project, led by CDC, will develop, implement, and evaluate multisectoral and multilevel interventions for underserved children aged 2–12 years and their families. The project uses an integrated model of primary care and public health approaches to lower the risk for obesity in racial and ethnic minority communities.

Lead/participating agencies: CDC, HRSA, Administration for Children and Families (ACF), AHRQ, NIH
Timeline: Starting in FY 2011

Goal IV: Advance Scientific Knowledge

*   *Develop, implement, and test strategies to increase the adoption and dissemination of interventions based on patient-centered outcomes research among racial and ethnic minority populations.* Patient-centered outcomes research informs healthcare decisions by providing evidence on the effectiveness, benefits, and harms of different treatment options. By working collaboratively with research and healthcare institutions, HHS can develop, implement, and test strategies to increase the adoption and dissemination of interventions based on patient-centered outcomes research among racial and ethnic minority populations. Targeted health conditions will include diabetes mellitus, asthma, arthritis, and cardiovascular diseases including stroke and hypertension.

Lead/participating agencies: NIH, AHRQ, Assistant Secretary for Planning and Evaluation (ASPE), OASH/OMH
Timeline: Starting in FY 2011

*   *Promote community-based participatory research (CBPR) approaches to increase cancer awareness, prevention, and control to reduce health disparities.* The NIH is supporting various CBPR approaches that integrate the complex and multilevel determinants of health to reduce the burden of disease such as cancer, cardiovascular diseases, and diabetes within communities. This initiative will fund new cooperative agreements through the existing National Cancer Institute (NIH/NCI) Community Networks Program centers to increase knowledge of, access to, and utilization of biomedical and behavioral procedures for reducing cancer disparities. Such efforts range from prevention through early detection, diagnosis, treatment, and survivorship in racial and ethnic minorities and other underserved populations. The centers also provide an opportunity for training health disparity researchers (particularly new and early-stage investigators) in CBPR approaches and cancer health disparities.

Lead/participating agencies: NIH
Timeline: Starting in FY 2011

Source: US Department of Health and Human Services. HHS Strategic Plan. Available at http://www.hhs.gov/strategic-plan/priorities.html, accessed January 12, 2015; US Department of Health and Human Services. HHS Action Plan to Reduce Racial and Ethnic Health. Available at http://www.minorityhealth.hhs.gov/npa/files/Plans/HHS/HHS_Plan_complete.pdf, accessed February 4, 2015.

APPENDIX 4.2: NIH

NIH Institutes

National Cancer Institute (NCI)—Est. 1937

NCI leads a national effort to eliminate the suffering and death due to cancer. Through basic and clinical biomedical research and training, NCI conducts and supports research that will lead to a future in which we can prevent cancer before it starts, identify cancers that do develop at the earliest stage, eliminate cancers through innovative treatment interventions, and biologically control those cancers that we cannot eliminate so they become manageable, chronic diseases.

National Eye Institute (NEI)—Est. 1968

The NEI's mission is to conduct and support research, training, health information dissemination, and other programs with respect to blinding eye diseases, visual disorders, mechanisms of visual function, preservation of sight, and the special health problems and requirements of the blind.

National Heart, Lung, and Blood Institute (NHLBI)—Est. 1948

The NHLBI provides global leadership for a research, training, and education program to promote the prevention and treatment of heart, lung, and blood diseases and enhance the health of all individuals so that they can live longer and more fulfilling lives. The NHLBI stimulates basic discoveries about the causes of disease, enables the translation of basic discoveries into clinical practice, fosters training and mentoring of emerging scientists and physicians, and communicates research advances to the public.

National Human Genome Research Institute (NHGRI)—Est. 1989

NHGRI is devoted to advancing health through genome research. The institute led NIH's contribution to the Human Genome Project, which was successfully completed in 2003 ahead of schedule and under budget. Building on the foundation laid by the sequencing of the human genome, NHGRI's work now encompasses a broad range of research aimed at expanding understanding of human biology and improving human health. In addition, a critical part of NHGRI's mission continues to be the study of the ethical, legal, and social implications of genome research.

National Institute on Aging (NIA)—Est. 1974

NIA leads a national program of research on the biomedical, social, and behavioral aspects of the aging process; the prevention of age-related diseases and disabilities; and the promotion of a better quality of life for all older Americans.

National Institute on Alcohol Abuse and Alcoholism (NIAAA)—Est. 1970

NIAAA conducts research focused on improving the treatment and prevention of alcoholism and alcohol-related problems to reduce the enormous health, social, and economic consequences of this disease.

National Institute of Allergy and Infectious Diseases (NIAID)—Est. 1948

NIAID research strives to understand, treat, and ultimately prevent the myriad infectious, immunologic, and allergic diseases that threaten millions of human lives.

National Institute of Arthritis and Musculoskeletal and Skin Diseases (NIAMS)—Est. 1986

NIAMS supports research into the causes, treatment, and prevention of arthritis and musculoskeletal and skin diseases, the training of basic and clinical scientists to carry out this research, and the dissemination of information on research progress in these diseases.

National Institute of Biomedical Imaging and Bioengineering (NIBIB)—Est. 2000

The mission of the NIBIB is to improve health by leading the development and accelerating the application of biomedical technologies. The institute is committed to integrating the physical and engineering sciences with the life sciences to advance basic research and medical care.

Eunice Kennedy Shriver **National Institute of Child Health and Human Development (NICHD)**—Est. 1962

NICHD research on fertility, pregnancy, growth, development, and medical rehabilitation strives to ensure that every child is born healthy and wanted and grows up free from disease and disability.

National Institute on Deafness and Other Communication Disorders (NIDCD)—Est. 1988

NIDCD conducts and supports biomedical research and research training on normal mechanisms as well as diseases and disorders of hearing, balance, smell, taste, voice, speech, and language that affect 46 million Americans.

National Institute of Dental and Craniofacial Research (NIDCR)—Est. 1948

NIDCR provides leadership for a national research program designed to understand, treat, and ultimately prevent the infectious and inherited craniofacial–oral–dental diseases and disorders that compromise millions of human lives.

National Institute of Diabetes and Digestive and Kidney Diseases (NIDDK)—Est. 1950

The mission of the NIDDK is to conduct and support medical research and research training and to disseminate science-based information on diabetes and other endocrine and metabolic diseases; digestive diseases, nutritional disorders, and obesity; and kidney, urologic, and hematologic diseases, to improve people's health and quality of life.

National Institute on Drug Abuse (NIDA)—Est. 1974

NIDA leads the nation in bringing the power of science to bear on drug abuse and addiction through strategic support and conduct of research across a broad range of disciplines and through rapid and effective dissemination and use of the results of that research to significantly improve prevention and treatment and to inform policy as it relates to drug abuse and addiction.

National Institute of Environmental Health Sciences (NIEHS)—Est. 1969

The mission of the NIEHS is to discover how the environment affects people in order to promote healthier lives.

National Institute of General Medical Sciences (NIGMS)—Est. 1962

The NIGMS supports basic research that increases understanding of biological processes and lays the foundation for advances in disease diagnosis, treatment, and prevention. NIGMS-funded scientists investigate how living systems work at a range of levels, from molecules and cells to tissues, whole organisms, and populations. The institute also supports research in certain clinical areas, primarily those that affect multiple organ systems. To assure the vitality and continued productivity of the research enterprise, NIGMS provides leadership in training the next generation of scientists, in enhancing the diversity of the scientific workforce, and in developing research capacities throughout the country.

National Institute of Mental Health (NIMH)—Est. 1949

NIMH provides national leadership dedicated to understanding, treating, and preventing mental illnesses through basic research on the brain and behavior, and through clinical, epidemiological, and services research.

National Institute on Minority Health and Health Disparities (NIMHD)—Est. 1993

The mission of NIMHD is to lead scientific research to improve minority health and eliminate health disparities. To accomplish its mission, NIMHD plans, reviews, coordinates, and evaluates all minority health and health disparities research and activities of the National Institutes of Health; conducts and supports research in minority health and health disparities; promotes and supports the training of a diverse research workforce; translates and disseminates research information; and fosters innovative collaborations and partnerships.

National Institute of Neurological Disorders and Stroke (NINDS)—Est. 1950

The mission of NINDS is to seek fundamental knowledge about the brain and nervous system and to use that knowledge to reduce the burden of neurological disease. To accomplish this goal, the NINDS supports and conducts basic, translational, and clinical research on the normal and diseased nervous system. The institute also fosters the training of investigators in the basic and clinical neurosciences, and seeks better understanding, diagnosis, treatment, and prevention of neurological disorders.

National Institute of Nursing Research (NINR)—Est. 1986

The mission of the NINR is to promote and improve the health of individuals, families, communities, and populations. NINR supports and conducts clinical and basic research and research training on health and illness across the life span to build the scientific foundation for clinical practice, prevent disease and disability, manage and eliminate symptoms caused by illness, and improve palliative and end-of-life care.

National Library of Medicine (NLM)—Est. 1956

NLM collects, organizes, and makes available biomedical science information to scientists, health professionals, and the public. The Library's web-based databases, including PubMed/Medline and MedlinePlus, are used extensively around the world. NLM conducts and supports research in biomedical communications; creates information resources for molecular biology, biotechnology, toxicology, and environmental health; and provides grant and contract support for training, medical library resources, and biomedical informatics and communications research.

NIH Centers

Center for Information Technology (CIT)—Est. 1964

CIT incorporates the power of modern computers into the biomedical programs and administrative procedures of the NIH by focusing on three primary activities: conducting computational biosciences research, developing computer systems, and providing computer facilities.

Center for Scientific Review (CSR)—Est. 1946

The CSR is the portal for NIH grant applications and their review for scientific merit. CSR organizes the peer review groups or study sections that evaluate the majority (70%) of the research grant applications sent to NIH. CSR also receives all grant applications for NIH, as well as for some other components of the US Department of Health and Human Services (HHS). Since 1946, the CSR mission has remained clear and timely: to see that NIH grant applications receive fair, independent, expert, and timely reviews—free from inappropriate influences—so NIH can fund the most promising research.

Fogarty International Center (FIC)—Est. 1968

FIC promotes and supports scientific research and training internationally to reduce disparities in global health.

National Center for Advancing Translational Sciences (NCATS)—Est. 2011

The mission of NCATS is to catalyze the generation of innovative methods and technologies that will enhance the development, testing, and implementation of diagnostics and therapeutics across a wide range of human diseases and conditions.

National Center for Complementary and Alternative Medicine (NCCAM)—Est. 1999

The mission of NCCAM is to define, through rigorous scientific investigation, the usefulness and safety of complementary and alternative medicine (CAM) interventions and their roles in improving health and health care.

NIH Clinical Center (CC)—Est. 1953

The NIH Clinical Center, America's research hospital, provides a versatile clinical research environment enabling the NIH mission to improve human health by investigating the pathogenesis of disease; conducting first-in-human clinical trials with an emphasis on rare diseases and diseases of high public health impact; developing state-of-the-art diagnostic, preventive, and therapeutic interventions; training the current and next generations of clinical researchers; and ensuring that clinical research is ethical, efficient, and of high scientific quality.

REFERENCES

Abrahamson JK, Gofin R, Hopp C, Gofin J, Donchin M, Habib J. Evaluation of a community program for the control of cardiovascular risk factors: The CHAD program in Jerusalem. *Israel J Med Sci.* 1981;17:201–212.

Adamo KB, Ferraro ZM, Brett KE. Can we modify the intrauterine environment to halt the intergenerational cycle of obesity? *Int J Environ Res Public Health.* 2012;9(4):1263–1307.

American Association for Cancer Research. AACR Cancer Progress Report 2014. *Clin Cancer Res.* 2014;20(Suppl 1):SI-S112.

American Cancer Society. Skin Cancer Facts, 2013. Available at http://www.cancer.org/cancer/cancercauses/sunanduvexposure/skin-cancer-facts, accessed January 7, 2015.

American Cancer Society. Stay Away from Tobacco Resource Page, Available at http://www.cancer.org/healthy/stayawayfromtobacco/index, accessed January 7, 2015.

American Diabetes Association. CheckUp America. Available at http://www.diabetes.org/are-you-at-risk/lower-your-risk/cua.html, accessed January 7, 2015.

American Diabetes Association. DKA (ketoacidiosis) & Ketones. Available at http://www.diabetes.org/living-with-diabetes/complications/ketoacidosis-dka.html, accessed December 23, 2014.

American Diabetes Association. Economic costs of diabetes in the U.S. in 2012. *Diabetes Care.* 2012;36:1033–1046.

American Diabetes Association. Press Release. The American Diabetes Association Applauds Stronger Screening Guidelines for Type 2 Diabetes, October 7, 2014a. Available at http://www.diabetes.org/newsroom/press-releases/2014/uspstf-type2-screening.html, accessed December 23, 2014.

American Diabetes Association. Diagnosis and classification of diabetes mellitus. *Diabetes Care.* 2014b;37 (Suppl 1):S81–S90.

American Diabetes Association. Diabetes Care. Standards of Medical Care in Diabetes—2015. *Diabetes Care.* 2015a;38(Suppl 1). Available at http://care.diabetesjournals.org/content/suppl/2014/12/23/38.Supplement_1.DC1/January_Supplement_Combined_Final.6-99.pdf, accessed February 4, 2015.

American Diabetes Association. Diabetes Care. Standards of Medical Care in Diabetes—2015. *Diabetes Care.* 2015b;38(Suppl 1):S70–S76. Available at http://care.diabetesjournals.org/content/37/Supplement_1/S14/T5.expansion.html, accessed December 23, 2014.

American Heart Association. My Life Check homepage. Available at http://mylifecheck.heart.org, accessed September 30, 2014.

Basen-Engquist K, Chang M. Obesity and cancer risk: Recent review and evidence. *Curr Oncol Rep.* 2011;13(1):71–76.

Beltrán-Sánchez H, Harhay MO, Harhay MM, McElligott S. Prevalence and trends of metabolic syndrome in the adult U.S. population, 1999–2010. *J Am Coll Cardiol.* 2013;62(8):697–703.

Boney CM, Verma A, Tucker R, Vohr BR. Metabolic syndrome in childhood: Association with birth weight, maternal obesity, and gestational diabetes mellitus. *Pediatrics.* 2005;115:e290–e296.

Boyle JP, Thompson TJ, Gregg EW, Barker LE, Williamson DF. Projection of the year 2050 burden of diabetes in the US adult population: Dynamic modeling of incidence, mortality, and prediabetes prevalence. *Popul Health Metr.* 2010;8:29.

Brännström I, Weinehall L, Persson LA, Wester PO, Wall S. Changing social patterns of risk factors for cardiovascular disease in a Swedish community intervention programme. *Int J Epidemiol.* 1993;22:1026–1037.

Carleton RA, Lasater TM, Assaf AR, Feldman HA, McKinlay S. The Pawtucket Heart Health Program: Community-wide education effects assessed by changes in cardiovascular disease risk. *Am J Public Health.* 1995;85:777–785.

Centers for Disease Control and Prevention. Cancer Prevention and Control. Health Disparities in Cancer, 2013a. Available at http://www.cdc.gov/cancer/healthdisparities/index.htm, accessed January 7, 2014.

Centers for Disease Control and Prevention. Cancer Prevention and Control. Lung Cancer Awareness, 2013b. Available at http://www.cdc.gov/cancer/dcpc/resources/features/lungcancer, accessed January 7, 2015.

Centers for Disease Control and Prevention. CDC health disparities and inequalities report—United States, 2011. *MMWR*. 2011b;60(Suppl). Available at http://www.cdc.gov/mmwr/pdf/other/su6001.pdf, accessed January 7, 2015.

Centers for Disease Control and Prevention. Current cigarette smoking among adults—United States, 2005–2012. *MMWR*. 2014d;63(2):29–34.

Centers for Disease Control and Prevention. Division of Cancer Prevention and Control (DCPC) homepage. Available at http://www.cdc.gov/cancer, accessed December 15, 2015.

Centers for Disease Control and Prevention. Division for Health Disease and Stroke Prevention. Sodium Reduction in Communities Program (SRCP). Last updated April 24, 2014. Available at http://www.cdc.gov/dhdsp/programs/sodium_reduction.htm, accessed September 30, 2014.

Centers for Disease Control and Prevention. Division of Heart Disease and Stroke Prevention (DHDSP) homepage. Available at http://www.cdc.gov/DHDSP/index.htm, accessed December 15, 2014.

Centers for Disease Control and Prevention. Division of Nutrition, Physical Activity, and Obesity homepage. Available at http://www.cdc.gov/nccdphp/dnpao/index.html, accessed December 15, 2014.

Centers for Disease Control and Prevention. Healthy Communities Program homepage. Available at http://www.cdc.gov/nccdphp/dch/programs/healthycommunitiesprogram/index.htm, accessed January 7, 2015.

Centers for Disease Control and Prevention. Heart Disease Facts. Available at http://www.cdc.gov/heartdisease/facts.htm, accessed January 12, 2015.

Centers for Disease Control and Prevention. Mortality in the United States, 2013. *NCHS Data Brief*. No. 178, December 2014a. Available at http://www.cdc.gov/nchs/data/databriefs/db178.htm, accessed December 23, 2014.

Centers for Disease Control and Prevention. National Center for Health Statistics, National Vital Statistics System. Deaths, % of Total Deaths, and Death Rates for the 15 Leading Causes of Death in 5-Year Age Groups, by Race and Sex: United States, 2010. Available at http://www.cdc.gov/nchs/data/dvs/LCWK1_2010.pdf, accessed January 7, 2015.

Centers for Disease Control and Prevention. National Comprehensive Cancer Control Program (NCCCP) homepage. Available at http://www.cdc.gov/cancer/ncccp, accessed January 7, 2015.

Centers for Disease Control and Prevention. *National Diabetes Fact Sheet: National Estimates and General Information on Diabetes and Prediabetes in the United States, 2011*. U.S. Department of Health and Human Services, Centers for Disease Control and Prevention, 2011a. Available at http://www.cdc.gov/diabetes/pubs/pdf/ndfs_2011.pdf, accessed January 7, 2015.

Centers for Disease Control and Prevention. National Diabetes Prevention Program homepage. Available at http://www.cdc.gov/diabetes/prevention/index.htm, accessed January 7, 2015.

Centers for Disease Control and Prevention. National Diabetes Statistics Report, 2014c. Last updated July 28, 2014. Available at http://www.cdc.gov//diabetes/pubs/statsreport14.htm, accessed September 26, 2014.

Centers for Disease Control and Prevention. National Diabetes Statistics Report, 2014: Data Sources, Methods, and References for Estimates of Diabetes and Its Burden in the United States. Available at http://www.cdc.gov/diabetes/pdfs/data/2014-report-national-diabetes-statistics-report-data-sources.pdf, accessed December 23, 2014.

Centers for Disease Control and Prevention. *National Diabetes Statistics Report: Estimates of Diabetes and Its Burden in the United States, 2014*. Atlanta, GA: U.S. Department of Health and Human Services, 2014b. Available at http://www.cdc.gov/diabetes/pubs/statsreport14/national-diabetes-report-web.pdf, accessed December 23, 2014.

Centers for Disease Control and Prevention. *New REACH Demonstration Projects*. National Center for Chronic Disease Prevention and Health Promotion, Division of Community Health, 2013a. Available at http://www.cdc.gov/nccdphp/dch/programs/reach/current_programs/reach-demo.htm, accessed January 7, 2015.

Centers for Disease Control and Prevention. Prevalence of overweight and obesity among adults with diagnosed diabetes—United States, 1988–1994 and 1999–2002. *MMWR*. 2004;53:1066–1068.

Centers for Disease Control and Prevention. Skin Cancer. What Can I Do to Reduce My Risk? Available at http://www.cdc.gov/cancer/skin/basic_info/prevention.htm, accessed January 7, 2015.

Centers for Disease Control and Prevention. Sodium Reduction in Communities. Division for Heart Disease and Stroke Prevention. Available at http://www.cdc.gov/dhdsp/programs/sodium_reduction.htm, accessed January 7, 2015.

Centers for Disease Control and Prevention. Vital signs: Awareness and treatment of uncontrolled hypertension among adults—United States, 2003–2201. *MMWR*. 2012;61(35):703–709. Available at http://www.cdc.gov/mmwr/preview/mmwrhtml/mm6135a3.htm, accessed September 30, 2014.

Centers for Disease Control and Prevention. WISEWOMAN homepage. Available at http://www.cdc.gov /wisewoman/, accessed January 7, 2015.

Dabelea D, Mayer-Davis EJ, Saydah S et al. Prevalence of type 1 and type 2 diabetes among children and adolescents from 2001 to 2009. *JAMA.* 2014;311(17):1778–1786.

Dalleck LC, Kjelland EM. The prevalence of metabolic syndrome and metabolic syndrome risk factors in college-aged students. *Am J Health Promot.* 2012;27(1):37–42.

Diabetes Prevention Program. National Diabetes Information Clearing House. Updated September 9, 2013. Available at http://diabetes.niddk.nih.gov/dm/pubs/preventionprogram/, accessed December 23, 2014.

Ervin RB. Prevalence of metabolic syndrome among adults 20 years of age and over, by sex, age, race and ethnicity, and body mass index: United States, 2003–2006. *National Health Statistics Reports.* No. 13, 2009. Available at http://www.cdc.gov/nchs/data/nhsr/nhsr013.pdf, accessed January 7, 2015.

Eyre H, Kahn R, Robertson RM et al. Preventing cancer, cardiovascular disease, and diabetes: A common agenda for the American Cancer Society, the American Diabetes Association, and the American Heart Association. *CA Cancer J Clin.* 2004;54:190–207.

Farquhar JW, Fortmann SP, Flora JA et al. Effect of community-wide education on cardiovascular disease risk factors: The Stanford Five-City Project. *JAMA.* 1990;264:359–365.

Fernandes J, Lofgren IE. Prevalence of metabolic syndrome and individual criteria in college students. *J Am Coll Health.* 2011;59(4):313–321.

Flegal KM, Carroll MD, Kit BK, Ogden CL. Prevalence of obesity and trends in the distribution of body mass index among U.S. adults, 1999–2010. *JAMA.* 2012;307(5):491–497.

Food Research and Action Center. Relationship between Poverty and Overweight or Obesity. Available at http://frac.org/initiatives/hunger-and-obesity/are-low-income-people-at-greater-risk-for-overweight-or -obesity/, accessed December 23, 2014.

Ford ES, Giles WH, Dietz WH. Prevalence of the metabolic syndrome among U.S. adults: Findings from the Third National Health and Nutrition Examination Survey. *JAMA.* 2002;287(3):356–359.

Ford ES, Mokdad AH, Giles WH, Brown DW. The metabolic syndrome and antioxidant concentrations: Findings from the Third National Health and Nutrition Examination Survey. *Diabetes.* 2003;52:2346–2352.

Ford ES, Bergmann MM, Kroger J, Schienkiewitz A, Weikert C, Boeing H. Healthy living is the best revenge: Findings from the European prospective investigation into cancer and nutrition—Potsdam study. *Arch Intern Med.* 2009;169(5):1355–1362.

Freedman DS, Ogden CL, Flegal KM, Khan LK, Serdula MK, Dietz WH. Childhood overweight and family income. *MedGenMed.* 2007;9(2):26. Available at http://www.ncbi.nlm.nih.gov/pmc/articles/PMC 1994830, accessed January 7, 2015.

GCP Study Group. The German Cardiovascular Prevention (GCP) study: Design and methods. *Eur Heart J.* 1988;10:629–646.

Go AS, Mozaffarian D, Roger VL et al. Heart disease and stroke statistics—2013 update: A report from the American Heart Association. *Circulation.* 2013;127:e6–e245.

Go AS, Mozaffarian D, Roger VL et al. Heart disease and stroke statistics—2014 update: A report from the American Heart Association. *Circulation.* 2014;129:e28–e292.

Goran MI, Ball GDC, Cruz ML. Obesity and risk of type 2 diabetes and cardiovascular disease in children and adolescents. *J Clin Endocrin Metab.* 2003;88:1417–1427.

Harjutsala V, Sund R, Knip M, Groop P-H. Incidence of type 1 diabetes in Finland. *JAMA.* 2013;310 (4):427–428.

Healthy People 2020. Healthy People 2020 Summary of Objectives: Health Communication and Health IT. Available at http://www.healthypeople.gov/2020/topics-objectives/topic/health-communication-and-health -information-technology, accessed January 7, 2015.

Healthy People 2020. Heart Disease and Stroke. National Snap Shot. Hypertension. Available at http://www .healthypeople.gov/2020/topics-objectives/topic/heart-disease-and-stroke/national-snapshot, accessed January 12, 2015.

Healthy People 2020. Heart Disease and Stroke Objectives. HDS-2 Reduce coronary heart disease deaths. Available at http://www.healthypeople.gov/2020/topics-objectives/topic/heart-disease-and-stroke/objec tives, accessed January 7, 2015.

Heidenreich PA, Trogdon JG, Khavjou OA et al. Forecasting the future of cardiovascular disease in the United States: A policy statement from the American Heart Association. *Circulation.* 2011;123:933–944.

Hoyert DL, Xu J. Deaths: Preliminary data for 2011. *National Vital Statistics Reports.* 2012;61(6). Available at http://www.cdc.gov/nchs/data/nvsr/nvsr61/nvsr61_06.pdf, accessed January 7, 2015.

Huang TT, Kempf AM, Strother ML, Li C, Lee RE, Harris KJ, Kaur H. Overweight and components of the metabolic syndrome in college students. *Diabetes Care.* 2004;27:3000–3001.

Jemal A, Siegel R, Xu J, Ward E. Cancer Statistics, 2010. *CA Cancer J Clin.* 2010;60(5):277–300.

Johnson WD, Kroon JJ, Greenway FL, Bouchard C, Ryan D, Katzmarzyk PT. Prevalence of risk factors for metabolic syndrome in adolescents: National health and nutrition examination survey (NHANES), 2001–2006. *Arch Pediatr Adolesc.* 2009;163(4):371–377.

Joslin Diabetes Center & Joslin Clinic. *Clinical Nutrition Guideline for Overweight and Obese Adults with Type 2 Diabetes, Prediabetes or Those at High Risk for Developing Type 2 Diabetes.* Joslin Diabetes Center, 2011. Available at http://www.joslin.org/bin_from_cms/Nutrition_Guidelines-8.22.11(1).pdf, accessed January 7, 2015.

Kaufman F. Preventing type 2 diabetes in children—A role for the whole community. *Diabetes Voice.* 2007;52:35–38.

Kaufman FR. Type 2 diabetes mellitus in children and youth: A new epidemic. *J Pediatr Endocrinol Metab.* 2002;15(Suppl 2):737–744.

Key TJ. Fruit and vegetables and cancer risk. *Br J Cancer.* 2011;104:6–11.

Knowler WC, Barrett-Connor E, Fowler SE, Hamman RF, Lachin JM, Walker EA, Nathan DM. Diabetes Prevention Program Research Group. Reduction in the incidence of type 2 diabetes with lifestyle intervention or metformin. *N Engl J Med.* 2002;346:393–403.

Kochanek KD, Murphy SL, Xu H, Arias W. Mortality in the United States, 2013. *NCHS Data Brief.* No. 178, December 2014. Available at http://www.cdc.gov/nchs/data/databriefs/db178.htm, accessed January 7, 2015.

Koh HK, Graham G, Glied SA. Reducing racial and ethnic disparities: The action plan from the Department of Health and Human Services. *Health Affairs.* 2011;30(10):1822–1829.

Kruger J, Yore MM, Solera M, Moeti R. Prevalence of fruit and vegetable consumption and physical activity by race/ethnicity—United States, 2005. *MMWR.* 2007;56(13):301–304. Available at http://www.cdc.gov/mmwr/preview/mmwrhtml/mm5613a2.htm#tab, accessed January 7, 2015.

Kushi LH, Doyle C, McCullough M et al. American Cancer Society guidelines on nutrition and physical activity for cancer prevention. *CA Cancer J Clin.* 2012;62:30–67.

Labarthe D, Grove B, Galloway J et al. *The Public Health Action Plan to Prevent Heart Disease and Stroke: Ten-Year Update.* Washington, DC: National Forum for Heart Disease and Stroke Prevention, 2014. Available at http://nationalforum.org/sites/default/files/Action%20Plan%20-%20Ten%20Year%20Update%20April%202014.pdf, accessed February 4, 2015.

LaVeist TA, Gaskin DJ, Richard P. *The Economic Burden of Health Inequalities in the United States.* The Joint Center for Political and Economic Studies, 2009. Available at https://www.ndhealth.gov/heo/publications/The%20Economic%20Burden%20of%20Health%20Inequalities%20in%20the%20United%20States.pdf, accessed December 23, 2014.

Let's Move! Available at http://www.letsmove.gov, accessed January 7, 2015.

Li C, Ford ES, McGuire LC, Mokdad AH. Increasing trends in waist circumference and abdominal obesity among U.S. adults. *Obesity.* 2007;15(1):216.

Lipman T, Levitt Katz L, Ratcliffe S et al. Increasing incidence of type 1 diabetes in youth. Twenty years of the Philadelphia Pediatric Diabetes Registry. *Diabetes Care.* 2013;36(6):1597–1603.

Liu LL, Yi JP, Beyer J et al. Type 1 and type 2 diabetes in Asian and Pacific Islander U.S. youth. *Diabetes Care.* 2009;32(Suppl 2):S133–S140.

Liu LL, Lawrence JM, Davis C et al. Prevalence of overweight and obesity in youth with diabetes in USA: The SEARCH for diabetes in youth study. *Pediatr Diabetes.* 2010;11(1):4–11.

Luepker RV, Murray DM, Jacobs DR Jr. et al. Community education for cardiovascular disease prevention: Risk factor changes in the Minnesota Heart Health Program. *Am J Public Health.* 1994;84:1383–1393.

MacDorman MF, Mathews TJ. QuickStats: Infant mortality rates, by race and Hispanic ethnicity of mother—United States, 2000, 2005, and 2009. *MMWR.* 2013;62(5):90. Available at http://www.cdc.gov/mmwr/preview/mmwrhtml/mm6205a6.htm, accessed January 7, 2015.

Mayer-Davis EJ, Bell RA, Dabelea D et al. The many faces of diabetes in American youth: Type 1 and type 2 diabetes in five race and ethnic populations: The SEARCH for diabetes in youth study. *Diabetes Care.* 2009;32(Suppl 2):S99–S101.

Million Hearts. *About Heart Disease & Stroke: Consequences & Costs.* Centers for Disease Control and Prevention. Available at http://millionhearts.hhs.gov/abouthds/cost-consequences.html, accessed January 7, 2015.

Murphy SL, Xu JQ, Kochanek KD. Deaths: Final data for 2010. *National Vital Statistics Reports.* 2013;61(4). Available at http://www.cdc.gov/nchs/data/nvsr/nvsr61/nvsr61_04.pdf, accessed January 7, 2015.

National Cancer Institute. SEER. 2014. Available at http://seer.cancer.gov/about/overview.html, accessed February 4, 2015.

National Center for Health Statistics. *Health, United States, 2012: With Special Feature on Emergency Care*, Tables 68–69, 2013a. Available at http://www.cdc.gov/nchs/data/hus/hus12.pdf, accessed January 7, 2015.

National Center for Health Statistics. *Health, United States, 2012: With Special Feature on Emergency Care*, Table 67, 2013b. http://www.cdc.gov/nchs/data/hus/hus12.pdf, accessed January 7, 2015.

National Forum for Heart Disease and Stroke Prevention. Who We Are. Available at http://www.national forum.org/organization, accessed September 30, 2014.

National Institutes of Health. About NIH. Available at http://www.nih.gov/about/organization.htm, accessed January 12, 2015.

National Institutes of Health, National Heart Lung, and Blood Institute. *Morbidity & Mortality: 2012 Chart Book on Cardiovascular, Lung, and Blood Diseases*. National Institutes of Health, 2012. Available at https://www.nhlbi.nih.gov/files/docs/research/2012_ChartBook_508.pdf, accessed January 7, 2015.

Office of the Surgeon General (US); Office of Disease Prevention and Health Promotion (US); Centers for Disease Control and Prevention (US); National Institutes of Health (US). *The Surgeon General's Call to Action to Prevent and Decrease Overweight and Obesity*. Rockville, MD: Office of the Surgeon General, 2001. Available at http://www.ncbi.nlm.nih.gov/books/NBK44206/, accessed December 23, 2014.

Ogden CL, Flegal KM. Changes in terminology for childhood overweight and obesity. *National Health Statistics Reports*. No. 25, 2010. Available at http://www.cdc.gov/nchs/data/nhsr/nhsr025.pdf, accessed January 7, 2015.

Ogden CL, Carroll MD, Kit BK, Flegal KM. Prevalence of obesity in the United States, 2009–2010. *NCHS Data Brief*. No. 82, 2012a. Available at http://www.cdc.gov/nchs/data/databriefs/db82.pdf, accessed January 7, 2015.

Ogden CL, Carroll MD, Kit BK, Flegal KM. Prevalence of obesity and trends in body mass index among US children and adolescents, 1999–2010. *JAMA*. 2012b;307(5):483–490.

Pekka P, Pirjo P, Ulla U. Influencing public nutrition for non-communicable disease prevention: From community intervention to national programme—Experiences from Finland. *Public Health Nutr*. 2002; 5(S):245–251.

Proper KI, Singh AS, van Mechelen W, Chinapaw MJM. Sedentary behaviors and health outcomes among adults: A systematic review of prospective studies. *Am J Prev Med*. 2011;40(2):174–182.

Prospective Studies Collaboration. Body-mass index and cause-specific mortality in 900,000 adults: Collaborative analyses of 57 Prospective studies. *Lancet*. 2009;373:1083–1096.

Renehan AG, Tyson M, Egger M, Heller RF, Zwahlen M. Body-mass index and incidence of cancer: A systematic review and meta-analysis of prospective observational studies. *Lancet*. 2008;371:569–578.

Rewers A, Klingensmith G, Davis C et al. Presence of diabetic ketoacidosis at diagnosis of diabetes mellitus in youth: The search for diabetes in youth study. *Pediatrics*. 2008;121:e1258–e1266.

Roger VL, Go AS, Lloyd-Jones DM et al. Heart disease and stroke statistics—2012 update: A report from the American Heart Associatoin. *Circulation*. 2012;125:e2–e220.

Sacks FM, Svetkey LP, Vollmer WM et al. Effects on blood pressure of reduced dietary sodium and the Dietary Approaches to Stop Hypertension (DASH) diet. DASH-Sodium Collaborative Research Group. *N Engl J Med*. 2001;344(1):3–10.

Strengthening Families Program. Available at http://www.strengtheningfamiliesprogram.org/index.html, accessed January 7, 2015.

Task Force on Community Preventive Services. Recommendations to increase physical activity in communities. *Am J Prev Med*. 2002;22(4S):67–72. Available at http://www.thecommunityguide.org/pa/pa-ajpm -recs.pdf, accessed January 7, 2015.

The Henry R. Kaiser Family Foundation. Disparities Policy. Disparities in Health and Health Care: Five Key Questions and Answers, November 30, 2012. Available at http://kff.org/disparities-policy/issue-brief/dis parities-in-health-and-health-care-five-key-questions-and-answers/, accessed January 12, 2015.

The SEARCH for Diabetes in Youth Study Group. The burden of diabetes mellitus among US youth: Prevalence estimates from the SEARCH for diabetes in youth study. *Pediatrics*. 2006;118:1510–1518.

The SEARCH for Diabetes in Youth Study Group. *Phase 3 Protocol*. Centers for Disease Control and Prevention, 2010. Available at https://www.searchfordiabetes.org/public/SEARCH_Phase_3_Protocols.pdf, accessed January 7, 2015.

The SEARCH Writing Group. SEARCH for diabetes in youth: A multi-center study of the prevalence, incidence and classification of diabetes mellitus in youth. *Control Clin Trials*. 2004;25:458–471.

The Writing Group for the SEARCH for Diabetes in Youth Study Group. Incidence of diabetes in youth in the United States. *JAMA*. 2007;297(24):2716–2724.

US Cancer Statistics Working Group. *United States Cancer Statistics: 1999–2011 Incidence and Mortality Web-Based Report*. U.S. Department of Health and Human Services, Centers for Disease Control and Prevention and National Cancer Institute, 2014. Available at http://www.cdc.gov/uscs, accessed January 7, 2015.

US Department of Agriculture. ChooseMyPlate.gov. Food Groups Overview. Available at http://www.choosemyplate.gov/food-groups/, accessed January 12, 2015.

US Department of Agriculture. ChooseMyPlate.gov. Selected Messages for Consumers. Available at http://www.choosemyplate.gov/print-materials-ordering/selected-messages.html, accessed January 12, 2015.

US Department of Agriculture. SNAP-Ed Connection Resource Library. Body & Soul: A Celebration of Health Eating & Living. Available at http://snap.nal.usda.gov/foodstamp/resource_finder_details.php?id=409, accessed January 7, 2015.

US Department of Agriculture. *What We Eat in America*, NHANES 2011–2012, Table 1. Nutrient Intakes from Food and Beverages. Mean Amounts Consumed per Individual. Available at http://www.ars.usda.gov/services/docs.htm?docid=18349, accessed January 7, 2015.

US Department of Health and Human Services. Control Your Diabetes: For Life. National Diabetes Education Program. Available at http://ndep.nih.gov/partners-community-organization/campaigns/ControlYourDiabetesForLife.aspx, accessed January 7, 2015.

US Department of Health and Human Services. *Diabetes: A National Plan for Action. Steps to a Healthier U.S.*, 2004. Available at http://aspe.hhs.gov/health/NDAP/NDAP04.pdf, accessed December 15, 2014.

US Department of Health and Human Services. *Effective Public Health Strategies to Prevent and Control Diabetes: A Compendium*. Centers for Disease Control and Prevention, 2013. Available at http://www.cdc.gov/diabetes/pubs/pdf/PublicHealthCompedium.pdf, accessed January 7, 2015.

US Department of Health and Human Services. *HHS Action Plan to Reduce Racial and Ethnic Disparities: A Nation Free of Disparities in Health and Health Care*. Washington, DC: U.S. Department of Health and Human Services, April 2011b.

US Department of Health and Human Services. *HHS Action Plan to Reduce Racial and Ethnic Health Disparities*. Office of Minority Health, 2011c. Available at http://minorityhealth.hhs.gov/npa/files/Plans/HHS/HHS_Plan_complete.pdf, accessed January 7, 2014.

US Department of Health and Human Services. HHS Organizational Chart. Available at http://www.hhs.gov/about/orgchart/index.html, accessed January 12, 2015.

US Department of Health and Human Services. HHS Strategic Plan and Secretary's Strategic Initiatives. Available at http://www.hhs.gov/strategic-plan/priorities.html, accessed January 12, 2015.

US Department of Health and Human Services. National Institutes of Health. About NIH. Mission. Available at http://www.nih.gov/about/mission.htm, accessed December 23, 2014.

US Department of Health and Human Services. National Institute on Minority Health and Health Disparities. About NIMHD. Available at http://www.nimhd.nih.gov/about/visionMission.html, accessed December 23, 2014.

US Department of Health and Human Services. *NIH Health Disparities Strategic Plan and Budget, Fiscal Years 2009–2013*. National Institutes of Health, 2011a. Available at http://www.nimhd.nih.gov/documents/NIH%20Health%20Disparities%20Strategic%20Plan%20and%20Budget%202009-2013.pdf, accessed January 7, 2015.

US Department of Health and Human Services. Small Steps. Big ReStrengthening Families Program. Available at http://www.strengtheningfamiliesprogram.org/index.html, accessed January 7, 2015.

US Department of Health and Human Services. Small Steps. Big Rewards: Prevent Type 2 Diabetes. National Diabetes Education Program. Available at http://www.ndep.nih.gov/campaigns/SmallSteps/SmallSteps_index.htm, accessed December 26, 2014.

US Department of Health and Human Services. *The Health Consequences of Smoking—50 Years of Progress: A Report of the Surgeon General*. Atlanta, GA: U.S. Department of Health and Human Services, Centers for Disease Control and Prevention, National Center for Chronic Disease Prevention and Health Promotion, Office on Smoking and Health, 2014.

US Department of Health and Human Services. *Update to A Public Health Action Plan to Prevention Heart Disease and Stroke*. Centers for Disease Control and Prevention, 2008. Available at http://www.cdc.gov/dhdsp/action_plan/pdfs/2008_Action_Plan_Update.pdf, accessed January 7, 2015.

US Department of Health and Human Services, Centers for Disease Control and Prevention. *REACH U.S.—Finding Solutions to Health Disparities: At a Glance, 2010*. National Center for Chronic Disease Prevention and Health Promotion, 2010. Available at http://www.cdc.gov/chronicdisease/resources/publications/aag/pdf/2010/REACH-AAG.pdf, accessed January 7, 2015.

US Department of Health and Human Services, Office of Minority Health. *Heart Disease Data/Statistics*. Office of Minority Health, 2012. Available at http://minorityhealth.hhs.gov/omh/browse.aspx?lvl=4&lvlid=19, accessed January 7, 2015.

US Department of Health and Human Services; Public Health Service; National Institutes of Health; National Heart, Blood, and Lung Institute. *Third Report of the National Cholesterol Education Program Expert Panel on Detection. Evaluation, and Treatment of High Blood Cholesterol in Adults (Adult Treatment Panel III): Final Report*. NIH Publication No. 02-5215, September 2002. Available at http://www.nhlbi.nih.gov/guidelines/cholesterol/atp3full.pdf, accessed December 26, 2014.

US Government Accountability Office. Healthcare: Approaches to address racial and ethnic disparities. GAO-03-862R, 2003. Available at http://www.gao.gov/new.items/d03862r.pdf, accessed February 4, 2015.

US Renal Data System. *USRDS 2012 Annual Data Report: Atlas of Chronic Kidney Disease and End-Stage Renal Disease in the United States*, Vol. II. National Institutes of Health, National Institute of Diabetes and Digestive and Kidney Diseases, 2012, chap. 1. Available at http://www.usrds.org/2012/view/v2_01.aspx, accessed January 7, 2015.

VERB™ homepage. Available at http://www.cdc.gov/youthcampaign/index.htm. Accessed January 7, 2015.

Weiss R, Dziura J, Burgert TS et al. Obesity and the metabolic syndrome in children and adolescents. *N Engl J Med*. 2004;350:2362–2374.

Whelton PK, He J, Appel LJ et al. Primary prevention of hypertension: Clinical and public health advisory from The National High Blood Pressure Education Program. *JAMA*. 2002;288:1882–1888.

Women's Heart Foundation. Women and Heart Disease Facts. Available at http://www.womensheart.org/content/HeartDisease/heart_disease_facts.asp, accessed December 23, 2014.

World Cancer Research Fund and American Institute for Cancer Research. *Food, Nutrition and the Prevention of Cancer: A Global Perspective*. Washington, DC: American Institute for Cancer Research, 1997.

World Cancer Research Fund and American Institute for Cancer Research. *Food, Nutrition, Physical Activity, and the Prevention of Cancer: A Global Perspective*. Washington, DC: AICR, 2007.

World Health Organization. *A Global Brief on Hypertension*. World Health Organization, 2013. Available at http://www.who.int/cardiovascular_diseases/publications/global_brief_hypertension/en/, accessed January 7, 2015.

5 Weight Control
Challenges and Solutions

Watermelon—it's a good fruit. You eat, you drink, you wash your face.

Enrico Caruso (1873–1921)

INTRODUCTION*

In 2001, then US Surgeon General Satcher described overweight and obesity as having reached "nationwide epidemic proportions," noting that approximately 300,000 deaths a year in the United States are currently associated with these conditions. Health risks associated with obesity include type 2 diabetes, heart disease, stroke, hypertension, sleep apnea, psychological disorders such as depression, some cancers, and premature death. Dr. Satcher called for the prevention and treatment of overweight and obesity and their associated health problems by

- Promoting the recognition of overweight and obesity as major public health problems.
- Helping people balance healthful eating with regular physical activity to achieve and maintain a healthy or healthier body weight.
- Identifying effective and culturally appropriate interventions to prevent and treat overweight and obesity.
- Encouraging environmental changes that help prevent overweight and obesity.
- Developing and enhancing public–private partnerships to help implement these goals (US Department of Health and Human Services 2001).

To start, we describe the extent of the problem. The high prevalence of overweight and obesity—as indicated by national surveys—impacts not only individual health but also national healthcare costs, levels of work productivity, and social interactions. Then we review the potential sources of the problem; the built environment, economic environment, US farm policy, advertising, the food environment (such as increased snacking and portion sizes), and the lack of physical activity have all been implicated in our escalating national weight. Finally, we look at solutions ranging from individual dietary changes to federally implemented education campaigns and policies in community, school, and workplace settings.

EXTENT OF THE PROBLEM

DEFINING OVERWEIGHT AND OBESITY

Adults

The body mass index (BMI) is a quick and reliable indicator of body fatness for most people and is used to screen for overweight and obesity. BMI is calculated as weight in kilograms divided by height in meters squared. The National Institutes of Health (NIH) defines a healthy weight in adults as a BMI of 18.5–24.9 kg/m², overweight as a BMI of 25–29.9 kg/m², obesity as a BMI equal to or greater than 30 kg/m², and extreme obesity as a BMI of at least 40 kg/m². Figure 5.1 is a BMI chart.

---

* Kate O'Connor and Megan Trusdell contributed primary research and prepared draft versions of portions of this chapter.

Body Mass Index Table

Body weight (pounds) — Categories: BMI 19–24 Normal; BMI 25–29 Overweight; BMI 30–39 Obese; BMI 40–54 Extreme obesity

Height (inches) \ BMI	19	20	21	22	23	24	25	26	27	28	29	30	31	32	33	34	35	36	37	38	39	40	41	42	43	44	45	46	47	48	49	50	51	52	53	54
58	91	96	100	105	110	115	119	124	129	134	138	143	148	153	158	162	167	172	177	181	186	191	196	201	205	210	215	220	224	229	234	239	244	248	253	258
59	94	99	104	109	114	119	124	128	133	138	143	148	153	158	163	168	173	178	183	188	193	198	203	208	212	217	222	227	232	237	242	247	252	257	262	267
60	97	102	107	112	118	123	128	133	138	143	148	153	158	163	168	174	179	184	189	194	199	204	209	215	220	225	230	235	240	245	250	255	261	266	271	276
61	100	106	111	116	122	127	132	137	143	148	153	158	164	169	174	180	185	190	195	201	206	211	217	222	227	232	238	243	248	254	259	264	269	275	280	285
62	104	109	115	120	126	131	136	142	147	153	158	164	169	175	180	186	191	196	202	207	213	218	224	229	235	240	246	251	256	262	267	273	278	284	289	295
63	107	113	118	124	130	135	141	146	152	158	163	169	175	180	186	191	197	203	208	214	220	225	231	237	242	248	254	259	265	270	278	282	287	293	299	304
64	110	116	122	128	134	140	145	151	157	163	169	174	180	186	192	197	204	209	215	221	227	232	238	244	250	256	262	267	273	279	285	291	296	302	308	314
65	114	120	126	132	138	144	150	156	162	168	174	180	186	192	198	204	210	216	222	228	234	240	246	252	258	264	270	276	282	288	294	300	306	312	318	324
66	118	124	130	136	142	148	155	161	167	173	179	186	192	198	204	210	216	223	229	235	241	247	253	260	266	272	278	284	291	297	303	309	315	322	328	334
67	121	127	134	140	146	153	159	166	172	178	185	191	198	204	211	217	223	230	236	242	249	255	261	268	274	280	287	293	299	306	312	319	325	331	338	344
68	125	131	138	144	151	158	164	171	177	184	190	197	203	210	216	223	230	236	243	249	256	262	269	276	282	289	295	302	308	315	322	328	335	341	348	354
69	128	135	142	149	155	162	169	176	182	189	196	203	209	216	223	230	236	243	250	257	263	270	277	284	291	297	304	311	318	324	331	338	345	351	358	365
70	132	139	146	153	160	167	174	181	188	195	202	209	216	222	229	236	243	250	257	264	271	278	285	292	299	306	313	320	327	334	341	348	355	362	369	376
71	136	143	150	157	165	172	179	186	193	200	208	215	222	229	236	243	250	257	265	272	279	286	293	301	308	315	322	329	338	343	351	358	365	372	379	386
72	140	147	154	162	169	177	184	191	199	206	213	221	228	235	242	250	258	265	272	279	287	294	302	309	316	324	331	338	346	353	361	368	375	383	390	397
73	144	151	159	166	174	182	189	197	204	212	219	227	235	242	250	257	265	272	280	288	295	302	310	318	325	333	340	348	355	363	371	378	386	393	401	408
74	148	155	163	171	179	186	194	202	210	218	225	233	241	249	256	264	272	280	287	295	303	311	319	326	334	342	350	358	365	373	381	389	396	404	412	420
75	152	160	168	176	184	192	200	208	216	224	232	240	248	256	264	272	279	287	295	303	311	319	327	335	343	351	359	367	375	383	391	399	407	415	423	431
76	156	164	172	180	189	197	205	213	221	230	238	246	254	263	271	279	287	295	304	312	320	328	336	344	353	361	369	377	385	394	402	410	418	426	435	443

FIGURE 5.1 BMI chart. (From US Department of Health and Human Services. National Heart, Lung, and Blood Institute. Body Mass Index Table. Available at http://www.nhlbi.nih.gov/health/educational/lose_wt/BMI/bmi_tbl.pdf, accessed February 2, 2015.)

The math and metric conversions have already been calculated. To use the table, find the appropriate height in the left-hand column. Move across the row to the given weight. The number at the top of the column is the BMI for that height and weight (National Institutes of Health, http://www.nhlbi.nih.gov/guidelines/obesity/ob_gdlns.htm).

Children

Unlike adults, children's heights and weights grow at various rates based on age and sex, and thus a BMI of 20 kg/m² is interpreted differently for a 5-, 10-, and 15-year-old girl and boy. For BMI to be meaningful in children, it must be compared to a reference standard that accounts for age and sex. BMI z-scores (also called BMI standard deviation scores) and BMI percentiles provide this relative measure based on an external reference group. BMI z-scores are primarily used for statistical analysis, whereas BMI percentiles are used in clinical practice (Must and Anderson 2006).

To determine BMI percentiles, BMI-for-age growth charts are used to plot a child's BMI for his/her age and sex. In 2000, the Centers for Disease Control and Prevention (CDC) introduced charts representing BMI-for-age for children and adolescents, by gender, ages 2–20 years, portrayed in Figures 5.2 and 5.3.

The 2000 CDC growth charts represent the revised version of the 1977 National Center for Health Statistics (NCHS) growth charts. Most of the data used to construct these charts come from the CDC's National Health and Nutrition Examination Survey (NHANES), which has periodically collected height and weight and other health information on the American population since the early 1960s.

The BMI-for-age charts are used to assess childhood underweight, overweight, and obesity. According to the CDC, a child with a BMI-for-age that is at the 85th to below the 95th percentile indicates overweight, whereas a child with a BMI-for-age that is equal to or greater than the 95th percentile is considered to be obese. Children below the 5th percentile BMI-for-age are considered underweight (Ogden and Flegal 2010). CDC's BMI Percentile Calculator for Child and Teen is available on the agency's website (http://apps.nccd.cdc.gov/dnpabmi/), as are numerous clinical growth charts (http://www.cdc.gov/growthcharts/clinical_charts.htm).

PREVALENCE OF OBESITY IN THE UNITED STATES

Data indicate that the prevalence of obesity has significantly increased among the US population since the 1960s (Flegal et al. 1998). Recent studies in the United States have found high levels of obesity among adults and children, with one-third of adults and 17% of children obese; however, the rate appears to have leveled off between 2003–2004 and 2009–2010 (Ogden et al. 2014). Obesity among young people aged 2–19 is about 17% as of 2011–2012 and has not changed significantly since 2003–2004 (Centers for Disease Control and Prevention 2011–2012).

Estimates of rates of overweight and obesity in the United States differ based on whether heights and weights are self-reported or are measured by trained personnel. Self-reported weights tend to be lower than weights measured by survey personnel. Therefore, surveys that rely on measured weights produce higher calculated BMIs than surveys using self-reported weights. However, surveys that rely on measured weights and heights may be limited by the fact that some people, such as the extremely obese, are less likely to submit to examinations (Baskin et al. 2005). Nevertheless, national examination surveys that use measured weight and height data provide the best opportunity to track BMI trends.

Obesity Prevalence among Children

In the 1960s, less than 5% of children 6–19 years of age were obese (Ogden et al. 2002). As of 2010, about 12% of 2- to 5-year-olds and 18% of 6- to 19-year-olds were obese (Ogden et al. 2012). Taking into consideration those deemed overweight, the 2010 percentages show that over one-quarter (27%) of preschoolers ages 2–5 years and one-third (33%) of youth ages 6–19 years are exceeding a healthy

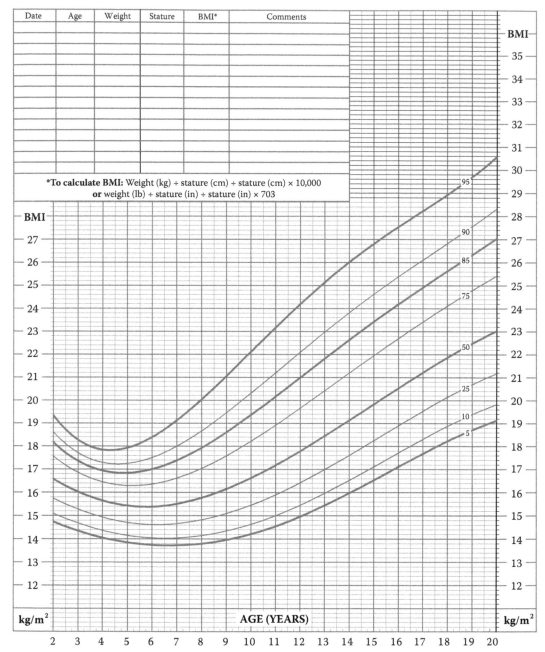

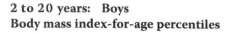

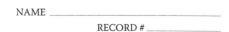

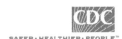

FIGURE 5.2   BMI-for-age growth chart for boys. (From Centers for Disease Control and Prevention. Clinical Growth Charts. Available at http://www.cdc.gov/growthcharts/clinical_charts.htm, accessed February 2, 2015.)

2 to 20 years: Girls
Body mass index-for-age percentiles

NAME _____

RECORD # _____

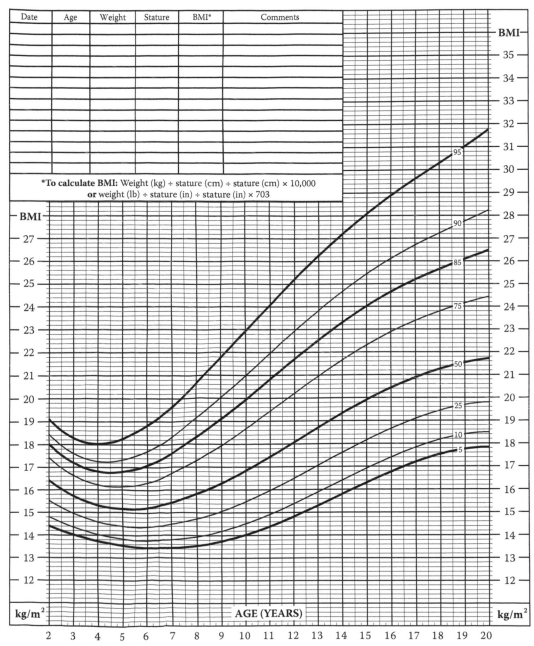

*To calculate BMI: Weight (kg) ÷ stature (cm) ÷ stature (cm) × 10,000
or weight (lb) ÷ stature (in) ÷ stature (in) × 703

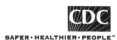

SAFER·HEALTHIER·PEOPLE™

FIGURE 5.3   BMI-for-age growth chart for girls. (From Centers for Disease Control and Prevention. Clinical Growth Charts. Available at http://www.cdc.gov/growthcharts/clinical_charts.htm, accessed February 2, 2015.)

weight. Among children of color, the rates are even higher, with 33% of Mexican American children ages 2–5 years and 41% of Mexican American and non-Hispanic black youth ages 6–19 years considered overweight or obese (Ogden et al. 2012). Although rates are high, the good news is that some decreases in the prevalence of obesity have been reported in some populations of youth in the United States, such as in low-income preschool-aged children in certain states participating in federal nutrition programs from 2008 to 2011 (Ogden et al. 2014).

Longitudinal data suggest an overweight future for overweight children. In the Pediatric Nutrition Surveillance System (PedNSS) study discussed in the following section on surveys, data on 380,518 low-income children from birth to age 59 months born between 1985 and 1990 indicate that overweight during infancy persists through the preschool years (Mei et al. 2003). In another study, data on 2610 children ages 2–17 years of age in 1973 who were followed to ages 18–37 years in 1996 (the mean follow-up was 17.6 years) indicate that childhood levels of both BMI and triceps skinfold thickness were associated with adult levels of BMI and adiposity. The magnitude of these longitudinal associations increased with childhood age, and the BMI levels of even the youngest children were moderately associated with adult adiposity. Overweight 2- to 5-year-olds were more than four times as likely to become overweight adults as were children with a BMI below the 50th percentile (Freedman et al. 2005). In sum, many overweight children will become overweight adults.

Impact of Socioeconomic Status and Ethnicity on Obesity Prevalence

Socioeconomic status (SES) categorizes individuals based on economic or social factors or according to occupational prestige and power. Occupation and income are frequently used as indicators of SES (Liberatos et al. 1998). Traditionally it was held that there exists an inverse relationship between obesity and SES in developed countries (that is, obesity increases as income level decreases), particularly among women, and a positive relationship between obesity and SES in developing countries (Sobal and Stunkard 1989).

Nevertheless, coincident with the increase in obesity in the United States over the past three decades, epidemiologists have observed that the relationship between BMI and SES has weakened. Analysis of data from NHANES I–III (1971–1994) and NHANES (1999–2000) indicates that high-SES groups are manifesting a significant *catch-up* in the prevalence of obesity (Zhang and Wang 2004). More recent data from NHANES 2005–2008 show that, in men, obesity prevalence is generally similar at all income levels, with slightly higher rates at higher income levels among non-Hispanic black and Mexican American men. Among women, those with a higher income are less likely to be obese, though the majority of obese women do not have low income. Regarding education, there is no significant trend between education level and obesity prevalence in men; however, among women, obesity prevalence increases as education decreases (Ogden et al. 2010a).

Additionally, the view that there is a positive relationship of obesity to SES in societies in developing countries has been disputed (Monteiro et al. 2004). In Brazil, for example, obesity is increasing faster among the groups with lower incomes (Monteiro et al. 2002).

Among children, NHANES data from 2005 to 2008 indicate that low-income adolescents were at a higher risk for obesity compared to their higher income peers (Ogden et al. 2010b). However, this relationship differed by race and ethnicity. Among non-Hispanic white girls and boys, there was a significant inverse association between income and obesity. Yet no significant trend in obesity prevalence by income level was found for either non-Hispanic black or Mexican American girls or boys. Likewise, there was a significant inverse relationship between overall obesity prevalence and education of the head of household for both girls and boys. Stratifying by race and ethnicity revealed that, among non-Hispanic white and black girls, the prevalence of obesity was significantly lower in households headed by college graduates than by those with less than a high school degree. No significant relationships were found among Mexican American girls or among boys of any racial or ethnic group (Ogden et al. 2010b).

National Health and Nutrition Examination Survey

The NHANES is a program of studies designed to assess the health and nutritional status of the US population. (The appendix to Chapter 1 provides a more detailed description of NHANES origins and methodology.) Among the data obtained are measured heights and weights, which allow for BMI calculation and classification. The third NHANES (NHANES III), conducted from 1988 to 1994, was designed to obtain nationally representative information on the health and nutritional status of the US population. Approximately 31,000 civilian, non-institutionalized individuals aged 2 months and older received direct physical examinations, including measurements of height and weight. Based on these data, it is estimated that 22.5% of the adult population were obese during this time (Flegal et al. 1998).

In 1999, NHANES became a continuous survey, with data published in 2-year cycles. BMI was calculated from measured heights and weights from 4115 adults in 1999–2000 (Hedley et al. 2004), 4390 adults in 2001–2002 (Baskin et al. 2005), 4431 adults in 2003–2004, 4356 adults in 2005–2006 (Centers for Disease Control and Prevention, http://www.cdc.gov/nchs/data/hestat /overweight/overweight_adult.htm), 5555 adults in 2007–2008 (Flegal et al. 2010), 5926 adults in 2009–2010 (Flegal et al. 2012), and 5181 adults in 2011–2012 (Fryar et al. 2014). As illustrated in Table 5.1, between 1999 and 2010, the age-adjusted prevalence of overweight (BMI ≥ 25) increased from 64.5% to 68.8%, and obesity (BMI ≥ 30) from 30.5% to 35.7% (Flegal et al. 2012). In 2011–2012, 34.9% of adults were obese, which is not significantly different from that obtained in 2009–2010 (Ogden et al. 2013).

Behavioral Risk Factor Surveillance System

The Behavioral Risk Factor Surveillance System (BRFSS) is a cross-sectional telephone survey conducted monthly by state health departments with assistance from the CDC. Self-reported data in BRFSS from 1991 to 1994 showed a prevalence of obesity of 12–14.4%. Thus, as noted above concerning self-reported data, the NHANES figures are more than 50% higher than the BRFSS estimates (Flegal et al. 1998).

TABLE 5.1
Age-Adjusted Prevalence of Overweight and Obesity for US Adults Aged 20 Years and Older, 1999–2012 (NHANES)

	Overweight (BMI ≥ 25)	Obesity (BMI ≥ 30)
NHANES 1999–2000[a] (n = 4115)	64.5% (SE 1.6)	30.5% (SE 1.5)
NHANES 2001–2002[a] (n = 4390)	65.7% (SE 0.6)	30.6% (SE 1.1)
NHANES 2003–4004[b] (n = 4431)	66.3% (SE 1.1)	32.2% (SE 1.2)
NHANES 2005–2006[c] (n = 4356)	67.0% (SE not published)	34.3% (SE not published)
NHANES 2007–2008[d] (n = 5555)	68.0% (95% CI 66.3–69.8)	33.8% (95% CI 31.6–36.0)
NHANES 2009–2010[e] (n = 5296)	68.8% (95% CI 65.9–71.5)	35.7% (95% CI 33.8–37.7)
NHANES 2011–2012[f] (n = 5181)	68.5% (95% CI 65.2–71.6)	34.9% (95% CI 32.0–37.9)

Source: [a]Data from Hedley AA et al., *JAMA*, 291(23):2847–50, 2004; [b]Data from Ogden CL et al., *JAMA*, 295(13):1549–55, 2006; [c]Data from NCHS Health E-Stats. Prevalence of overweight, obesity and extreme obesity among adults: United States, trends 1976–1980 through 2005–2006. Hyattsville, MD: National Center for Health Statistics, December 2008. Available at http://www .cdc.gov/nchs/data/hestat/overweight/overweight_adult.pdf, accessed January 20, 2015; [d]Data from Flegal KM et al., *JAMA*, 303(3):235–41, 2010; [e]Data from Flegal KM et al., *JAMA*, 307(5):491–7, 2012; [f]Data from Ogden CL et al., *JAMA*, 311(8):806–14, 2014.

TABLE 5.2

Overweight and Obesity Prevalence Rate, by State

State	Overweight (BMI 25.0–29.9 kg/m²)	Obese (BMI ≥ 30 kg/m²)	Overweight + Obese (BMI ≥ 25.0 kg/m²)
Nationwide (States, DC, and Territories)	35.4	28.9	64.3
Nationwide (States and DC)	35.4	29.4	64.8
Alabama	35.7	32.4	68.1
Alaska	37.7	28.4	66.1
Arizona	35.1	26.8	61.9
Arkansas	35.3	34.6	69.9
California	36.0	24.1	60.1
Colorado	35.1	21.3	56.4
Connecticut	37.6	25.0	62.6
Delaware	33.5	31.1	64.6
District of Columbia	30.9	22.9	53.8
Florida	36.4	26.4	62.8
Georgia	36.5	30.3	66.8
Guam	36.5	27.0	63.5
Hawaii	33.6	21.8	55.4
Idaho	35.4	29.6	65.0
Illinois	35.3	29.4	64.7
Indiana	35.4	31.8	67.2
Iowa	35.7	31.3	67.0
Kansas	35.3	30.0	67.3
Kentucky	34.1	33.2	67.3
Louisiana	34.3	33.1	67.4
Maine	36.0	28.9	64.9
Maryland	35.9	28.3	64.3
Massachusetts	34.4	23.6	58.0
Michigan	34.7	31.5	66.2
Minnesota	35.6	25.5	61.1
Mississippi	34.2	35.1	69.3
Missouri	35.1	30.4	65.5
Montana	36.8	24.6	61.4
Nebraska	35.9	29.6	65.5
Nevada	36.3	26.2	62.5
New Hampshire	35.0	26.7	61.7
New Jersey	36.5	26.3	62.8
New Mexico	36.3	26.4	62.7
New York	35.9	25.4	61.3
North Carolina	36.7	29.4	66.1
North Dakota	36.6	31.0	67.6
Ohio	34.7	30.4	65.1
Oklahoma	35.4	32.5	67.9
Oregon	33.4	26.5	59.9
Pennsylvania	34.5	30.0	64.5
Puerto Rico	38.7	27.9	66.6
Rhode Island	37.3	27.3	64.6

(Continued)

TABLE 5.2 (CONTINUED)
Overweight and Obesity Prevalence Rate, by State

State	Overweight (BMI 25.0–29.9 kg/m²)	Obese (BMI ≥ 30 kg/m²)	Overweight + Obese (BMI ≥ 25.0 kg/m²)
South Carolina	34.7	31.7	66.4
South Dakota	37.1	29.9	67.0
Tennessee	34.7	33.7	68.4
Texas	35.3	30.9	66.2
Utah	35.0	24.1	59.1
Vermont	37.2	24.7	61.9
Virginia	36.8	27.2	64.0
Washington	34.3	27.2	61.5
West Virginia	33.7	35.1	68.8
Wisconsin	36.7	29.8	66.5
Wyoming	36.6	27.8	64.4

Source: Centers for Disease Control and Prevention. Office of Surveillance, Epidemiology, and Laboratory Services. Behavioral Risk Factor Surveillance System. Prevalence and Trends Data: Overweight and Obesity (BMI)—2013. Available at http://apps.nccd.cdc.gov/brfss/index.asp, accessed January 20, 2015.

In 2013, self-reported data collected through the BRFSS indicated a 35.4% prevalence of overweight nationwide (states, District of Columbia, and territories) among US adults and a 28.9% prevalence of obesity. West Virginia had the highest rate of obesity (35.1%), and Colorado had the lowest (21.3%) (Centers for Disease Control and Prevention, http://apps.nccd.cdc.gov/brfss). Trends in state-specific obesity for the year 2013, the most recent BRFSS data available as of January 2015, appear in Table 5.2. The most recent available state-specific and national prevalence data may be found on the BRFSS interactive website at http://apps.nccd.cdc.gov/brfss/.

Youth BRFSS

From 1991 to 2013, the Youth BRFSS (YBRFSS) has collected data from more than 2.6 million high school students in more than 1100 separate surveys. The YBRFSS was developed in 1990 to monitor priority health-risk behaviors that contribute markedly to the leading causes of death, disability, and social problems among youth and adults in the United States. These behaviors include those that contribute to unintentional injuries and violence; sexual behaviors that contribute to unintended pregnancy and sexually transmitted infections, including HIV, alcohol, drug use, and tobacco use; unhealthy dietary behavior; and inadequate physical activity. The YBRFSS also monitors the prevalence of obesity and asthma. The CDC (http://www.cdc.gov/healthyyouth/yrbs/pdf/system_overview_yrbs.pdf) conducts a national survey every 2 years, but states and local jurisdictions may also conduct surveys.

The 2013 YBRFSS is the most recent data available as of the writing of this chapter. A national school-based survey was conducted by the CDC, as well as 42 state surveys, 5 territorial surveys, 2 tribal government surveys, and 21 local surveys. A total of 13,633 questionnaires were completed for the national survey. The school and student response rates were 77% and 88%, respectively; thus, there was an overall 68% response rate (the school response rate multiplied by the student response rate).

The September 2012–December 2013 survey period reported a nationwide obesity prevalence of 13.7% in students and overweight prevalence of 16.9%. Although obesity prevalence has increased since 1999 (10.6%), it did not rise significantly between 2011 and 2013; similarly, although the prevalence of overweight has increased since 1999 (14.1%), it did not show a significant rise from 2011 (Centers for Disease Control and Prevention 2014).

In 2005, the questions about fruit and vegetable consumption referenced servings; in 2013, the questions referenced the number of times per day fruit or vegetables were consumed. In 2013, 21.9% of students reported consuming fruit or 100% fruit juice three or more times, and 15.7% reported consuming vegetables three or more times a day.

Pediatric Nutrition Surveillance System

PedNSS was a cross-sectional survey of health records of low-income children from birth to 4 years old enrolled in the Special Supplemental Nutrition Program for Women, Infants, and Children (WIC) and other federally funded programs. PedNSS was discontinued by the CDC in 2012. An analysis of PedNSS data for 2- to 4-year-old children indicates increases in obesity between 1998 and 2008 (Sharma et al. 2009).

Obesity was defined as BMI-for-age ≥ 95th percentile based on the 2000 CDC sex-specific growth charts. From 1998 to 2008, the overall prevalence of obesity increased from 12.4% to 14.6% in the low-income preschool population. In 2008, rates were highest among American Indian/Alaska Native (21.2%) and Hispanic (18.5%) children, and lowest among non-Hispanic white (12.6%), Asians/Pacific Islanders (A/PI; 12.3%), and non-Hispanic black (11.8%) children. Table 5.3 shows the prevalence of obesity reported by selected areas. The only two reporting states that had obesity prevalence in low-income preschool children at or below 10% in 2008 were Colorado and Hawaii, and two federally funded Indian tribal organizations had obesity prevalences in this population at greater than 20%.

However, growth in obesity prevalence appears to be stabilizing over time: obesity prevalence increased 0.43 percentage points per year during 1998–2003, but only 0.02 percentage points per year during 2003–2008 (Sharma et al. 2009). These findings may indicate that prevention and intervention efforts in the United States are working to reverse the rising trend of childhood obesity.

TABLE 5.3

Selected Area Prevalences of Obesity in Low-Income Preschool Children (PedNSS)

State/Tribe	% Obese			Average % Change per Year	
	1998	2003	2008	1998–2003	2003–2008
Hawaii	10.3	10.1	9.3	NS	–0.16
Colorado	–	9.4	9.4	–	NS
Pennsylvania	10.7	12.4	11.5	0.34	–0.18
New Mexico	7.6	9.7	12.0	0.42	0.46
Ohio	10.4	11.6	12.2	0.24	0.12
Idaho	9.8	11.2	12.3	0.28	0.22
Cheyenne River Sioux Tribe (SD)	22.1*	17.5	18.4	NS	NS
Rosebud Sioux Tribe (SD)	16.4	17.3	19.2	NS	NS
Three Affiliated Tribes (ND)	–	–	19.6	–	–
Inter-Tribal Council of Arizona	19.8	20.9	23.5	NS	0.52
Standing Rock Sioux Tribe (ND)	–	20.1	25.0	–	NS

Source: Adapted from Sharma AJ et al., *MMWR*, 58(28):769–73, 2009.

Note: (*) Data from subsequent year used; (–) data not submitted; (NS) no significant change in obesity prevalence.

Racial and Ethnic Approaches to Community Health Risk Factor Surveys

In 2001, the CDC began to conduct annual risk factor surveys in minority communities to monitor the health of black, Hispanic, A/PI, and American Indians/Alaska Natives. The risk factor surveys are part of the Racial and Ethnic Approaches to Community Health (REACH) 2010 project, launched in 1999. REACH 2010 is the CDC's cornerstone initiative aimed at eliminating disparities in health status experienced by ethnic minority populations in key health indicators (Liao et al. 2004). For a more complete discussion of diet-related health disparities, please refer to Chapter 4.

Data from the 2001–2002 REACH 2010 Risk Factor Survey reveal that residents in minority communities bear greater risks for disease compared with the general population, with the median prevalence of obesity ranging from a low of 2.9% for men and 3.6% for women in A/PI communities to a high of 39.2% for men and 38.0% for women in American Indian communities. The prevalence of obesity was substantially higher among both men and women in American Indian communities and among women in black communities compared with national 2001 BRFSS data. Overall, more than one-third of American Indian men and women and black women were obese in the surveyed communities, whereas approximately one-fifth of adults were obese in the national BRFSS survey. Obesity was rare in A/PI communities at that time (Liao et al. 2004).

IMPACT ON PUBLIC HEALTH

A combination of poor diet, sedentary lifestyle, and overweight/obesity not only undermine quality of life, life expectancy, and productivity; they also contribute to between one-fifth and one-third of annual deaths in the United States (Danaei et al. 2009; Mokdad et al. 2004).

Specific diseases and conditions, such as cardiovascular disease, hypertension, and diabetes, are linked to diet. Overweight and obesity in adults increase blood pressure and cholesterol levels, and increase the risk of developing type 2 diabetes, heart disease, and gallstones (Field et al. 2001). Overweight children and teenagers are also at greater risk for developing type 2 diabetes and risk factors for heart disease at an earlier age, though several decades may pass for the effects of the present childhood obesity epidemic to manifest themselves as health problems in adults (Kelsey et al. 2014).

Lack of physical activity is likewise associated with a number of conditions, including type 2 diabetes, overweight and obesity, cardiovascular disease, and certain cancers (Kesaniemi et al. 2001; Rankinen and Bouchard 2002). In 2010, only about 65% of adults and 17% of high school students reported being physically active (Centers for Disease Control and Prevention 2010).

COSTS OF OVERWEIGHT AND OBESITY

Escalating rates of obesity in the United States have resulted in higher direct and indirect economic costs. Direct medical costs include prevention, diagnosis, and treatment related to obesity. Indirect costs are further subdivided into morbidity and mortality costs. Morbidity costs represent lost income from reduced productivity, restricted physical activity, absenteeism, and bed days. Mortality costs encompass lost future income due to premature death (Lehnert et al. 2013).

Using the 1998 and 2006 Medical Expenditure Panel Survey (MEPS) and the National Health Expenditure Accounts (NHEA) estimates, Finkelstein et al. (2009) computed per capita and total medical spending attributable to both overweight (BMI of 25.0–29.9 kg/m^2) and obesity (BMI $\geq$ 30.0 kg/m^2). In 2006, obese persons had per capita medical spending that was $1429 (41.5%) more than spending for healthy-weight individuals. Annual obesity-attributable medical spending ranged from $86 billion (MEPS data) to $147 billion (NHEA data), with 9.1% of medical spending for the US adult population attributable to obesity. Private insurers finance the majority of the overweight- and obesity-attributable medical spending, though the amount spent by the public sector (via Medicare and Medicaid) remains substantial (Finkelstein et al. 2009). Tsai et al.'s (2011) review of the literature, with its finding that 5.0–10% of health spending in the United States is attributable to overweight and obesity, essentially corroborates Finkelstein et al.'s figure of 9.1%.

Obesity-attributable healthcare costs are not confined to a single point in time but rather persist over a lifetime due to increased risk of disease and treatment. Finkelstein et al. (2008) estimate that, for a 20-year-old with a BMI between 30 and 34.9 kg/m², lifetime healthcare costs attributable to obesity range from $5340 for black women to $21,500 for white women. For 20-year-olds with a BMI > 35 kg/m², lifetime costs range from $14,580 for black men to $29,460 for white women (Finkelstein et al. 2008). Yet rising healthcare costs are not the only economic burdens associated with increased obesity prevalence. Wolf and Colditz observe that "indirect costs have a greater effect at the individual and societal levels because they reflect the value of lost health and vitality caused by morbidity" (Wolf and Colditz 1996). In a later study, Wolf notes that roughly 27% of the labor force in the United States has a BMI ≥ 29 kg/m². She cites numerous studies that evaluated decreased productivity (days missed due to illness), increased restricted activity, and impact on long-term disability due to obesity and concludes, "The evidence is quite strong that obesity impacts productivity and potentially all indirect morbidity outcomes" (Wolf 2002).

A 2008 review of the literature by Trogdon et al. (2008) reveals the following indirect cost estimates for the United States:

- Costs of obesity-attributable absenteeism—time away from work due to obesity—range from $3.38 billion (approximately $79 per obese person) to $6.38 billion ($132 per obese person).
- Costs associated with lost earnings due to premature mortality are nearly 10 times larger than those associated with increased life insurance costs ($30 billion or $625 per obese person vs. $2.53 billion or $59 per obese person).
- Costs of obesity-attributable presenteeism—reduced productivity at work—are estimated at $9.1 billion (or $350 per obese employee).
- Total indirect costs attributable to obesity (including absenteeism, disability, and premature mortality) are estimated at $65.67 billion ($1627 per obese person).

However, the authors do warn that these estimates may be inflated, as it cannot be said with certainty that obesity, rather than some other factor, is the underlying cause of the increased costs (Trogdon et al. 2008).

GLOBALIZATION AND OBESITY

The obesity epidemic is not confined to the United States—it is increasing worldwide. In fact, since 1980, global obesity has more than doubled, reaching rates of more than 13% of the world's adult population in 2014 (World Health Organization 2015). Low- and middle-income countries are facing a double burden of disease, whereby the prevalence of overweight and obesity is often found to exist simultaneously with undernutrition in the same country, community, or even household. Children in low- and middle-income countries are more vulnerable to inadequate nutrition during the prenatal, infant, and early childhood years, yet are exposed to energy-dense, nutrient-poor foods that are relatively lower in cost. Coupled with reduced physical activity, these dietary patterns result in weight gain and obesity even while undernutrition remains an unresolved issue. Still, overweight and obesity are associated with more deaths worldwide than underweight. Most of the world's population live in countries where overweight and obesity lead to higher mortality rates than underweight (World Health Organization 2015).

The World Health Organization (WHO) estimates that 36 million of the 57 million deaths (63%) that occurred globally in 2008 were due to noncommunicable disease (NCD), including cardiovascular disease, cancer, chronic respiratory disease, and diabetes caused by tobacco use, unhealthy diet, physical inactivity, and excessive alcohol consumption. Without changes to programs, policies, and practices, the total annual number of deaths from NCDs is projected to increase to 55 million by 2030 (World Health Organization 2013).

Indigenous cuisine and traditional food habits are being supplanted by a Westernized, energy-dense diet with its unhealthy concentration on soft drinks and meat consumption. A sharp decline in the cost of vegetable oils and sugar has put them in direct competition with cereals as the least expensive food ingredients worldwide. This in turn has reduced the proportion of the diet derived from grain and grain products and greatly increased world average energy consumption of sugar and oil, although this increase is not evenly distributed throughout the world's population. Taken together, this transition towards foods of animal origin, increased fats, and refined foods, along with the more sedentary lifestyle that accompanies urbanization, contributes to the current global epidemics of obesity, diabetes, and cardiovascular disease. The pace of change for both diet and physical activity has accelerated to varying degrees in different regions of the world. The shift of countries and large populations into the stage of development characterized by high prevalence of these nutrition-related NCDs is known as the *nutrition transition* (Caballero and Popkin 2002; Drewnowski 2000; Popkin 2001).

Nutrition Transition and Its Repercussions

In 2001, representatives from Africa, the Mideast, Europe, and the Americas met in Bellagio, Italy, to discuss the health implications of the nutrition transition. The Bellagio Declaration, which summarizes the findings of this meeting, states that although the control and prevention of undernutrition remains a challenge in many developing countries, nutrition-related NCDs have become the main causes of disability and death (Bellagio Declaration 2002).

The WHO and many national governments also recognize that the patterns of disease throughout the developing world are changing rapidly. Changes in food systems and patterns of work and leisure, and therefore in diets and physical activity, are causing overweight, obesity, diabetes, high blood pressure, cardiovascular disease (including stroke), and increasingly cancer, even in the poorest countries. Malnutrition early in life, followed by inappropriate diets and physical inactivity in childhood and adult life, increases vulnerability to chronic diseases.

In many developing countries, nutrition-related NCDs prematurely disable and kill a large proportion of economically productive people, a preventable loss of precious human capital. This includes countries where HIV/AIDS is a dominant problem. Four out of five deaths from nutrition-related NCDs occur in middle- and low-income countries. The incidence of new cases of diabetes is larger in India than in any other country, and when combined with China comprises the majority of new cases of diabetes in the world (Popkin 2002).

Low-income communities appear to be especially vulnerable to nutrition-related chronic diseases, once thought to be diseases only of affluence. The Bellagio Declaration concluded that immediate action to prevent and control nutrition-related chronic diseases is not only a public health imperative but also a political, economic, and social necessity. Successful programs integrate strategies to promote healthful diets and regular physical activity throughout life into all relevant policies and programs, including those designed to combat undernutrition. In addition, they must be multidisciplinary and include government, industry, the health professions, the media and civil society, and international agencies as partners. Community empowerment and action are crucial to overcome the environmental, social, and economic constraints to improvement in dietary quality and reduction of a sedentary lifestyle.

Successful programs in a few developed countries such as Finland and Norway have demonstrated that chronic diseases are preventable. Programs in developing countries include massive community participation in physical activity encouraged by *Agita São Paulo* in Brazil, protection of the traditional low-fat/high-vegetable diet in South Korea through strong support from home economics and dietetic professionals and infrastructure, selective price policies promoting consumption of soy products in China, and development of food-based dietary guidelines in several countries based on local disease patterns and available foods. School-based programs to promote healthy diets and physical activity provide additional opportunities for early prevention, aimed at protecting health over the life span. Examples include Brazil's national school food program that provides fresh, unprocessed food to school children and Thailand's national physical activity program (Bellagio Declaration 2002; Popkin 2002).

FACTORS CONTRIBUTING TO THE PROBLEM OF OBESITY

ENVIRONMENTAL DETERMINANTS OF OVERWEIGHT AND OBESITY

While it is true that overweight and obesity result from an energy imbalance caused by consuming too many calories relative to one's energy needs, body weight more realistically depends on a complex amalgam of genetics, metabolism, behavior, culture, economics, and SES. A public health perspective is most concerned with the social–ecological factors influencing individual choices that lead to overweight. There is a growing awareness that we have inadvertently created what has been described as an *obesogenic* environment, which discourages physical activity while encouraging overeating (Swinburn et al. 1999). Table 5.4 lists some of the environmental causes of obesity.

Environmental strategies include interventions that address energy intake and energy expenditure at different levels and settings throughout the built environment. Because it may take years to achieve the long-term population goal of reducing the prevalence of obesity, environmental modifications offer the best opportunity for the prevention and treatment of obesity. The Institute of Medicine (IOM) suggests these intermediate environmental goals:

- *Food access and availability.* Increase the access to and affordability of fruits and vegetables for low-income populations.
- *Opportunities for physical activity.* Increase the following: (1) availability of outlets that sell healthful foods and beverages located within walking distance of the communities they serve, (2) the number of children who can safely walk and bike to school, (3) the play and physical activity opportunities in the neighborhood, and (4) the availability and use of community recreational facilities.
- *Policies that connect energy intake and expenditure to the built environment.* Change institutional and environmental policies to support energy balance (Koplan et al. 2005).

Unfortunately, increasingly obesogenic environments, reinforced by many of the cultural changes associated with globalization, make the adoption of healthy lifestyles, especially by children and adolescents, more and more difficult. Contributors to obesogenic environments include the built environment, economic environment, US farm policy, advertising, the food environment, and school food.

Built Environment

Aspects of the environment that can potentially affect health include physical and social factors, such as housing, urban development, land use, transportation, industry, and agriculture. Environmental health refers to assessing and controlling these factors that comprise the *built environment* (Srinivasan et al. 2003).

The built environment encompasses all buildings and spaces created or modified by humans. It includes homes, neighborhoods, restaurants and food supermarkets, schools, workplaces, parks and recreation areas, greenways, business areas, and transportation systems. It extends overhead in the form of electric transmission lines, underground in the form of waste disposal sites and subway trains, and across the country in the form of highways. It includes land-use planning and policies that impact our communities in urban, rural, and suburban areas. The built environment influences obesity through food access and availability, opportunities for physical activity, and policies that support healthy eating and active lifestyles. Urban communities, particularly those of lower SES, typically have limited access to safe outdoor activities or to healthy food choices, whereas residents of suburban neighborhoods suffer from a heavy reliance on automobiles (Box 5.1).

TABLE 5.4
Environmental Causes of Obesity

Location	Environmental Factors
Home	Food access and availability • Increase in ready-made foods for meal preparation. • Limited time to cook. Opportunities for physical activity • Increased competition from attractive passive entertainment activities, such as television, smart phone, video/DVD, video/computer games, Internet. • Increase in the use of modern appliances (e.g., microwaves, dishwashers, washing machines, vacuum cleaners).
Work	Food access and availability • Employee lunchrooms and cafeterias that do not make nutritious food available. • Vending machines that are not stocked with nutritious snacks. Opportunities for physical activity • Increase in sedentary occupational lifestyles due to technology, increase in computerization. • Long work hours and commute times decrease time available for physical activity.
Public places	Food access and availability • Food courts in shopping malls. • Availability of food items in nonfood retail outlets. Opportunities for physical activity • Increase in the use of elevators, escalators, and even automatic doors.
Urban	Food access and availability • Paucity of supermarkets in low-income neighborhoods. Opportunities for physical activity • Limited open areas or recreation facilities for physical activity. Policies that connect energy intake and expenditure to the built environment • Fear of crime in urban areas.
Suburban	Policies that connect energy intake and expenditure to the built environment • Increase number of neighborhoods that depend on private automobiles for mobility. • Rise in car ownership. • Increase in driving shorter distances.
Community	Food access and availability • Unreasonably large portions of food served in restaurants. • Food outlets with low availability of low-calorie and/or nutritionally dense food items. • Relatively inexpensive food sources, such as fast food. • Fund-raising events that promote high-calorie foods, such as cookie and candy sales. • Advertising of unhealthy food items. Opportunities for physical activity • Few opportunities for physical activity in communities.
School	Food access and availability • School breakfast and lunch program meals that do not meet national standards. • Using food as a reward. • Availability of high-calorie low-nutrition competitive foods in school vending machines and on à la carte lines. Opportunities for physical activity • Low level of required physical education. Policies that connect energy intake and expenditure to the built environment • Crowded lunchrooms, short lunch period, long lunch lines. • Limited safe walking routes to school.

Source: Compiled from various sources, primarily "The Surgeon General's Call to Action to Prevent and Decrease Overweight and Obesity, 2001." Available at http://www.surgeongeneral.gov/library/calls/obesity/index.html, accessed January 20, 2015.

BOX 5.1   HEALTH AND COMMUNITY DESIGN

In their 2003 book, *Health and Community Design: The Impact of the Built Environment on Physical Activity*, L.D. Frank, P.O. Engelke, and T.L. Schmid maintain that the American iconization of the automobile has had dire consequences for the built environment, curtailing our physical and aesthetic existence.

The authors carefully explore the history and development of community design, the changing nature of physical activity in daily life, and the devastating impact of the one upon the other. In the beginning, cities grew *organically*—unplanned and as the need arose. Streets were winding and close together as befitted the primary mode of transportation: walking. Although large, rich civilizations such as the Roman Empire planned cities, their grid pattern continued to accommodate the pedestrian. More recently, as violent epidemics of typhus and cholera ripped through crowded slums, the close proximity of people to people and of homes to commerce was seen as antithetic to the public health. A belief in the benefits of space, light, and trees in combination with the advent of the automobile gave birth to the modern suburban development and changed the nature of our cities.

The authors posit the concepts of *proximity* (nearness of homes, businesses, shops, and schools to each other) and *connectivity* (ease of moving between homes, businesses, shops, and schools) in the context of the basic activities of walking and biking. They argue that reductions in proximity (for example, by zoning for single use and placing residences far from commerce) as well as decreases in connectivity (by thinking of roadways as deadly, high-speed, car-centric arteries leading to isolated residential dead ends) have made it unappealing if not impossible for inhabitants to engage in walking or biking for transport, thus eliminating much needed physical activity and contributing to obesity.

Economic Environment

An individual's food choices are naturally impacted by an individual's SES; however, the economic environment as it impacts food choices includes the larger economic situation and parameters of the country that the individual lives in, including federal and state policies regulating agriculture and advertising.

Food Insecurity: Energy Dense Food Choices and Weight

Food insecurity, as defined in 1989 by the Expert Panel of the American Institute of Nutrition, means "the limited or uncertain availability of nutritionally adequate and safe foods or limited or uncertain ability to acquire acceptable foods in socially acceptable ways" (Kendall et al. 1996; Townsend et al. 2001). Food insecurity is associated with lower food expenditures, low fruit and vegetable consumption, and lower-quality diets (Drewnowski and Darmon 2005; Drewnowski and Specter 2004). Frequency of consumption of fruit, salad, carrots, and vegetables declined significantly as food insecurity increased (Kendall et al. 1996). Some US policymakers have doubted the existence of food insecurity because of the prevalence of overweight in lower income groups (Townsend et al. 2001). Excess body weight and inadequate food supply do seem paradoxical, yet research shows that women who experience food insecurity are more likely to be overweight or obese than women who are food secure (Dinour et al. 2007; Larson and Story 2011).

Fresh fruits and vegetables are often perceived as luxury items and are not always easily accessible. As incomes diminish, households first consume less expensive foods to maintain energy intakes, but at a lower cost; and only when incomes diminished even further did energy intakes decrease (Drewnowski and Specter 2004). An important strategy used by low-income consumers is to stretch the food budget by consuming energy-dense foods (Box 5.2).

Energy-dense foods are frequently less expensive than foods that are not energy-dense, allowing for higher energy consumption at a lower cost. In other words, there is an inverse relationship between energy density (kilocalories per gram) and energy cost (kilocalories per dollar) (Drewnowski and Specter 2004). Although cost is a key predictor of dietary choice (Glanz et al. 1998), there has been little emphasis on the low economic cost of becoming obese (Drewnowski and Specter 2004). In other words, obesity may be a more likely outcome if low amounts are spent on food. For example, the Thrifty Food Plan (TFP), developed by the United States Department of Agriculture (USDA) to aid low-income householders in shopping for food, becomes more expensive when healthier, lower-fat options are included (Box 5.3).

Cost constraints reduce the proportion of energy contributed by fruits, vegetables, meat, and dairy and increase the proportion of energy contributed by cereals, added fats, and sweets. The low cost of energy-dense foods may in turn promote overconsumption. Income disparities affect diet quality more than total energy intake does (Drewnowski and Specter 2004). Nutrient intake was found to be lower for the food insecure for all nutrients except vitamin A and fat (Kendall et al. 1996).

BOX 5.2   ENERGY DENSITY: VOLUME VS. CALORIES

All foods have a certain number of calories within a given amount (volume). Some foods, such as desserts, candies, and processed foods, have a high energy density. This means that a small volume of that food has a large number of calories. For example, one cup of raisins delivers more than 400 calories.

Alternatively, some foods, such as vegetables and fruit, have a low energy density. These foods provide a larger portion size with a fewer number of calories. For example, one cup of grapes has about 82 calories.

Three factors play an important role in determining energy density: water, fiber, and fat.

- *Water.* Many fruits and vegetables are high in water, which provides volume but not calories. Grapefruit, for example, is about 90% water and has just 37 calories in half a fruit. Raw fresh carrots are about 88% water, and a medium carrot has only 25 calories.
- *Fiber.* High-fiber foods, such as vegetables, fruits, and whole grains, not only provide volume but also take longer to digest, leading to a sense of satiety for a longer period of time. For example, air-popped popcorn, a whole grain, contains only 30 calories per cup.
- *Fat.* Fat, by nature, is energy dense. As a comparison, one pat of butter contains nearly the same number of calories as two cups of raw broccoli. Choosing lower fat meats and dairy products over their higher-fat counterparts will decrease the energy density of the food.

Source: MayoClinic.com. Weight loss: feel full on fewer calories. Available at http://www.mayoclinic.org/healthy
-living/weight-loss/in-depth/weight-loss/art-20044318, accessed January 20, 2015.

BOX 5.3   THE THRIFTY FOOD PLAN

The standard Thrifty Food Plan (TFP) market basket is a low-cost meal plan developed by the USDA that demonstrates how people on a modest budget can meet minimum USDA food and nutrition recommendations. The TFP serves as the basis for market basket studies and the maximum allotment for the Supplemental Nutrition Assistance Program (SNAP, formerly Food Stamps). The TFP market baskets have been revised over time to reflect updated dietary guidance, food composition data, food habits, and food price information.

The 2006 TFP, the most recent revision as of the writing of this chapter, contains 1-week quantities of 29 food categories by age and gender. For the 2006 revision, the market baskets for each age–gender group had to meet 100% or more of the group's 1997–2005 recommended dietary allowances (RDAs) or adequate intakes (A/Is), but not exceed tolerable upper intake levels (ULs), for vitamin A, vitamin C, vitamin B6, vitamin B12, thiamin, riboflavin, niacin, calcium, phosphorus, magnesium, iron, folate, zinc, copper, and fiber. TFP market baskets also had to fall within the acceptable macronutrient distribution range (AMDR) for linoleic acid, alpha-linolenic acid, protein, carbohydrate, and total fat, as well as meet the food group intake requirements for the five major food groups (including subgroups, such as whole grains and non-juice fruit) and for oils. Additionally, recommended saturated fat and cholesterol limits were met. The 2006 TFP market baskets do not, however, meet the vitamin E and potassium recommendations for some age–gender groups, and exceed the sodium recommendation for many age–gender groups.

Source: Carlson A, Lino M, Juan W-Y, Hanson K, Basiotis PP. *Thrifty Food Plan, 2006.* CNPP-19. US Department of Agriculture, Center for Nutrition Policy and Promotion. April 2007. Available at http://www.cnpp.usda.gov/sites/default/files/usda_food_plans_cost_of_food/TFP2006Report.pdf, accessed January 20, 2015.

US Agricultural Policies

The Institute for Agriculture and Trade Policy (IATP) argues that an often overlooked but nonetheless significant contributor to obesity in the United States is the government's farm policy. Over the past five decades, while the price of fruits and vegetables has continued to rise, government support has consistently kept the price of a few commodities such as corn and soybeans low, encouraging their use as ingredients in numerous food products. Not coincidentally, these commodities fall into the dietary categories of added fats and sugars linked to obesity. Low-cost, processed foods high in added fats and sugars are often more available and more affordable than healthier choices (Box 5.4) (Schoonover and Muller 2006).

Farmers, as well as the public health sector, have been negatively affected by policies that favor the production of low-value bulk crops over those of higher value. While farmers struggle to stay in business by growing low-value grains and oilseeds, US consumers are becoming ever more dependent on imports of high-value crops. Governmental inertia supports the status quo, yet consumers have begun to seek other routes to healthier foods such as direct purchasing from farmers. Schools and workplaces are also establishing policies to supply cafeterias with fresh, local food, and food councils and farm-to-table networks are becoming more commonplace (Schoonover and Muller 2006).

Advertising

Food manufacturers spent roughly $1.79 billion on food marketing to youth in 2009, 35% of which was spent on television and 7% (a small but growing amount) on new media outlets, such as company-sponsored websites, Internet, digital, word-of-mouth, and viral marketing (Leibowitz et al.

BOX 5.4   US FOOD CONSUMPTION TRENDS

- Americans' average daily calorie intake was 400 calories higher in 2007 than in 1985 and 600 calories higher than in 1970.
- The United States is the largest corn producer in the world, with only about 20% of the total crop exported to other countries. About 4.7% of the total corn crop is used to produce high-fructose corn syrup (HFCS).
- Between 1970 and 2007, calories from corn (from corn flour, corn meal, hominy, and corn starch) increased by 191%, while added sugar intake (for cane and beet sugar, honey, syrups, and corn sweeteners) rose by 14%. Calories from corn sweeteners alone increased by 359% to 246 calories per day.
- By 2005–2006, the average American child drank 172 calories from sugar-sweetened beverage (SSB) every day, many of those sweetened with HFCS.
- The United States is also the largest producer of soybeans, producing 20.6 billion lb. of soy oil in 2008, only 7% of which was exported to other countries.
- From 1970 to 2007, average daily calories from added fats and oils rose by 69%. The leading sources of fats are soy oil (70%) and corn oil (8%).
- Fewer than 10% of Americans consume recommended levels of fruits and vegetables. To meet recommended levels, Americans would need to increase daily consumption of fruit by 132% and vegetables by 31%.
- Yet, the US food system supplies 24% fewer servings per person than the recommended five daily vegetable servings (based on a 2000 calorie diet). More specifically, the United States produces only half of the recommended servings of dark green vegetables, one-third of the orange vegetables, and one-quarter of the recommended legumes.

Source: Wallinga D. Agricultural policy and childhood obesity: A food systems and public health commentary. *Health Aff.* 2010;29(3):405–10.

2012). Food product categories with the highest advertising intensity tend to be highly processed and expensively packaged items that are overconsumed in the United States relative to federal dietary recommendations, such as fast food, sweetened beverages, and candy and sweet snacks, as illustrated in Table 5.5 (Harris et al. 2010; Leibowitz et al. 2012).

Television Advertising Targeting Children

An examination of data on 13,000 children who participated in the National Health Examination Survey (NHES, a precursor to NHANES) found that among 12- to 17-year-olds, the prevalence of obesity increased by 2% for each additional hour of television viewed (Dietz and Gortmaker 1985). The authors suggest that 29% of the cases of obesity could be prevented by reducing television viewing to less than one hour per week (Dietz and Gortmaker 1993). Similarly, an analysis of NHANES III (1988–1994) data indicates that among 8- and 16-year-old youth, those who watched the most television had higher BMIs than those who watched less. The prevalence of obesity is lowest among children watching one or fewer hours of television a day, and highest among those watching four or more hours of television a day (Crespo et al. 2001).

Although increased television viewing is associated with increased BMI in children (Proctor et al. 2003) and altering this behavior affects weight gain (Gortmaker et al. 1999; Robinson 1999), there is no incontrovertible evidence that watching television commercials in particular causes pediatric obesity (Robinson 1998). Nevertheless, children are the target of intense and aggressive food marketing

TABLE 5.5

Youth (Ages 2–17)-Directed Marketing Expenditures by Food Manufacturers, 2009

Product Category	$ Thousands	Percentage Share
Restaurant foods	714,298	40.0%
Carbonated beverages	395,128	22.1%
Breakfast cereal	186,085	10.4%
Snack foods	123,285	6.9%
Juice and noncarbonated beverages	121,156	6.8%
Candy/frozen desserts	79,006	4.4%
Dairy products	78,457	4.4%
Prepared foods and meals	65,987	3.7%
Baked goods	16,893	0.9%
Fruits and vegetables	7160	0.4%
Total	1,787,455	100.0%

Source: Leibowitz J et al., A review of food marketing to children and adolescents: Follow-up report. Federal Trade Commission. December 2012. Available at: http://www.ftc.gov/sites/default/files/documents/reports/review-food-marketing-children-and-adolescents-follow-report/121221foodmarketingreport.pdf, accessed January 20, 2015.

and advertising efforts, and television advertising is the most prevalent form of food and beverage marketing to children (Leibowitz et al. 2012). Low-income children are exposed to the most advertising because they watch more television than their more affluent counterparts (Koplan et al. 2005).

A review of the research on the role of media in childhood obesity indicates that television food advertisements influence the food choices children make (Kaiser Family Foundation 2004). The amount of time children spend watching television has been shown to be a significant predictor of how often they request products in the grocery store, and as many as three-quarters of these requests were for products seen in television advertisements. In addition, preschoolers preferred specific foods that appeared in a video they were shown as compared to children in a control group who had not seen the video (Borzekowski and Robinson 2001). Despite these findings, exactly how media contributes to childhood obesity has not been conclusively documented. Several mechanisms have been proposed, such as (1) increased sedentary activity and displacement of physical activities; (2) unhealthy eating practices learned from television programs and advertisements for unhealthy foods; (3) increased snacking behaviors during viewing time; and (4) interference with normal sleep patterns (Council on Communications and Media 2011). The likely main mechanism may be through children's exposure to billions of dollars' worth of food advertising and marketing (Kaiser Family Foundation 2004).

New Media Advertising Targeting Children

Between 2006 and 2009, food companies increased spending by 50% to reach youth through new media forms, such as online display advertising, food company websites (including *advergames*), mobile advertising, and viral marketing (Leibowitz et al. 2012). These tactics are a growing area of concern, given that as of fall 2013, 76% of children 8 years and under have a computer in their household, and 69% live in a house with high-speed Internet access. In addition, 72% of children 8 and under have used a *smart* mobile device, such as a smartphone or tablet, for playing games, watching videos, or using apps (Rideout 2013).

Research in the area of food marketing using new media outlets is still developing, though studies have documented the content and tactics used to market to children in this way (Henry and Story 2009; Montgomery and Chester 2009; Weber et al. 2006). For example, analysis of 130 food and beverage brand websites reveals that 62 (48%) feature a *designated children's area* within two links of the brand's home page (Weber et al. 2006). Yet only 8 of the 62 brands with a designated children's area on their website meet a full set of nutrition criteria developed by the National Alliance for Nutrition and Activity (NANA) (Center for Science in the Public Interest, http://www.cspinet.org/nutritionpolicy/nana.html). Between July 2009 and June 2010, more than 3 billion display advertisements for food and beverages were viewed on popular children's websites. Although three-quarters of the advertisements promoted brands identified by food companies as healthier dietary choices, 84% of these ads nonetheless promoted foods high in fat, sugar, and sodium (Ustjanauskas et al., http://www.yaleruddcenter.org/resources/upload/docs/what/advertising/banner_ads_ijpo_7.13.pdf).

Food Environment

The types of foods available to an individual at home, at school, at work, or in one's neighborhood comprise the food environment. Availability of food is affected by both accessibility and affordability.

Food Away from Home

Americans are eating more meals away from home (43.1% in 2012) (Economic Research Service and US Department of Agriculture 2013), and eating frequently in restaurants is one of the behaviors associated with poor diet quality and obesity (Binkley et al. 2000; Bowman and Vinyard 2004; French et al. 2000; Ma et al. 2003; Mancino et al. 2010; McCrory et al. 1999; Todd et al. 2010).

- The share of total food expenditure that Americans spend on food away from home (FAFH) has nearly doubled from 27.7% in 1962 to 49.5% in 2012 (US Department of Agriculture, http://www.ers.usda.gov/data-products/food-expenditures.aspx#.U3zzpy8hkzw).
- The number of fast-food restaurants in the United States doubled between 1997 and 2006, while the number of full-service restaurants remained relatively constant. In 2006, fast-food restaurants accounted for nearly 30% of all restaurants, compared to 17% in 1997 (Powell et al. 2007).
- Between 1977–1978 and 2005–2008, consumption of FAFH increased from 17.7% to 31.6% of total calories (Lin and Guthrie 2012).
- Compared to home-cooked foods, foods eaten away from home are calorically denser (Variam 2005). FAFH meals and snacks contain more calories per eating occasion. FAFH is higher in total fat, saturated fat, cholesterol, and sodium on a per-calorie basis than at-home food. Conversely, FAFH contains less dietary fiber and calcium on a per-calorie basis than at-home food (Lin and Guthrie 2012).

Portion Sizes

The size of food portions has increased over time and exceeds federal standards as defined by the USDA in MyPlate and the Food and Drug Administration (FDA) for food labels. (See US Department of Health and Human Services, NIH, Portion Distortion at http://www.nhlbi.nih.gov/health/public/heart/obesity/wecan/eat-right/portion-distortion.htm.) Larger portions contain more calories and simultaneously encourage people to eat more (Young and Nestle 2002).

In 1916, Coca Cola came in 6.5 oz. bottles. By the 1950s, 10 and 12 oz. *king-sized* bottles were available; however, the 6.5 oz. size still accounted for 80% of sales. Currently, soft drinks marketed for individual consumption come for the most part in 20 and 32 oz. bottles. The 20 oz. size has

TABLE 5.6
Portion Size Inflation

Food	Portion Size in 1960	Portion Size in 2000
Bagel	2–3 oz.	4–6 oz.
Muffin	2–3 oz.	5–7 oz.
Coca-Cola, bottle	6.5 fl. oz.	20 fl. oz.
Chocolate bar	1 oz.	1.5–8 oz.
Potato chips, bag	1 oz.	2–4 oz.
McDonald's hamburger	1.5 oz.	1.5–8 oz.
McDonald's soda	7 fl. oz.	12–42 fl. oz.
McDonald's French fries	2.4 oz.	2.4–7.1 oz.
Pasta entrée	1.5 cups	3 cups
Beer, can	12 fl. oz.	12–24 fl. oz.

Source: Young L. *The Portion Teller.* New York: Morgan Road Books; 2005, p 9.

replaced the 12 oz. size in vending machines and at convenience stores. This portion size inflation is pervasive, as illustrated in Table 5.6. An analysis of 66 restaurants showed a 12% increase in menu offerings described as *king size* or *queen size* between 1988 and 1993 (French et al. 2001). Between 1998 and 2006, national fast-food chains such as Burger King and Wendy's continued to increase food and beverage portion sizes, with *large* or *king sizes* reaching 6.9 oz. French fries, 12 ounce hamburger patties, and 42 fluid ounce fountain sodas (Young and Nestle 2007).

Analysis of nationally representative data of children and adolescents 2–18 years old from the Nationwide Food Consumption Survey (NFCS, 1977–1978), the Continuing Survey of Food Intake by Individuals (CSFII, 1994–1996 and 1998), and the pooled NHANES 2003–2004 and 2005–2006 indicates that, with the exception of desserts, portion sizes (calories/portion) of all key foods studied (salty snacks, soft drinks, fruit drinks, French fries, hamburgers, cheese-burgers, pizzas, Mexican fast foods, and hot dogs) increased significantly between 1977–1978 and 2003–2006. During this time, portion sizes of Mexican fast food increased by 48 g (149 calories/portion), pizza by 41 g (131 calories/portion), and hamburgers and cheeseburgers by 31 and 22 g (90 calories/portion), respectively. Significant portion-size increases were observed for soft drinks purchased from stores, restaurants, and fast-food restaurants; pizza purchased from stores and fast-food restaurants; and French fries purchased from fast-food restaurants (Piernas and Popkin 2011).

Snacking

Analysis of nationally representative data of adults 19 years and older from the NFCS (1977–1978), the CSFII (1989–1991 and 1994–1996), and the pooled NHANES 2003-2004 and 2005-2006 indicates that snacking prevalence over a 2-day period increased from 71% in 1977 to 97% in 2003–2006. The number of snacking occasions increased by about one additional snack during this time, and the percentage of total energy intake from snacking occasions increased from 18% to 24% (Piernas and Popkin 2010a). Similar trends in snacking have been found in children (Piernas and Popkin 2010b).

School Food: Federal Programs

In the latter half of the twentieth century, the federal government developed and expanded a set of measures to combat the problems of domestic hunger and malnutrition. Congress passed the National School Lunch Act in 1946 (now known as the Richard B. Russell National School Lunch

Act) as a measure of national security, to safeguard the health and well-being of the nation's children, and to encourage the domestic consumption of nutritious agricultural commodities. The bill made permanent the National School Lunch Program (NSLP), under which all students receive low-cost lunches and low-income students receive them at reduced or no cost. The School Breakfast Program (SBP) began as a pilot program in 1966 and was expanded into a permanent program in 1975.

School breakfasts must provide, on average over each school week, at least one-fourth of the daily RDAs for protein, iron, calcium, and vitamins A and C. Lunches must provide, on average over each school week, at least one-third of the daily RDAs of these nutrients. Local schools make the choice of which foods to serve and how the foods are prepared and presented.

Since the inception of school lunch in 1946, Congress has improved the child school nutrition program to better serve children and families and adjust to changes in nutrition recommendations and guidelines, families, workplaces, schools, and communities. The Healthy Meals for Children Act (Public Law 104–149 §1, May 29, 1996, 110 Stat. 1379), effective 1997, established that to be eligible for federal reimbursement by the USDA, schools must serve breakfasts and lunches consistent with the applicable recommendations of the most recent *Dietary Guidelines for Americans* (see Chapters 9 and 11).

Through Team Nutrition, USDA (Food and Nutrition Service, http://www.fns.usda.gov/tn/team -nutrition) provides schools with technical training and assistance to help school service personnel prepare meals that meet federal guidelines. Team Nutrition also offers nutrition education to help children understand the link between diet and health.

The Child Nutrition and WIC Reauthorization Act of 2004 (Public Law 108-265) requires each local education authority to establish a School Wellness Policy for participating schools. The policy must include goals for nutrition education, physical activity, and other school-based activities designed to promote health and prevent obesity (see Chapter 11).

Most recently, the Healthy, Hunger-Free Kids Act of 2010 (HHFKA) (Public Law 111-296) requires the USDA to update the meal patterns and nutrition standards for school lunches and breakfasts to reflect the recommendations issued by the Food and Nutrition Board of the National Research Council of the National Academies of Science, part of the IOM (US Government Publishing Office 2010). Table 5.7 summarizes many of the resultant shifts made to the school lunch and breakfast meal patterns, the first major changes made to school meals in 15 years.

Competitive Food in Schools

Historically, most schools have allowed food to be sold outside of the official food service, through à la carte sales in school cafeterias or through other outlets, such as vending machines, school stores, snack bars, and fund raisers. These *competitive foods* have been criticized as providing many children with unneeded calories (from fat and sugar), supplanting the more nutritionally dense foods available through the federal food programs.

Although they have long been a source of concern to nutritionists, supporters contend that competitive foods, particularly those sold through vending machines, generate significant revenues that fund special activities or items not covered in a school's budget. Beverage companies, which offer bonuses to schools for signing contracts that permit exclusive use of their particular brand, have been a major source of funds for school districts. The schools receive cash and other incentives, and the beverage company receives the right to sell sodas in vending machines and to advertise on scoreboards, in hallways, on book covers, and other places. Such *pouring rights* have been available on college campuses since the early 1990s and have more recently appeared in schools for children of all ages (Nestle 2000).

During the school year 2009–2010, 13% of elementary schools, 67% of middle schools, and 85% of high schools made vending machines available to students (US Department of Agriculture et al. 2012). On an average school week, schools collected $925 per 1000 students in revenue from sales

TABLE 5.7

Previous and HHFKA Regulatory Requirements for NSLP and SBP Meal Patterns

Food Group	Previous Requirements K-12	Requirements K-12 July 1, 2012
	National School Lunch Program Meal Pattern	
Fruits and vegetables	1/2–3/4 cup fruits and vegetables combined per day	3/4–1 cup vegetables and 1/2–1 cup fruits per day
	No specifications on vegetable subgroup	Weekly requirement for • Dark green. • Red/orange. • Beans/peas (legumes). • Starchy. • Other (defined by 2010 Dietary Guidelines).
Meat/meat alternate	1.5–2 oz. eq. (daily minimum)	Daily minimum and weekly ranges: • Grades K-5: 1 oz. eq. min daily (8–10 oz. weekly). • Grades 6–8: 1 oz. eq. min daily (9–10 oz. weekly). • Grades 9–12: 2 oz. eq. min daily (10–12 oz. weekly).
Grains	8 servings per week (minimum of 1 serving per day)	Daily minimum and weekly ranges: • Grades K-5: 1 oz. eq. min daily (8–9 oz. weekly). • Grades 6–8: 1 oz. eq. min daily (8–10 oz. weekly). • Grades 9–12: 2 oz. eq. min daily (10–12 oz. weekly).
Whole grains	Encouraged	At least half of grains must be whole grain-rich beginning July 1, 2012. Beginning July 1, 2014, all grains must be whole-grain rich.
Milk	1 cup	1 cup
	Variety of fat contents allowed; flavor not restricted	Must be fat-free (unflavored/flavored) or 1% low fat (unflavored)
Calories	Minimum only	Minimum and maximum
	Traditional menu planning: • Grades K-3: 633. • Grades 4–12: 785. • Optional grades 7–12: 825. Enhanced or nutrient-based menu planning: • Grades K-6: 664. • Grades 7–12: 825. • Optional grades K-3: 633.	• Grades K-5: 550–650. • Grades 6–8: 600–700. • Grades 9–12: 750–850.
	School Breakfast Program Meal Pattern	
Fruit	1/2 cup per day (vegetable substitution allowed)	1 cup per day (vegetable substitution allowed)
Grains and meat/meat alternate	2 grains or 2 meat/meat alternates or 1 of each per day	Daily minimum and weekly ranges for grains: • Grades K-5: 1 oz. eq. min daily (7–10 oz. weekly). • Grades 6–8: 1 oz. eq. min daily (8–10 oz. weekly). • Grades 9–12: 1 oz. eq. min daily (9–10 oz. weekly).
Whole grains	Encouraged	At least half of grains must be whole grain-rich beginning July 1, 2013. Beginning July 1, 2014, all grains must be whole-grain rich.

(Continued)

TABLE 5.7 (CONTINUED)
Previous and HHFKA Regulatory Requirements for NSLP and SBP Meal Patterns

Food Group	Previous Requirements K-12	Requirements K-12 July 1, 2012
	School Breakfast Program Meal Pattern	
Milk	1 cup	1 cup
	Variety of fat contents allowed; flavor not restricted	Must be fat-free (unflavored/flavored) or 1% low fat (unflavored)
Calories	Minimum only	Minimum and maximum
	• Grades K-12: 554.	• Grades K-5: 350–500.
	• Optional grades 7–12: 774.	• Grades 6–8: 400–550.
	Nutrient-based menu planning:	• Grades 9–12: 450–600.
	• Grades K-12: 554.	
	• Optional grades 7–12: 618.	

Source: Food and Nutrition Service. United States Department of Agriculture. Comparison of Previous and Current Regulatory Requirements under Final Rule "Nutrition Standards in the National School Lunch and School Breakfast Programs" (published January 26, 2012). Available at http://www.gpo.gov/fdsys/pkg/FR-2012-01-26/pdf/2012-1010.pdf, accessed January 20, 2015.

of à la carte foods and beverages, though the amounts were more than three times higher in middle and high schools compared to elementary schools ($1618 and $1647 per 1000 students, respectively, vs. $495 per 1000 students). Overall, vending machines in middle schools allocated more space to 100% juice and water than to other beverages, such as carbonated sodas, energy/sports drinks, juice drinks, and chocolate drinks (58% vs. 41%, respectively). In high schools, more space was allocated to other beverages than to 100% juice and water (52% vs. 44%, respectively). Schools with snack machines allocated an average of 85% of the available space to snack foods (such as snack chips, candy, and crackers) compared to baked goods and other types of foods (US Department of Agriculture et al. 2012).

Studies indicate that the availability and consumption of competitive foods are associated with increased calorie, fat, and sugar consumption and decreased fruit, vegetable, and milk intake (Fried and Simon 2007; Story et al. 2009). Additionally, studies suggest that exposure to competitive food is associated with higher BMIs in adolescents (Fox et al. 2009; Story et al. 2009). Preliminary small-scale studies suggest that the presence of competitive foods in schools is related to a decrease in fruit and vegetable consumption and an increase in calories obtained from fat. A small study examining the behaviors of 598 seventh-grade students found that, on average, students in schools with à la carte programs consumed fewer fruits and vegetables and obtained more of their daily calories from total fat and saturated fat than students in schools without à la carte programs (Kubik et al. 2003). In another study, changes in food and beverage consumption were examined over time for two student cohorts of a total of 594 middle school students. In year 1, fourth graders in the experimental group had access only to the school lunch program but gained snack bar access in year 2 when they transitioned to the fifth grade. Compared to the control group, average consumption of fruits, regular vegetables, and milk decreased, and average consumption of high-fat vegetables and sweetened beverages increased for students moving from fourth to fifth grade. These middle school students who gained access to school snack bars consumed fewer healthy foods compared with the previous school year when they were in elementary school and had access only to lunch meals served at school. Snack bar access may have played a role in some of the observed changes (Cullen and Zakeri 2004).

In response to concerns over the school food environment, including competitive foods, the Child Nutrition and WIC Reauthorization Act of 2004 (Public Law 108-265) requires school districts to establish their own local wellness policies regarding competitive foods, among other things (see Chapter 11). In the years since, several large school districts—including the New York City Department of Education and the Los Angeles Board of Education—have enacted policies to restrict competitive foods beyond federal regulations, which until July 1, 2014 only restricted foods of minimal nutritional value (FMNV) (Box 5.5).

Likewise, a number of individual schools across the United States have taken actions to restrict competitive foods in schools beyond federal, state, and school board regulations. These actions include removing all food from vending machines except water and juice, removing soda and candy from vending machines and replacing them with juices and cereal bars, removing all vending machines selling soda and snack food, and removing sodas and other nutrient-poor foods from vending machines. Yet research has found that not all local wellness policies are comprehensive or powerful, as many districts recommend or encourage, rather than require, competitive food guidelines (Metos and Nanney 2007; Probart et al. 2008; School Nutrition Association and School Nutrition Foundation 2007). School districts that do mandate stricter guidelines may actually be maintaining the status quo by repeating regulations already required by other entities, such as a State Board of Education (Metos and Nanney 2007; Probart et al. 2008).

HHFKA provided the USDA with the authority to establish nutrition standards for competitive foods. In June 2013, the USDA published interim final rules that include minimum nutrition standards for all foods and beverages sold to students on school campuses during the school day, other than meals reimbursable under the NSLP and SBP. These nutrition standards, listed in Table 5.8, took effect on July 1, 2014. To help schools determine whether foods and beverages conform to the new standards, the Alliance for a Healthier Generation created a *Smart Snack Product Calculator*, found at https://schools.healthiergeneration.org/focus_areas/snacks_and_beverages/smart_snacks/alliance_product_calculator/. Additional resources, including background information regarding competitive foods and guidelines for implementation of nutrition standards, are available through the USDA (http://www.fns.usda.gov/school-meals/smart-snacks-school) and Team Nutrition (http://healthymeals.nal.usda.gov/smartsnacks).

BOX 5.5   FOODS OF MINIMAL NUTRITIONAL VALUE

Prior to July 1, 2014, federal regulations restricted only a subset of competitive foods—known as foods of minimal nutritional value (FMNV)—from being sold during mealtimes in food service areas. FMNV means (1) in the case of artificially sweetened foods, a food that provides less than 5% of the reference daily intake (RDI) for each of the eight specified nutrients per serving, and (2) in the case of all other foods, a food that provides less than 5% of the RDI of each of the eight specified nutrients per serving. The eight nutrients to be assessed for this purpose are protein, vitamin A, vitamin C, niacin, riboflavin, thiamine, calcium, and iron. The categories of FMNV include soda water, water ices, chewing gum, certain candies, hard candy, jellies and gums, marshmallow candies, fondant, licorice, spun candy, and candy-coated popcorn.

Source: Competitive Food Service and Standards, 7 CFR § 210.11. Revised as of June 28, 2013. Categories of Foods of Minimal Nutritional Value, 7 CFR § 210.App B. Revised as of June 28, 2013. Available at http://www.ecfr.gov/cgi-bin/text-idx?c=ecfr&rgn=div5&view=text&node=7:4.1.1.1.1&idno=7, accessed January 20, 2015.

TABLE 5.8
Nutrition Standards for Competitive Foods

Food/Nutrient	Standard	Exemptions to Standard
General requirements	To be allowed, a competitive food must 1. Meet all proposed nutrient standards (see below); and 2. Be a grain product with at least 50% whole grains by weight or have whole grains as first ingredient*; or 3. Have as first ingredient* a nongrain food group: fruits, vegetables, dairy, or protein foods (meat, beans, eggs, poultry, seafood, nuts, etc.); or 4. Be a combination food containing at least ¼ cup fruits and/or vegetables; or 5. Contain 10% of the daily value of calcium, potassium, vitamin D, or dietary fiber. (As of July 1, 2016, this criterion may not be used to qualify as a competitive food.) *If water is the first ingredient, the second ingredient must be an item from 2–4 above.	• Fresh fruits and vegetables with no added ingredients except water. • Canned and frozen fruits with no added ingredients except water, or packed in 100% juice, extra light syrup, or light syrup. • Canned vegetables with no added ingredients except water or those containing a small amount of sugar for processing purposes to maintain vegetable quality and structure.
NSLP/SBP entrée items sold à la carte	Any entrée item offered as part of the NSLP or SBP is exempt from all competitive food standards *if* it is sold as a competitive food on the day of service or the day after service in the lunch or breakfast program.	
Total fats	≤35% calories from total fat as served	• Reduced fat cheese (including part-skim mozzarella). • Nuts and seeds and nut/seed butters. • Products consisting of only dried fruit with nuts and/or seeds with no added nutritive sweeteners or fats. • Seafood with no added fat • Combination foods are *not* exempt and must meet all nutrient standards.
Saturated fats	<10% calories from saturated fat as served	• Reduced fat cheese (including part-skim mozzarella). • Nuts and seeds and nut/seed butters. • Products consisting of only dried fruit with nuts and/or seeds with no added nutritive sweeteners or fats. • Combination foods are *not* exempt and must meet all nutrient standards.
Trans fat	Zero grams of trans fat as served (≤0.5 g per portion)	

(Continued)

TABLE 5.8 (CONTINUED)
Nutrition Standards for Competitive Foods

Food/Nutrient	Standard	Exemptions to Standard
Sugar	≤35% of weight from total sugar as served	• Dried whole fruits or vegetables (or pieces); and dehydrated fruits or vegetables with no added nutritive sweeteners. • Dried whole fruits, or pieces, with nutritive sweeteners that are required for processing and/or palatability purposes (i.e., cranberries, tart cherries, or blueberries). • Products consisting of only exempt dried fruit with nuts and/or seeds with no added nutritive sweeteners or fats.
Sodium	Snack items and side dishes sold à la carte: ≤230 mg sodium per item as served (effective July 1, 2016, the limit changes to ≤200 mg sodium per item as served, including any accompaniments) Entrée items sold à la carte: ≤480 mg sodium per item as served, including any accompaniments	
Calories	Snack items and side dishes sold à la carte: ≤200 calories per item as served, including any accompaniments Entrée items sold à la carte: ≤350 calories per item as served, including any accompaniments	Entrée items served as an NSLP or SBP entrée are exempt on the day of or day after service in the program meal
Accompaniments	Use of accompaniments is limited when competitive food is sold to students in school. The accompaniment must be included in the nutrient profile as part of the food item served and meet all proposed standards	
Caffeine	Elementary and middle school: foods and beverages must be caffeine-free with the exception of trace amounts of naturally occurring caffeine substances High school: foods and beverages may contain caffeine	
Beverages	Elementary school • Plain water or plain carbonated water (no size limit). • Low-fat milk, unflavored (≤8 fl. oz.). • Nonfat milk, flavored or unflavored (≤8 fl. oz.), including nutritionally equivalent milk alternatives as permitted by school meal requirements. • 100% fruit/vegetable juice (≤8 fl. oz.). • 100% fruit/vegetable juice diluted with water (with or without carbonation), and no added sweeteners (≤8 fl. oz.)	

(Continued)

TABLE 5.8 (CONTINUED)
Nutrition Standards for Competitive Foods

Food/Nutrient	Standard	Exemptions to Standard
Beverages	Middle school	

Middle school
- Plain water or plain carbonated water (no size limit).
- Low-fat milk, unflavored (≤12 fl. oz.).
- Nonfat milk, flavored or unflavored (≤12 fl. oz.), including nutritionally equivalent milk alternatives as permitted by school meal requirements.
- 100% fruit/vegetable juice (≤12 fl. oz.).
- 100% fruit/vegetable juice diluted with water (with or without carbonation), and no added sweeteners (≤12 fl. oz.).

High school
- Plain water or plain carbonated water (no size limit).
- Low-fat milk, unflavored (≤12 fl. oz.).
- Nonfat milk, flavored or unflavored (≤12 fl. oz.), including nutritionally equivalent milk alternatives as permitted by school meal requirements.
- 100% fruit/vegetable juice (≤12 fl. oz.).
- 100% fruit/vegetable juice diluted with water (with or without carbonation), and no added sweeteners (≤12 fl. oz.).
- Other flavored and/or carbonated beverages (≤20 fl. oz.) that are labeled to contain ≤5 calories per 8 fl. oz., or ≤10 calories per 20 fl. oz.
- Other flavored and/or carbonated beverages (≤12 fl. oz.) that are labeled to contain ≤40 calories per 8 fl. oz., or ≤60 calories per 12 fl. oz.

Source: US Department of Agriculture, Food and Nutrition Service. Nutrition Standards for All Foods Sold in School. Available at http://www.fns.usda.gov/sites/default/files/allfoods_summarychart.pdf, accessed February 2, 2015.

OBESITY PREVENTION

Ideally, the treatment of obesity should parallel its prevention: "increasing physical activity, improving diet, then sustaining these lifestyle changes can reduce both body weight and risk of diabetes" (Mokdad et al. 2003). This is, of course, easier said than done. Several studies have found that only a small fraction of the US population adheres to a healthy lifestyle. Reeves and Rafferty defined four healthy lifestyle characteristics (HLC)—nonsmoking, healthy weight, fruit and vegetable consumption, and regular physical activity—that together serve as a single healthy lifestyle indicator. Using data from the 2000 BRFSS, they determined that only 3.0% of US adults practiced all four healthful lifestyle behaviors (Reeves and Rafferty 2005). A subsequent study by King et al., using five HLCs (nonsmoking, healthy weight, fruit and vegetable consumption, regular physical activity, and moderate alcohol consumption), compared data from NHANES III (1988–1994) and NHANES 2001–2006 (Box 5.6). They found that, over the 18-year time span, adherence to all five HLCs significantly declined from 15% to 8% ($p < .05$) among adults aged 40–74 years. The authors conclude, "These findings should provide new motivation for an increasing commitment to promoting healthy lifestyles for the public good" (King et al. 2009).

BOX 5.6   ACTIVE LIVING BY DESIGN

In 2001, the Robert Wood Johnson Foundation (RWJF) created the Active Living by Design Program to support comprehensive approaches that encourage people to be more physically active in their daily lives. The RWJF provided each of 25 diverse communities across the United States with 5-year $200,000 grants to increase *active living* (a way of life that integrates physical activity into daily routines). In addition to the grant, each community received technical assistance to address community design, land use, transportation, architecture, trails, parks, and other issues that influence healthier lifestyles. The communities developed interdisciplinary partnerships to collaborate among a variety of organizations in public health and other disciplines, such as city planning, transportation, architecture, recreation, crime prevention, traffic safety and education, as well as key groups concentrating on land use, public transit, nonmotorized travel, public spaces, parks, trails, and architectural practices that advance physical activity. Each grantee was expected to establish innovative approaches to increase physical activity through community design and communications strategies.

Evaluation of the 8-year program indicates that community partnerships spearheaded or contributed to 188 projects, 115 policies, and 115 new or expanded programs that create, support, or encourage active living. Projects most commonly focused on street improvements to support walking and bicycle travel, such as new crosswalks, sidewalks, and bike lanes and parking. Policies included local ordinances, policies, or guidelines that promote walking and bicycling; funding for pedestrian and bike transportation enhancements; and creation of local active living advisory boards. Examples of programs include walking clubs, programs encouraging children to walk or bike to school, and bicycle recycling and education.[1]

Two communities, Somerville, Massachusetts, and Columbia, Missouri, received additional awards to evaluate behavior change as a result of their Active Living by Design interventions. In Somerville, high school students were 1.61 times more likely, and adult residents 2.36 times more likely, to report meeting physical activity guidelines at the end of the intervention in 2008 compared to baseline in 2002. In addition, when compared to a control community (Everett, Massachusetts), Somerville adults were 1.1 times more likely than Everett adults to report meeting physical activity guidelines in 2008.[2] In Columbia, there were greater bicyclist counts in July 2009 compared to either 2007 or 2008, and increased pedestrian counts in July 2009 and October 2009 compared to 2007 and 2008. The authors note that as the increased physical activity behavior was seen in 2009, 6 years after the initiation of the Active Living by Design intervention, "behavior change may occur slowly following an intervention."[3]

Though Active Living by Design funding ended in 2008, as of April 2011, many partnerships remained active, though some with expanded or modified focus. In communities where the partnership ended, the new policies, infrastructure, and norms developed as a result of the partnership continued to encourage and support physical activity. The lessons learned from the Active Living by Design Program helped inform a new, $33 million RWJF program called Healthy Kids, Healthy Communities. Launched in 2008, the program's focus is to expand local opportunities for physical activity and access to healthy, affordable foods.[1]

Source: [1]Data from Robert Wood Johnson Foundation. Executive Summary: Active Living by Design. Last updated February 4, 2013, available at http://www.rwjf.org/content/dam/farm/reports/program_results_reports/2013/rwjf71184/subassets/rwjf71184_1, accessed January 20, 2015.
[2]Data from Chomitz VR, McDonald JC, Aske DB et al. Evaluation results from an active living intervention in Somerville, Massachusetts. *Am J Prev Med.* 2012;43(5S4):S367–S378.
[3]Data from Sayers SP, LeMaster JW, Thomas IM, Petroski GF, Ge B. Bike, walk, and wheel: A way of life in Columbia, Missouri, revisited. *Am J Prev Med.* 2012;43(5S4):S379–S383.

DIETING: INDIVIDUAL PREVENTION

With nearly one-half of adults trying to lose weight over the course of a year (QuickStats 2008), Americans seek the one perfect diet. Of these, the low-carbohydrate, high-fat diet popularized by Dr. Robert Atkins had a stunning run of popularity. Why? The basic philosophy of the diet—that fat calories do not matter and that carbohydrates are bad—contradicts the tenets of the less glamorous, hard-working, high-carbohydrate diet where weight loss can only occur if caloric expenditure exceeds intake (Blackburn et al. 2001; Tapper-Gardzina et al. 2002). True, the fantasy low-carbohydrate, high-fat diet of steak and bacon results in fairly rapid, early weight loss; however, by 12 months there is no appreciable difference in results (Blackburn et al. 2001). In its favor, the low-carbohydrate diet raises high-density lipoprotein (HDL) and lowers triglyceride levels but does so at the expense of the rest of the lipoprotein profile (Foster et al. 2003). Through the alchemy of ketosis, the low-carbohydrate advocates claim excess fat *melts* away. Unfortunately, the long-term effects of ketosis—such as possible kidney and liver damage—are not resolved. Similar discord arises in discussions of insulin resistance (Blackburn et al. 2001).

No weight-loss diet is easy to adhere to. There are many well-accepted methods to reduce initial body weight by 7–10%, but long-term maintenance of that lost weight is more problematic. On average, among treatment-seeking populations, approximately one-third of lost weight is regained by 1 year; by 5 years most or all previously lost weight is regained (Tapper-Gardzina et al. 2002). Only about 20% of overweight individuals are successful at maintaining long-term weight loss (defined as maintaining a 10% loss of initial body weight for at least 1 year) (Wing and Phelan 2005). An ongoing registry using a convenience sample of long-term weight loss maintainers is providing valuable information about behaviors endorsed by those with long-term success. As indicated by the National Weight Control Registry (http://www.nwcr.ws), those who achieve long-term success at weight loss often report that they engage in high levels of physical activity, consume a diet that is low in calories and fat, eat breakfast, self-monitor weight regularly, maintain a consistent eating pattern, and identify *slips* before they lead to larger regains of weight (Wing and Phelan 2005). In essence, people who are successful at losing weight and who maintain their lower weight status are always dieting (Shick et al. 1998), or so it seems to their overweight counterparts (Box 5.7).

PROPOSED OBESITY PREVENTION STRATEGIES AND POLICIES

The WHO published the following recommendations for developing strategies to reduce obesity: (Diet, Nutrition and the Prevention of Chronic Diseases 2003)

- Strategies should be comprehensive and address all major dietary and physical activity risks for chronic diseases together, alongside other risks (such as tobacco use) from a multi-sectoral perspective.
- Each country should select what will constitute the optimal mix of actions that are in accord with national capabilities, laws, and economic realities.
- Governments have a central steering role in developing strategies, ensuring that actions are implemented, and monitoring their impact over the long term.
- Ministries of health have a crucial convening role—bringing together other ministries needed for effective policy design and implementation.
- Governments need to work together with the private sector, health professional bodies, consumer groups, academics, the research community, and other nongovernmental bodies if sustained progress is to occur.
- A life-course perspective on chronic disease prevention and control is critical. This starts with maternal and child health, nutrition, and care practices, and carries through to school and workplace environments and access to preventive health and primary care, as well as community-based care for the elderly and disabled people.

BOX 5.7   STRATEGIES FOR SUCCESSFUL WEIGHT LOSS MAINTENANCE

Successful weight loss maintainers enrolled in the National Weight Control Registry (NWCR) consistently report six strategies they use to maintain their weight loss:

- *Consuming a low-calorie, low-fat diet.* It is estimated that registry members eat about 1800 calories per day, with about one-quarter of calories from fat. Registry members report consuming 2.5 meals per week in restaurants and 0.74 meals per week in fast food establishments, much less frequently than the national average.
- *Engaging in high levels of physical activity for about 1 hour per day.* Three-quarters of the respondents walk briskly every day; other activities engaged in most frequently include weight lifting, cycling, and aerobics.
- *Self-weighing on a regular basis.* Almost half of the respondents weigh themselves every day, and about a third report weighing themselves at least once a week. This frequent monitoring of weight allows these individuals to catch small weight gains and hopefully initiate corrective behavior changes.
- *Consuming breakfast daily.* Over three-quarters of registry members report eating breakfast daily, and only 4% report never eating breakfast.
- *Maintaining a consistent diet.* Registry members who report consuming a consistent diet over the course of a full week are 1.5 times more likely to maintain their weight within 5 lb. than respondents who diet more strictly on weekdays compared to weekends. Similarly, respondents who allow themselves more dietary flexibility on holidays are more likely to regain weight.
- *Catching slips before they turn into larger relapses.* Only about one-in-ten registry members report recovering from even minor weight gains of 1–2 kg (2.2–4.4 lb.). Those that regain the least amount of weight appear most likely to reverse the relapse.

Source: Wing RR, Phelan S. Long-term weight loss maintenance. *Am J Clin Nutr.* 2005;82(suppl):222S–5S.

- Strategies should explicitly address equality and diminish disparities; they should focus on the needs of the poorest communities and population groups. This requires a strong role for government.
- Strategies should be gender sensitive, as women generally make decisions about household nutrition.

In the United States, the CDC has also developed resource guides for nutrition (Centers for Disease Control and Prevention 2011a), physical activity (Centers for Disease Control and Prevention 2011b), and breastfeeding interventions (Centers for Disease Control and Prevention 2013) to prevent and control obesity and other chronic diseases. Each guide includes a number of strategies to improving fruit and vegetable consumption, increasing physical activity, and supporting breastfeeding mothers and babies, respectively (Box 5.8).

In the following, we describe various obesity prevention strategies and policies proposed in the United States.

Regulating Advertising to Children

Legislators, consumer advocates, and health groups have focused on the significant number of food advertisements seen by children. According to a 2007 report by the Kaiser Family Foundation, children ages 2–7 years view an average of 12 food advertisements a day on television, and those

BOX 5.8 CDC STRATEGIES TO PREVENT OBESITY
AND OTHER CHRONIC DISEASES

Increasing Fruit and Vegetable Access[1]
- Promote food policy councils at the state and local levels.
- Improve access to retail stores that sell high-quality fruits and vegetables, or increase the availability of high-quality fruits and vegetables at retail stores in underserved areas.
- Start or expand farm-to-institution programs in schools, hospitals, workplaces, etc.
- Start or expand farmers' markets in all settings.
- Start or expand community-supported agriculture programs in all settings.
- Ensure access to fruits and vegetables in workplace cafeterias and other food service venues.
- Ensure access to fruits and vegetables at workplace meetings and events.
- Support and promote community and home gardens.
- Establish policies to incorporate fruit and vegetable activities into schools.
- Include fruits and vegetables in emergency food programs.

Increasing Physical Activity[2]
- Community-wide campaigns.
- Point-of-decision prompts to encourage stair use.
- Individually adapted health behavior change programs.
- Enhanced school-based physical education.
- Social support interventions in community settings.
- Creation of or enhanced access to places for physical activity combined with informational outreach activities.
- Street-scale urban design and land-use policies.
- Community-scale urban design and land-use policies.
- Active transport to school.
- Transportation and travel policies and practices.

Increasing Breastfeeding[3]
- Maternity care practices.
- Professional education.
- Access to professional support.
- Peer support programs.
- Support for breastfeeding in the workplace.
- Support for breastfeeding in early care and education.
- Access to breastfeeding education and information.
- Social marketing.
- Addressing the marketing of infant formula.

Source: [1]Data from Centers for Disease Control and Prevention. Strategies to Prevent Obesity and Other Chronic Diseases: The CDC Guide to Strategies to Increase the Consumption of Fruits and Vegetables. Atlanta: US Department of Health and Human Services; 2011. Available at http://www.cdc.gov/obesity/downloads/fandv_2011 _web_tag508.pdf, accessed January 20, 2015.
[2]Data from Centers for Disease Control and Prevention. Strategies to Prevent Obesity and Other Chronic Diseases: The CDC Guide to Strategies to Increase Physical Activity in the Community. Atlanta: US Department of Health and Human Services; 2011, available at http://www.cdc.gov/obesity/downloads/PA_2011_WEB.pdf, accessed January 20, 2015.
[3]Data from Centers for Disease Control and Prevention. Strategies to Prevent Obesity and Other Chronic Diseases: The CDC Guide to Strategies to Support Breastfeeding Mothers and Babies. Atlanta: US Department of Health and Human Services; 2013. Available at http://www.cdc.gov/breastfeeding/pdf/BF-Guide-508.PDF, accessed January 20, 2015.

8–12 years old see 21 per day. Half of all the advertising time on children's television shows is for food. Of these, a third were for candy and snacks, over a quarter were for cereal, and one-tenth promoted fast food. Only 4% advertised dairy products and none promoted fruits and vegetables. Most advertisements were for foods that health officials and government agencies say should be limited or consumed in moderation (Gantz et al. 2007). According to the American Psychological Association (APA), children under the age of 8 are unable to critically comprehend televised advertising messages and are prone to accept advertiser messages as truthful, accurate, and unbiased, which can lead to unhealthy eating habits (Wilcox et al. 2004). As sugared cereals, candies, sweets, sodas, and snack foods are the most common products marketed to children, advertising of unhealthy food products to young children may be a variable in the current epidemic of pediatric overweight. Similarly, an IOM committee found that "Television advertising influences the food preferences, purchase requests, and diets, at least of children under age 12 years, and is associated with the increased rates of obesity among children and youth" (National Research Council 2006).

Research on children's commercial recall and product preferences confirms that advertising does typically get young consumers to buy products. A series of studies on product choices demonstrates that children not only recall content from the advertisements to which they have been exposed but also exhibit preferences for a product with as little as a single commercial exposure, a preference that is strengthened with repeated exposures. These product preferences can affect children's product purchase requests, putting pressure on parents' purchasing decisions and instigating parent–child conflicts when parents deny requests (Wilcox et al. 2004). In fact, research from food and beverage companies confirm that food marketing to kids is effective in generating *pester power* (Leibowitz et al. 2012). One company found that food advertisements and packaging were key to children asking for a food item, and 75% of parents bought a product for the first time because their child requested it (Leibowitz et al. 2012).

The American Public Health Association (APHA) has a long history of supporting legislation to limit television advertising aimed at children. For example, in 1977 it supported regulation of sugared snacks advertisements to children. Since 2003, the APHA supports congressional action to eliminate television food advertising aimed at young children (American Public Health Association 2003). At present, the Federal Communications Commission (FCC) allows 10.5 minutes of commercials to be broadcast per hour of children's television shows or digital video programming aired on weekends, and 12 minutes per hour on weekdays. These requirements apply to television broadcasters, cable operators, and satellite providers, and limitations are prorated for programs shorter than 1 hour in duration. The programming at issue for the commercial time limits is programming originally produced and aired primarily for an audience of children 12 years old and younger. The FCC also bars children's television programs from displaying an Internet website address during a show unless

- The website is substantially noncommercial and has *bona fide program-related* content.
- The website is not primarily intended for advertising or selling of products or services.
- The website's home page and linked menu pages are clearly labeled to distinguish between commercial and noncommercial sections.
- The displayed website address does not direct viewers to a page with commercial material and is not used for advertising or sales of products or services.

Furthermore, the FCC's rule barring *host selling* prohibits the characters of children's television shows (i.e., actors, animated figures, or costumed characters) from being used in commercials during or adjacent to the program featuring that character. The rule also regulates host selling on websites where the website address is displayed during a children's program (Federal Communications Commission, http://www.fcc.gov/guides/childrens-educational-television).

However, the accumulation of evidence on advertising to children is compelling enough to warrant further regulatory action by the government. APA recommends that restrictions be placed on

BOX 5.9   FIRST AMENDMENT, US CONSTITUTION

Congress shall make no law respecting an establishment of religion, or prohibiting the free exercise thereof; or abridging the freedom of speech, or of the press; or the right of the people peaceably to assemble, and to petition the Government for a redress of grievances. First Amendment rights are the foundation of democracy in the United States. They help to create an open society in which people have the ability to share and discuss differing opinions and beliefs. The First Amendment was written precisely to protect controversial and/or offensive speech and ideas (other speech and ideas would not have to be protected). It covers spoken and written words, as well as pictures, art, and other forms of expression of ideas and opinions, such as armbands and insignia. *It is a restriction on the power of government* rather than on individuals or private businesses. There are times when the government can regulate the time, place, and manner of speech, but—generally—it cannot censor the *content* of protected expression. Most advertising is considered commercial speech. Commercial speech does receive First Amendment protection, although the government may restrict commercial speech that is false, is misleading, or promotes a product, service, or conduct that is illegal. For example, broadcast media (television, radio) has been highly regulated through licenses granted by the Federal Trade Commission.

advertising to children too young to recognize its persuasive intent, a policy that would bring the United States alongside Australia, Canada, Sweden, and Great Britain, which have already adopted regulations prohibiting advertising on programs whose audiences are young children (Wilcox et al. 2004).

As expected, the advertising industry opposes any such regulation, citing its long history of self-regulation. The private organization Children's Advertising Review Unit (CARU, http://www .caru.org/guidelines/guidelines.pdf) has developed self-regulating guidelines for advertisers to follow when advertising to children. The voluntary nature of the program has drawn criticism, and the guidelines have been criticized for focusing on advertising techniques rather than the nature of the foods and beverages being promoted (Center for Science in the Public Interest, http://www .cspinet.org/new/pdf/limitingfood_marketing.pdf). First Amendment free speech protection is also frequently invoked (Box 5.9).

Industry spokespersons claim that advertising's role in preventing obesity is in adhering to the marketing principles outlined in the Children's Advertising Review Unit (CARU) guidelines for advertising directed to children under 12 years of age. They also tout activities such as their childhood obesity campaign, which aims to "provide clear, consistent, research-based messages to children and parents on the importance of practicing a healthier lifestyle and offer them the means to do it" (Ad Council, http://www.healthychildrencoalition.org/index.html).

Although television watching may contribute to childhood obesity, use of the media may also provide opportunities to positively affect the problem. Leading policy options include reducing or regulating food advertisements targeted to children, expanding public education campaigns to promote healthy eating and exercise, and incorporating messages about healthy eating into television storylines.

Sugar-Sweetened Beverage Taxes and Portion Size Limitations

SSBs—including sugar-sweetened sodas, juice drinks, and sports drinks—have been identified by public health professionals as one of the key targets for reducing caloric intake, body weight, and obesity-related conditions (Brownell et al. 2009; Vartanian et al. 2007). Based on the success of tobacco taxes in reducing smoking prevalence, taxation of SSBs has been proposed to both reduce consumption (and thus lower healthcare costs) as well as generate funds to support health promotion programs (Brownell et al. 2009). As of January 1, 2014, 34 states and the District of Columbia levied sales taxes (average of 5.2%) to sugar-sweetened sodas sold at food stores, and 39 states and the District of Columbia applied sales taxes (average of 5.3%) to sugar-sweetened sodas sold via vending machines (Chirqui et al. 2014). However, these sales taxes have been criticized for being too low to have meaningful impacts on overall consumption and weight. In addition, sales taxes are collected at the point of purchase—rather than incorporated into the shelf price— and thus consumers do not know about the tax until the final cash register receipt is provided. Instead, many SSB taxation advocates support an excise tax per ounce of beverage or per gram of added sugar that would be levied before the point of purchase, so that consumers will see a shelf price difference between SSBs and sugar-free beverages (and ultimately make the cheaper, lower-calorie choice) (Brownell et al. 2009; Chirqui et al. 2014).

A tax of one cent per ounce of beverage is predicted to increase the cost of a 20 oz. soda by 15–20%, leading to a conservative estimate of a 10% reduction in calorie consumption from SSBs (20 calories per person per day). Such a tax at the national level would raise $14.9 billion in the first year, which can then be used for childhood nutrition and/or obesity prevention programs (Brownell et al. 2009). The Center for Science in the Public Interest (CSPI) has developed a Soft Drink Tax Calculator (https://www.cspinet.org/liquidcandy/sugarydrinktaxes.html) to estimate the potential revenue generated from a sales or excise tax at the state or federal level.

Another proposed strategy to reduce consumption of SSBs is to regulate portion size. In September 2012, the New York City Board of Health passed a one-of-a-kind proposal that set a 16 oz. maximum size for SSBs sold by restaurants, mobile food vendors, and snack bars at movie the-aters and stadiums. However, the following month, the American Beverage Association, National Restaurant Association, National Association of Theatre Owners of New York State, and others filed a lawsuit to prevent the rule's enforcement (Farley et al. 2013; Grynbaum 2013). Although the cap was to become effective March 12, 2013, New York State Supreme Court Judge Milton Tingling suspended the cap as of March 11, 2013 on the grounds that it is unlawful and that the rule is "arbi-trary and capricious" because it excludes certain businesses, like convenience stores and bodegas (regulated by the state), and does not apply to all caloric beverages, such as dairy-based beverages (Grynbaum 2013). The city repealed the ruling in both Manhattan Court of Appeals (where Judge Tingling's decision was upheld in July 2013) and the New York State Court of Appeals, where the rule was ultimately defeated in June 2014 (Grynbaum 2014).

Supporters of the rule, including a number of physicians and public health groups, viewed the portion size cap as a necessary step toward shifting social norms about SSB portion sizes and improving the health of all New Yorkers (New York City Department of Health and Mental Hygiene 2014). Opponents claimed that the rules discriminate against minorities and the poor, are harm-ful to small businesses, and limit individual choice (New York City Department of Health and Mental Hygiene, http://www.nyc.gov/html/doh/downloads/pdf/cdp/sugary-drink-facts.pdf). Similar proposals have been introduced in Los Angeles and Cambridge, Massachusetts, but to date, a cap on SSB portion size has yet to be implemented in the United States.

Menu Labeling

As mandated by Section 4205 of the Patient Protection and Affordable Care Act (Public Law 111-148), calories must be posted on menus and menu boards (including drive-through menu boards) at res-taurants and similar retail food establishments with 20 or more outlets nationwide. The law also requires vending machine operators who own or operate 20 or more vending machines to disclose calorie content for certain items. Additional nutrient information—such as fat, saturated fat, choles-terol, sodium, and sugar—must be made available in writing upon request. Any individual restau-rant, chain, or vending operator that is not covered by this law may voluntarily elect to comply with the requirements and register with the FDA. This national law was preceded by a growing number of cities, counties, and states that implemented similar menu labeling policies in an effort to help consumers make informed choices when eating out. Studies suggest that menu labeling may lead to modest improvements in food choices (Auchincloss et al. 2013; Bassett et al. 2008; Krieger et al. 2013) as well as offerings (Bruemmer et al. 2012; Namba et al. 2013).

Nutrition Facts Labeling

The FDA has proposed updates to the Nutrition Facts box that are relevant to weight control. The proposed update would place a greater emphasis on calories and serving sizes by making both more prominent. The caloric content of foods will be highlighted by bolding and increasing the type size of the font. Serving size requirements will change to reflect how people eat and drink today. Packaged foods, including drinks, typically eaten in one sitting must be labeled as a single serving and that calorie and nutrient information be declared for the entire package. For example, a 20 oz. bottle of soda, typically consumed in a single sitting, would be labeled as one serving. Dual-column labels must indicate both *per serving* and *per package* calories and nutrient information for certain packages that could be consumed in one sitting or multiple sittings, such as a 24 oz. bottle of soda or a pint of ice cream. Additionally, the proposed label would require information about added sugars and remove the "calories from fat" as a highlighted category because research shows that the type of fat is more important than the amount (but "Total Fat," "Saturated Fat," and "Trans Fat" would be kept) (US Food and Drug Administration 2014). In 2014, the FDA proposed a new food label, which appears in Figure 5.4.

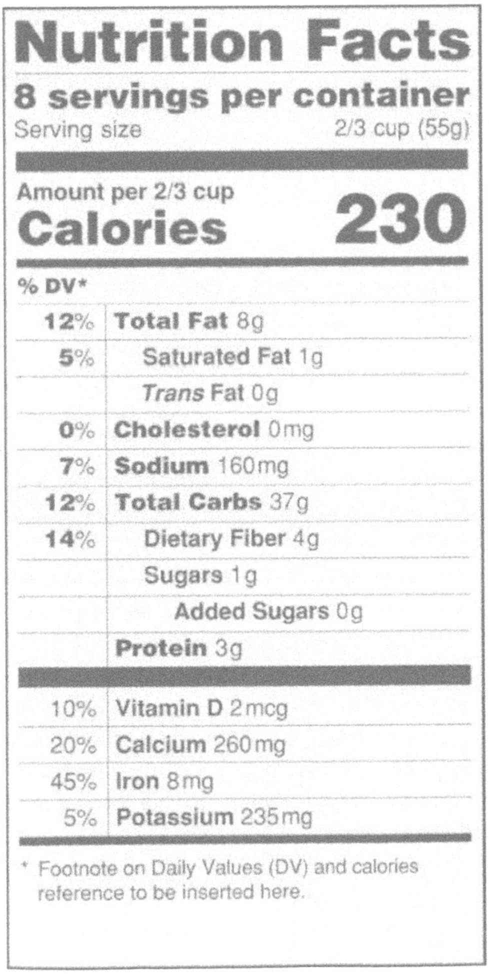

FIGURE 5.4 Proposed Nutrition Facts Label. (From *Federal Register*. 2014;79[41, March 3]:11882.)

SCHOOL-BASED PROGRAMS

Schools play a critical role in promoting student health, preventing childhood obesity, and combating problems associated with poor nutrition and physical inactivity.

School Wellness Policies

To formalize and encourage the critical role schools play in promoting student health, the Child Nutrition and Reauthorization Act of 2004 (Public Law 108-265) required each school district participating in the NSLP and/or SBP to establish a local wellness policy by the start of the 2006 school year. HHFKA expands the scope of local school wellness policies; allows for additional stakeholders to be involved in policy development, implementation, and review; and requires public updates on the content and implementation of the wellness policies (Box 5.10).

Significant online support for developing school wellness policies is available from the USDA (http://healthymeals.nal.usda.gov/local-wellness-policy-resources/school-nutrition-environment -and-wellness-resources-0) and NANA (http://www.schoolwellnesspolicies.org). The USDA provides guidance on local wellness policy requirements, information on creating a policy, examples of extant policies, implementation tools and resources, and sources of funding for supporting policy implementation.

NANA's site makes available resources related to their six priority areas: strengthening NSLP, other foods sold in schools, and other child nutrition programs; strengthening school wellness policies; promoting healthier food choices in public locations; supporting physical education and activity in schools; supporting national menu labeling; and strengthening national and state nutrition, physical activity, and obesity programs (Center for Science in the Public Interest, http://cspinet.org /nutritionpolicy/nana.html).

BOX 5.10   COMPONENTS OF A LOCAL WELLNESS POLICY

As required by law, a local wellness policy, at a minimum, must

- *Include goals for nutrition promotion and education, physical activity, and other school-based activities* that promote student wellness.
- *Include nutrition guidelines for all foods available* on each school campus under the local educational agency during the school day, with the objectives of promoting student health and reducing childhood obesity.
- *Allow parents, students, representatives of the school food authority, physical education teachers, school health professionals, and the general public* to participate in the development, implementation, and review/update of the local wellness policy.
- *Inform and update the public about the content, implementation, and assessment of local wellness policies.*
- *Be measured periodically,* including the extent to which schools are in compliance with the local wellness policy, the extent to which the local education agency's local wellness policy compares to model policies, and the progress made in reaching the goals of the local wellness policy.

Source: Food and Nutrition Service, US Department of Agriculture. Team Nutrition: Local School Wellness Policy Requirements. Available at http://www.fns.usda.gov/tn/local-school-wellness-policy-requirements, accessed January 20, 2015.

Healthy Schools Programs

In 2005, the American Heart Association and the William J. Clinton Foundation teamed up to form the Alliance for a Healthier Generation to combat the spread of childhood obesity and associated morbidities such as heart disease and diabetes. Alliance programs focus on healthy schools, industry, physical activity in children, and healthcare. In 2006, the Alliance announced the Healthy Schools Program (Alliance for a Healthier Generation, https://schools.healthiergeneration.org/), an initiative to collaborate with schools to help them create environments that foster healthy lifestyles and ultimately prevent overweight and obesity among students. Upon launch, the Healthy Schools Program reached 231 schools in 13 states. Since 2006, the program includes more than 20,000 schools in all 50 states, the District of Columbia, and Puerto Rico. The Healthy Schools Program has been made possible through the support of the RWJF (http://www.rwjf.org/), who has awarded the Alliance over $51 million. RWJF is self-described as the nation's largest philanthropy devoted exclusively to improving the health and healthcare of all Americans. In addition to its support of the Alliance for a Healthier Generation, the foundation has initiated Healthy Eating Research (Robert Wood Johnson Foundation, http://www.healthyeatingresearch.org/), a national program to support research that identifies, analyzes, and evaluates environmental and policy approaches to increasing healthy eating among children.

FEDERAL PROGRAMS AND RESOURCES FOR OBESITY PREVENTION

The federal government has implemented programs directly addressing solving obesity as well as providing resources and technical support designed to facilitate the implementation of obesity prevention programs and policies. Highlighted in the following are select programs initiated by the Obama Administration, the USDA, the CDC, and the NIH.

Obama Administration: Let's Move!

Launched by First Lady Michelle Obama on February 9, 2010, the comprehensive *Let's Move!* Health initiative (http://www.letsmove.gov) is "dedicated to solving the problem of obesity within a generation, so that children born today will grow up healthier and able to pursue their dreams" (http://www.letsmove.gov/about). In addition to healthy eating, *Let's Move!* aims to increase opportunities for physical activity. A *Let's Move!* five simple steps message encourages children to

1. Move every day!
2. Try new fruits and veggies.
3. Drink lots of water.
4. Do jumping jacks to break up TV time.
5. Help make dinner.

At the initiative's launch, President Barack Obama signed a Presidential Memorandum that created the first Task Force on Childhood Obesity. The Task Force was charged with reviewing all child nutrition and physical activity-related programs and policies, and developing a national action plan for working toward the goal of *Let's Move!* The Task Force recommendations are illustrated by the five focus areas of *Let's Move!*:

- Creating a healthy start for children.
- Empowering parents and caregivers.
- Providing healthy food in schools.
- Improving access to healthy, affordable foods.
- Increasing physical activity (Let's Move!, http://www.letsmove.gov/about).

Parents and caregivers, policymakers, healthcare professionals, schools, faith-based organizations, communities, and private sector companies are being encouraged to establish programs and policies that support behavior changes and encourage healthier lifestyle choices.

A number of *Let's Move!* programs engage these various stakeholders.

- *Let's Move! Cities, Towns, and Counties* requires participating local elected officials to commit, as of July 2012, to five goals, namely, (1) to provide children with a healthier start by helping early care and education program providers incorporate best practices for nutrition, physical activity, and screen time into their programs; (2) to empower parents and caregivers through displaying MyPlate in all municipally- or county-owned or operated venues that offer or sell food/beverages; (3) to provide healthy food to children and youth by expanding access to meal programs; (4) to improve access to healthy, affordable foods by aligning food service with the *Dietary Guidelines for Americans* in all municipally- or county-owned or operated venues that offer or sell food/beverages; and (5) to increase physical activity through mapping local playspaces, completing a needs assessment, developing an action plan, and launching a minimum of three recommended policies, programs, or initiatives aimed at increasing access to play (National League of Cities, http://www .healthycommunitieshealthyfuture.org/the-five-lmctc-goals).
- *Chefs Move to Schools* matches chefs with school districts to help schools improve health and nutrition. Chefs teach new techniques and recipes for healthier meals and engage youth in learning about nutrition and making healthy choices (Let's Move!, http://www.letsmove .gov/chefs-move-schools). Chefs also help schools participate in the *HealthierUS School Challenge* (HUSSC), a voluntary initiative established by the USDA in 2004 to recognize schools participating in the National School Lunch Program that promote nutrition and physical activity, described in more detail in the next section on USDA initiatives.
- *Let's Move Faith and Communities* engages faith-based and community-based organizations to promote healthy living. Organizations are encouraged to provide wellness leadership through simple messages and guidance (available in the MyPlate community toolkit), to organize by identifying a Wellness Ambassador and supporting the creation and activities of a Wellness Council or Ministry through development of an action plan and commitment to appropriate activities that can improve community wellness (Let's Move!, http://www.letsmove.gov /wellness-leadership). Suggested ideas for action include using the MyPlate, hosting nutrition education classes, starting a garden, hosting summer meal programs for children, and hosting weekly exercise activities (Let's Move!, http://www.letsmove.gov/ideas-action). Additional resources are available in a toolkit: http://www.letsmove.gov/faith-communities-toolkit.
- *Let's Move Outside* provides links to search for nearby nature and outdoor events, forests and parks, and local playgrounds, as well as ideas to inspire fun, affordable physical activities. *Let's Move! Outside* allows users to search for nearby nature trails and outdoor events, forests and parks, pools and outdoor water sports, and local playgrounds (Let's Move!, http://www.letsmove.gov/lets-move-outside).
- *Let's Move in the Clinic* encourages healthcare providers to conduct five simple steps, namely: (1) join *Let's Move* (http://www.letsmove.gov/health-care-providers), (2) make BMI screening a standard part of care, (3) talk to patients about breastfeeding and first foods, (4) prescribe activity and healthy habits, and (5) be a community leader.

USDA Initiatives

Started in 2004, the HUSSC is a voluntary, nationwide award program established by the USDA to recognize those schools that have created healthier school environments by promoting nutritious food, nutrition education, and physical activity. Schools are eligible to apply if they participate in the NSLP or SBP, or if they are a USDA Team Nutrition school. Four award levels, each with a corresponding monetary award, are available depending on the level of criteria met: Bronze

($500), Silver ($1000), Gold ($1500), and Gold Award of Distinction ($2000) (US Department of Agriculture and Food and Nutrition Service 2012). As of January 21, 2015, 7022 schools in 50 states and the District of Columbia are certified. Application materials and award criteria are available online (http://www.fns.usda.gov/hussc/healthierus-school-challenge-application-materials-0). The USDA's National Institute of Food and Agriculture also funds a Childhood Obesity Prevention program (US Department of Agriculture, http://www.nifa.usda.gov/funding/rfas/afri.html). The USDA's Agricultural Research Service also funds obesity research, one example being a Community Nutrition and Physical Activity Program in Grand Forks, North Dakota, that began September 1, 2011 and is scheduled to end August 31, 2016. This project aims to evaluate the efficacy and sustainability of diet and physical activity interventions to maintain healthy body weight and reduce risk factors for obesity-related chronic disease in a community setting (US Department of Agriculture, http://www.ars.usda.gov/research/projects/projects.htm?ACCN_NO=421980).

CDC Initiatives

The CDC has extensive experience in population-based prevention efforts through schools and worksites, the communications and marketing fields, and the nation's public health system. The CDC's Division of Nutrition, Physical Activity, and Obesity (DNPAO) addresses three important risk factors for illness, disability, and premature death by aiming to

1. Improve dietary quality to support healthy child development and reduce chronic disease
2. Increase physical activity for people of all ages
3. Decrease prevalence of obesity through prevention of weight gain and maintenance of healthy weight (Centers for Disease Control and Prevention, http://www.cdc.gov/nccdphp/dnpao/aboutus/index.html)

Between 2008 and 2013, the DNPAO funded numerous programs addressing overweight and obesity, including programs focusing on active transportation, school physical education, urban environment design and policies, access to regionally grown produce, food policy councils, retail access to fruits and vegetables, maternity care practices (including breastfeeding), supporting breastfeeding in the workplace, limiting access to sugar sweetened beverages, promoting menu labeling policies and restaurant programs, applying nutrition policies in child care, school, and workplace settings, and addressing obesity in child-care settings. Program highlights are available at http://www.cdc.gov/obesity/stateprograms/highlights.html.

As of 2015, the DNPAO is focusing on environmental approaches to make good nutrition and physical activity easier and more convenient for Americans, and is currently funding the State Public Health Actions to Prevent and Control Diabetes, Heart Disease, Obesity and Associated Risk Factors and Promote School Health (State Public Health Actions) Program.

State Public Health Actions is a national program that provides a base level of funding to all 50 states and the District of Columbia to focus on underlying strategies that address all of the disease names in the full title of the program. Each states' key action strategies must include the following two DNPAO priorities:

1. Promote the adoption of food service guidelines and nutrition standards, including sodium
2. Promote the adoption of physical activity in early child-care centers, schools, and work sites

Thirty-two states receive additional resources to implement more intensive interventions that include the following three additional DNPAO priorities as strategies:

1. Increase access to healthy foods and beverages
2. Increase physical activity access and outreach
3. Increase access to breastfeeding friendly environments (Centers for Disease Control and Prevention, http://www.cdc.gov/obesity/stateprograms/funded-state-local-programs.html)

The DNPAO is also funding a focused program on reducing obesity in high-obesity areas by awarding $4.2 million to land grant universities in the following states with counties that have more than 40% prevalence of adult obesity: Alabama, Kentucky, South Dakota, Tennessee, Texas, and West Virginia. This project seeks to improve access to healthy foods and physical activity opportunities. Universities will conduct intervention strategies through existing cooperative extension outreach services at the county level, aiming to improve physical activity and nutrition, reduce obesity, and prevent and control diabetes, heart disease, and stroke (Centers for Disease Control and Prevention, http://www.cdc.gov/obesity/stateprograms/funded-state-local-programs.html).

The DNPAO has launched a website on Healthy Food Service Guideline to help make healthier choices more available at workplaces, or other community settings such as hospitals, parks, and recreation areas (see http://www.cdc.gov/obesity/strategies/food-serv-guide.html).

In addition to conducting surveys, CDC's REACH 2010 also funded programs addressing health disparities. REACH 2010 was funded until 2006, and since then, additional REACH funding opportunities have been made available to state and local health departments, tribes, universities, and community-based organizations, as listed in Table 5.9.

TABLE 5.9
REACH Award History

Program	Funding Years	Purpose	Number of Awards
REACH 2010	1999–2006	Supported projects focused on a coalition-based approach targeting racial/ethnic minorities within six health priority areas: cardiovascular disease (CVD), immunizations, breast and cervical cancer screening and management, diabetes, HIV/AIDS, and infant mortality.	40
REACH US	2007–2012	Funded 18 Centers of Excellence in the Elimination of Disparities and 22 Action Communities and used community-oriented participatory approaches to address racial and ethnic health disparities in one or more of seven designated areas: CVD, diabetes mellitus, infant mortality, asthma, hepatitis B, HIV/AIDS, adult immunization, and tuberculosis.	40
REACH National Organizations	2009–2014	Enables national organizations to share evidence- and practice-based programs related to specific health disparity areas with their local affiliates and chapters.	6
REACH CORE	2010–2012	Funds communities to organize, implement, and evaluate evidence-based interventions that eliminate racial and ethnic health disparities in chronic diseases. This program supports the transition of communities from the analysis of intervention results to the use of these results in eliminating health disparities.	10
REACH	2012–2017[a]	Funds organizations to implement sustainable evidence- and practice-based strategies impacting health disparities.	6
REACH Demonstration Project	2012–2015	Funds awardees to develop and implement strategies that reduce obesity and hypertension in populations experiencing health disparities.	2

Source: Centers for Disease Control and Prevention. National Center for Chronic Disease Prevention and Health Promotion. Division of Community Health. Investments in Community Health: Racial and Ethnic Approaches to Community Health (REACH). Available at http://www.cdc.gov/nccdphp/dch/programs /reach/pdf/2-reach_factsheet-for-web.pdf, accessed January 20, 2015.

[a] Funding years may vary, up to 5 years.

Currently, the Boston Public Health Commission and the Community Health Councils, Inc. are the recipients of the 3-year REACH Obesity and Hypertension Demonstration Projects. These two awardees will apply strategies to prevent obesity and hypertension and increase the evidence around programs that are effective in racial and ethnic communities in Boston, Massachusetts, and West Adams Baldwin Hills and South Los Angeles, California, respectively. Approximately $12.3 million will fund these REACH Demonstration Projects until 2015 (Centers for Disease Control and Prevention, http://www.cdc.gov/nccdphp/dch/programs/reach/current_programs/reach-demo.htm).

Other general physical activity and nutrition programs sponsored by the CDC include "BAM! Body and Mind," a kid-friendly website that provides information on how to make healthy lifestyle choices from the CDC's Division of Population Health. The site targets youth ages 9–13 years through interactive games and quizzes that focus on food and nutrition, physical activity, disease, media literacy, and other health-related topics (http://www.cdc.gov/bam/index.html). The CDC is also the lead government agency and primary health authority behind the "Fruits and Veggies—More Matters" health initiative: a national effort to increase the daily per capita consumption of fruits and vegetables (http://www.fruitsandveggiesmorematters.org/).

NIH Initiatives

"Ways to Enhance Children's Activity and Nutrition" (We Can!)

To help families adopt healthier lifestyles, in 2005, the National Heart, Lung, and Blood Institute (NHLBI) of the NIH launched a national public education program targeting parents and caregivers of children ages 8–13. We Can! provides resources for parents, caregivers, and communities to help 8- to 13-year-old children stay at a healthy weight by encouraging healthy eating, increased physical activity, and reduced screen time (US Department of Health and Human Services, http://www.nhlbi.nih.gov/health/educational/wecan/about-wecan/index.htm). For example, the program focuses on the following topics to help guide behavior change for parents and children:

- Eat a sufficient amount of a variety of fruits and vegetables every day.
- Energy balance: E in = E out—the calories you burn in activities should equal the calories you eat.
- Choose small portions at home and at restaurants.
- GO/SLOW/WHOA foods—GO foods can be eaten almost anytime; SLOW foods several times a week; and WHOA foods only once in a while, as outlined in Table 5.10.
- Substitute water or fat-free or low-fat milk for sweetened beverages such as sodas.
- Engage in at least 60 minutes of moderate physical activity on most, preferably all, days of the week.
- Reduce recreational screen time to no more than 2 hours per day (We Can! 2005).

Because achieving and maintaining a healthy weight is a universal chronic disease prevention goal, the program is promoted by the NHLBI in collaboration with three other NIH Institutes: NIDDK, the National Cancer Institute (NCI), and the National Institute of Child Health and Human Development, as well as several national private sector organizations (US Department of Health and Human Services, http://www.nhlbi.nih.gov/health/educational/wecan/about-wecan/index.htm).

EatPlayGrow

EatPlayGrow is a new health educational curriculum created through an innovative public–private partnership between the NIH and the Children's Museum of Manhattan (CMOM) and is a spin-off of We Can's parent program, which was originally geared to parents of children ages 8–13. EatPlayGrow aims to teach children ages 2–5 and their parents how to make healthy nutrition and physical activity choices (US Department of Health and Human Services, http://www.nhlbi.nih.gov/health/educational/wecan/tools-resources/eatplaygrow.htm).

TABLE 5.10

GO, SLOW, WHOA Foods from the *We Can!* Parent Handbook

Food Group	GO (Almost Anytime Foods) Nutrient-Dense	SLOW (Sometimes Foods) ← →	WHOA (Once in a While Foods) Calorie-Dense
Description	Lowest in fat and added sugar; relatively low in calories	Higher in fat, added sugar, and calories than GO foods	Highest in fat and added sugar, and low in nutrients
Vegetables	Almost all fresh, frozen, and canned vegetables without added fat and sauces	All vegetables with added fat and sauces; oven-baked French fries; avocado	Fried potatoes, like French fries or hash browns; other deep-fried vegetables
Fruits	All fresh, frozen, canned (in juice)	100% fruit juice; fruits canned in light syrup; dried fruits	Fruits canned in heavy syrup
Breads and cereals	Whole-grain breads, pita bread, tortillas, and pasta; brown rice; hot and cold unsweetened whole-grain breakfast cereals	White refined flour bread, rice, and pasta; French toast; taco shells; cornbread; biscuits; granola; waffles and pancakes	Croissants; muffins; doughnuts; sweet rolls; crackers made with trans fats; sweetened breakfast cereals
Milk and milk products	Fat-free or 1% reduced-fat milk; fat-free or low-fat yogurt; part-skim, reduced fat, and fat-free cheese; low-fat or fat-free cottage cheese	2% low-fat milk; processed cheese spread	Whole milk; full-fat American cheddar, Colby, Swiss, cream cheese; whole-milk yogurt
Meats, poultry, fish, eggs, beans, and nuts	Trimmed beef and pork; extra lean ground beef; chicken and turkey without skin; tuna canned in water; baked, broiled, steamed, grilled fish and shellfish; beans, split peas, lentils, tofu; egg whites and egg substitutes	Lean ground beef, broiled hamburgers; ham, Canadian bacon; chicken and turkey with skin; low-fat hot dogs; tuna canned in oil; peanut butter; nuts; whole eggs cooked without added fat	Untrimmed beef and pork; regular ground beef; fried hamburgers; ribs; bacon; fried chicken, chicken nuggets; hot dogs; lunch meats, pepperoni, sausage; fried fish and shellfish; whole eggs cooked with fat
Sweets and snacks[a]	Ice milk bars; frozen fruit juice bars; low-fat frozen yogurt and ice cream; fig bars, ginger snaps; baked chips; low-fat microwave popcorn; pretzels		Cookies and cakes; pies; cheese cake; ice cream; chocolate; candy; chips; buttered microwave popcorn
Fats	Vinegar; ketchup; mustard; fat-free creamy salad dressing; fat-free mayonnaise; fat-free sour cream; vegetable oil, olive oil, and oil-based salad dressing[b]	Low-fat creamy salad dressing; low-fat mayonnaise; low-fat sour cream	Butter, margarine; lard; salt pork; gravy; regular creamy salad dressing; mayonnaise; tartar sauce; sour cream; cheese sauce; cream sauce; cream cheese dips
Beverages	Water, fat-free milk, or 1% reduced-fat milk; diet soda; diet iced teas and lemonade	2% low-fat milk; 100% fruit juice; sports drinks	Whole milk; regular soda; sweetened iced teas and lemonade; fruit drinks with less than 100% fruit juice

Source: Adapted from CATCH: Coordinated Approach to Child Health, 4th Grade Curriculum, University of California and Flaghouse, Inc., 2002.

[a] Though some of the foods in this row are lower in fat and calories, all sweets and snacks need to be limited so as not to exceed one's daily calorie requirements.

[b] Vegetable and olive oils contain no saturated or trans fats and can be consumed daily, but in limited portions, to meet daily calorie needs (about 6 teaspoons a day for the 2000-calorie level). (HHS/USDA *Dietary Guidelines for Americans.*)

Go4Life

Go4Life is an exercise and physical activity campaign designed to help older adults include more exercise and physical activity into their daily lives. Developed by the National Institute on Aging at NIH, *Go4Life* offers an evidence-based exercise guide, motivational tips, exercise video, success stories, activity tracker, and other online resources in English and Spanish to motivate older adults to become physically active for the first time, return to exercise after a period of non-activity, or build more physical activity into current routines (US Department of Health and Human Services, http://go4life.nia.nih.gov/).

The President's Challenge

The President's Challenge is a long-standing program of the President's council on Fitness, Sports, and Nutrition that is aimed at motivating Americans to lead active lifestyles. Several challenges are available, including the Presidential Youth Fitness Program (providing a model for fitness education in schools), the Adult Fitness Test (covering aerobic fitness, muscular strength and endurance, flexibility, and body composition), the Presidential Active Lifestyle Award (awarding commitment to daily physical activity and healthy eating), and the Presidential Champions challenge (aimed at individuals who are already physically active but want to do more) (The Office of the President's Council on Fitness, Sports and Nutrition, https://www.presidentschallenge.org/index.shtml).

Federal Resources for Facilitating Obesity Prevention Programs and Policies

A selection of material designed by the federal government to facilitate implementation of obesity prevention programs and policies is highlighted in the following.

- *Making It Happen—School Nutrition Success Stories*, a joint product of HHS, USDA, and the Department of Education, provides case studies of 32 schools and school districts that have implemented innovative strategies to improve the nutritional quality of foods and beverages offered and sold on school campuses. The most consistent theme emerging from these vignettes is that students will buy and consume healthful foods and beverages—and schools can make money from healthful options (Food and Nutrition Service et al. 2005).
- *School Health Guidelines to Promote Healthy Eating and Physical Activity*, developed by the CDC, offers nine guidelines that serve as the foundation for developing, implementing, and evaluating school-based healthy eating and physical activity policies and practices. Each guideline includes a set of strategies for implementation and additional resources (Centers for Disease Control and Prevention 2011c).
- *The Health Education Curriculum Analysis Tool* is a user-friendly checklist designed by the CDC to help schools select or develop curricula based on the extent to which they have characteristics that research has identified as being critical for leading to positive effects on youth health behaviors (Centers for Disease Control and Prevention 2012a). The companion *Physical Education Curriculum Analysis Tool* will help school districts develop state-of-the-art physical education curriculum based on insights gained from research and best practice (Centers for Disease Control and Prevention 2006).
- *Media Smart Youth: Eat, Think, and Be Active!* is a curriculum with supporting materials developed by the National Institute of Child Health and Human Development for youth ages 11–13 years. It is designed to create awareness of the role that media plays in shaping values concerning physical activity and nutrition, while building skills to encourage critical thinking, healthy lifestyle choices, and informed decision making, now and in their future (National Institute of Child Health and Human Development 2013).
- The *School Health Index (SHI): Self-Assessment and Planning Guide* was developed by CDC in partnership with school administrators and staff and nongovernmental agencies in order to enable schools to identify strengths and weaknesses in their health and safety

policies and programs; help schools develop an action plan for improving student health, which can be incorporated into the School Improvement Plan; and engage stakeholders (teachers, parents, students, the community) in promoting health-enhancing behaviors and better health. The 2012 edition of the SHI covers physical activity and physical education, nutrition, tobacco use prevention, asthma, safety (unintentional injury and violence prevention), and sexual health (including HIV, other STDs, and pregnancy prevention). CDC has developed guidelines for schools to address each of these risk behaviors, which are typically established during childhood and adolescence. Additional health topics will be added in the future (Centers for Disease Control and Prevention 2012b).

- *Fruit and Vegetables Galore: Helping Kids Eat More*, developed in 2004 by USDA in collaboration with HHS, provides strategies for school foodservice professionals on planning, purchasing, preparing, presenting, and promoting fruits and vegetables in school food programs. The program also includes suggestions for working with teachers by providing them with teaching tools and by supporting their educational efforts (making daily meal offerings competitive with other commercial options available to students) and motivating students to choose a more healthful diet (Food and Nutrition Service and US Department of Agriculture 2004).

WORKPLACE WELLNESS PROGRAMS

As the prevalence of chronic disease in working-aged adults has grown over time, employers have become increasingly concerned about rising healthcare costs and decreased employee productivity. As such, employers are implementing a variety of health promotion and disease prevention strategies, referred to as workplace wellness programs. In fact, roughly half of US employers with 50 or more employees offer wellness programs (Mattke et al. 2013). Such programs may include screening activities to identify health risks, preventive interventions to address health risks (lifestyle management) and improve control of chronic conditions (disease management), and health promotion activities to support healthy lifestyles (Mattke et al. 2013).

Employee wellness programs that account for both individual and environmental influences can improve the health status of the workforce and quantifiably reduce healthcare costs. One evaluation found that, compared to matched nonparticipants, participants of employee wellness programs had statistically significant and clinically meaningful improvements in exercise frequency, smoking behavior, and weight control (Mattke et al. 2013). According to a meta-analysis of the literature, there is an average reduction of $3.27 in healthcare costs for each dollar spent on wellness programs, and absenteeism costs fall by about $2.73 for every dollar spent (Baicker et al. 2010).

Successful workplace health promotion programs share a set of common characteristics, including the use of one or more of the following: involving employees' supervisors in workplace health promotion programs, targeting organizational and/or environmental factors to influence behavior, screening employees prior to intervention, and individually tailoring programs to address participant needs (Box 5.11) (Cancelliere et al. 2011).

A number of legislative efforts have been taken at the state level to induce behavioral change through the workplace; businesses receiving a tax credit and reduced healthcare costs would have a stake in sustaining a wellness program. A listing of such bills introduced in 2009–2010 can be found at the National Conference of State Legislatures website: http://www.ncsl.org/research /health/wellness-legislation-2010.aspx.

At the federal level, the Patient Protection and Affordable Care Act of 2010 (Public Law 111-148) (US Government Publishing Office 2010) expands existing wellness program policies and creates new incentives to promote and encourage employer wellness programs and healthier workplaces (US Department of Labor, http://www.dol.gov/ebsa/newsroom/fswellnessprogram.html). The final rule (Federal Register 2013), which took effect on January 1, 2014, supports the continuance of

---

**BOX 5.11   *HEALTHY PEOPLE 2020* WORKSITE
WELLNESS-RELATED OBJECTIVES**

Educational and Community-Based Programs
- *Objective ECBP-8:* Increase the proportion of worksites that offer an employee health promotion program to their employees.
- *Objective ECBP-9:* Increase the proportion of employees who participate in employer-sponsored health promotion activities.

Environmental Health
- *Objective EH-2:* Increase use of alternative modes of transportation for work (e.g., bicycling, walking).

Maternal, Infant, and Child Health
- *Objective MICH-22:* Increase the proportion of employers that have worksite lactation support programs.

Nutrition and Weight Status
- *Objective NWS-7:* Increase the proportion of worksites that offer nutrition or weight management classes or counseling.

Physical Activity
- *Objective PA-12:* Increase the proportion of employed adults who have access to and participate in employer-based exercise facilities and exercise programs.

Tobacco Use
- *Objective TU-12:* Increase the proportion of persons covered by indoor worksite policies that prohibit smoking.
- *Objective TU-13:* Establish laws in States, District of Columbia, Territories, and Tribes on smoke-free indoor air that prohibit smoking in public places and worksites.

Source: Healthy People 2020. Available at http://www.healthypeople.gov/2020/topics-objectives/2020-Topics-and -Objectives-Objectives-A-Z, accessed January 20, 2015.

"participatory wellness programs," which are made available to individuals without regard to health status or medical history. Such programs may include reimbursement for fitness center membership fees, provision of incentives for attending a free health education seminar, or provision of rewards for completing a health screening. Participatory wellness programs must be made available to all similarly situated individuals, regardless of health status. The rules also amend standards for "health-contingent wellness programs" that require individuals to meet a specific health-related standard, such as those providing a reward for completing a diet or exercise program, abstaining or reducing tobacco use, or lowering cholesterol levels or weight. These programs must reasonably promote health or prevent disease and must be made available to all similarly situated individuals. Individuals eligible for these programs must be given the opportunity to qualify for the reward at least annually, and programs must provide notice to individuals of the opportunity to quality for the same reward through different means. The rules also increase the maximum allowed reward under a health-contingent wellness program from 20% to 30% of the cost of health coverage, and increase the maximum reward to up to 50% for tobacco prevention or reduction programs (Federal Register 2013).

State and federal incentives are not the only approach, nor likely the only solution, to promoting workplace wellness. The Wellness Council of America (WELCOA) has developed guidelines and resources to build and sustain worksite health promotion programs. Their website (http://www.welcoa.org) offers benchmarks to success, links to key resources, and recognition awards for successful programs.

CONCLUSION

Over the last 50 years, the rates of overweight and obesity in the United States have increased across all population categories to the point where they are now described as epidemic. In 2001, in response to this alarming trend, the Surgeon General published a call to action to prevent and decrease overweight and obesity. In 2010, Surgeon General Regina M. Benjamin recognized that some gains had occurred, but the prevalence and comorbidity remained too high, and announced a plan to strengthen and expand on the 2001 call to action. Dr. Benjamin's plan recognizes that just as overweight and obesity have no single, identifiable cause, they have no single solution. Critical opportunities for interventions can occur in multiple settings: home, child care, school, work place, healthcare, and community (US Department of Health and Human Services, http://www.surgeongeneral.gov/initiatives/healthy-fit-nation/obesityvision2010.pdf).

Action must be taken on all fronts, from the individual making informed health choices, to the federal government introducing and supporting effective policies. The built, economic, and food environments each play a role in inducing and reducing obesity. However, the impact of any undertaking will likely take several decades to become evident and comes with the risk that we will turn our attention elsewhere before such time.

ACRONYMS

A/I	Adequate intake
A/PI	Asians/Pacific Islanders
AMDR	Acceptable macronutrient distribution range
APA	American Psychological Association
APHA	American Public Health Association
BMI	Body mass index
BRFSS	Behavioral Risk Factor Surveillance System
CARU	Children's Advertising Review Unit
CDC	Centers for Disease Control and Prevention
CSFII	Continuing Survey of Food Intake by Individuals
CSPI	Center for Science in the Public Interest
DNPAO	Division of Nutrition, Physical Activity, and Obesity
FAFH	Food away from home
FCC	Federal Communication Commission
FDA	Food and Drug Administration
FMNV	Foods of minimal nutritional value
HDL	High-density lipoprotein
HFCS	High fructose corn syrup
HHFKA	Healthy, Hunger-Free Kids Act of 2010
HLC	Healthy lifestyle characteristics
HUSSC	HealthierUS School Challenge
IATP	Institute for Agriculture and Trade Policy
IOM	Institute of Medicine
MEPS	Medical Expenditure Panel Survey

NANA	National Alliance for Nutrition and Activity
NCD	Noncommunicable disease
NCHS	National Center for Health Statistics
NFCS	Nationwide Food Consumption Survey
NHANES	National Health and Nutrition Examination Survey
NHEA	National Health Expenditure Accounts
NHES	National Health Examination Survey
NHLBI	National Heart, Lung, and Blood Institute
NIH	National Institutes of Health
NSLP	National School Lunch Program
NWCR	National Weight Control Registry
PedNSS	Pediatric Nutrition Surveillance System
RDA	Recommended dietary allowance
RDI	Reference daily intake
REACH 2010	Racial and Ethnic Approaches to Community Health 2010
RWJF	Robert Wood Johnson Foundation
SBP	School Breakfast Program
SES	Socioeconomic status
SHI	School health index
SNAP	Supplemental Nutrition Assistance Program
SSB	Sugar-sweetened beverage
TFP	Thrifty Food Plan
UL	Tolerable upper intake limit
USDA	United States Department of Agriculture
WELCOA	Wellness Council of America
WHO	World Health Organization
WIC	Special Supplemental Nutrition Program for Women, Infants, and Children
YBRFSS	Youth Behavior Risk Factor Surveillance System

STUDENT ASSIGNMENTS AND ACTIVITIES DESIGNED TO ENHANCE LEARNING AND STIMULATE CRITICAL THINKING

1. Research the most recent obesity prevalence rates for children and adults. Have these rates changed significantly from prior years? If so, how?
2. How does the obesity rate in your state compare to neighboring states and the country as a whole? What programs and/or policies have been implemented in your state to address obesity?
3. Research and describe waist circumference, a measurement used to estimate abdominal fat. What is the rationale for using body mass index (BMI) rather than waist circumference to identify adults who are overweight and obese?
4. How would you suggest preventing and reducing obesity in preschool-aged children? Be sure to support your answer with evidence.
5. The Boston Public Health Commission and the Community Health Councils, Inc. are the recipients of the 3-year REACH Obesity and Hypertension Demonstration Projects (ending 2015). Research these two awardees and describe how they have applied strategies to prevent obesity and hypertension and increase the evidence around programs that are effective in their respective communities.
6. Your friend's 13-year-old daughter, Alicia, has recently been seen by her primary care physician, who recommended that Alicia see a dietitian. Alicia's BMI history is listed below. Using the female growth chart in Figure 7.3, plot Alicia's BMI history. Based on the growth chart, describe Alicia's BMI changes over time. What is Alicia's current weight

status (underweight, normal weight, overweight, or obese)? What recommendations would you give your friend?

Age	BMI
2	15
3	15.2
4	16.7
7	19.9
11	24.1
13	27.7

7. Walk around the community you live in and assess the built environment. Using a camera, capture a photo image of five community characteristics that are *obesogenic* and five characteristics that promote a healthy weight. Describe the barriers and facilitators that you have visually framed and discuss the real and potential impact(s) that these characteristics have on the health and weight status of those who live nearby. Based on your assessment, what are three possible and achievable environmental modifications that can be made in your community to prevent or reverse obesity?

8. Review the box describing US Food Consumption Trends. Go to the supermarket and record each cereal brand that features a cartoon character or celebrity on the box. Buy one of these cereal boxes and bring it home. In a regular bowl, pour out the amount of cereal you would normally eat. Next, use a measuring cup to determine how many cups of cereal are in your portion. Then, read the nutrition label on the box to determine the amount of sugar per serving. Based on the serving size listed, calculate the amount of sugar contained in your cereal portion. Finally, divide this amount by 4 to get the number of teaspoons of sugar in your portion of cereal. Be sure to show all your work.

   In order to visualize the amount of sugar in your cereal portion, measure out the same number of teaspoons of sugar into a cup (if you do not have sugar, you can use another finely granulated substance, such as salt, garlic, sand, etc.). Compare this to a 12 oz. cola, which contains 30 g (7.5 teaspoons) of sugar. Describe what you learned from this exercise.

9. Watch a children's television program for 1 hour and count the number of commercials you view. Classify the food commercials based on the categories listed in Table 5.8. How many of the commercials are food commercials? Of the food commercials, how many advertise processed foods? What category was most represented by the commercials you viewed? What category was least represented? What do you conclude from this exercise?

10. SNAP benefits are allotted to eligible households based on the Thrifty Food Plan. Find the most current average weekly cost of the Thrifty Food Plan based on your age–gender group (see http://www.cnpp.usda.gov/USDAFoodCost-Home.htm). Then, determine the weekly quantity of the 29 food categories, in pounds, allotted to the Thrifty Food Plan market basket for your age–gender group (see Table ES-1 in http://www.cnpp.usda.gov/sites/default /files/usda_food_plans_cost_of_food/TFP2006Report.pdf). Using supermarket circulars or price checks at supermarkets, *shop* for the allotted quantity of each food category, staying as close to the weekly cost as possible. Keep a log of the food category, food item, weight (in pounds), and cost. Describe and reflect on your experiences with this activity. Do you believe you were able to *purchase* foods that support a healthy, nutrient-dense diet? Defend your answer.

11. Visit a local vending machine, and list all items it contains. Using the Alliance Product Calculator for Smart Snacks (https://schools.healthiergeneration.org/focus_areas/snacks

_and_beverages/smart_snacks/alliance_product_calculator/), determine whether these 10 items are compliant with the USDA standards for snacks in schools (Table 5.8). What percentage of the vending machine items met the standards? Did any of the item assessments surprise you? In other words, did you feel that one or more of the items deemed compliant should not be sold in schools? Conversely, did one or more of the items deemed noncompliant seem as if they should be allowed? Describe your reasoning(s).

12. Read the following documents:
    - Centers for Disease Control and Prevention. *Body Mass Index Measurement in Schools: Executive Summary.* Available at http://www.cdc.gov/HealthyYouth/obesity/bmi/pdf/BMI_execsumm.pdf.
    - Eating Disorders Coalition. *Talking Points: BMI.* Available at http://www.eatingdisorderscoalition.org/documents/TalkingpointsBMI.pdf.
    - Flaherty MR. "Fat letters" in public schools: Public health versus pride. *Pediatrics.* 2013;132(3):403–5. Available at http://www.usnews.com/pubfiles/0819childletters.pdf.
    - Kantor J. As obesity fight hits cafeteria, many fear a note from school. *New York Times.* January 8, 2007. Available at http://query.nytimes.com/gst/fullpage.html?res=9801E4DA1530F93BA35752C0A9619C8B63&smid=pl-share.

    What are the arguments for and against mandatory BMI reporting of school-aged children to their parents? What position do you take, and why?
13. Search the Internet and published literature for more about sugar sweetened beverage (SSB) taxation. What groups are opposed to such a tax, and what are their objections? What actions have these groups taken to stymie the passage of SSB tax policies at the local, state, and federal levels? How can supporters of SSB tax policies address these objections and actions?
14. Research and describe the fate of the New York City SSB Portion Cap Rule. Has any other government body succeeded in passing a similar policy? What other initiatives have been proposed to reduce the consumption of SSBs among Americans?
15. Obtain a local wellness policy from a school district, and compare it to the model policy developed by the Yale Rudd Center for Food Policy and Obesity (http://www.yaleruddcenter.org/resources/upload/docs/what/communities/Model_Wellness_Policy.pdf). What are the areas of particular strength in the district policy you obtained? What are some additions or changes that could be made to the district policy that would further protect and promote student health?

REFERENCES

Ad Council. Coalition for Healthy Children: Combating Childhood Obesity. Available at http://www.healthychildrencoalition.org/index.html, accessed January 20, 2015.

Alliance for a Healthier Generation. Healthy Schools Program. Available at https://schools.healthiergeneration.org/, accessed January 20, 2015.

American Public Health Association. Policy Statement Database. Food Marketing and Advertising Directed at Children and Adolescents: Implications for Overweight. Policy #200317, November 18, 2003. Available at http://www.apha.org/policies-and-advocacy/public-health-policy-statements/policy-database/2014/07/24/16/35/food-marketing-and-advertising-directed-at-children-and-adolescents-implications-for-overweight, accessed January 20, 2015.

Auchincloss AH, Mallya GG, Leonberg BL, Ricchezza A, Glanz K, Schwarz DF. *Am J Prev Med.* 2013;45(6):710–719.

Baicker K, Butler D, Song Z. Workplace wellness programs can generate savings. *Health Affairs.* 2010;29(2):304–311.

Baskin ML, Ard J, Franklin F, Allison DB. Prevalence of obesity in the United States. *Obes Rev.* 2005;6(1):5–7.

Bassett MT, Dumanovsky T, Huang C et al. Purchasing behavior and calorie information at fast-food chains in New York City, 2007. *Am J Public Health.* 2008;98(8):1457–1459.

Bellagio Declaration. Nutrition and health transition in the developing world: The time to act. *Pub Health Nutr.* 2002;5(1A):279–280.

Binkley JK, Eales J, Jekanowski M. The relation between dietary change and rising US obesity. *Int J Obes Relat Metab Disord.* 2000;24(8):1032–1039.

Blackburn GL, Phillips JCC, Morreale S. Physician's guide to popular low-carbohydrate weight-loss diets. *Cleve Clin J Med.* 2001;68:761–774.

Borzekowski DLG, Robinson TN. The 30-second effect: An experiment revealing the impact of television commercials on food preferences of preschoolers. *J Am Diet Assoc.* 2001;101(1):42–46.

Bowman SA, Vinyard BT. Fast food consumption of US adults: Impact on energy and nutrient intakes and overweight status. *J Am Coll Nutr.* 2004;23(2):163–168.

Brownell KD, Farley T, Willett WC, Popkin BM, Chaloupka FJ, Thompson JW, Ludwig DS. The public health and economic benefits of taxing sugar-sweetened beverages. *N Engl J Med.* 2009;361(16):1599–1605.

Bruemmer B, Krieger J, Saelens BE, Chan N. Energy, saturated fat, and sodium were lower in entrees at chain restaurants at 18 months compared with 6 months following the implementation of mandatory menu labeling regulation in King County, Washington. *J Acad Nutr Diet.* 2012;112(8):1169–1176.

Caballero B, Popkin BM, eds. *The Nutrition Transition: Diet and Disease in the Developing World.* London: Academic Press, 2002.

Cancelliere C, Cassidy JD, Ammendolia C, Côté P. Are workplace health promotion programs effective at improving presenteeism in workers? A systematic review and best evidence synthesis of the literature. *BMC Public Health.* 2011;11:395. doi:10.1186/1471-2458-11-395.

Center for Science in the Public Interest. Limiting Food Marketing to Children. Available at http://www.cspinet .org/new/pdf/limitingfood_marketing.pdf, accessed January 20, 2015.

Center for Science in the Public Interest. National Alliance for Nutrition and Activity. Available at http://www .cspinet.org/nutritionpolicy/nana.html, accessed January 20, 2015.

Centers for Disease Control and Prevention. *Childhood Obesity Facts. Prevalence of Childhood Obesity in the United States, 2011–2012.* Available at http://www.cdc.gov/obesity/data/childhood.html, accessed January 20, 2015.

Centers for Disease Control and Prevention. Funded DNPAO State and Local Programs. Available at http:// www.cdc.gov/obesity/stateprograms/funded-state-local-programs.html, accessed February 2, 2015.

Centers for Disease Control and Prevention. *Physical Education Curriculum Analysis Tool.* Atlanta, GA: CDC, 2006. Available at http://www.cdc.gov/healthyyouth/pecat/index.htm, accessed January 20, 2015.

Centers for Disease Control and Prevention. Prevalence of overweight, obesity and extreme obesity among adults: United States, trends 1976–1980 through 2005–2006. *NCHS Health E-Stat.* Available at http:// www.cdc.gov/nchs/data/hestat/overweight/overweight_adult.htm, accessed January 20, 2015.

Centers for Disease Control and Prevention. Racial and Ethnic Approaches to Community Health (REACH). New REACH Demonstration Projects. Available at http://www.cdc.gov/nccdphp/dch/programs/reach /current_programs/reach-demo.htm, accessed January 20, 2015.

Centers for Disease Control and Prevention. School health guidelines to promote health eating and physical activity. *MMWR.* 2011c;60(5):1–80. Available at http://www.cdc.gov/mmwr/pdf/rr/rr6005.pdf, accessed January 20, 2015.

Centers for Disease Control and Prevention. *State Indicator Report on Physical Activity, 2010.* Atlanta, GA: US Department of Health and Human Services, 2010. Available at http://www.cdc.gov/physicalactivity /downloads/PA_State_Indicator_Report_2010.pdf, accessed January 20, 2015.

Centers for Disease Control and Prevention. *Strategies to Prevent Obesity and Other Chronic Diseases: The CDC Guide to Strategies to Increase the Consumption of Fruits and Vegetables.* Atlanta, GA: US Department of Health and Human Services, 2011a. Available at http://www.cdc.gov/obesity/downloads /fandv_2011_web_tag508.pdf, accessed January 20, 2015.

Centers for Disease Control and Prevention. *Strategies to Prevent Obesity and Other Chronic Diseases: The CDC Guide to Strategies to Increase Physical Activity in the Community.* Atlanta, GA: US Department of Health and Human Services, 2011b. Available at http://www.cdc.gov/obesity/downloads/PA_2011 _WEB.pdf, accessed January 20, 2015.

Centers for Disease Control and Prevention. *Strategies to Prevent Obesity and Other Chronic Diseases: The CDC Guide to Strategies to Support Breastfeeding Mothers and Babies.* Atlanta, GA: US Department of Health and Human Services, 2013. Available at http://www.cdc.gov/breastfeeding/pdf/BF-Guide-508 .pdf, accessed January 20, 2015.

Centers for Disease Control and Prevention. *Health Education Curriculum Analysis Tool, 2012.* Atlanta, GA: CDC, 2012a. Available at http://www.cdc.gov/healthyyouth/HECAT/index.htm, accessed January 20, 2015.

Centers for Disease Control and Prevention. *School Health Index: Self-Assessment and Planning Guide, 2012.* Atlanta, GA: CDC, 2012b. Available at http://www.cdc.gov/HealthyYouth/SHI/, accessed January 20, 2015.

Centers for Disease Control and Prevention. Youth risk behavior surveillance system: Overview. Available at http://www.cdc.gov/healthyyouth/yrbs/pdf/system_overview_yrbs.pdf, accessed February 2, 2015.

Centers for Disease Control and Prevention. Youth risk behavior surveillance—United States, 2013. *MMWR. Surveill Summ.* 2014;63(4). Available at http://www.cdc.gov/mmwr/pdf/ss/ss6304.pdf, accessed February 2, 2015.

Centers for Disease Control and Prevention. Division of Nutrition, Physical Activity, and Obesity. Available at http://www.cdc.gov/nccdphp/dnpao/aboutus/index.html, accessed January 20, 2015.

Centers for Disease Control and Prevention. Office of Surveillance, Epidemiology, and Laboratory Services. Behavioral Risk Factor Surveillance System. *Prevalence and Trends Data.* Available at http://apps.nccd.cdc.gov/brfss, accessed January 20, 2015.

Children's Advertising Review Unit. Self-Regulatory Program for Children's Advertising. Available at http://www.caru.org/guidelines/guidelines.pdf, accessed January 20, 2015.

Chirqui JF, Eidson SS, Chaloupka FJ. *State Sales Taxes on Regular Soda (as of January 1, 2014)—Bridging the Gap Fact Sheet.* Chicago, IL: Bridging the Gap Program, Health Policy Center, Institute for Health Research and Policy, University of Illinois at Chicago, 2014. Available at http://www.bridgingthegap research.org/_asset/s2b5pb/BTG_soda_tax_fact_sheet_April2014.pdf, accessed January 20, 2015.

Council on Communications and Media. From the American Academy of Pediatrics: Policy statement—Children, adolescents, obesity, and the media. *Pediatrics.* 2011;128(1):201–208.

Crespo CJ, Smit E, Troiano RP, Bartlett SJ, Macera CA, Andersen RE. Television watching, energy intake, and obesity in US children: Results from the third National Health and Nutrition Examination Survey, 1988–1994. *Arch Pediatr Adolesc Med.* 2001;155(3):360–365.

Cullen KW, Zakeri I. Fruits, vegetables, milk, and sweetened beverages consumption and access to à la carte/snack bar meals at school. *Am J Public Health.* 2004;94:463–467.

Danaei G, Ding EL, Mozaffarian D, Taylor B, Rehm J, Murray CJL, Ezzati M. The preventable causes of death in the United States: Comparative risk assessment of dietary, lifestyle, and metabolic risk factors. *PLoS Med.* 2009;6(4):1–23.

Dietz W, Gortmaker S. Do we fatten our children at the TV set? Obesity and television viewing in children and adolescents. *Pediatrics.* 1985;75(5):807–812.

Dietz W, Gortmaker S. TV or not TV: Fat is the question. *Pediatrics.* 1993;91(2):499–500.

Dinour LM, Bergen D, Yeh M-C. The food–insecurity–obesity paradox: A review of the literature and the role food stamps may play. *J Am Diet Assoc.* 2007;107(11):1952–1961.

Drewnowski A. Nutrition transition and global dietary trends. *Nutrition.* 2000;16(7–8):486–487.

Drewnowski A, Specter SE. Poverty and obesity: The role of energy density and energy costs. *Am J Clin Nutr.* 2004;79(1):6–15.

Drewnowski A, Darmon N. The economics of obesity: Dietary energy density and energy cost. *Am J Clin Nutr.* 2005;82(Suppl):265S–273S.

Economic Research Service, US Department of Agriculture. *Food Consumption and Demand: Food Away From Home Briefing Room,* 2013. Available at http://www.ers.usda.gov/topics/food-choices-health/food-consumption-demand/food-away-from-home.aspx, accessed January 20, 2015.

Economic Research Service, US Department of Agriculture. *Food Expenditures. Table 10—Food Away from Home as a Share of Food Expenditures.* Available at http://www.ers.usda.gov/data-products/food-expenditures.aspx#.U3zzpy8hkzw, accessed January 20, 2015.

Farley T, Kansagra S, Merrill T. From Supersize to Human-Size: Shrinking Sugary Drink Portions. New York City Department of Health and Mental Hygiene. Webinar: Center for Science in the Public Interest, January 15, 2013. Available at http://cspinet.org/liquidcandy/CSPI-Webinar-NYC-DHMH-presentation.pdf, accessed January 20, 2015.

Federal Communications Commission. Children's Educational Television. Available at http://www.fcc.gov/guides/childrens-educational-television, accessed January 20, 2015.

Field AE, Coakley EH, Must A et al. Impact of overweight on the risk of developing common chronic diseases during a 10-year period. *Arch Intern Med.* 2001;161(13):1581–1586.

Finkelstein EA, Trogdon JG, Brown DS, Allaire BT, Dellea PS, Kamal-Bahl SJ. The lifetime medical cost burden of overweight and obesity: Implications for obesity prevention. *Obesity.* 2008;16(8):1843–1848.

Finkelstein EA, Trogdon JG, Cohen JW, Dietz W. Annual medical spending attributable to obesity: Payer- and service-specific estimates. *Health Affairs.* 2009;28(5):w822–w831.

Flegal KM, Carroll MD, Kuczmarski RJ, Johnson CL. Overweight and obesity in the United States: Prevalence and trends, 1960–1994. *Int J Obes Relat Metab Disord.* 1998;22(1):39–47.

Flegal KM, Carroll MD, Ogden CL, Curtin LR. Prevalence and trends in obesity among US adults, 1999–2008. *JAMA*. 2010;303(3):235–241.

Flegal KM, Carroll MD, Kit BK, Ogden CL. Prevalence of obesity and trends in the distribution of body mass index among US adults, 1999–2010. *JAMA*. 2012;307(5):491–497.

Food and Nutrition Service, US Department of Agriculture. *Fruits & Vegetables Galore: Helping Kids Eat More*. FNS-365, February 2004. Available at http://www.fns.usda.gov/tn/fruits-vegetables-galore-helping -kids-eat-more, accessed January 20, 2015.

Food and Nutrition Service, US Department of Agriculture, Centers for Disease Control and Prevention, US Department of Health and Human Services, US Department of Education. *Making It Happen! School Nutrition Success Stories*. FNS-374, January 2005. Available at http://www.fns.usda.gov/tn/making-it -happen-school-nutrition-success-stories, accessed January 20, 2015.

Foster GD, Wyatt HR, Hill JG et al. A randomized trial of low-carbohydrate diet for obesity. *N Engl J Med*. 2003;348(21):2082–2090.

Fox MK, Dodd AH, Wilson A, Gleason PM. Association between school food environment and practices and body mass index of US public school children. *J Am Diet Assoc*. 2009;109(2):S108–S117.

Freedman DS, Khan LK, Serdula MK, Dietz WH, Srinivasan SR, Berenson GS. The relation of childhood BMI to adult adiposity: The Bogalusa Heart Study. *Pediatrics*. 2005;115(1):22–27.

French SA, Harnack L, Feffery RW. Fast food restaurant use among women in the Pound of Prevention study: Dietary, behavioral and demographic correlates. *Int J Obes*. 2000;24:1353–1359.

French SA, Story M, Jeffery RW. Environmental influences on eating and physical activity. *Annu Rev Public Health*. 2001;22(1):309–335.

Fried EJ, Simon M. The competitive food conundrum: Can government regulations improve school food? *Duke Law J*. 2007;56:1491–1539.

Fryar CD, Carroll MD, Ogden CL. Prevalence of overweight, obesity, and extreme obesity among adults: United States, 1960–1962 through 2011–2012. *Health E-Stat*, September 2014. Available at http://www .cdc.gov/nchs/data/hestat/obesity_adult_11_12/obesity_adult_11_12.pdf, accessed January 20, 2015.

Gantz W, Schwartz N, Angelinie JR, Rideout V. *Food for Thought: Television Food Advertising to Children in the United States*. A Kaiser Family Foundation Report. Menlo Park, CA: The Henry J. Kaiser Family Foundation, 2007. Available at http://kaiserfamilyfoundation.files.wordpress.com/2013/01/7618.pdf, accessed January 20, 2015.

Glanz K, Basil M, Maibach E, Goldberg J, Snyder D. Why Americans eat what they do: Taste, nutrition, cost, convenience, and weight control concerns as influences on food consumption. *J Am Diet Assoc*. 1998;98(10):1118–1126.

Gortmaker SL, Peterson K, Wiecha J et al. Reducing obesity via a school-based interdisciplinary intervention among youth: Planet health. *Arch Pediatr Adolesc Med*. 1999;153(4):409–418.

Grynbaum MM. Judge blocks New York City's limits on big sugary drinks. *New York Times*, March 11, 2013. Available at http://www.nytimes.com/2013/03/12/nyregion/judge-invalidates-bloombergs-soda-ban.html? _r=0, accessed January 20, 2015.

Grynbaum MM. New York's ban on big sodas is rejected by final court. *New York Times*, June 26, 2014. Available at http://www.nytimes.com/2014/06/27/nyregion/city-loses-final-appeal-on-limiting-sales-of -large-sodas.html?_r=0, accessed January 20, 2015.

Harris JL, Weinberg ME, Schwartz MB, Ross C, Ostroff J, Brownell KD. *Trends in Television Food Advertising: Progress in Reducing Unhealthy Marketing to Young People?* Rudd Center for Food Policy and Obesity, Yale University, April 2010. Available at http://www.yaleruddcenter.org/resources/upload/docs/what /reports/RuddReport_TVFoodAdvertising_2.10.pdf, accessed January 20, 2015.

Healthy, Hunger-Free Kids Act of 2010, Public Law 111-296, 124 Stat.(2010): 3183–3266. Available at http:// www.gpo.gov/fdsys/pkg/PLAW-111publ296/pdf/PLAW-111publ296.pdf, accessed January 26, 2014.

Hedley AA, Ogden CL, Johnson CL, Carroll MD, Curtin LR, Flegal KM. Prevalence of overweight and obesity among US children, adolescents, and adults, 1999–2002. *JAMA*. 2004;291(23):2847–2850.

Henry AE, Story M. Food and beverage brands that market to children and adolescents on the Internet: A content analysis of branded web sites. *J Nutr Educ Behav*. 2009:41(5):353–359.

Incentives for Nondiscriminatory Wellness Programs in Group Health Plans, Final Rule, 78 Fed. Reg. 33157– 33192, June 3, 2013. Available at https://www.federalregister.gov/articles/2013/06/03/2013-12916/incen tives-for-nondiscriminatory-wellness-programs-in-group-health-plans, accessed January 20, 2015.

Kaiser Family Foundation. The Role of Media in Childhood. Issue Brief. Report No. 7030, February 2004. Available at http://kff.org/other/issue-brief/the-role-of-media-in-childhood-obesity/, accessed January 20, 2015.

Kelsey MM, Zaepfel A, Bjornstad P, Nadeau KJ. Age-related consequences of childhood obesity. *Gerontology*. 2014;60(3):222–228.

Kendall A, Olson CM, Frongillo EA. Relationship of hunger and food insecurity to food availability and consumption. *J Am Diet Assoc.* 1996;96(10):1019–1024.

Kesaniemi YA, Danforth E Jr., Jensen MD, Kopelman PG, Lefebvre P, Reeder BA. Dose–response issues concerning physical activity and health: An evidence-based symposium. *Med Sci Sport Exerc.* 2001;33(6 Suppl):S531–S538.

King DE, Mainous AG III, Carnemolla M, Everett CJ. Adherence to healthy lifestyle habits in US adults, 1988–2006. *Am J Med.* 2009;122(6):528–534.

Koplan JP, Liverman CT, Kraak VI, eds. Committee on Prevention of Obesity in Children and Youth. *Preventing Childhood Obesity: Health in the Balance.* Washington, DC: The National Academies Press, 2005, p. 4.

Krieger JW, Chan NL, Saelens BE, Ta ML, Solet D, Fleming DW. Menu labeling regulations and calories purchased at chain restaurants. *Am J Prev Med.* 2013;44(6):595–604.

Kubik MY, Lytle LA, Hannan PJ, Perry CL, Story M. The association of the school food environment with dietary behaviors of young adolescents. *Am J Public Health.* 2003;93:1168–1173.

Larson NI, Story MT. Food insecurity and weight status among US children and families: A review of the literature. *Am J Prev Med.* 2011;40(2):166–173.

Lehnert T, Sonntag D, Konnopka A, Riedel-Heller S, Konig H-H. Economic costs of overweight and obesity. *Best Pract Res Clin Endocrinol Metab.* 2013;27(2):105–115.

Leibowitz J, Rosch JT, Ramirez E, Brill J, Ohlhausen M. *A Review of Food Marketing to Children and Adolescents: Follow-Up Report.* Federal Trade Commission, December 2012. Available at http://www .ftc.gov/sites/default/files/documents/reports/review-food-marketing-children-and-adolescents-follow -report/121221foodmarketingreport.pdf, accessed January 20, 2015.

Let's Move! About Let's Move! Available at http://www.letsmove.gov/about, accessed January 20, 2015.

Let's Move! Chefs Move to Schools. Available at http://www.letsmove.gov/chefs-move-schools, accessed January 20, 2015.

Let's Move! Health Care Providers. Available at http://www.letsmove.gov/health-care-providers, accessed January 20, 2015.

Let's Move! Ideas for Action. Available at http://www.letsmove.gov/ideas-action, accessed February 2, 2015.

Let's Move! Let's Move Outside. Available at http://www.letsmove.gov/lets-move-outside, accessed February 2, 2015.

Let's Move! Wellness Leadership. Available at http://www.letsmove.gov/wellness-leadership, accessed February 2, 2015.

Liao Y, Tucker P, Okoro CA, Giles WH, Mokdad AH, Harris VB. REACH 2010 surveillance for health status in minority communities—United States, 2001–2002. *MMWR Surveill Summ.* 2004;53(SS06):1–36. Available at http://www.cdc.gov/mmwr/preview/mmwrhtml/ss5306a1.htm, accessed January 20, 2015.

Liberatos P, Link BG, Kelsey JL. The measurement of social class in epidemiology. *Epidemiol Rev.* 1998;10(1):87–121.

Lin B-H, Guthrie J. *Nutritional Quality of Food Prepared at Home and Away from Home, 1977–2008.* EIB-105. US Department of Agriculture, Economic Research Service, December 2012. Available at http://www .ers.usda.gov/publications/eib-economic-information-bulletin/eib105.aspx#.U3z1qS8hkzw, January 20, 2015.

Ma Y, Bertone ER, Stanek EJ III et al. Association between eating patterns and obesity in a free-living US adult population. *Am J Epidemiol.* 2003;158(1):85–92.

Mancino L, Todd J, Guthrie J, Lin B-H. *How Food Away from Home Affects Children's Diet Quality.* ERR-104. US Department of Agriculture, Economic Research Service, October 2010. Available at http://www.ers .usda.gov/publications/err-economic-research-report/err104.aspx#.U3zv9S8hkzy, accessed January 20, 2015.

Mattke S, Liu H, Caloyeras JP, Huang CY, Van Busum KR, Khodyakov D, Shier V. *Workplace Wellness Programs Study: Final Report.* Santa Monica, CA: RAND Corporation, 2013. Available at http://www .dol.gov/ebsa/pdf/workplacewellnessstudyfinal.pdf, accessed January 20, 2015.

McCrory MA, Fuss PJ, Hays NP, Vinken AG, Greenberg VS, Roberts SB. Overeating in America: Association between restaurant food consumption and body fatness in healthy adult men and women ages 19 to 80. *Obes Res.* 1999;7(6):564–571.

Mei Z, Grummer-Strawn LM, Scanlon KS. Does overweight in infancy persist through the preschool years? An analysis of CDC Pediatric Nutrition Surveillance System data. *Soz Praventivmed.* 2003;48(3):161–167.

Metos J, Nanney MS. The strength of school wellness policies: One state's experience. *J Sch Health.* 2007;77(7):367–372.

Mokdad AH, Ford ES, Bowman BA, Dietz WH, Vinicor F, Bales VS, Marks JS. Prevalence of obesity, diabetes, and obesity-related health risk factors, 2001. *JAMA.* 2003;289(1):76–79.

Mokdad AH, Marks JS, Stroup DF, Gerberding JL. Actual causes of death in the United States, 2000. *JAMA*. 2004;291(10):1238–1245.

Monteiro CA, Conde WL, Popkin BM. Is obesity replacing undernutrition? Evidence from different social classes in Brazil. *Public Health Nutr.* 2002;5(1A):105–112.

Monteiro CA, Moura EC, Conde WL, Popkin BM. Socioeconomic status and obesity in adult populations of developing countries: A review. *Bull World Health Org.* 2004;82(12):940–946.

Montgomery KC, Chester J. Interactive food and beverage marketing: Targeting adolescents in the digital age. *J Adolesc Health.* 2009;45(3 Suppl):S18–S29.

Must A, Anderson SE. Body mass index in children and adolescents: Considerations for population-based applications. *Int J Obesity.* 2006;30(4):590–594.

Namba A, Auchincloss A, Leonberg BL, Wootan MG. Exploratory analysis of fast-food chain restaurant menus before and after implementation of local calorie-labeling policies, 2005–2011. *Prev Chronic Dis.* 2013;10:E101.

National Heart, Lung, and Blood Institute. EatPlayGrow™. Available at http://www.nhlbi.nih.gov/health/edu cational/wecan/tools-resources/eatplaygrow.htm, accessed February 2, 2015.

National Heart, Lung, and Blood Institute, National Institutes of Health, US Department of Health and Human Services. About We Can! Available at http://www.nhlbi.nih.gov/health/educational/wecan/about-wecan /index.htm, accessed January 20, 2015.

National Institute on Aging, National Institutes of Health, US Department of Health and Human Services. Go4Life. Available at http://go4life.nia.nih.gov/, accessed January 20, 2015.

National Institute of Child Health and Human Development. *Media Smart Youth: Eat, Think, and Be Active*, May 2013. Available at http://www.nichd.nih.gov/msy/Pages/index.aspx, accessed January 20, 2015.

National Institutes of Health, National Heart, Lung, and Blood Institute. Classification of Overweight and Obesity by BMI, Waist Circumference and Associated Disease Risks. Available at http://www.nhlbi.nih .gov/guidelines/obesity/ ob_gdlns.htm, accessed January 20, 2015.

National Research Council. *Food Marketing to Children and Youth: Threat or Opportunity?* Washington, DC: The National Academies Press, 2006.

Nestle M. Soft drink "pouring rights": Marketing empty calories to children. *Public Health Rep.* 2000;115(4): 308–319.

New York City Department of Health and Mental Hygiene. Statements from Health Commissioner Mary T. Bassett and Supporters of New York City's Sugary Drink Portion Rule, June 4, 2014. Available at http:// www.nyc.gov/html/doh/downloads/pdf/press/sugary-drinks-statement.pdf, accessed January 20, 2015.

New York City Department of Health and Mental Hygiene. Sugary Drink Portion Cap Rule: Fact vs. Fiction. Available at http://www.nyc.gov/html/doh/downloads/pdf/cdp/sugary-drink-facts.pdf, accessed January 5, 2015.

Ogden CL, Flegal KM. Changes in terminology for childhood overweight and obesity. *Natl Health Stat Rep.* 2010;(25):1–5.

Ogden CL, Flegal KM, Carroll MD, Johnson CL. Prevalence and trends in overweight among US children and adolescents, 1999–2000. *JAMA*. 2002;288(14):1728–1732.

Ogden CL, Lamb MM, Carroll MD, Flegal KM. Obesity and socioeconomic status in adults: United States, 2005–2008. *NCHS Data Brief.* 2010a;(50):1–8.

Ogden CL, Lamb MM, Carroll MD, Flegal KM. Obesity and socioeconomic status in children and adolescents: United States, 2005–2008. *NCHS Data Brief.* 2010b;(51):1–8.

Ogden CL, Carroll MD, Kit BK, Flegal KM. Prevalence of obesity and trends in body mass index among US children and adolescents, 1999–2010. *JAMA*. 2012;307(5):483–490.

Ogden CL, Carroll MD, Kit BK, Flegal KM. Prevalence of obesity among adults: United States, 2011–2012. *NCHS Data Brief* No. 131. Hyattsville, MD: National Center for Health Statistics, October 2013. Available at http://www.cdc.gov/nchs/data/databriefs/db131.pdf, accessed January 20, 2015.

Ogden CL, Carroll MD, Kit BK, Flegal KM. Prevalence of childhood and adult obesity in the United States, 2011–2012. *JAMA*. 2014;311(8):806–814.

Patient Protection and Affordable Care Act, Pub. L. no. 111–148, 124 Stat. 119 (2010). Available at http://www .gpo.gov/fdsys/pkg/PLAW-111publ148/html/PLAW-111publ148.htm, accessed January 20, 2015.

Piernas C, Popkin BM. Snacking increased among US adults between 1977 and 2006. *J Nutr.* 2010a;140(2): 325–332.

Piernas C, Popkin BM. Trends in snacking among US children. *Health Affairs.* 2010b;29(3):398–404.

Piernas C, Popkin BM. Food portion patterns and trends among US children and the relationship to total eating occasion size, 1977–2006. *J Nutr.* 2011;141(6):1159–1164.

Popkin BM. The nutrition transition and obesity in the developing world. *J Nutr.* 2001;131(Suppl):871S–873S.

Popkin BM. An overview on the nutrition transition and its health implications: The Bellagio meeting. *Pub Health Nutr.* 2002;5(1A):93–103.

Powell LM, Chaloupka FJ, Bao Y. The availability of fast-food and full-service restaurants in the United States: Associations with neighborhood characteristics. *Am J Prev Med.* 2007;33(4 Suppl):S240–S245.

Probart C, McDonnell E, Weirich JE, Schilling L, Fekete V. Statewide assessment of local wellness policies in Pennsylvania public school districts. *J Am Diet Assoc.* 2008;108(9):1497–1502.

Proctor MH, Moore LL, Gao D, Cupples LA, Bradlee ML, Hood MY, Ellison RC. Television viewing and change in body fat from preschool to early adolescence: The Framingham Children's Study. *Int J Obes Relat Metab Disord.* 2003;27(7):827–833.

QuickStats: Percentage of adults aged ≥ 20 years who said they tried to lose weight during the preceding 12 months, by age group and sex—National Health and Nutrition Examination Survey, United States, 2005–2006. *MMWR.* 2008;57(42):1155. Available at http://www.cdc.gov/mmwr/preview/mmwrhtml /mm5742a4.htm, accessed January 20, 2015.

Rankinen T, Bouchard C. Dose–response issues concerning the relations between regular physical activity and health. President's Council on Physical Fitness and Sports. *Res Dig.* 2002;3(18):1–8.

Reeves MJ, Rafferty AP. Healthy lifestyle characteristics among adults in the United States. *Arch Intern Med.* 2005;165;854–857.

Rideout V. Zero to Eight: Children's Media Use in America 2013. *Common Sense Media,* Fall 2013. Available at https://www.commonsensemedia.org/research/zero-to-eight-childrens-media-use-in-america-2013, accessed January 20, 2015.

Robert Wood Johnson Foundation. Healthy Eating Research. Available at http://www.healthyeatingresearch .org/, accessed January 20, 2015.

Robinson TN. Does television cause childhood obesity? *JAMA.* 1998;279(12):959–960.

Robinson TN. Reducing children's television viewing to prevent obesity: A randomized controlled trial. *JAMA.* 1999;282(16):1561–1567.

School Nutrition Association, School Nutrition Foundation. From Cupcakes to Carrots: Local Wellness Policies One Year Later, September 2007. Available at https://schoolnutrition.org/uploadedFiles/5_News_and _Publications/4_The_Journal_of_Child_Nutrition_and_Management/Fall_2010/From_Cupcakes_to _Carrots.pdf, accessed January 20, 2015.

Schoonover H, Muller M. *Food without Thought: How US Farm Policy Contributes to Obesity.* Institute for Agriculture and Trade Policy: Environment and Agriculture Program, March 2006. Available at http:// www.iatp.org/files/421_2_80627.pdf, accessed January 20, 2015.

Sharma AJ, Grummer-Strawn LM, Dalenius K et al. Obesity prevalence among low-income, preschool-aged children—United States, 1998–2008. *MMWR.* 2009;58(28):769–773.

Shick SM, Wing RR, Klem ML, McGuire MT, Hill JO, Seagle H. Persons successful at long-term weight loss and maintenance continue to consume a low-energy, low-fat diet. *J Am Diet Assoc.* 1998;98:408–413.

Sobal J, Stunkard AJ. Socioeconomic status and obesity: A review of the literature. *Psychol Bull.* 1989;105(2):260–275.

Srinivasan S, O'Fallon LR, Dearry A. Creating healthy communities, healthy homes, healthy people: Initiating a research agenda on the built environment and public health. *Am J Public Health.* 2003;93;1446–1450.

Story M, Nanney MS, Schwartz MB. Schools and obesity prevention: Creating school environments and policies to promote healthy eating and physical activity. *Milbank Q.* 2009;87(1):71–100.

Swinburn B, Egger G, Raza F. Dissecting obesogenic environments: The development and application of a framework for identifying and prioritizing environmental interventions for obesity. *Prev Med.* 1999;29(6 Pt 1):563–570.

Tapper-Gardzina Y, Cotunga N, Vickery C. Should you recommend a low-carb, high-protein diet? *Nurse Pract.* 2002;27:52–59.

The Five LMCTC Goals. Available at http://www.healthycommunitieshealthyfuture.org/the-five-lmctc-goals, accessed January 20, 2015.

The President's Challenge. Available at https://www.presidentschallenge.org/index.shtml, accessed January 20, 2015.

Todd J, Mancino L, Lin B-H. *The Impact of Food Away from Home on Adult Diet Quality.* ERR-90. US Department of Agriculture, Economic Research Service, February 2010. Available at http://www.ers .usda.gov/publications/err-economic-research-report/err90.aspx#.U3zwDy8hkzw, accessed January 20, 2015.

Townsend MS, Peterson J, Love B, Achterberg C, Murphy SP. Food insecurity is positively related to overweight in women. *J Nutr.* 2001;131(6):1738–1745.

Trogdon JG, Finkelstein EA, Hylands T, Dellea PS, Kamal-Bahl SJ. Indirect costs of obesity: A review of the current literature. *Obes Rev.* 2008;9:489–500.

Tsai AG, Williamson DF, Glick HA. Direct medical cost of overweight and obesity in the USA: A quantitative systematic review. *Obes Rev.* 2011;12(1):50–61.

US Department of Agriculture. Agricultural Research Service. Available at http://www.ars.usda.gov/research /projects/projects.htm?ACCN_NO=421980, accessed February 2, 2015.

US Department of Agriculture, Food and Nutrition Service. HealthierUS School Challenge: Recognizing Excellence in Nutrition and Physical Activity. FNS-413, June 2012. Available at http://www.fns.usda .gov/sites/default/files/HUSSCbrochure2012.pdf, accessed January 20, 2015.

US Department of Agriculture, Food and Nutrition Service, Office of Research and Analysis. *School Nutrition Dietary Assessment Study IV, Vol. I: School Food Service Operations, School Environments, and Meals Offered and Served.* Alexandria, VA: Fox MK, Condon E, Crepinsek MK et al. Project Officer: Lesnett F, November 2012. Available at http://www.fns.usda.gov/sites/default/files/SNDA-IV_Vol1Pt1_0.pdf, accessed January 20, 2015.

US Department of Agriculture, Food and Nutrition Service. Team Nutrition. Available at http://www.fns.usda .gov/tn/team-nutrition, accessed January 20, 2015.

US Department of Agriculture. National Institute of Food and Agriculture. Available at http://www.nifa.usda .gov/funding/rfas/afri.html, accessed February 2, 2015.

US Department of Agriculture. Team Nutrition. School Nutrition Environment and Wellness Resources. Updated May 21, 2014. Available at http://healthymeals.nal.usda.gov/local-wellness-policy-resources /school-nutrition-environment-and-wellness-resources-0, accessed January 20, 2015.

US Department of Health and Human Services. Office of the Surgeon General. The Surgeon General's Vision for a Healthy and Fit Nation. Available at http://www.surgeongeneral.gov/initiatives/healthy-fit-nation /obesityvision2010.pdf, accessed February 2, 2015.

US Department of Health and Human Services. *The Surgeon General's Call to Action to Prevent and Decrease Overweight and Obesity.* Rockville, MD: US Department of Health and Human Services, Public Health Service, Office of the Surgeon General, 2001. Available at http://www.surgeongeneral.gov/library/calls /obesity/index.html, accessed January 20, 2015.

US Department of Health and Human Services. *We Can!:* Ways to Enhance Children's Activity & Nutrition. *Families Finding the Balance: A Parent Handbook.* NIH Publication 05-5273. National Institutes of Health, 2005. Available at http://www.nhlbi.nih.gov/files/docs/public/heart/parent_hb_en.pdf, accessed January 7, 2015.

US Department of Labor. Employee Benefits Security Administration Fact Sheet: The Affordable Care Act and Wellness Programs. Available at http://www.dol.gov/ebsa/newsroom/fswellnessprogram.html, accessed January 20, 2015.

Ustjanauskas AE, Harris JK, Schwartz MB. *Food and Beverage Advertising on Children's Websites.* Rudd Center for Food Policy and Obesity. Available at http://www.yaleruddcenter.org/resources/upload/docs /what/advertising/banner_ads_ijpo_7.13.pdf, accessed February 2, 2015.

Variam JN. The price is right: Economics and the rise in obesity. *Amber Waves.* 2005;3(1):20–27.

Vartanian LR, Schwartz MB, Brownell KD. Effects of soft drink consumption on nutrition and health: A systematic review and meta-analysis. *Am J Public Health.* 2007;97(4):667–675.

Weber K, Story M, Harnack L. Internet food marketing strategies aimed at children and adolescents: A content analysis of food and beverage brand web sites. *J Am Diet Assoc.* 2006;106(9):1463–1466.

Wilcox BL, Kunkel D, Cantor J, Dowrick P, Linn S, Palmer E. *Report of the APA Task Force on Advertising and Children.* American Psychological Association, 2004. Available at http://www.apa.org/pi/families /resources/advertising-children.pdf, accessed January 20, 2015.

Wing RR, Phelan S. Long-term weight loss maintenance. *Am J Clin Nutr.* 2005;82(Suppl):222S–225S.

Wolf AM. Economic outcomes of the obese patient. *Obes Res.* 2002;10(Suppl 1):58S–62S.

Wolf AM, Colditz GA. Social and economic effects of body weight in the United States. *Am J Clin Nutr.* 1996;63(Suppl):466S–469S.

World Health Organization. Diet, Nutrition and the Prevention of Chronic Diseases: Report of a Joint WHO/ FAO Expert Consultation. Geneva, January 28–February 1, 2002. WHO Technical Report Series 916. Geneva, Switzerland: WHO, 2003. Available at http://whqlibdoc.who.int/trs/WHO_TRS_916. pdf?ua=1, accessed January 20, 2015.

World Health Organization. *Global Action Plan for the Prevention and Control of Noncommunicable Diseases 2013–2020.* Geneva: WHO Press, 2013. Available at http://apps.who.int/iris/bitstream/10665 /94384/1/9789241506236_eng.pdf?ua=1, accessed January 20, 2015.

World Health Organization. Media Centre: Obesity and Overweight. Available at http://www.who.int/media centre/factsheets/fs311/en/, updated January 2015, accessed January 29, 2015.

Young LR, Nestle M. The contribution of expanding portion sizes to the US obesity epidemic. *Am J Public Health.* 2002;92(2):246–249.

Young LR, Nestle M. Portion sizes and obesity: Responses of fast-food companies. *J Public Health Policy.* 2007;28(2):238–248.

Zhang Q, Wang Y. Trends in the association between obesity and socioeconomic status in US adults: 1971 to 2000. *Obes Res.* 2004;12(10):1622–1632.

6 Special Populations*

It is very important to understand the following true thing: women are not a special population. They are *half* (more, actually) of the population.

Rippetoe and Kilgore (2008)

INTRODUCTION

This chapter examines three populations that are (or should be) of special interest to public health nutritionists: lactating mothers, people living with HIV/AIDS, and inmates in correctional facilities. We focus on these groups for diverse reasons:

- The incidence and duration of breastfeeding took a turn for the worse in the middle of the last century; public health has a mandate to reverse this trend.
- With the advent of highly active antiretroviral therapy (HAART; the combination of several antiretroviral medications, which slows the rate at which HIV multiplies in the body), the population that is HIV seropositive is living longer, turning HIV into a chronic disease requiring constant dietary vigilance.
- Inmates with chronic diseases who have not had access to nutritionally appropriate diets nor who have learned self-management techniques while incarcerated will reenter society in a health-compromised state and will be less able or likely to manage their health.

LACTATING MOTHERS AND BREASTFED INFANTS

According to the 2014 Centers for Disease Control and Prevention (CDC) Breastfeeding Report Card (Centers for Disease Control and Prevention 2014), babies born in 2011 were breastfed at rates that approached or exceeded the targets set by Healthy People 2010. A rate of 79% was reported for breastfeeding initiation, with a 49% continuation rate to 6 months and 27% at 1 year of age. Encouraged by these results, the Academy of Nutrition and Dietetics (AND) (American Dietetic Association 2009), the American Academy of Pediatrics (AAP) (2012), the World Health Organization (WHO) (2001), and the US Department of Health and Human Services (HHS) have all recommended increases in the proportion of mothers who breastfeed their babies. In particular, HHS's *Healthy People 2020* calls for an 81.9% breastfeeding initiation rate, a 60.6% continuation rate to 6 months, and a 34.1% rate at 1 year (US Department of Health and Human Services 2010).

In the United States, breastfeeding rates vary geographically and sociodemographically. To increase the initiation and duration of breastfeeding, public health measures should target the populations with the lowest breastfeeding rates and invest in institutional changes that will support this behavioral outcome.

BENEFITS OF BREASTFEEDING

The physiological benefits of breastfeeding to mother and child are well documented, yet other apparent benefits have not yet received unqualified support. In addition to these physiologic advantages, breastfeeding boasts several nonphysiological benefits that have major implications for public health.

---

* Ellen Passov contributed primary research and prepared draft versions of portions of this chapter.

Physiologic Benefits

The documented health benefits of breastfeeding for new mothers are decreased postpartum bleeding and more rapid uterine involution. For the infant, human milk feeding has been shown to decrease the incidence and/or severity of a wide range of infectious diseases, including bacterial meningitis, bacteremia, gastroenteritis, respiratory tract infection, necrotizing enterocolitis (NEC), otitis media, urinary tract infection, and late-onset sepsis in preterm infants. Three of these childhood diseases commonly afflict children under 2 years old:

- *Otitis media* is an inflammation of the ear and is the most frequently reported diagnosis for children under the age of 2 years. Breastfeeding reduces the incidence of otitis media; in the first year of life, infants who breastfed exclusively for at least 4 months have half as many episodes of acute otitis media as formula-fed infants.
- *Gastroenteritis* refers to vomiting or diarrhea as a discrete illness for a 24-hour period.
- *NEC* is the most common gastrointestinal tract disease in the neonatal intensive care unit (NICU), the leading cause of emergency surgical treatment in newborns, and a major cause of neonatal death. Over 90% of NEC cases affect premature infants. Incidence approaches 12% of all low birth weight (LBW) premature infants. The onset of NEC is usually within the first 10 days of life. Its incidence in exclusively breastfed LBW infants is 1%, compared with an incidence of 7% in formula-fed LBW infants (Steube 2009).

In addition to the known benefits of breastfeeding, there is preliminary evidence of its associations with decreased rates of sudden infant death syndrome (SIDS) in the first year of life, and with reductions in types 1 and 2 diabetes, lymphoma, leukemia, Hodgkin's disease, overweight and obesity, hypercholesterolemia, and asthma in older children and adults. Breastfeeding has also been associated with slightly enhanced tests of cognitive development.

Additional Benefits

Economic, family, and environmental benefits result from breastfeeding. These benefits include the potential for decreased environmental burden from reduced disposal of formula cans and bottles, decreased energy costs associated with the manufacture and transport of artificial feeding products, decreased medical bills due to a lessened incidence of childhood illness, and decreased employee absenteeism to care for sick children. An unknown proportion of the medical care savings would be offset by increased costs associated with lactation. These extra expenses would include consultations by physicians and others, and equipment associated with breastfeeding, such as breast pumps. With the passage of the Affordable Care Act in 2010 (ACA), all of these expenses must be fully covered by third-party reimbursement (US Health Resources and Services Administration, http://www.hrsa.gov/womensguidelines).

Healthcare costs, both direct and indirect, related to childhood illness are staggering. The annual cost of treating US children under 5 for otitis media alone is estimated at $5 billion per year (Bondy et al. 2000). Breastfeeding results in decreased national healthcare costs and decreased employee absenteeism to care for infants who are ill. Based on epidemiological studies that relate breastfeeding to the risk of otitis media, gastroenteritis, and NEC, and estimates of treatment costs, the United States Department of Agriculture (USDA) estimated that an increase in breastfeeding rates from the 1988 levels to the year 2010 targets of 75% at discharge and 50% at 6 months would save a minimum of $3.6 billion annually. The majority of these savings are attributable to preventing premature deaths due to NEC. Because this analysis represents savings from treating only three childhood illnesses, the $3.6 billion figure is probably an underestimation (Weimer, http://www.ers.usda.gov/publications/fanrr-food-assistance-nutrition-research-program/fanrr13.aspx). In fact, an updated analysis using the same methods but by different authors estimates the savings of increasing compliance to 90% at 6 months to comprise $13 billion a year (Bartick and Reinhold 2010).

As for the individual family, the cost savings in 1999 for breastfed infants when compared with formula-fed babies were estimated to be between $331 and $475 per child in a single year, based on less frequent episodes of otitis media, diarrhea, and lower respiratory tract infections (Ball and Wright 1999).

Breastfeeding contributes to the health of the environment in numerous ways. Human milk is a renewable natural resource manufactured at the cost of only 450 (Butte and King 2005) to 500 (Picciano 2003) kcal/day per infant during the first few months postpartum. Human milk is delivered at no cost at all or very inexpensively in terms of breast pumping and milk storage for later use. Unlike bottle feeding, breastfeeding consumes no energy associated with transportation, shipping, and disposing of containers (American Dietetic Association 2009).

BREASTFEEDING TRENDS

Despite its benefits, rates of breastfeeding in the United States declined dramatically during the mid-twentieth century. According to AND (American Dietetic Association 2009), almost all infants were breastfed in colonial America, but by the 1880s, mothers began to supplement breastfeeding with raw cow's milk and to wean their infants before they were 3 months old. Infants fed with raw cow's milk had higher mortality rates than their breastfed counterparts. The breastfeeding decline continued during the period when milk substitutes (evaporated cow's milk and infant formula) became widely available. These human milk substitutes were aggressively marketed as being both more convenient for the mother and more nutritious for her infant than human milk.

More than two-thirds of women born in the 1920s began breastfeeding their first child, and more than 40% were still breastfeeding at 6 months. Only about 25% of women born in the late 1940s began breastfeeding their first child, and less than 5% continued at 6 months. In other words, breast-feeding initiation had relatively precipitously declined over two generations to a low of 25% during the late 1960s/early 1970s (Hirschman and Butler 1981).

Breastfeeding initiation rose again to almost 66% in 1982, according to the Ross Mothers Survey conducted in 1988 (Ryan 1997), and after a dip in the late 1980s, continued to increase, reaching 70% in 2003 and 79% for babies born in 2011 (Centers for Disease Control and Prevention 2014).

However, the number of breastfeeding mothers and trends in breastfeeding vary widely across socioeconomic and cultural categories. Among the groups experiencing the most precipitous declines in breastfeeding levels from the late 1950s to the late 1970s were black women, women with less than 12 years of education, and women who never worked outside the home (US Department of Agriculture et al. 2004).

In the 1950s, black and Hispanic mothers were more likely to breastfeed their babies than white mothers. But during the decline in breastfeeding prevalence in the early 1970s, rates of breastfeeding dropped most dramatically for blacks and have not fully recovered. In contrast, breastfeeding rates among white and Hispanic mothers rose sharply beginning in the 1970s, and reached or exceeded 1950s levels by the late 1980s (Ryan and Zhou 2006). Historically, breastfeeding rates among Special Supplemental Nutrition Program for Women, Infants, and Children (WIC) participants have lagged behind those of non-WIC mothers. However, in 2012, for the first time, the number of participant mothers breastfeeding exceeded that of those who were not (US Department of Agriculture et al. 2013). As 53% of US infants participate in WIC (US Department of Agriculture, http://www.fns.usda.gov/wic/about-wic-wic-glance), unarguably, a goal of public health nutrition must be to help increase the initiation and duration of breastfeeding.

BREASTFEEDING SURVEILLANCE

A number of surveys and surveillance systems measure breastfeeding in the United States, each of which faces its own challenges and problems.

Ross Mothers Survey

Although flawed, the oldest data about breastfeeding in the United States come from the Ross Mothers Survey (RMS). Ross Products, a division of Abbott Laboratories, a US marketer of pediatric nutritionals, started conducting periodic surveys in 1955 to examine infant feeding patterns during the first year of life. Although until 1999 it did not differentiate between *any* breastfeeding and *exclusive* breastfeeding, it remains the only source of long-term infant-feeding trends available (Ryan 2004).

National Immunization Survey

The National Immunization Survey (NIS) is sponsored by the National Immunization Program (NIP) and conducted jointly by NIP and the CDC's National Center for Health Statistics (NCHS). The NIS is a random-digit dialing telephone survey of households with children 9–36 months of age (Zell et al. 2000). Since 2003, breastfeeding questions have been added to the survey in order to assess the population's breastfeeding practices. The questions were updated in 2004 and again in 2006. Starting in 2011, a cellular telephone sample was also conducted. Each survey year presents a cohort from prior birth years. For example, the 2012 survey includes data for births between January 2009 and May 2011. The 2012 survey included the following questions about breastfeeding (Centers for Disease Control and Prevention, http://www.cdc.gov/breastfeeding/data/nis_data /survey_methods.htm):

- Was [child's name] ever breastfed or fed breast milk?
- How old was [child's name] when [child's name] completely stopped breastfeeding or being fed breast milk?
- How old was [child's name] when [he/she] was first fed formula?
- This next question is about the first thing that [child's name] was given other than breast milk or formula. Please include juice, cow's milk, sugar water, or anything else that [child's name] may have been given, even water. How old was [child's name] when he/she was first fed anything other than breast milk or formula?

A study of the validity and reliability of maternal recall of breastfeeding history revealed that maternal recall is a valid and reliable estimate of breastfeeding initiation and duration, especially when the duration of breastfeeding is recalled after a short period of time (through 3 years). However, validity and reliability of maternal recall for the age at introduction of food and fluids other than breast milk are less satisfactory (Box 6.1) (Li et al. 2005).

Pregnancy Risk Assessment Monitoring System

Pregnancy Risk Assessment Monitoring System (PRAMS) is an ongoing state- and population-based surveillance system implemented in 40 states plus New York City as of 2014 (Centers for Disease Control and Prevention, http://www.cdc.gov/prams/). The goal of PRAMS is to improve the health of mothers and infants by reducing adverse outcomes. The system was designed to monitor selected maternal behaviors and experiences that occur before, during, and after pregnancy among women who deliver live-born infants. PRAMS employs a mixed mode data-collection methodology: up to

---

BOX 6.1   VALIDITY AND RELIABILITY

A test is valid when it measures what it is meant to measure. How valid a test is depends on its purpose—for example, a ruler may be a valid measuring device for length but is not valid for measuring volume. A test is reliable if it yields consistent results. A test can be both reliable and valid, one or the other, or neither.

three self-administered surveys are mailed to a sample of mothers, and nonresponders are followed up with telephone interviews. Self-reported survey data are linked to selected birth certificate data and weighted for sample design, nonresponse, and noncoverage to create the annual PRAMS analysis data sets. PRAMS can be used to produce statewide estimates of different perinatal health behaviors and experiences among women delivering live infants. PRAMS data can also be used to identify racial, ethnic, and socioeconomic disparities in critical maternal health-related behaviors.

PRAMS surveys women about breastfeeding initiation—a behavior for which substantial health disparities have been previously identified. Data are available for 29 states. Among women in those states, the overall prevalence of breastfeeding initiation as of 2008 was 77.1%, with state-specific prevalence estimates ranging from 49.5% in Mississippi to 93.8% in Oregon (initiation rates were generally lower in the southeastern states and higher in the western states). Twenty-eight states had 3 or more years of consecutive data available, and 24 of those states showed significant increasing trends in the prevalence of breastfeeding initiation. When viewed by the characteristic of age, the lowest rates of breastfeeding initiation occurred in women who were less than 20 years old. When viewed by race/ethnicity, the lowest rates of breastfeeding initiation occurred among black women. Finally, the rates were significantly lower among women who received Medicaid and those who participated in WIC as compared to those who did not. As the characteristic of low prevalence may vary by state, state-specific policies and programs may be critical.

States can use PRAMS data to identify populations at greatest risk for maternal behaviors that have negative consequences for maternal and infant health and to develop policies and plan programs that target populations at high risk. Although prevalence data cannot be used to identify causes or interventions to improve health outcomes, they do indicate the magnitude of disparities and identify populations that should be targeted for intervention. Additionally, the data produced by this study and others using PRAMS can serve as a baseline for use in measuring the impact of policies and programs on achieving policy goals, such as that of Healthy People 2020.

Sociodemographic Factors of Lactating Mothers

Understanding the sociodemographic characteristics of women who do and do not breastfeed is important for designing and implementing breastfeeding promotion campaigns. Before developing lactation programs, healthcare planners must know the age, income, and other demographic characteristics of the target population they hope to reach. When health educators are preparing lactation-related educational materials or activities, they need to know the demographic profile of the target audience, so that appropriate programs or efforts are made available.

The CDC (http://www.cdc.gov/breastfeeding/data/nis_data/) publishes updated NIS survey data on a rolling basis. As of November 2014, data were published with overall population estimates for the initiation, duration, and exclusivity of breastfeeding for children born between 2001 and 2011. It also provides geographic-specific and sociodemographic breastfeeding rates for babies born in birth cohorts from 2009 to 2011 and separately for birth cohorts 2000–2007. Table 6.1 provides 2011 sociodemographic breastfeeding rates.

Although the highest income women have for the most part the highest prevalence of any breastfeeding behaviors, all income groups have seen a healthy increase in exclusive breastfeeding at 6 months. The lowest breastfeeding rates are evident in women with one or more of the following characteristics: unmarried, under the age of 20 years, income below the poverty threshold, and a WIC participant. Understandably, these findings prompted WIC to concentrate on promoting breastfeeding. The WIC initiatives to increase the initiation and duration of breastfeeding are discussed later in this chapter.

Consistent with previous research, the NIS breastfeeding data reveal that non-Hispanic blacks, American Indians/Alaska Natives, and groups with low socioeconomic status (SES) have the lowest breastfeeding rates, while Asians, whites, and Latinas are the most likely to breastfeed exclusively for at least 3 months.

TABLE 6.1

Rates of Any and Exclusive Breastfeeding by Sociodemographics among Children Born in 2011 (Percentage ± Half 95% Confidence Interval)[a,b]

		Any Breastfeeding				Exclusive Breastfeeding	
Sociodemographic Factors	n	Ever Breastfed % ± Half 95% CI	Breastfed at 6 Months % ± Half 95% CI	Breastfed at 12 Months % ± Half 95% CI	n	Exclusive Breastfeeding through 3 Months % ± Half 95% CI	Exclusive Breastfeeding through 6 Months % ± Half 95% CI
US National	14,456	79.2 ± 1.2	49.4 ± 1.5	26.7 ± 1.3	14,131	40.7 ± 1.5	18.8 ± 1.2
Gender							
Male	7481	79.5 ± 1.6	49.6 ± 2.1	25.9 ± 1.9	7312	40.5 ± 2.1	18.4 ± 1.7
Female	6975	78.9 ± 1.7	49.3 ± 2.2	27.6 ± 1.9	6819	40.9 ± 2.2	19.2 ± 1.7
Race/Ethnicity							
Hispanic	2801	83.8 ± 2.4	48.4 ± 3.8	24.8 ± 3.3	2756	38.3 ± 3.8	17.1 ± 2.9
Non-Hispanic white	8382	81.1 ± 1.4	52.3 ± 1.8	28.4 ± 1.6	8162	44.8 ± 1.8	20.3 ± 1.4
Non-Hispanic black	1414	61.6 ± 4.1	35.0 ± 3.9	16.4 ± 3.3	1386	26.9 ± 3.8	13.7 ± 3.2
Non-Hispanic Asian	648	90.9 ± 3.0	71.2 ± 7.1	47.3 ± 7.8	634	52.5 ± 7.6	26.6 ± 7.0
Non-Hispanic Hawaiian Pacific Islander	67	75.0 ± 21.7	49.8 ± 22.0	25.7 ± 16.4	67	41.1 ± 20.4	21.0 ± 17.5
Non-Hispanic American Indian/ Alaska Native	221	77.1 ± 8.3	37.3 ± 11.8	25.0 ± 9.7	216	45.5 ± 14.7	15.6 ± 7.4
2 or more races	923	75.0 ± 5.3	48.4 ± 5.8	29.3 ± 5.0	910	40.1 ± 5.5	19.6 ± 4.3
Maternal Education							
Less than high school	1582	69.1 ± 3.7	34.4 ± 4.0	19.7 ± 3.4	1555	27.3 ± 4.2	13.5 ± 3.1
High school graduate	2622	69.2 ± 2.8	38.2 ± 3.2	19.6 ± 2.8	2573	32.6 ± 3.3	15.8 ± 2.6
Some college or technical school	3859	81.0 ± 2.3	46.1 ± 2.9	23.6 ± 2.6	3776	41.8 ± 3.0	16.5 ± 2.3
College graduate	6393	91.2 ± 1.1	68.3 ± 2.1	38.1 ± 2.2	6227	53.5 ± 2.2	25.5 ± 1.9
Maternal Age							
Under 20	201	66.9 ± 10.6	19.4 ± 8.2	13.1 ± 7.1	201	19.3 ± 8.7	5.6 ± 5.0
20–29	5559	73.6 ± 2.1	39.1 ± 2.4	18.8 ± 2.0	5458	36.4 ± 2.5	15.2 ± 1.7
30 or older	8696	84.2 ± 1.3	58.8 ± 1.9	33.6 ± 1.9	8472	45.0 ± 2.0	22.2 ± 1.7
Poverty Income Ratio[c]							
Less than 100	3690	70.5 ± 2.5	37.8 ± 2.9	20.3 ± 2.5	3627	31.2 ± 2.9	14.2 ± 2.2
100–199	2919	77.9 ± 2.6	45.5 ± 3.1	24.7 ± 2.7	2843	39.3 ± 3.1	18.0 ± 2.5
200–399	3732	85.8 ± 1.9	57.7 ± 2.9	32.1 ± 2.7	3633	49.2 ± 2.9	22.0 ± 2.4
400–599	2237	87.1 ± 2.2	61.9 ± 3.4	34.9 ± 3.5	2200	49.0 ± 3.6	25.2 ± 3.3
600 or greater	1878	90.6 ± 2.2	67.9 ± 4.0	33.5 ± 4.4	1828	50.9 ± 4.6	23.1 ± 3.8
Marital Status[d]							
Married	10,371	86.7 ± 1.2	60.1 ± 1.8	33.3 ± 1.7	10,102	47.7 ± 1.8	22.6 ± 1.5
Unmarried	4085	67.1 ± 2.4	32.1 ± 2.6	16.1 ± 2.2	4029	29.4 ± 2.6	12.7 ± 1.9

(Continued)

TABLE 6.1 (CONTINUED)

Rates of Any and Exclusive Breastfeeding by Sociodemographics among Children Born in 2011 (Percentage ± Half 95% Confidence Interval)[a,b]

Sociodemographic Factors	n	Any Breastfeeding			n	Exclusive Breastfeeding	
		Ever Breastfed	Breastfed at 6 Months	Breastfed at 12 Months		Exclusive Breastfeeding through 3 Months	Exclusive Breastfeeding through 6 Months
		% ± Half 95% CI	% ± Half 95% CI	% ± Half 95% CI		% ± Half 95% CI	% ± Half 95% CI
Geographic Location[e]							
Metropolitan	2907	83.5 ± 2.4	54.9 ± 3.2	30.6 ± 3.0	2841	43.2 ± 3.3	21.7 ± 2.8
Nonmetropolitan	892	71.4 ± 5.2	42.2 ± 5.6	25.9 ± 5.0	870	37.6 ± 5.6	17.0 ± 4.3
Birth Order							
First born	8841	78.5 ± 1.6	50.0 ± 2.0	27.7 ± 1.8	8634	41.3 ± 2.0	19.0 ± 1.6
Not first born	5615	80.3 ± 1.8	48.4 ± 2.3	25.2 ± 2.1	5497	39.8 ± 2.3	18.5 ± 1.8
Receiving WIC[f]							
Yes	6519	71.8 ± 1.9	37.8 ± 2.2	19.7 ± 1.8	6408	31.7 ± 2.2	13.9 ± 1.6
No, but eligible	987	83.4 ± 4.4	56.1 ± 5.6	32.8 ± 5.1	954	50.3 ± 5.6	26.5 ± 4.9
Ineligible	6883	89.8 ± 1.1	66.0 ± 2.0	36.2 ± 2.1	6708	53.0 ± 2.2	24.9 ± 1.9

Source: National Immunization Survey, Centers for Disease Control and Prevention, Department of Health and Human Services. Available at http://www.cdc.gov/breastfeeding/data/nis_data/rates-any-exclusive-bf-socio-dem-2011.htm, accessed January 9, 2015.

[a] Breastfeeding rates presented in this table are based on dual-frame (landline and cellular telephone) samples from 2012 and 2013 NIS. See survey methods for details on study design.

[b] Exclusive breastfeeding is defined as ONLY breast milk—NO solids, no water, and no other liquids.

[c] Poverty income ratio = ratio of self-reported family income to the federal poverty threshold value depending on the number of people in the household.

[d] Unmarried includes never married, widowed, separated, divorced.

[e] Metropolitan area is defined by the Census Bureau.

[f] WIC = Special Supplemental Nutrition Program for Women, Infants, and Children.

As of November 2014, the NIS Breastfeeding Data and Statistics for children born in 2007 reveals that 26 states achieved the Healthy People 2010 objective of 75% of mothers initiating breastfeeding. Sixteen states achieved the objective of 50% of mothers breastfeeding their children at 6 months of age. Twelve states achieved the objective of having 25% of infants still breastfeeding at 12 months of age. In addition, 9 states had a greater than 20% rate of infants being breastfed without supplemental foods or liquids for the first 6 months of life, which is known as *exclusive breastfeeding* and consistent with the AAP's breastfeeding recommendation (Centers for Disease Control and Prevention, http://www.cdc.gov/breastfeeding/data/NIS_data/2007/state_any.htm).

OVERCOMING BARRIERS TO BREASTFEEDING

A number of factors act as barriers to breastfeeding initiation and continuation. The major deterrents to breastfeeding include aggressive formula product marketing, lack of social support, lack of role models, lack of proper guidance from healthcare providers, lack of timely and postpartum follow-up care, disruptive hospital maternity care practices, and an increasing number of women in the workforce. An examination of these factors appears in the next two sections. The discussion is based on the CDC's *Guide to Strategies to Support Breastfeeding Mothers and Babies*, the 2013 update to the CDC's 2005 *Guide to Breastfeeding Interventions*.

Social Support

According to the CDC (*The CDC Guide to Strategies to Support Breastfeeding Mothers and Babies* 2013), social networks influence women's decision-making processes. Networks can be either barriers or points of encouragement for breastfeeding. New mothers' preferred resource for concerns about child rearing is other mothers (such as advice from a friend). Perceived social support has also been found to predict success in breastfeeding.

Peer support represents a cost-effective, individually tailored, and culturally competent (see Chapter 7) way to promote and support breastfeeding for women of varying socioeconomic backgrounds, especially when peer mothers have similar sociocultural backgrounds as those whom they support.

The goal of peer support is to encourage and support pregnant women and those who currently breastfeed. Peer support, provided by mothers who are currently breastfeeding or who have done so in the past, includes individual counseling and mother-to-mother support groups. Peer mothers provide support and counseling to help women address their barriers to breastfeeding and assist them in preventing and managing breastfeeding problems. Peer support includes psycho-emotional support, encouragement, education about breastfeeding, and help with solving problems. Women who provide peer support undergo specific training and may work in an informal group or one on one through telephone calls or visits in the home, clinic, or hospital.

In 1997, as part of the WIC National Breastfeeding Promotion Project of the late 1990s, the USDA's Food and Nutrition Service (FNS) introduced *Loving Support Makes Breastfeeding Work* using social marketing techniques (mass media, participant education materials) and staff training. A follow-up effort in 2002, called *Using Loving Support to Build a Breastfeeding-Friendly Community*, provided training and technical assistance to selected WIC state agencies to build state-specific breastfeeding promotion programs, also using social marketing techniques to raise public awareness, acceptance, and support of breastfeeding. In 2004, FNS launched a national peer counseling initiative developed specifically for WIC: *Using Loving Support to Implement Best Practices in Peer Counseling* (US Department of Agriculture 2010).

This program helped institutionalize peer counseling as a core service. While many WIC state agencies already provided successful peer counseling programs, new programs were implemented as part of this national effort. After receiving extensive training, WIC peer counselors work primarily from home to provide telephone support to pregnant and breastfeeding mothers. In many WIC programs, peer counselors also provide clinic-based counseling, make home visits during the early postpartum period, lead prenatal breastfeeding classes and postpartum support groups, and provide one-to-one support in the hospital setting (US Department of Agriculture 2010).

Education

In the United States, most new mothers do not have direct, personal knowledge of breastfeeding, and many find it hard to rely on family members for consistent, accurate information and guidance about infant feeding. Further, although many women have a general understanding of the benefits of breastfeeding, they lack exposure to sources of information regarding how breastfeeding is actually carried out. The CDC found that *prenatal breastfeeding education is the single most effective intervention for increasing breastfeeding initiation and short-term duration.*

The goal of educating mothers is to influence their attitudes toward breastfeeding as well as to increase their breastfeeding knowledge and skills. Breastfeeding education occurs most often during the prenatal and intrapartum (childbirth) periods and should be taught by someone with expertise or training in lactation management.

Prenatal instruction typically occurs within an informally structured small group setting but may be given one to one. This education primarily includes information and resources. The target audience is usually pregnant or breastfeeding women but may also include fathers and others who support the breastfeeding mother.

Intrapartum breastfeeding education is time sensitive. This type of education is often less formal than education provided during pregnancy, is generally conducted individually, and almost always occurs within a hospital setting. Intrapartum education usually focuses on immediate issues, such as fostering appropriate latch and positioning, adequate milk removal, stability of the infant, and comfort of the mother. It also provides an opportunity to reassure and support a concerned mother or family member, provides mothers and family members with referral information for further postpartum support, and allows the reiteration of signs of success or potential problems in the first few days after hospital discharge. All hospitals that routinely handle births should have staff with adequate training and knowledge to address and facilitate routine, standard breastfeeding education in the intrapartum period for all breastfeeding mothers and infants.

The professional member of the healthcare team for complex breastfeeding problems and lactation management is generally the international board-certified lactation consultant (IBCLC). Other health professionals with expertise in breastfeeding support include dietitians, physicians, and nurses who specialize in lactation. Since 2008, the International Board of Certified Lactation Examiners (http://www.iblce.org/) has administered an examination process to credential individuals trained in lactation support. To date, over 27,000 individuals have been certified worldwide.

Maternity Care Practices

Breastfeeding is a time-sensitive relationship. Experiences with breastfeeding in the first hours and days of life influence an infant's later feeding. Because of its inextricable relationship with the birth experience, breastfeeding must be supported throughout the maternity hospital stay, not delayed until the infant goes home. The hospital stay, although short, is a critical period for the establishment of breastfeeding. Many of the experiences of mothers and newborns in the hospital and the practices in place there affect how likely breastfeeding is to be established.

Prenatal education on breastfeeding can affect a mother's decision to even consider it as a feeding option. Medications and procedures administered to the mother during labor affect the infant's behavior at the time of birth, which in turn affects the infant's ability to suckle in an organized and effective manner at the breast. Infants who are put to the breast within the first few hours after birth continue breastfeeding longer than those whose first breastfeeding is delayed. Mothers who are able to have their infants in their room will have more opportunities to practice breastfeeding because of the infant's proximity.

Maternity care practices supportive of breastfeeding include developing a written policy on breastfeeding, providing all staff (e.g., nurses, physicians, radiology staff, pharmacy staff, food service, and housekeeping staff) with education and training, encouraging early breastfeeding initiation, supporting cue-based feeding, restricting supplements and pacifiers for breastfed infants, and providing for postdischarge follow-up. The use of medications during labor and cesarean birth has been shown to have a negative effect on breastfeeding, whereas providing continuous support during labor and maintaining skin-to-skin contact between mother and baby after birth has a positive effect on breastfeeding.

Baby-Friendly Hospital Initiative

The Baby-Friendly Hospital Initiative (BFHI) is a global United Nations International Children's Emergency Fund/WHO (UNICEF/WHO)-sponsored effort to promote breastfeeding. Launched in 1991, the initiative is based on 10 policy or procedure statements, known as Ten Steps, jointly developed and published in 1989 by UNICEF and WHO in consultation with international experts. In 1990, the Ten Steps were accepted as the central theme of the Innocenti Declaration and, later that year, endorsed at the World Summit on Children. The Innocenti Declaration (http://www.unicef

.org/programme/breastfeeding/innocenti.htm), stated in Appendix 6.1, has four targets: government involvement, participation of maternity facilities in the Ten Steps, enforcement of principles guiding the marketing of breast-milk substitutes, and legislative enforcement of rights of breastfeeding women in the workplace. In 2005, the Declaration was updated to address breastfeeding challenges in the face of the HIV pandemic, gender inequalities, and environmental contaminants (UNICEF, http://www.unicef-irc.org/publications/435), and the training on accomplishing the Ten Steps was updated in 2009 to address the challenges faced by HIV-infected pregnant and nursing women (World Health Organization, http://www.who.int/nutrition/topics/bfhi/en/).

A maternity facility can be designated baby-friendly when it does not accept free or low-cost breast-milk substitutes, feeding bottles, or nipples, (i.e., conforming to the International Code of Breastmilk Substitutes) and has implemented these 10 specific steps to support successful breastfeeding (Baby-Friendly USA, https://www.babyfriendlyusa.org/about-us/baby-friendly-hospital-initiative/the-ten-steps).

1. Have a written breastfeeding policy that is routinely communicated to all healthcare staff.
2. Train all healthcare staff in skills necessary to implement this policy.
3. Inform all pregnant women about the benefits and management of breastfeeding.
4. Help mothers initiate breastfeeding within a half-hour of birth.
5. Show mothers how to breastfeed and how to maintain lactation even if they should be separated from their infants.
6. Give newborn infants no food or drink other than breast milk, unless medically indicated.
7. Practice rooming-in—allow mothers and infants to remain together—24 hours a day.
8. Encourage breastfeeding on demand.
9. Give no artificial teats or pacifiers to breastfeeding infants.
10. Foster the establishment of breastfeeding support groups and refer mothers to them on discharge from the hospital or clinic.

As of 2006, more than 20,000 healthcare facilities in more than 150 countries around the world have achieved Baby-Friendly certified status through implementation of the Ten Steps and termination of the practice of distributing free or low-cost breast-milk substitutes (Box 6.2) (Abrahams and Labbok 2009).

The BFHI is considered one of the most successful international efforts ever undertaken to protect, promote, and support breastfeeding. It helps mothers to initiate exclusive nursing. Even when mothers do not achieve (or aspire to) the widely accepted goal of approximately 6 months of exclusive breastfeeding, the initiation of exclusive nursing supports any breastfeeding goal (Naylor 2001).

Boston Medical Center (BMC) reported that breastfeeding initiation rates rose from 58% in 1995 before implementation of their program to 87% in 1999 after the policies were in place, including an increase in breastfeeding initiation among US-born African American mothers from 34% to 74% (Philipp et al. 2001). BMC's NICU reported that improvement in breastfeeding initiation and any breastfeeding at 2 weeks of age for NICU infants has continued 10 years after Baby-Friendly designation, with initiation increased from 74% in 1999 to 85% in 2009, and any breast milk at 2 weeks of age increased from 66% to 80%. The authors also report that breastfeeding initiation increased among black mothers from 68% in 1999 to 86% in 2009 (Parker et al. 2013).

In 2007, only 2.9% of US births occurred in Baby-Friendly designated facilities. As of the end of 2014, the BFHI is implemented in 229 facilities in the United States, accounting for 10.44% of US births (Baby-Friendly USA 2014). The Healthy People 2020 goal of 8.1% births has been met—and exceeded (US Department of Health and Human Services, http://www.healthypeople.gov/2020/topics objectives2020/TechSpecs .aspx?hp2020id=MICH-24).

As described by the BMC breastfeeding committee, becoming a Baby-Friendly institution entails strategic planning, implementing, and maintaining change throughout an entire institution, staff education at all levels, cooperation between many departments, the support of senior staff members, and expense. Persuading a large institution to pay for infant formula, which most US

BOX 6.2 INTERNATIONAL CODE OF MARKETING OF BREAST MILK

The WHO/UNICEF International Code of Marketing of Breast-Milk Substitutes was adopted in 1981 by Resolution WHA34.22 of the World Health Assembly (WHA) to promote infant health by protecting and supporting breastfeeding. The Code bans all *promotion* of bottle-feeding and establishes requirements for labeling and information on infant feeding products. The Code pertains to all products that are marketed in a manner suggesting they should replace breastfeeding. The products include but are not limited to infant formula, follow-up formula, baby foods, juices (for infants under 4 months of age), and infant feeding paraphernalia such as bottles, nipples, bottles with collapsible liners, and so on. Resolutions updating or clarifying the Code have been adopted every 2 years since 1982, closing many of the loop-holes capitalized on by the baby food industry.

The International Code and its resolutions do not ban breast-milk substitutes, but they set out how companies are permitted to market them. These stipulations are regarded as the minimum requirement for effective action to promote breastfeeding. In particular, baby food companies may not engage in the following:

- Promote their products in hospitals, shops, or to the general public.
- Give free samples to mothers or free or subsidized supplies to hospitals or maternity wards.
- Give gifts to health workers or mothers.
- Promote their products to health workers: any information provided by companies must contain only scientific and factual matters.
- Promote foods or drinks for babies.
- Give misleading information.

Thirty years after its endorsement, only 37 out of 199 countries reporting (19%) have passed laws reflecting all of the recommendations of the WHO/UNICEF International Code of Marketing of Breast-Milk Substitutes Code; however, 69 countries (35%) fully prohibit advertising of breast-milk substitutes; 62 (31%) completely prohibit free samples or low-cost supplies; 64 (32%) completely prohibit gifts of any kind from relevant manufacturers to health workers; and 83 (42%) require a message about the superiority of breastfeeding on breast-milk substitute labels.

Source: Country Implementation of the International Code of Marketing of Breast-Milk Substitutes. Status Report: 2011. Available at http://apps.who.int/iris/bitstream/10665/85621/1/9789241505987_eng.pdf, accessed January 9, 2015.

hospitals receive for free from infant formula manufacturers, was cited as an especially difficult barrier to overcome (Merewood and Philipp 2000).

To comply fully with the BFHI, an institution must pay fair market price for all formula and infant feeding supplies that it uses; it cannot accept free or heavily discounted formula and supplies. Hospitals have problems achieving this step to being designated Baby-Friendly. When a hospital is already receiving free formula, it seems illogical to persuade administrators to reverse a trend and pay for a product that is usually free. The BMC researchers caution that any facility interested in pursuing the Baby-Friendly designation must consider the ramifications of this added expense. Nevertheless, they encourage facilities to apply for the certificate of intent and begin work, even if it is not immediately clear where funds for the formula to be paid for will originate.

Each of the Ten Steps takes the hospital along an important course, is never wasted effort, and increases the number of breastfeeding mothers (thereby reducing formula costs). Demonstrating a willingness to invest time and energy for the benefit of patients and the institution as a whole is valuable when requesting support for formula payment. Hospital administrators, who may make the final decision regarding formula payment, will be more willing to listen to breastfeeding advocates if they have already accomplished significant goals within the institution and have collected supporting data. The authors conclude that although for BMC not accepting free formula was the most difficult barrier to overcome on the path to Baby-Friendly designation, it was not insurmountable.

Furthermore, rejecting the practice of giving away free formula samples to mothers is a step that can be taken even if the hospital is not fully certified as Baby-Friendly. Ban the Bags is a nonprofit organization and national campaign started in Massachusetts in 2006 to address the aggressive formula company marketing tactics in hospitals. In December 2005, the state's Public Health Council passed regulations that stopped the practice of hospitals passing along formula company gift bags to new mothers. These regulations were promulgated after extensive testimony and public review, and garnered support from physician groups and public health organizations. However, then Governor Mitt Romney overturned the ban in February of 2006. The Public Health Council voted to revisit the issue in 3 months; Romney's office removed two council members who supported the ban immediately before the scheduled vote. The outcome proved positive, nonetheless. After debate about the proposed ban drew national attention, leading Massachusetts hospitals voluntarily changed policies (Ban the Bags, http://banthebags.org/about/), and as of July 2012, the last maternity hospitals that were still offering the free gift bags have decided to ban the practice. All 49 Massachusetts birth facilities have voluntarily eliminated the formula giveaways, following the lead of Rhode Island, the first state to do so in November 2011 (Kotz 2012).

Keep Formula Marketing Out of Health Care Facilities is another national campaign aimed at this practice, and assisted by the United States Breastfeeding Committee to coordinate with local breastfeeding coalitions. Public Citizen's campaign using research, advocacy at the hospital, legal and policy level, and communications strategy is aimed at supporting local initiatives, focusing public attention on state and national leading hospitals and targeting formula manufacturers directly. Public Citizen has published a report of case studies documenting success in numerous regions and highlighting strategies that can be used to help inform advocacy work elsewhere. In general, effective strategies and tactics employed by advocacy groups to change hospital practices include (Public Citizen, http://www.citizen.org/documents/report-successful-initiatives-formula-marketing.pdf)

- Developing presentations, fact sheets, and other educational materials documenting in-hospital formula marketing's correlation with lower exclusive breastfeeding rates; the correlating negative health and economic effects on women, infants and families; and the potential legal risks associated with formula sample distribution.
- Educating hospital personnel on the common misconception that hospitals are obligated to distribute formula company-sponsored bags to mothers if they receive free formula supplies from sponsoring formula manufacturers.
- Showing under-resourced hospitals, unable to immediately undergo the process of Baby-Friendly designation, that ending formula marketing is one important step toward improving breastfeeding support.
- Engaging governmental health departments and prominent doctors to encourage hospitals to end formula marketing through letter writing campaigns, model policy development, and regulatory enforcement.
- Engaging a diverse range of local and national groups in advocacy efforts while using both internal and external pressure to urge change.
- Taking advantage of regional hospital competition by publicly acknowledging and awarding hospitals that have ended or limited formula marketing.
- Publicly singling out hospitals that have failed to end formula marketing, where the majority of competing state and city-wide hospitals have already done so.
- Presenting the case to nurse leaders at perinatal forums.
- Reaching out to communications channels including blogs and press to publicize the issue.

LEGISLATIVE EFFORTS: STATE AND FEDERAL

In recent years, the practice of breastfeeding has expanded. As a consequence of this trend, 46 states, the District of Columbia (DC), and the Virgin Islands (VI) have laws that specifically allow breastfeeding to occur in any public or private location. Twenty-nine states, DC, and VI exempt breastfeeding from public indecency laws; 25 states, DC, and Puerto Rico have laws relating to breastfeeding in the workplace (National Conference of State Legislatures, http://www.ncsl.org/research/health/breast feeding-state-laws.aspx).

The laws vary considerably in their scope and in their coverage. Initially, legislation concerned itself with issues about breastfeeding in public, clarifying that mothers have a right to breastfeed their babies wherever they go. Since then, other issues have arisen, such as exempting breastfeeding mothers from jury duty or protecting breastfeeding mothers when they return to work. Maine and Michigan have enacted laws that require courts in family law cases (divorce or separation) to consider breastfeeding in making custody and visitation or parenting time decisions. Maryland became the first state to provide an exemption from the sales tax laws for breastfeeding accessories, such as pumps, shields, and other paraphernalia used by breastfeeding mothers. State laws may be generally classified into five broad categories: permitting a mother to breastfeed in any public or private location where the mother is legally entitled to be; exempting breastfeeding from public indecency laws; laws related to breastfeeding in the workplace; exempting breastfeeding mothers from jury duty; and laws implementing or encouraging the development of breastfeeding awareness programs (Weimer 2009).

Federal Breastfeeding Laws

In March 2010, the Patient Protection and Affordable Care Act, which contains breastfeeding provisions, was passed into law. Until this time, federal laws regarding breastfeeding were limited to allowing breastfeeding on federal property and breastfeeding promotion through WIC.

Table 6.2 is a legislative history of breastfeeding promotion requirements in WIC. These statutes are more symbolic than utilitarian. They demonstrate to the nation the intent of Congress, expecting that state governments will follow suit. Indeed, as noted earlier in this text, 46 states have enacted laws that specifically sanction breastfeeding in public places. The ACA, however, provides more substantial rights relevant to breastfeeding including granting nonexempt workers an appropriate place (other than a bathroom) and time to express breast milk during the workday up until a child's first birthday and mandating insurance coverage for lactation support and the cost of breastfeeding equipment (United States Breastfeeding Committee, http://www.usbreastfeeding.org/Employment /WorkplaceSupport/WorkplaceSupportinFederalLaw/tabid/175/Default.aspx).

Additional federal legislation on breastfeeding continues to be introduced in Congress. Since 2003, at least 20 bills related to breastfeeding have been introduced, only one of which has emerged from the Committee. HR 5462 passed the House after Amendment but did not proceed further. The following list provides the details on the proposed bills (http://www.Congress.gov).

Proposed Federal Legislation since 2003 Promoting Breastfeeding

- S 418: 108th Congress (2003–2004). Pregnancy Discrimination Act Amendments of 2003. Amends the Civil Rights Act of 1964 to include breastfeeding (including expression of milk by a lactating woman) within the definitions of "because of sex" or "on the basis of sex" for purposes of the discrimination prohibitions of such Act. Introduced.
- HR 2790: 108th Congress (2003–2004). Breastfeeding Promotion Act. Amends the Civil Rights Act of 1964 to include lactation (breastfeeding, including expression of milk) as protected conduct under such Act. Amends the Internal Revenue Code (IRC) to allow a limited credit to employers for expenses incurred in enabling employed nursing mothers to breastfeed. Safe and Effective Breast Pumps Act—Directs the Secretary of Health and Human Services to: (1) put into effect a performance standard for breast pumps irrespective

TABLE 6.2
Legislative History of Breastfeeding Promotion Requirements in WIC

Year	Legislation
1972	P.L. 92-443. Congress authorized a 2-year pilot project to serve pregnant and lactating women, infants, and children up to age 4. In addition to meeting the income guidelines, participants were required to be at nutritional risk.
1975	P.L. 94-105. WIC officially became a permanent national health and nutrition program. Congress explicitly used the term *breastfeeding* in the legislation. Breastfeeding women were defined as women who breastfed their infants up to 1 year of age. Non-breastfeeding postpartum women could participate up to 6 months postpartum. Eligibility for children was extended to age 5.
1989	P.L. 101-147. Further increased emphases on breastfeeding promotion WIC by requiring the following:

- That the USDA define the term *breastfeeding* and develop standards to ensure adequate breastfeeding promotion and support at state and local levels.
- Authorization of the use of WIC nutrition services and administrative (NSA) funds to purchase breastfeeding aids such as breast pumps that directly support the initiation and continuation of breastfeeding.
- The addition of an expert in breastfeeding promotion and support to the National Advisory Council on Maternal, Infant, and Fetal Nutrition.
- That WIC state agencies.
  - Spend annually, at a minimum, their share of $8 million specifically targeted for breastfeeding promotion and support.
  - Make a yearly evaluation of breastfeeding promotion/support activities (rescinded in 1996).
  - Provide nutrition education and breastfeeding materials in languages other than English as appropriate.
  - Include plans to provide nutrition education and breastfeeding promotion and to coordinate operations with local agency programs for breastfeeding promotion.
  - Designate a breastfeeding coordinator to provide training to local staff.

Year	Legislation
1992	P.L. 102-342. Required the Secretary of Agriculture to establish a national breastfeeding promotion program to promote breastfeeding as the best method of infant nutrition, foster wider public acceptance of breastfeeding in the United States, and assist in the distribution of breastfeeding equipment to women. To do so, the secretary may develop or assist others to develop appropriate materials. Authorized the USDA to enter into cooperative agreements with federal, state, local, or other entities to carry out a breastfeeding promotion program and authorized USDA to solicit and accept outside donations for establishing a breastfeeding promotion program.
1994	P.L. 103-448. Revised the formula for determining the amount of funds to be expended for WIC breastfeeding promotion and support; required WIC state agencies to spend $21 per pregnant and breastfeeding woman in support of breastfeeding promotion; required each WIC state agency to collect data on the incidence and duration of breastfeeding among participants and report this information to Congress every 2 years.
1996	P.L. 104-193. Eliminated the state agency requirement for annually evaluating breastfeeding promotion and support activities.
1998	P.L. 105-336. Authorized WIC state agencies to use food funds for the purchase or rental of breast pumps.
2004	P.L. 108-265. Child Nutrition and WIC Reauthorization Act of 2004. Earmarked up to $20 million annually for special nutrition education such as peer breastfeeding counseling and other activities to help achieve breastfeeding goals.
2010	P.L. 111-296. Healthy, Hunger Free Kids Act of 2010. Sec. 231: Amends the Child Nutrition Act of 1966 to include breastfeeding support and promotion as goals of the WIC program. Requires that annual breastfeeding performance measures be compiled and published for each WIC state and local agency, that exemplary breastfeeding support practices at local agencies or clinics participating in the WIC program be recognized, and performance bonuses to up to 15 state WIC agencies that have the highest proportion of breastfed infants or show the greatest improvement in the proportion of such infants. Requires funds be set aside for FY2010–FY2015 for WIC infrastructure, special projects to promote breastfeeding and to improve WIC services, management information systems, and special nutrition education. Sec. 232: requires the scientific review of the supplemental foods available under the WIC program at least once every 10 years.

Source: USDA Food and Nutrition Service. Women, Infants and Children (WIC) Legislative History of Breastfeeding Promotion Requirements in WIC. Available at http://www.fns.usda.gov/wic/legislative-history-breastfeeding-promotion-requirements-wic, accessed January 8, 2015. Breastfeeding and WIC keyword search. Available at http://www.congress.gov, January 9, 2015.

of the class to which the breast pumps have been classified under the Federal Food, Drug, and Cosmetic Act; and (2) issue a compliance policy guide which will assure that women who want to breastfeed a child are given full and complete information respecting breast pumps. Expands the IRC definition of medical care to include qualified breastfeeding equipment and services. Introduced.

- HR 2122: 109th Congress (2005–2006). Pregnancy Discrimination Act Amendments of 2005. Same as HR 2790 above but also includes consultation services relating to breastfeeding in the business tax credit provision. Introduced.
- S 1074: 109th Congress (2005–2006). HeLP America Act. "Healthy Lifestyles and Prevention America Act or the HeLP America Act" provides for the establishment of the BFHI to certify a hospital as a baby friendly hospital/center for breastfeeding excellence. Introduced.
- S 403 (Resolution): 109th Congress (2005–2006). Urges states to take steps to (1) protect a mother's right to breastfeed and (2) remove the barriers faced by women who breastfeed. Introduced.
- HR 2236: 110th Congress (2007–2008) Breastfeeding Promotion Act of 2007. Same as HR 2122 and HR 2790 above. Introduced.
- S 1342: 110th Congress (2007–2008) Healthy Lifestyles and Prevention America Act. (aka HeLP America Act). Provides for the establishment of the BFHI to certify a hospital as a baby friendly hospital/center for breastfeeding excellence and amends the Family and Medical Leave Act of 1993 to require employers to provide lactation periods and lactation facilities to permit employees to breastfeed eligible children. Introduced.
- HR 2633: 110th Congress (2007–2008) Provides for the establishment of the BFHI to certify a hospital as a baby friendly hospital/center for breastfeeding excellence and amends the Family and Medical Leave Act of 1993 to require employers to provide lactation periods and lactation facilities to permit employees to breastfeed eligible children. Introduced.
- HR 2819/S 1244: 111th Congress (2009–2010) Breastfeeding Promotion Act of 2009. Mostly the same as HR 2790 but includes some modification to the tax credit proposal. Expands the tax deduction for medical expenses to include expenses for breastfeeding equipment and consultation services. Amends the Fair Labor Standards Act to require employers with 50 or more employees to provide their breastfeeding employees with break time and private areas to express breast milk for their nursing children. Introduced.
- HR 3626/S 3132: 111th Congress (2009–2010) Exemplary Breastfeeding Support Act. Amends the Child Nutrition Act of 1966 to direct the Secretary of Health and Human Services (HHS) to implement programs in support of breastfeeding in the special supplemental nutrition program for women, infants, and children (WIC). Introduced.
- HR 5462/S 3479 111th Congress (2009–2010) Birth Defects Prevention Risk Reduction, and Awareness Act of 2010. Requires the Secretary of Health and Human Services (HHS), acting through the Director of the CDC, to establish and implement a birth defects prevention and public awareness program, which includes (1) a nationwide media campaign to increase awareness among healthcare providers and at-risk populations about pregnancy and breastfeeding information services; (2) grants for the provision of, or campaigns to increase awareness about, pregnancy and breastfeeding information services; and (3) grants for the conduct or support of surveillance of or research on maternal exposures that may influence the risk of adverse pregnancy outcomes and maternal exposures that may influence health risks to a breastfed infant, or of networking to facilitate such surveillance or research. Introduced; Passed House (Amended).
- S 174: 112th Congress (2011–2012) HeLP America Act. Provisions to promote breastfeeding among working women. Introduced.
- HR 2029/S 1131: 112th Congress (2011–2012) Birth Defects Prevention Risk Reduction, and Awareness Act of 2011. See HR 5462/S 3479. Introduced.

- HR 2758/S 1463: 112th Congress (2011–2012) Breastfeeding Promotion Act of 2011. Amends the Civil Rights Act of 1964 to include lactation (i.e., breastfeeding or the expressing of milk from the breast) as protected conduct under such Act (specifically, an amendment to such Act commonly known as the Pregnancy Discrimination Act). Amends the Fair Labor Standards Act of 1938 to extend the requirement that certain employers provide reasonable break time for an employee to express breast milk for her nursing child to bona fide executive, administrative, or professional capacity employees or outside salesmen who are exempt from federal labor laws that limit the number of hours in a workweek. Introduced.
- S 39: 113th Congress (2013–2014) HeLP America Act. Provisions to promote breastfeeding among working women. Introduced.
- HR 4492/S 1994: 113th Congress (2013–2014) TRICARE Moms Improvement Act of 2014. Requires the contracts entered into by the Secretary of Defense (DOD) for medical care for military dependents (e.g., TRICARE) to provide for breastfeeding support, supplies, and counseling as appropriate during pregnancy and the postpartum period. Introduced.

Federal Breastfeeding Policy

Since 1989, the federal government has produced sweeping legislation and policy statements regarding the promotion of breastfeeding:

- *1989–1998*: WIC breastfeeding initiatives are ramped up through enactment of various legislative actions.
- *2000*: Publication of *Blueprint for Action on Breastfeeding* by the Surgeon General of the United States presents a plan for breastfeeding based on education, training, awareness, support, and research. The *Blueprint* offers action steps for the healthcare system, families, the community, employers, and researchers. Its recommendations include training on breastfeeding counseling for healthcare professionals who provide maternal and childcare; ensuring that women who return to work after childbirth can continue breastfeeding; the creation of social support and information resources; and supporting research.
- *2001*: The US Breastfeeding Committee publishes *Breastfeeding in the U.S.: A National Agenda* that calls for (1) access to comprehensive, current, and culturally appropriate lactation care and services for all women, children, and families; (2) recognition of breastfeeding as the normal and preferred method of feeding infants and young children; (3) all federal, state, and local laws relating to child welfare and family law to recognize and support the importance and practice of breastfeeding; and increase protection, promotion, and support for breastfeeding mothers in the workforce (Centers for Disease Control and Prevention 2014).
- *2001*: *Healthy People 2010* outlines the measurable objectives regarding changes sought in the initiation and duration of breastfeeding. The targets are for 75% of new mothers to be breastfeeding when discharged from the hospital; 50% breastfeeding by the time the baby is 6 months of age; and 25% breastfeeding when the child is 12 months of age.
- *2005*: Publication of *The Guide to Breastfeeding Interventions* by the CDC, which describes successful breastfeeding interventions: maternity care practices, workplace support, peer support, educating mothers, professional support, and media and social marketing. Professional education, public acceptance, and hotlines and other information resources were found to be only marginally successful.
- *2009*: US Breastfeeding Committee restates strategic plan for 2009–2013.

- *2010*: *Healthy People 2020* updated the 2010 objectives regarding changes sought in the initiation and duration of breastfeeding. The targets are for 81% of new mothers to be breastfeeding when discharged from the hospital; 61% breastfeeding by the time the baby is 6 months of age; and 34% breastfeeding when the child is 12 months of age.
- *2010*: The Patient Protection and Affordable Care Act requires employers to provide suitable place and time for lactation for mothers of children up to 12 months of age. In addition, the act requires insurance coverage for lactation support and equipment.
- *2011*: The US Breastfeeding Committee restates strategic plan for 2009–2013 and updates to place greater emphasis on counteracting the marketing of breast-milk substitutes, as detailed in Appendix 6.2.
- *2013*: CDC publishes *Guide to Strategies to Support Breastfeeding Mothers and Babies.* This is an update to CDC's 2005 *Guide to Breastfeeding Interventions* publication.

Special Supplemental Nutrition Program for Women, Infants, and Children (WIC)

The federal laws regarding breastfeeding in the WIC program are of great practical and public health significance as half of the babies born in the United States participate in WIC. WIC operates under the broad goal of improving the health of women, infants, and children by providing supplemental foods, nutrition and breastfeeding education, and access to health services. Since the program began in 1974, WIC program staff have counseled and encouraged women, both before and after delivery, regarding breastfeeding and infant care. Annual NIS data consistently show low rates of breastfeeding among WIC participants. As a result, breastfeeding promotion and support programs have been strengthened over the years, as detailed in Table 6.2 noted previously, and over time, program and funding changes have enabled WIC state agencies to provide breastfeeding aids, offer an enhanced food package to women who breastfeed exclusively, and designate a staff person to coordinate breastfeeding promotion activities at the state level (Box 6.3).

Beginning in 1989, Congress began designating a specific portion of each state's WIC budget allocation to be used exclusively for the promotion and support of breastfeeding among its participants. The Child Nutrition and WIC Reauthorization Act of 2004 earmarked up to $20 million per year for special nutrition education such as breastfeeding peer counseling and related activities to help achieve the breastfeeding goals, increasing the proportion of mothers who breastfeed their babies to 75% in the early postpartum period and to 50% at 6 months.

In 2006 WIC food packages were redesigned to promote the benefits of breastfeeding. The final rule was published on March 4, 2014. Mother–infant pairs who rely on breastfeeding as the primary feeding method are provided with greater amounts and a wider variety of foods than before. The WIC food package for primarily breastfeeding mothers includes more milk, eggs, cheese, and whole grains than the packages for women who formula-feed. The packages for older infants who are given no formula contain twice the amount of baby food, fruits, and vegetables than the packages for their formula-fed counterparts.

As of June 2010, the *Loving Support* Peer Counseling model had been adopted by 50 states, the District of Columbia, and 34 Indian Tribal Organizations and Territories, and 2010 USDA appropriations had increased annual program funding from $15 million to $80 million (US Department of Agriculture 2010).

State agencies use these funds to implement or expand peer counseling programs in accordance with the FNS Model for a Successful Peer Counseling Program. An extensive collection of breastfeeding support materials is also available at the WIC Program website, http://www.fns.usda.gov /wic/women-infants-and-children-wic (Box 6.4).

Workplace Initiatives

As indicated in the CDC's 2013 *Guide to Strategies to Support Breastfeeding Mothers and Infants* (2013), mothers are the fastest-growing segment of the US labor force. Approximately 60% of

BOX 6.3   WIC BREASTFEEDING PROMOTION ACTIVITIES CARRIED OUT BY THE STATES AND AGENCIES

- Each state agency designates a breastfeeding promotion coordinator to coordinate breastfeeding promotion efforts identified in the state plan.
- The state plan must include the state agency's nutrition education goals and action plans, including a description of the methods that will be used to promote breastfeeding.
- A breastfeeding mother and her infant shall be placed in the highest priority level for which either is qualified, and certified at intervals of approximately 6 months and ending with the breastfed infant's first birthday.
- Fully breastfeeding food packages are for mothers and their babies who do not receive formula from WIC and are considered to be breastfeeding exclusively. Mothers and infants may receive this package until the infant is 12 months of age. For mothers, this package provides the largest quantity and variety of foods. For infants, this package provides twice the amount of infant food fruits and vegetables as the package for infants who receive formula, and also provides infant food meat.
- Partially breastfeeding food packages are for mothers and their infants who mostly breastfeed but also receive some formula from WIC after the first month postpartum. Mothers and infants may receive this package until the infant is 12 months of age. For mothers, this package provides extra quantities and varieties of foods—more than for mothers who mostly formula-feed. For infants, formula amounts are kept to a minimum to help mothers continue to successfully breastfeed.
- Routine issuance of infant formula in the first month is not authorized to partially breastfeeding mothers to allow the establishment of successful breastfeeding.
- Women who are not breastfeeding or only breastfeeding a minimal amount receive a WIC basic food package. Minimally breastfeeding women whose infants greater than 6 months of age receive more formula from WIC than is allowed for a partially breastfeeding infant do not receive a food package. They may receive other WIC benefits, however, such as breastfeeding support and breast pumps, nutrition education, and referrals to health and social services.

NUTRITION EDUCATION

State agencies perform the following activities in carrying out nutrition education responsibilities:

- Provide training on the promotion and management of breastfeeding to staff at local agencies who will provide information and assistance on this subject to participants.
- Identify or develop resources and educational materials for use in local agencies, including breastfeeding promotion and instruction materials, taking reasonable steps to include materials in languages other than English in areas where a significant number of or proportion of the populations need the information in a language other than English.
- Establish standards for breastfeeding promotion and support that include, at a minimum, (1) a policy that creates a positive clinic environment that endorses breastfeeding as the preferred method of infant feeding; (2) a requirement that each local agency designate a staff person to coordinate breastfeeding promotion and support activities; (3) a requirement that each local agency incorporate task-appropriate breastfeeding promotion and support training into orientation programs for new staff involved in direct contact with WIC clients; and (4) a plan to ensure that women have

access to breastfeeding promotion and support activities during the prenatal and postpartum periods.

- All pregnant participants shall be encouraged to breastfeed unless contraindicated for health reasons.

Source: US Department of Agriculture. Breastfeeding Promotion in WIC: Current Federal Requirements. Food and Nutrition Service. Available at http://www.fns.usda.gov/wic/breastfeeding-promotion-wic-current-federal -requirements, accessed January 8, 2015.

BOX 6.4   US DEPARTMENT OF AGRICULTURE FOOD AND NUTRITION SERVICE

MODEL FOR A SUCCESSFUL PEER COUNSELING PROGRAM

A *peer counselor* is a paraprofessional, recruited and hired from the target population, who is available to WIC clients outside usual clinic hours and outside the WIC clinic environment.

Adequate Program Support from State and Local Management

- Designated breastfeeding peer counseling program managers and/or coordinators at the state and/or local level.
- Defined job parameters and job descriptions for peer counselors.
- Adequate compensation and reimbursement of peer counselors.
- Training of appropriate WIC state/local peer counseling management and clinic staff.
- Establishment of standardized breastfeeding peer counseling program policies and procedures at the state and local level as part of agency nutrition education plan.
- Adequate supervision and monitoring of peer counselors.
- Establishment of community partnerships to enhance the effectiveness of a WIC peer counseling program.

Adequate Program Support of Peer Counselors

- Adequate training and continuing education of peer counselors.
- Timely access to breastfeeding coordinators and other lactation experts for assistance with problems outside of peer counselor scope of practice.
- Regular, systematic contact with supervisor.
- Participation in clinic staff meetings and breastfeeding in-service opportunities as part of the WIC team.
- Opportunities to meet regularly with other peer counselors.

Source: United States Department of Agriculture. WIC Works Learning Center. Available at http://www.nal.usda .gov/wicworks/Learning_Center/FNS_model.pdf, accessed January 9, 2015.

---

mothers of infants are employed. About one-third of employed mothers return to work within 3 months after birth and two-thirds return within 6 months. Working outside the home is related to a shorter duration of breastfeeding, and intentions to work full time are significantly associated with lower rates of breastfeeding initiation and shorter duration. Low-income women are more likely than their higher-income counterparts to return to work earlier and to hold jobs that compromise their ability to continue breastfeeding. Given the substantial presence of new mothers in the workforce, there is a need to establish lactation support in the workplace.

Support for breastfeeding in the workplace includes these employee benefits and services:

- Flexible work schedules to provide time for milk expression.
- Access to a private location for milk expression.
- Access to a nearby clean and safe water source and sink for washing hands and rinsing out any breast-pump equipment.
- Access to high-quality breast pumps and hygienic storage options for the mother to store her breast milk.

As of 2014, 46 states (92%) have enacted some type of breastfeeding laws, as described in Appendix 6.3. Legislation to protect breastfeeding mothers when they return to work has been enacted in 25 states, the District of Columbia, and Puerto Rico.

In 1993, the World Alliance for Breastfeeding Action (WABA, http://www.waba.org.my/what wedo/womenandwork/mfwi.htm) launched the Mother-Friendly Workplace Initiative (MFWI) to take baby friendliness outside the hospital and into women's work environments. The initiative aims to help women continue breastfeeding after returning to work. States such as Texas and California used the WABA model to create their own mother-friendly workplaces. With the passage of Assembly Bill 1025 in 2001, the state of California became one of the first states to reduce a major barrier to breastfeeding by enacting legislation requiring employers to provide unpaid break time and a private space to express breast milk during the workday. This right is now available in all states due to the ACA.

PEOPLE LIVING WITH HIV/AIDS

Human immunodeficiency virus (HIV) kills or damages cells of the body's immune system, progressively destroying the body's ability to fight infections and certain cancers. People living with HIV progress to the diagnosis of acquired immunodeficiency syndrome (AIDS) when they develop life-threatening diseases called opportunistic infections (OIs). These infections occur more frequently, and are more severe, in individuals that have weakened immune systems, such as people with HIV (Centers for Disease Control and Prevention, http://www.cdc.gov/hiv/living/opportunistic infections.html).

Since the first cases of AIDS were reported in 1981, infection with HIV has grown to pandemic proportions, resulting in an estimated 78 million infections and 39 million deaths. During 2013, an estimated 1.5 million persons died from AIDS, 2.1 million were newly infected with HIV, and more than 35 million were living with HIV/AIDS worldwide (Foundation for Aids Research, http://www .amfar.org/About-HIV-and-AIDS/Facts-and-Stats/Statistics—Worldwide). In the United States, at the end of 2012, an estimated 1,201,100 persons were living with HIV infection, and during 2012, almost 48,000 people were diagnosed with HIV infection and almost 28,000 with AIDS (Centers for Disease Control and Prevention, http://www.cdc.gov/hiv/statistics/basics/ataglance.html).

HIV/AIDS drug therapies, such as antiretroviral therapy (ART), are prolonging the lives of people with HIV/AIDS who have access to medical treatment, effectively rendering HIV a chronic disease. Between 2004 and 2010, the estimated number of persons in the United States living with HIV/AIDS tripled while the level of new infections remained stable. In 2006, it was reported that ART in the United States had prolonged life by an estimated 13 years (Walensky et al. 2006).

Early HIV treatment not only extends lives but also reduces the risk of transmission of HIV to an uninfected partner per the 2011 publication of findings from the HIV Prevention Trials Network (HPTN) 052 study. This randomized clinical trial study validated that early HIV treatment has a profound prevention benefit: results showed that by reducing the viral load of the infection, the risk of transmitting HIV to an uninfected partner was reduced by 96% (Centers for Disease Control and Prevention, http://www.cdc.gov/hiv/prevention/research/tap/). The December 2011 issue of *Science* named this study as "Breakthrough of the Year" (Cohen 2011). Although *prevention by treatment* is significant for public health efforts, appropriate healthcare treatment remains a challenge. Only 33% of people diagnosed with HIV remain in regular care and are prescribed ART. Only 25% are virally suppressed (The Henry J. Kaiser Family Foundation 2014). Comprehensive programs are needed to reach all persons who require treatment and to prevent transmission of new infections.

Good nutrition is essential to the management of HIV infection. People living with HIV/AIDS (PLWH/A) have special dietary requirements that must be managed in order to delay weight loss, wasting, and malnutrition. Nutritious food profoundly affects the immune system, may delay disease progression, increases tolerance of medical treatments, and can have a major impact on the quality of life.

NUTRITION AND HIV/AIDS

Nutritional status is strongly predictive of survival and functional status among PLWH/A (Nerad et al. 2003). Nutritional problems may occur at any stage of the disease and can contribute to impaired immune response, accelerate disease progression, increase the frequency and severity of OIs, and impede the effectiveness of medications. Many nutritional disturbances are preventable and manageable. Access to food, nutritional assessments, and nutrition interventions such as counseling and therapy can have a positive impact on morbidity, mortality, and quality of life (Box 6.5).

Nutritional interventions can also decrease or delay hospitalizations, emergency room visits, and costly and invasive treatments. The primary care setting offers an important opportunity to help prevent and mitigate nutrition-related complications. Yet, nutritional services are not always integrated into the primary care framework. Care teams sometimes do not include anyone with expertise in nutrition in HIV/AIDS. As a result, many nutrition-related problems go undiagnosed and untreated.

Preventing, diagnosing, and treating nutritional disturbances require providers to navigate a complex and cyclical web of cause and effect. The systems that regulate nutrient intake and absorption are affected by—and, in turn, affect—HIV disease itself, OIs associated with the disease, and the effects of drugs used to fight HIV and HIV-induced illnesses. Inadequate nutrition makes it difficult for PLWH/A to preserve their already weakened immune systems, increasing the risk of OIs and reducing the effectiveness of treatment. Infections can further compromise nutritional status and the strength of the immune system. Finally, HIV medications involve numerous food–drug interactions, so successful treatment adherence requires specific timing of medication doses and complicated dietary regimens.

BOX 6.5   FOOD ASSISTANCE

Three types of food assistance are available to PLWH/A: groceries, congregate meals, and home-delivered meals.

- *Pantry bags (groceries) and food vouchers* allow PLWH/A with limited financial resources access to nutritious food. In conjunction with nutrition services, PLWH/A are able to increase their levels of independence by preparing meals and making their own food choices.
- *Congregate meals* are served in community locations fostering access to healthcare, prevention, and supportive services, while meeting the nutritional needs of PLWH/A. Many participants who use the congregate meal programs are indigent, homeless, or in marginal housing, which lack kitchen facilities and food preparation equipment.
- *Home-delivered meals* help to maintain or improve the health and well-being of home-restricted individuals by providing calorie- and protein-rich, therapeutically tailored meals and snacks. For PLWH/A who lack the ability to shop for and prepare food, home-delivered meals fulfill a critical need, often allowing them to leave the hospital sooner and remain in the community longer.

The medical and physiological sources of nutritional problems associated with HIV/AIDS may be grouped into three general categories: inadequate intake, poor absorption, and altered metabolism. An additional nutritional problem is AIDS wasting and lipodystrophy.

Inadequate Intake

Many factors affect whether PLWH/A can ingest enough calories and nutrients to maintain health. Reduced nutrient intake can lead to weight loss as well as protein, vitamin, and mineral deficiencies. It generally results from loss of appetite caused by nausea, vomiting, altered sense of taste, fatigue, OIs in the gastrointestinal (GI) tract, or depression caused by receiving a diagnosis that is positive for HIV.

Altered Absorption

Malabsorption is a common manifestation of HIV infection, which may be secondary to lactose intolerance or GI infections. Even early on, HIV disease can directly damage the GI tract and interfere with nutrient absorption, resulting in depleted levels of micronutrients, particularly the carotenoids, B-vitamins, vitamin C, selenium, and zinc. As HIV disease progresses, OIs, including intestinal parasites and candidiasis, can further impair intestinal absorption. Malabsorption may also appear as a side effect of medication.

Altered Nutrient Metabolism

Metabolic abnormalities alter the way the body uses, stores, and excretes nutrients and may result in an increased need for calories and protein. Metabolic problems include impaired regulation of glucose and lipid abnormalities that may arise from immune dysfunction, medication side effects, OIs, hormonal alterations, or the direct effects of HIV itself.

AIDS Wasting and Lipodystrophy

Although the efficacy of ART has reduced the incidence of some HIV-related nutritional problems, new nutrition-related challenges have emerged in their place. In some cases, the problems are complications of medical progress—either the direct result of treatment advances or simply a function of prolonged survival. Among the most important nutritional disturbances are AIDS wasting syndrome (AWS) and lipodystrophy.

AWS is characterized by involuntary weight loss of more than 10% of body weight along with either chronic diarrhea or weakness and fever. AWS incidence fell after the introduction of HAART. However, weight loss and muscle wasting remain significant concerns, even in people with access to treatment. For example, lesser degrees of weight loss, such as dropping 5% of body weight within 6 months, although not included in the technical definition of AWS, are associated with increased morbidity and mortality. Unlike starvation-induced weight loss, HIV-associated wasting results in loss primarily of lean body mass (LBM), which increases the likelihood of OIs and is an independent predictor of increased morbidity and mortality, even if total body weight is preserved.

People on ART who develop AWS may not exhibit the symptoms characteristic of the pre-HAART era. Monitoring of weight and physical appearance may be insufficient measurements for assessing the development of AWS, particularly in people with lipodystrophy, which may camouflage depletion of LBM. Therefore, routine monitoring of changes in weight, body mass, and body composition is essential.

Lipodystrophy is characterized by two types of changes in body fat distribution, which may occur alone or in combination: (1) the loss of fat in certain areas, particularly in the cheeks, temples, buttocks, arms, and legs; and (2) isolated fat deposits, most commonly at the back of the neck and shoulders and around the abdomen. These changes to body shape can interfere with daily activities, such as exercising, sleeping, and even breathing. Lipodystrophy has been associated with increased risk for high blood pressure and dyslipidemia (abnormal cholesterol or triglyceride levels). The cause of lipodystrophy is not known but may be related to HAART because the syndrome was identified only after the use of HAART became widespread.

Nutritional Care and HIV/AIDS

As nutritional changes can occur early in HIV infection, nutrition intervention should begin soon after diagnosis (Nerad et al. 2003). Nutrition screening and a complete baseline nutrition assessment should be part of every care plan, as should ongoing reassessment. The key components of nutritional care risk are screening, comprehensive baseline evaluation or assessment, and ongoing monitoring and treatment—including self-care training, nutrition education, and various interventions.

Screening and Referral

Screening for nutritional status is a critical part of early intervention to identify and treat nutrition problems. At a minimum, it should include patient history, basic body measurements, and laboratory tests. Ideally, nutrition screening is conducted by a registered dietitian (RD) with experience in HIV/AIDS, but all HIV/AIDS providers should be able to identify nutrition-related problems and know when and how to refer clients for further evaluation and treatment.

Various online resources are available to guide providers in assessing risk in their HIV-positive clients. This includes the tools contained in *HealthCare and HIV: Nutritional Guide for Providers and Clients*, developed by the AIDS Education and Training Centers (AETC) Program of the Ryan White Care Act (TARGET Center Tools for the Ryan White Community, https://careacttarget.org /library/health-care-and-hiv-nutritional-guide-providers-and-clients).

A recommended protocol for referrals to an RD for medical nutrition therapy (MNT) developed in the late 1990s/early 2000s as detailed in the article by Nerad et al., cited above, was based on criteria published by the Los Angeles County Commission on HIV Health Services and the American Dietetic Association, now the Academy of Nutrition and Dietetics (AND). As of 2010, AND recommends that all people with HIV infection be referred for MNT based on nutritional risk. The timeline for referral of patients categorized by nutritional risk is as follows: high risk, to be seen by an RD within 1 week; moderate risk, to be seen by an RD within 1 month; low risk, to be seen by an RD at least annually. The RD should collaborate with any relevant parties to ensure that all people with HIV infection are screened for nutrition-related problems at every visit, as people with HIV infection can be at nutritional risk at any time point during the course of their illness.

Risk levels are defined as follows (Nerad et al. 2003; Academy of Nutrition and Dietetics 2014):

1. *High risk*, for example, greater than 10% unintentional weight loss over 4–6 months, severely dysfunctional psychosocial situation, and two or more medical comorbidities (including poorly controlled DM and pregnancy) should be evaluated by an RD within 1 week.
2. *Moderate risk*, including obesity, hypertension, lipid abnormality, gastrointestinal problems, disordered eating, unstable psychosocial situation, possible food allergies, intolerances, or food–drug–nutrient interactions, should be evaluated by an RD within 1 month.
3. *Low risk*, for example, lacking manifestations of nutrition-related problems, should be seen by an RD as needed (but at least annually).

Medical Nutrition Therapy

The major goals of MNT for persons living with HIV were described by the Los Angeles County Commission on HIV Health Services (2002) as follows:

- Optimize nutrition status, immunity, and overall well-being.
- Prevent the development of specific nutrient deficiencies.
- Prevent loss of weight and LBM.
- Reduce risk for onset or complications of comorbidities such as diabetes and cardiovascular, kidney, and liver diseases.

- Maximize effectiveness of medical and pharmacological treatments.
- Minimize healthcare cost.

In 2010, the AND (2010), based on the work of the organization's HIV/AIDS expert working group, defined the primary goals of MNT for individuals with HIV/AIDS as follows:

- To delay HIV disease progression.
- To prevent and treat malnutrition.
- To maximize food and water safety practices.
- To minimize the impact of other comorbidities on the progression of HIV.

In general, the shift in causes of death from acute OIs to causes found in the rest of the US population—such as diabetes and heart disease—also indicates a shift in focus in nutritional therapy promulgated by AND. For example, the shocking weight loss and wasting that commonly manifested in the early years of the HIV/AIDS epidemic meant that the first nutritional priority was often simply increased energy intake over dietary quality; but in 2009, obesity was reported to be higher in one HIV positive study population than was wasting syndrome (Hendricks et al. 2009).

The AND comments that a shift in causes of death from acute OIs to other causes, such as diabetes and heart disease, indicates the need for a more comprehensive approach to healthy living for people with HIV. With the advances in medical research and medication therapy, the model of HIV care has changed into one of a chronic, manageable condition; thus AND (http://www.eatright.org /Public/content.aspx?id=5546) encourages individuals who have the HIV virus under control to follow the same principles of healthy eating that are recommended for everyone and to seek a referral for an RD nutritionist from their doctor (Box 6.6).

**BOX 6.6   NUTRITION EDUCATION PRIORITIES
FOR PEOPLE LIVING WITH HIV DISEASE AND AIDS**

Information and guidance should be provided on the following topics:

- Consumption of a healthy diet.
- Maintaining or increasing lean body mass.
- Achieving and maintaining normal growth in children.
- Management of metabolic complications related to HIV and ART.
- Management of medication–food interactions.
- Management of gastrointestinal side effects of medications.
- Cultural and ethnic beliefs related to food and diet.
- Exercise.
- Management of nausea and diarrhea.
- Substance abuse and nutrition.
- Nutrition during acute illnesses.
- Food safety.
- Nutrition during pregnancy.
- Access to food, including infant formula.
- Breastfeeding and HIV transmission.
- Use of herbal and nutritional supplements.
- Community sources of food and nutrition support.

Source: Adapted from Nerad, J. et al., *Clin Infect Dis.* 36(Suppl. 2), S52–S62, 2003.

LEGISLATIVE AND COMMUNITY SUPPORT

In 2010, the United States adopted a national HIV/AIDS strategy designed to reduce the incidence of infection; increase access to care and improve health outcomes; and decrease HIV-related health disparities (The White House, http://www.whitehouse.gov/sites/default/files/uploads/NHAS.pdf). The Ryan White HIV/AIDS Treatment Extension Act of 2009, aspects of the 2010 ACA, and various community programs support these efforts.

The Ryan White HIV/AIDS Treatment Extension Act

The Ryan White HIV/AIDS Treatment Extension Act of 2009 (RWA) is federal-level legislation that addresses the unmet health needs of PLWH/A by funding primary healthcare and support services. It is the largest discretionary investment solely devoted to the care of PLWH/A in the United States, reaching more than 500,000 people a year in all 50 states, the District of Columbia, Puerto Rico, and the US territories. Funding is provided to cities, states, territories, providers, and other organizations. The program is administered through the HIV/AIDS Bureau of the Health Resources and Services Administration (HRSA) within HHS. Originally passed in 1990, the legislation is named after Ryan White, an Indiana teenager infected with the illness after a blood transfusion, who died shortly before the act was passed. The program considers MNT as a core service (New Mexico Community Planning and Action Group, http://www.nmcpag.org/pdf/ryan_white_program_defs .pdf).

RWA legislation, which must be reauthorized every 5 years, was extended in 1996 (by P.L. 104-146), 2000 (P.L. 106-345), 2006 (P.L. 109-415), and 2009 (P.L. 111-87). Adjustments to RWA may be made at each authorization. For example, the 2006 reauthorization allowed for the funding of early intervention services, including nutrition counseling (Health Resources and Services Administration 2006).

RWA includes four parts (A-D) and three special programs as follows: (A) emergency relief; (B) HIV care and AIDS Drug Assistance Program (ADAP); (C) early intervention; (D) women, infants, children, and youth; AIDS Education Training Centers Programs (AETC); Dental Program and Special Projects of National Significance. Roughly 58% of the budget is allocated for HIV care, 28% for emergency relief, and 17% for the remaining programs. The bill was due for reauthorization in September 2013, but by January 2015, it had not yet received Congressional action in part due to healthcare changes brought about by the ACA (National Alliance of State and Territorial AIDS Directors 2013).

Nevertheless, the program was funded for about $2.3 billion in 2014. A separate act of Congress appropriates the money on a yearly basis. Adjusting for inflation, funding has remained relatively steady for the past decade despite a 33% increase in the number of people living with HIV (Kaiser Family Foundation 2013). Part B, HIV care, includes funding for ADAP. The standard of care for a majority of those living in the United States with HIV is HAART, which can cost $12,000 or more per year. More people are living longer with HIV, and more public support is required (HRSA, http://hab.hrsa.gov/abouthab/partbdrug.html).

Affordable Care Act

The Affordable Care Act of 2010 (ACA) increases access to healthcare services and insurance coverage and includes a number of provisions that will specifically benefit PLWH/A (HRSA, http://hab.hrsa.gov/affordablecareact/keyprovisions.pdf). These include guaranteed availability of coverage and fair health insurance premiums regardless of preexisting conditions. In addition, the ACA establishes a new Medicaid eligibility category for low-income adults 19–64 years of age. If a state expands its Medicaid program, people who are living with HIV and who meet these criteria will no longer have to wait for an AIDS diagnosis to be eligible for benefits. These changes may alter the need for the *last resort* programs of the Ryan White Act, and it is for this reason that reauthorization remains pending.

The Association of Nutrition Services Agencies (ANSA) collaborates with other national organizations working on nutrition and/or HIV/AIDS as a core issue to help ensure the long-term sustainability of their members' programs and to move the entire field of nutrition services forward with a unified voice. ANSA advocates for (1) Ryan White Act reauthorization, (2) new funding for non-HIV/AIDS critically ill populations, and (3) building a national coalition—the National Nutrition Collaborative—composed of national organizations with hunger and nutrition as core issues. ANSA is an alliance of more than 85 nonprofit organizations working on behalf of the acutely ill and began in 1994 with a small gathering of US programs feeding people with HIV/AIDS. Community Servings (http://www.servings.org/about/history.cfm), one such organization, started in 1989 as a small neighborhood meals program delivering a hot dinner to 30 individuals struggling with HIV/AIDS and has grown to a regional program serving free, nutritionally tailored meals—over 5.5 million since 1990—and providing nutrition education to thousands of acutely ill people per year across Massachusetts, regardless of illness.

A similar program, New York's God's Love We Deliver, grew out of a visit by a hospice volunteer named Ganga Stone to an AIDS patient in 1985. Realizing that the patient, Richard Sayles, was too ill to cook for himself, Ganga prepared and brought a meal on the next visit, and then realized the severity of the situation demanded something more than just food; nutritionally tailored meals that would support an individual's specific medical treatment were necessary. Over 12 million meals have been served; meals nutritionally tailored for those homebound and suffering from cancer, Alzheimer's, MS, and other debilitating diseases as well as from HIV/AIDS (God's Love We Deliver, https://www.glwd.org/press/kit.jsp).

AND reports that the nutrition support funded through RWA can be cost-effective, as a nutritionally tailored diet might cost around $20 per day, whereas a hospital stay might cost upwards of $4000 per day. A study by the Metropolitan Area Neighborhood Nutrition Alliance in Philadelphia found that the average monthly healthcare costs for HIV/AIDS clients in the 6 months following initiation of food and nutrition services went from an average of roughly $50,000 per month to approximately $17,000 per month after the initiation of food and nutrition services (Academy of Nutrition and Dietetics, http://www.eatrightwashington.org/docs/Policy/2013/Issue%20Brief%20 Ryan%20White%20PPW%202013.pdf).

In 2010, 59% of those individuals helped by RWA had incomes at or below the poverty level (HRSA 2010). PLWH/A who are food-insecure report more missed appointments for primary care visits than those who do not have difficulties obtaining enough food (Aidala et al. 2011). The potential negative health outcome of such missed appointments might include failure to prevent further nutrition-related complications, or an inability to monitor how well a patient is adhering to medication therapy. Food and nutrition security, assistance, and counseling are important cornerstones for HIV/AIDS treatments (Academy of Nutrition and Dietetics 2014).

JAIL AND PRISON INMATES

In the United States, incarceration occurs in a number of different settings: federal prisons, state prisons, and local jails, as well as juvenile correctional facilities. Jails are locally operated correctional facilities that confine persons before or after adjudication. Inmates sentenced to jail usually have a sentence of a year or less, although jails also incarcerate persons in a wide variety of other categories. Prisons, on the other hand, are federal or state facilities that house felons who must serve a sentence longer than 1 year.

State and federal prison authorities had in custody 1.574 million inmates at year-end 2013, with a slight decline in federal numbers of almost 2000 persons (the first decline since 1980) and an increase in state numbers of just over 6000 persons (the first increase since 2009) (Carson 2014). Since 2004, the number of persons awaiting trial or serving a sentence in local jails has been in excess of 700,000 (731,208 as of mid-year 2013) (Golinelli and Minton 2013). It is important to note that this population is consistently renewing, because at any given moment, most of the at least

700,000 people in local jails have not been convicted and are in jail because they cannot make bail and are being held before trial, or because they have just been arrested and will make bail in the next few hours or days (Wagner and Sakala 2014). Almost 12 million people, according to the Bureau of Justice, cycle through local jails each year (Minton 2013).

If incarceration rates remain unchanged, 6.6% of US residents born in 2001 will go to prison at some time during their lifetime, up from 5.2% in 1991 and up from 1.9% in 1974 (US Department of Justice 1974–2001).

FEDERAL DETENTION

The Federal Bureau of Prisons (BOP) was responsible for the custody and care of approximately 219,000 federal offenders in 2013, over 80% of whom were confined in bureau-operated correctional institutions and detention centers. The rest are confined in privately operated prisons, detention centers, community corrections centers, and juvenile facilities, as well as facilities operated by state or local governments. The federal prison system is a nationwide system of prisons and detention facilities for the incarceration of inmates who have been sentenced to imprisonment for federal crimes and the detention of individuals awaiting trial or sentencing in federal court; the system is also responsible for incarcerating the District of Columbia's sentenced felon inmate population. The BOP places most inmates in community corrections centers (halfway houses) prior to their release from custody to help them adjust to life in the community after their release (Federal Bureau of Prisons, http://www.bop.gov/). At year-end 2011, the federal system was 38% overcapacity. Parole is no longer available for federal offenders, and BOP has limited ability to adjust sentences (US Government Accountability Office 2012).

STATE DETENTION

In addition to the federal system, each state has its own department of corrections (New York has both a New York State and a New York City Department of Corrections). The largest state systems at year-end 2013 were Texas (168,280), California (135,981), and Florida (103,028). In 2013, five states imprisoned at least 600 persons per 100,000 state residents: Louisiana (847 prisoners per 1,000,000 state residents), Mississippi (692), Oklahoma (659), Alabama (647), and Texas (602). The states with the lowest incarceration rates were Maine (148 inmates per 100,000 state residents), Minnesota (189) Rhode Island (194), Massachusetts (192), and North Dakota (211). At year-end 2013, 19 state prison systems were operating at or above their highest capacity (Carson 2014).

PRISON HEALTH AND SAFETY RIGHTS AND STANDARDS

One of the most contested aspects of imprisonment is access to healthcare. The United States is unique among Western countries in that it has no general governmental oversight of prisons and jails. Therefore, it is left to the courts to develop the minimum standards for treatment of prisoners.

Bernard P. Harrison, J.D., and B. Jaye Anno, PhD, introduced the concepts of national standards and voluntary accreditation as a means to upgrade healthcare in correctional facilities. Their work marked the beginning of the field known as correctional health. In the early 1970s, Harrison and Anno brought to the nation's attention the tremendous inadequacy of healthcare for the incarcerated, spearheading efforts to survey and research the state of healthcare in correctional healthcare facilities. They demonstrated the gravity of health problems of inmates, the risk that these problems posed to the health of the public beyond jails and prisons, and the inadequacy of care that was being provided to inmates. Along with key organizations and constituencies, they increased awareness of the problem and sought to improve standards for health services in prisons. Attributed to their work was a subsequent fourfold increase in the detection of previously undiagnosed and untreated illnesses among inmates and a Supreme Court ruling requiring states to ensure that an inmate's basic needs are met, including healthcare.

Beginning in the early 1970s, a series of cases was decided in the federal courts that served to further clarify the scope and extent of inmates' Eighth Amendment rights to medical treatment. As a result of these decisions, prisoners are the only Americans with a constitutional right to healthcare. In Estelle v. Gamble, 429 US 97 (1976), the Supreme Court ruled that "deliberate indifference" to a prisoner's health was "cruel and unusual punishment," which is prohibited by the Eighth Amendment to the Constitution. In this case, the Court interpreted the Eighth Amendment protections to require that healthcare for convicted felons must meet a standard equal to that in the community. Although the Eighth Amendment is the usual focus of a discussion of prisoners' rights, any official actions rising to a violation of a prisoner's civil liberties may impact their Fourteenth Amendment right to equal protection under the law, as well as their right to due process.

In 1981, Anno and Harrison founded the National Commission on Correctional Health Care (NCCHC), a nonprofit organization dedicated to improving healthcare in the nation's jails, prisons, and juvenile detention and confinement facilities. The organization has created a certification program for correctional health personnel, sets standards for health services in correctional facilities, and provides a voluntary accreditation program for facilities that meet NCCHC (http://www.ncchc .org/accreditation-facility-services) standards. However, no data have been published establishing the effectiveness of these standards. In 2009, citing emerging work in quality improvement in community healthcare, a group at John Jay College in New York published a new set of standards focused on patient safety in prisons (Stern et al. 2010).

Demographic Trends in Correctional Populations

Race and Ethnicity

Cities have more poor people, more people of color, and higher crime rates than suburban and rural areas; thus, urban populations are overrepresented in the nation's jails and prisons. As a result, US incarceration policies and programs have a disproportionate impact on urban black and Latino communities (Freudenberg 2001). At year-end 2013, about 37% of imprisoned males were black, 32% white, and 22% Hispanic. Almost 3% of black male US residents of all ages were imprisoned on December 31, 2013, compared to 1.0% of Hispanics and 0.5% of white males. The disparity shows most greatly in the youngest adult population; black males of ages 18–19 are more than nine times more likely to be imprisoned than white males of the same age (1092 inmates per 100,000 black males, as compared to 115 inmates per 100,000 white males) (Carson 2014).

Gender

Although the number of incarcerated women is substantially less than the number of incarcerated men, women make up the fastest growing segment of the US incarcerated population, increasing at rates 50% higher than men for a period of time after 1980. At the end of 2004, 96,125 women were serving state or federal prison sentences—almost nine times the number in prison in 1977 (Greene and Pranis, http://66.29.139.159/institute/hardhit/part1.htm).

As of 2013, the female inmate population was in excess of 111,000. Although the gap in rate of incarceration of females compared to men has decreased more recently, the average annual increase in numbers of females incarcerated during the 10-year period of 2003–2013 remained higher than for males, at 1.0%, compared to 0.7% for men. And, in 2013, some states with smaller prison populations saw increases greater than 10% in female prisoners: Arkansas (up 26%), Vermont (up 21%), and New Hampshire (up 15%). Black females were imprisoned at more than twice the rate of white females; 25% of female prisoners were serving time for drug offenses, compared to 15% of male prisoners. As in the case with males, black females ages 18–19 (33 inmates per 100,000) were almost five times more likely to be imprisoned than white females (7 inmates per 100,000) (Carson 2014).

Women's nutrition and health issues that must be addressed during incarceration include pregnancy. According to a 1998 national survey of US correctional systems, there were about 1900 pregnant females entering prison and more than 1400 gave birth (US Government Accountability Office 1999). The Bureau of Justice reported in 1991 and 1997 that 5–6% of women entered prison pregnant (Greenfeld and Snell 1999; Snell 1994). Issues that may have been present prior to incarceration such as suboptimal nutrition and prenatal care may become problematic during incarceration.

Aging Inmates

The past decade has seen a dramatic increase in the number of incarcerated elderly, due to mandatory minimum sentencing, longer sentences, and tighter parole policies. In 2013, an estimated 58% of male inmates and 61% of female inmates in state and federal prison were age 39 or younger, and conversely, roughly 42% of males and 39% of females were age 40 or older (Carson 2014).

It has been estimated that while within the correctional system, 30%–50% of inmates are diagnosed with a new chronic condition (Maruschak 2008), and the prevalence of chronic diseases of aging is expected to increase in prison (Williams et al. 2010). Corrections officials recognize that the cost of maintaining older prisoners is nearly triple that of other inmates, primarily due to the expense of healthcare. Poor living conditions in prison, inadequate medical treatment, and prior lifestyles (which accelerate aging and medical conditions) make older prisoners a unique population with special prerelease needs. Solutions to the aging inmate challenges that have been suggested include the establishment of private medical prisons; early release of nonviolent, low-risk older offenders; and the exploration of alternatives to incarceration (Williams et al. 2012).

Chronic Disease Burden

Jail and prison inmates have a higher burden of some chronic medical conditions than the general population even adjusting for sociodemographics and alcohol consumption (Binswanger et al. 2009). As of 2002, an estimated 80,000 inmates have diabetes and more than 280,000 have hypertension, with prevalence rates of about 5% and 18%, respectively (Hornung et al. 2002). In 2009, the age-standardized prevalence of diabetes in the incarcerated population was estimated at 11.1% (federal), 10.1% (state), and 8.1% (jail), and for hypertension, 29.5% (federal), 30.8% (state), and 27.9% (jail) (Wilper et al. 2009).

Prevalence rates for several diseases vary by race, gender, and age. For example, the prevalence of diabetes and hypertension is considerably higher for inmates 50 years or older than for younger prisoners. Diabetes is more common among black and Hispanic inmates than among white inmates, similar to patterns in the general population (Baillargeon et al. 2000).

The prevalence of diabetes and its related comorbidities and complications is likely to continue to increase in the prison population as current sentencing guidelines continue to increase the number of aging prisoners *and* as the incidence of diabetes in young people continues to increase. A 2010 survey of chronic medical conditions in Texas prisoners revealed that almost two-thirds of the population over 55 suffered from at least one chronic illness (Harzke et al. 2010).

Food Service in the Prison Systems

Federal System

The meals provided through the federal system meet recommended dietary allowances (RDAs). And, some of the meals served through the USDA's National School Lunch Program and School Breakfast Program go to juveniles and adolescents in state and local detention facilities. These meals, funded and regulated through the USDA, must meet the calories and nutrition standards of the lunch and breakfast programs. Special meals are available to accommodate inmates' religious and medical dietary requirements.

As part of settling a civil rights action, BOP initiated a Modified Common Fare Religious Diet Program in 1984, originally as a continuation of a pilot project. As initially described, the Common Fare Religious diet program serves foods that largely require no preparation, contain no pork or pork derivatives, do not mix meat or dairy products in the service of food items, and are served with utensils that have not come in contact with pork or pork derivatives (Al Shakir v. Carlson 1984).

In 2000, Congress passed the Religious Land Use and Institutionalized Persons Act (RLUIPA), which prohibits impositions of burdens on the ability of prisoners to worship, and also defines the term *religious exercise* as any exercise of religion, whether or not compelled by, or central to, a system of religious belief. Although case law has developed supporting a constitutional right and a statutory right under RLUIPA for inmates to receive a nutritious diet in keeping with their sincere religious beliefs, an inmate must demonstrate that the diet choices already provided to him/her by the prison substantially burden his/her religious practice. Cases brought to court may involve arguments over denials of requests for a religious diet, characterizations of what constitutes a religion and specific rules pertaining to that religion, and whether the removal of an inmate from a religious diet was appropriately conducted.

As of 2014, the BOP describes the religious diet program in an inmate orientation handbook as follows: The religious diet program, called the Alternative Diet Program, consists of two distinct components: one component provides for religious dietary needs through self-selection from the main line, which includes a no-flesh option.

The *no-flesh option* is available at all times to any inmate through the main line meal service; no meat from animals, fish, or birds will be served in any form, and any vegetables supplied through the main meal line, which are normally prepared with meat or meat by-products, also have an alternate no-flesh option (The Becket Fund for Religious Liberty 2007).

The other component accommodates dietary needs through nationally recognized, religiously certified processed foods and is available through the approval of Religious Services. For the religious diet, the bureau has a nationally approved menu, available to approved inmates at all institutions, and offers a prepackaged entrée, which is heavily supplemented to ensure sufficient calories are provided. Precise instructions are given to the institutions for the use, maintenance, and storage of utensils in addition to those for food preparation and services, including the provision of separate areas within the institutional kitchen for common fare food preparation and utensil storage. Inmates must be approved for participation. The institution chaplain verifies that an applying inmate holds a sincere religious conviction through an application and interview process. Inmates may voluntarily leave the program or be involuntarily removed from the program if they violate the program rules (The Becket Fund for Religious Liberty 2007).

State Systems

State correctional facility meals are not federally regulated. There are no federal regulations on the minimum standards for calorie intake in state prisons (Collins and Thompson 2012). State correctional facility meals are governed by state or country rules and facility officials; and any particular state nutrition or dietary legislative mandates or regulations may be revised from time to time, particularly when the state may be seeking cost-saving budget measures. Conversely, jurisdictions that take a long view on public health costs may seek to provide healthier diets.

Accordingly, corrections dietitians who participate in menu and recipe planning must be knowledgeable of religious diet restrictions as well as standards for the varying jurisdictions (such as state and local law and regulations and court rulings) and standards set by accrediting organizations, such as NCCHC or the American Correctional Food Service Association (Wakeen 2014). These standards are informed by US dietary guidance and the recommendations of national health organizations, but unless specifically regulated at the state or local level or tied to federal funding, state and local correctional facilities are not governed by these recommendations.

As an example of state regulation, California requires that "each inmate shall be provided a wholesome, nutritionally balanced diet. Nutrition levels shall meet the Recommended Dietary

Allowances (RDAs) and Dietary Reference Intakes (DRIs) as established by the Food and Nutrition Board of the Institute of Medicine, National Academy of Science" (California Department of Corrections and Rehabilitation 2014). Note that this regulation references nutritional standards (RDAs and DRIs) but does not reference the *Dietary Guidelines for Americans*, which provides recommendations on how to achieve nutritional standards. The California regulation does not require the provision of specific food groups (such as whole grains), except for the provision that "pregnant inmates shall receive two extra eight ounce cartons of milk or a calcium supplement if lactose intolerant, two extra servings of fresh fruit, and two extra servings of fresh vegetables daily. A physician may order additional nutrients as necessary."

Local regulations could consist of policy promulgated by food policy councils, or city and county governments. As an example of local regulation, in 2012, Santa Clara County in California promulgated nutrition standards for custodial populations that exceed California state mandates. The Santa Clara County Nutrition Standards are based on and follow the 2010 *Dietary Guidelines for Americans*. Under the Nutrition Standards, beverages provided to custodial populations may include only the following:

- Water.
- Carbonated water (no added caloric sweeteners).
- Nonsweetened coffee or tea (sugar may be provided as a condiment).
- Unflavored and unsweetened nonfat or 1% low-fat dairy milk, plant-derived milk ≤ 130 calories per 8 ounce serving.
- Low calorie beverages that do not exceed 40 calories per 8 ounce serving.
- 100% fruit or vegetable juice (limited to a maximum of 8 ounce container).

Custodial facilities were also directed to (County of Santa Clara, California 2012)

- Provide more fruits, vegetables, whole grains, and nonfat or low-fat dairy products.
- Minimize the use of processed foods that contains added sugar and sodium.
- Reduce the overall fat content by using healthy cooking techniques.
- Serve high-calorie items in smaller portions (e.g., mini muffins).
- Use low-sodium items wherever possible assuming cost neutrality, and work toward reducing the overall sodium content.

In some cases, federal standards for religious meals have been adopted by states, in whole or in part. In 2007, a survey of other state institutions' religious dietary practices was conducted in Florida. Forty-one states provided information, 38 states of which reported providing some alternate religious dietary accommodation; but only 22 states reported providing an alternate entrée, although most of the states offer vegetarian options. Twenty-five percent offered a lacto-ovo alternative. Pork-free meals were then available in state prisons in 18 states, and those states reported that, on average, they had done so for 10 years. At the time, 26 states offered a kosher menu, while only five offered a Muslim or halal meal. Most states replied that vegetarian or kosher menus are considered acceptable alternatives. Some states (18 at the time) have been court-mandated to provide religious meals (The Becket Fund for Religious Liberty 2007).

State Spending on Meals

The Bureau of Justice reported in 2001 that, on average nationwide, state departments of correction spent $2.62 per capita to feed inmates each day. Pennsylvania ($5.69) and Washington ($5.68) reported the largest amounts, followed by Maine ($5.03), Hawaii ($4.87), and Iowa ($4.81). North Carolina indicated the lowest cost ($0.52), followed by Alabama ($0.72), Mississippi ($0.81), and Louisiana ($0.96). States that reported low food costs often reflected the contribution of prisoner-operated farm and food processing operations. For example, facilities in Mississippi grew a wide variety of fruits, vegetables, and grains, and even raised livestock for other prisons in the state, whereas prison enterprises in North Carolina operated a cannery, a meat processing plant, warehouses, and trucks to deliver food and equipment to correctional facilities statewide (James 2004). (Although the history and social context of prison farms is a significant topic, it is unfortunately beyond the scope of this chapter [Box 6.7].)

Unfortunately, the Bureau of Justice has not reported recent state average costs per day to feed inmates, but the average amount may not be much different today than when it was reported in 2001. For example, as of 2014, it was reported that Florida spends $1.93 per inmate per day for the standard meal service (Controversy over Kosher Meals in Florida Prisons 2014). Kentucky reported in 2008 that regular meals cost $2.63 per day; this is the amount paid to a private contractor, Aramark Correctional Services (Upton and Harp, http://www.lrc.ky.gov/lrcpubs/rr373.pdf). Increasingly, correctional food service is subcontracted out to private contractors to reduce costs. While Aramark (http://www.Aramark.com/industries/correctionalinstitutions) is the largest player, serving over 600 facilities as of the end of 2014, others include A'Viands Food & Services Management, ABL Management, and Compass Group Canteen Correctional Services.

Menu Planning

Providing food at these costs is nutritionally and logistically challenging, as discussed in numerous *Insider* articles. Note that as of December 2014, the USDA (2014) estimates the cost of a "Thrifty Food Plan" for an adult male aged 19–50 at $43.20 for a week to be $6.17 a day. If it takes $6.17 a day for an adult male to achieve a nutritionally adequate diet based on US dietary guidance, correctional dietitians are faced with quite a challenge to do the same for much less, even accounting for the efficiencies of institutional purchasing power and preparation.

Researchers, noting the effect of the recent recession, comment that many states have sought cost-cutting measures, such as serving less food or serving only two meals on weekends. In light

---

BOX 6.7   PRISON FARMS AND FOOD BANKS

- San Diego's Richard J. Donovan Correctional Facility and Rehabilitation Meals program has set aside 3 acres of the prison grounds for growing produce. Twenty trained prison inmates will tend and harvest the garden with the help of prison staff gardeners and volunteers. The fresh produce will be used in the prison cafeteria, with surpluses donated to local food banks. The program also offers inmates the educational opportunity of developing gardening and farming skills and learning about healthy eating.

- Since partnering with Salvation Farms establishment in late 2012, Vermont Department of Corrections inmates helped to plant, grow, harvest, and process about 141,000 lb. of six different crops. The harvest is used in the prison cafeteria, food banks, schools, and other institutions in the area. By offering inmates an opportunity to develop farming skills, and hands-on food processing experience, the program hopes to reduce recidivism.

- The Oregon State Correctional Institution produces over 20,000 lb. of produce in their prison-grounds greenhouse. The harvest is split between the prison cafeteria and local food banks. The greenhouse program offers prisoners the opportunity to gain job-skills in sustainable agriculture and knowledge of ecology and conservation topics.

Source: Sustainable Cities Collective. Six U.S. Correctional Facilities with "Farm to Prison" Local Food Sourcing Programs. January 6, 2015. Available at http://sustainablecitiescollective.com/seedstock/1033746/six-us -correctional-facilities-farm-prison-local-food-sourcing-programs, accessed January 9, 2015.

of a 2004 news article that reported South Carolina costs of $1.13 per day compared to national average food of $3.32, these researchers analyzed menus served in two South Carolina correction facilities. They reported that, based on the menus, compared to US dietary guidance, equivalent amounts of meat and beans were served, but greater amounts of grains and lesser amounts of fruit, vegetables, and milk. Nutritionally, by using DRI values, the prison meals were low in vitamin E, magnesium, and potassium. The menus were also high in cholesterol, sodium, and vitamin A (Collins and Thompson 2012).

Although the cost for individuals to purchase and prepare food may naturally be higher than the cost of institutional procurement and preparation due to efficiencies of quantity, given the difference between what the USDA considers to be the bare minimum daily cost and what correctional institutions are spending, it is not surprising that food service has often been a cause of dissatisfaction among inmates. In addition to protesting quality or quantity, inmates have also protested that the food is not healthy, including a late 2014 lawsuit arguing that the standard high starch diet is unhealthy (Newell v. Asure 2014), as well as lawsuits in 2009 and 2011 arguing that the amount of soy (100 g and more per day) being used in the daily meals was not healthy (Alvarez 2011).

Corrections Dietitians

Corrections dietitians in the United States represent a minority in the field of nutrition and dietetics and food service management. The roles of the correctional dietitian vary, depending on the agency and facility, but this list represents an overview of the tasks that are performed:

- Promote the use of standardized menus and diets.
- Ensure compliance with standards and policies.
- Ensure nutritional adequacy of menus via computerized nutritional analysis.
- Review and approve menus annually and/or semiannually and make recommendations as needed.
- Write menus.
- Write medical diets or provide guidance for diets as requested. Typical therapeutic diets include the following types: low fat, diabetic, vegetarian, lactose-free, mechanical soft, religious (such as kosher and Muslim), allergy, and gluten-free.
- Set policy. Although there is general consensus that the DRIs and RDAs should be met, each system establishes its own standards regarding nutrients and energy provided in meals as well as the use of food in behavior management. The modification of food service, such as the use of the *Loaf* to control behavior, is an ongoing ethical debate in the corrections field. Another form of controlling behavior through food access is through limiting the amount of money that inmates can spend in the commissary (Box 6.8) (Newell v. Asure 2014).

Dietary Guidelines and Correctional Menus

With the publication of the 2010 *Dietary Guidelines for Americans*, corrections dietitians have been faced with the challenge of modifying corrections menus in order to meet the new meal pattern recommendations within the constraints of a limited budget (Wakeen 2011), and may need to do so once again when the 2015 *Dietary Guidelines for Americans* are published. In many ways, corrections dietitians face challenges similar to those faced by the school lunch programs:

- How are state and federal correction facilities modifying menus to meet these guidelines?
- How can sodium be reduced to 2300 mg when large caloric levels and processed foods are served, and when 2300 mg of sodium is considered a therapeutic level of sodium in many correctional facilities?
- What modifications are being made both to menus and by manufacturers to accommodate the fat, cholesterol, and saturated fat restrictions?
- Is meeting the DRIs and RDAs sufficient to be in compliance with agency standards?

BOX 6.8   *THE LOAF*: MODIFYING FOOD SERVICE TO CONTROL BEHAVIOR

The American Correctional Association standards preclude the use of food as a disciplinary measure. Inmates and staff, except those on special medical or religious diets, are expected to eat the same meals, and food should not be withheld as a disciplinary sanction. Though compliance to these standards is voluntary, they are viewed as valid and acceptable standards of operation within the industry.

Nevertheless, occasionally an inmate will be served a food product known as the *Loaf* (or variously, Special Management Meal, Behavioral Loaf, Nutri-Loaf, or Prison Loaf), which is designed to be nutritionally complete. Three loaves per day meet the basic nutritional needs of an adult inmate (2400–3900 calories with a distribution of approximately 10–15% protein, 50–79% carbohydrate, and 5–38% fat). The loaf is often served in a disposable container with no eating utensils and is accompanied by a beverage. This meal is a nutritionally complete, *albeit* tasteless alternative to the regular food service. The individual governing agency, warden, or jail administrator decides whether to use the loaf as either a reprimand for severe, deviant, antisocial behavior by the inmate or as a protective measure so that the inmate is less likely to injure himself.

There are no reliable statistics regarding how many facilities use the loaf. An informal survey indicated that it was used by half of the 19 facilities that responded for typically 1–3 days (but as many as 30). Respondents indicated that the loaf was used for discipline or behavior modification. In the majority of cases, administrative and/or medical personnel approved its use with strict monitoring procedures. Two respondents were sued; both cases were resolved in favor of the prison authority.

Source: Wakeen, B. and Montgomery, J.W. The "loaf"—part II. *ACFS Insider.* Summer 2003, pp. 19–20. Available at http://www.acfsa.org/cfppgm/pdfs/diet103.pdf, accessed August 9, 2006; Anno, B.J. Correctional HealthCare: Guidelines for the Management of an Adequate Delivery System, 2001 edition. National Commission on Correctional HealthCare, 2001.

- To help meet the dietary guidelines, will facilities accept menu modifications that include reducing overall calories, increasing meatless meals, and/or incorporating soy products into recipes to offset fat and cholesterol, offering skim milk, omitting and/or limiting non-nutritional items, such as sugar and coffee, and cooking without added salt?

In 2013, the *Insider* reported a trend in correctional institutions toward adopting heart healthy guidelines, including the reduction of calories, the use of low or reduced sodium products, the reduction of trans-fat, increased whole grain products and fiber, and limiting sugar use (through elimination of sugar packets but also through adoption of sugar-free desserts), but also including foods fortified with nutrients (Vanoni 2013). (Could future inmate lawsuits argue that a fortified beverage, although nutritionally appropriate, is not a meal?) Given that inmates are truly a captive audience, a broad transformation of the food environment could provide opportunities to evaluate if such food service changes will lead to improved health outcomes.

CORRECTIONAL HEALTH AS PUBLIC HEALTH

Health conditions overrepresented in incarcerated populations include substance abuse; HIV and other infectious diseases; perpetration of and victimization by violence; mental illness; chronic diseases; and reproductive health problems (Freudenberg 2001). Whereas the vast majority of individuals affected by these conditions develop them prior to incarceration, the period of incarceration provides a window of opportunity to serve the broad public health interest by providing testing, treatment, counseling, health education, and health promotion to an otherwise disenfranchised population prior to their ultimate release back into the community. Not only would it be cost effective to treat several of these diseases while individuals are incarcerated, but in quite a few instances it would also save money in the long run (National Commission on Correctional HealthCare 2002).

Prisons and jails offer a unique opportunity to establish better disease control in the community by providing improved healthcare and disease prevention to inmates before they are released. Unarguably, tens of thousands of inmates are being released into the community every year with undiagnosed or untreated communicable disease, chronic disease, and mental illness. The vast majority of the prison population is arrested in and returned to urban, low-income communities. The prison population has had little prior access to primary healthcare or health interventions, and many are returning to their communities without critical preventive health information and skills, appropriate medical services, and other necessary support (Box 6.9) (Hammett et al. 1998).

In 1997, Congress instructed the US Department of Justice (DOJ) to investigate the health status of soon-to-be-released inmates. At question was the extent that changes in correctional healthcare might be able to improve the public health of communities at large. NCCHC studied the problem and in 2002 released to Congress *The Health Status of Soon-to-Be-Released Inmates* (National Commission on Correctional HealthCare 2002).

This report found that although prisons and jails are channels to the community, corrections and public health maintain related, yet often uncoordinated, systems. In addition to public health benefits, coordinating health treatment approaches could also result in financial savings to taxpayers. Only 29 of the 41 systems reviewed indicated that inmates with chronic disease were given a supply of medication when released. Although many may view such care as outside the responsibility of publicly funded correctional agencies, inadequate access to care and follow-up services creates a cost burden (in dollars and in the potential development of resistance to treatment) for public health institutions once inmates are released (National Commission on Correctional HealthCare 2002).

Correctional systems can have a direct effect on the health of urban populations by offering targeted healthcare screenings and health promotion in jails and prisons (Binswanger et al. 2012), by

---

BOX 6.9   INNOVATION IN CORRECTIONAL HEALTH

Faced with explosive growth in its prison population and a legal mandate to improve medical care for incarcerated offenders, the state of Texas implemented a novel correctional managed healthcare program in 1994. The organizational structure of the program is based on a series of contractual relationships between the state prison system and two of the state's academic medical centers, which provide all medical, dental, and psychiatric care for the state's inmates. The health delivery system is composed of several levels of care, including primary ambulatory care clinics in each prison unit, infirmaries at strategic locations throughout the state, several regional medical facilities, and a dedicated prison hospital with a full range of services. Specialized treatment programs have been established at various units for patients with such chronic conditions as hypertension and diabetes mellitus.

Ten years after the managed care program was established, researchers reported significant positive health outcomes and millions of dollars saved. Significant changes in diet-related chronic conditions were reported from 1995 to 2003. The mean blood glucose level for patients with type 1 diabetes mellitus decreased from 230 to 188 mg/dL, the mean low-density lipoprotein cholesterol (LDL-C) level among patients with hyperlipidemia decreased from 174 to 132 mg/dL, and the proportion of inmates with essential hypertension (blood pressure $\geq 140/90$ mm/Hg) decreased from 83% to 51% (Carson 2014).

Source: Raimer, B.G. and Stobo, J.D., *JAMA.* 292, 485–489, 2004.

linking inmates to community services after release, and by assisting in the process of community reintegration. It is suggested that federal, state, and local reentry programs provide a three-phase, comprehensive assistance and support services approach from the (a) prerelease phase—with education, mental health, and substance abuse treatment, job training, and risk assessment, to the (b) transition phase prior to and immediately following offender release, and the (c) postrelease, sustained, long-term mentoring, counseling, and support phase (National Commission on Correctional HealthCare 2002). Without such support back to connections in the community, any gains in health status or nutritional status are likely to roll back; the development of post-incarceration transition clinic has been reported helpful in improving medical care during this time (Wang et al. 2010).

However, such post-incarceration clinics tend to focus on primary care, social service help, and substance use, rather than chronic disease outcomes (Conklin et al. 1998). A study of released prisoners found that retention in medical care and health outcome was worse for patients with diabetes than for those with HIV, with one possible reason that supportive services and housing options are more available to HIV patients. Comorbid substance use disorders and mental illness could be another confounding factor. Ultimately, medical care is necessary but not sufficient to control chronic diseases. Efforts to improve health outcomes for this population must also address the social conditions to which formerly incarcerated persons are exposed (Fox et al. 2014).

As an example, case managers with the New York City Link program are responsible for creating a community-services plan for inmates at the city's jail (Rikers Island), filing benefit applications on inmates' behalf and providing housing referrals. The program assists inmates in the application process and to secure access to benefits such as Medicaid, food stamps, and cash assistance after release. Under the program, a Medicaid application can be submitted up to 45 days before or within 7 days after release (Judge David L. Bazelon Center for Mental Health Law 2006).

Managing Nutrition-Related Chronic Diseases

People with diabetes, high blood pressure, and high blood cholesterol in correctional facilities should receive care that meets national standards; however, correctional institutions have unique circumstances that need to be considered so that all standards of care may be achieved. Policies must take into consideration issues such as security needs, transfer from one facility to another, and access to medical personnel and equipment.

NCCHC has adopted guidelines for disease management to help correctional healthcare professionals effectively manage diet-related chronic diseases commonly found in jails, prisons, and juvenile confinement facilities. NCCHC guidelines, updated in 2014, currently include ones for diabetes and hypertension, and obesity (for adolescents). The guidelines are adapted for the correctional environment from nationally accepted clinical guidelines prepared by the American Diabetes Association and the National Heart, Lung, and Blood Institute of the National Institutes of Health, and are written to specifically help correctional healthcare providers improve patient care outcomes. The guidelines encourage total disease management, which requires clear indicators of the degree of control of the patient's disease and, frequently, the more subtle distinction as to whether the condition is stable, improving, or deteriorating (National Commission on Correctional HealthCare, http://www.ncchc.org/guidelines).

Health Promotion through Correctional Food Access Policies

In addition to menu planning for nutritional adequacy, correctional dietitians can be involved in overall health promotion through food access policies. Correctional facilities vary as to the method of meal service (cafeteria or cell) and as to portion control (self-service or cafeteria staff served). Solutions that are acceptable for inmates with special dietary needs may also help improve health in the general prison population. For example, inmates with diabetes, hypertension, and/or hypercholesterolemia who have special dietary needs may benefit from simple solutions such as a reduced fat, reduced sodium salad bar that would relieve food service of the burden of preparing individual trays and would allow otherwise healthy prisoners to live outside of special units (Stoller

2000). Rules and policies also vary from facility to facility as to accessibility to vending machines, commissary foods, and cooking in cells. Adding healthy options to the commissary and vending machines while still stocking inmate favorites can allow and encourage inmates to exercise choice.

Nutrition Education

Prison programs incorporating nutrition education have been developed by corrections staff and outside agencies (Khavjou et al. 2007). A 2013 study of a voluntary nutrition workshop offered in a state prison found that a significantly greater proportion of participants (23.5%) than controls (3.2%) reported improved nutrition practices post workshop (Curd et al. 2013). In response to inmate complaints about obesity and the high-fat, high-energy meals being served, the South Dakota Women's Penitentiary in Pierre, South Dakota, developed a wellness education program that also included the provision of modified menu meals prepared in more healthful manners (such as baked chicken instead of fried). To be eligible for the low-energy meals, the inmates must commit to the program for at least 1 month. Nutrition analysis of food is posted so that the women may keep track of their intakes. The commissary began stocking more healthful snack options as well (Vitucci 1999).

A British Columbia center initiative involved incarcerated women themselves in program design, implementation, and evaluation of a 6-week nutrition and fitness pilot program. The program included a weekly nutrition presentation and group circuit exercise classes twice a day. The inmate research team designed preprogram and postprogram evaluation methods, which relied on responses to a self-administered questionnaire and body measurements. Sixteen women completed the pre- and post-questionnaires, reporting in general a decrease in weight and body measurements and improvement in energy, sleep, and stress levels. The fact that it was self-run was commented on: "Because it was organized and led by another woman in prison... she understands us... not someone coming in from the outside saying, you must do this because it is healthy for you" (Granger-Brown et al. 2012). Although prisoners may be the passive recipient of healthful changes to their food environment while incarcerated, providing food and nutrition education to prisoners can help support the adoption of improved personal habits upon release.

Correctional settings have unique challenges and constraints for nutrition and health intervention and promotion programming; and these will vary from setting to setting. Health needs and programming, including efforts at nutritional improvement, may vary for those with longer term sentences as compared to those with shorter ones. Nonetheless, correctional settings avail the unique opportunity to address the public health of our citizens; "as the vast majority of prison inmates are incarcerated for only a few months before returning to the community.... they are, over the long term, more appropriately regarded as 'citizens' than 'prisoners'" (Hellard and Aitken 2004).

RESOURCES AND PROFESSIONAL AFFILIATIONS

Correctional health nutrition professionals can join the American Correctional Food Service Association (ACFSA), and/or participate in the Corrections subunit Dietary Practice Group of AND, housed in the Dietetics in Health Care Communities (DHCC, http://www.dhccdpg.org) practice group. The Corrections subunit sponsors an electronic mailing list, and in 2004, its members published the *Correctional Foodservice and Nutrition Manual*, second edition. ACFSA (http://www.acfsa.org/about.php) is a nonprofit organization, formed in 1969, dedicated to the professional growth of correctional foodservice employees. ACFSA has a certification program, organizes training opportunities and conferences, and publishes a quarterly magazine called *The ACFSA Insider*. Articles of specific interest to dietitians are highlighted on the website (Association of Correctional Food Service Affiliates, http://www.acfsa.org/insider.php).

The NCCHC, a nonprofit organization dedicated to improving healthcare in the nation's jails, prisons, and juvenile detention and confinement facilities, has created a certification program for correctional health personnel, sets standards for health services in correctional facilities, and provides a voluntary accreditation program for facilities that meet NCCHC standards (Hellard and Aitken

2004). The NCCHC *Journal of Correctional HealthCare* is the only national, peer-reviewed journal to address correctional healthcare topics. This quarterly publication features original research, case studies, best practices, and literature reviews in the areas of health services administration, personnel and staffing, ethical issues, clinical and support services, medical records, continuous quality improvement, risk management, and medical-legal issues. As NCCHC develops clinical guidelines and position statements, these are also published in the journal.

Other associations for professional correctional health personnel include

- Academy of Correctional Health Professionals (http://www.correctionalhealth.org/).
- American Correctional Health Services Association (http://www.achsa.org).
- Corrections.com Healthcare Network (http://www.corrections.com/healthcare).
- American Correctional Association (http://www.aca.org).

CONCLUSION

This chapter has examined three distinctly different populations: breastfeeding mothers and infants, persons living with HIV/AIDS, and those who have been incarcerated. Combined, they comprise a substantial (though sometimes overlapping) portion of our population. Increasing the number of women who breastfeed and the duration of breastfeeding among all economic and ethnic strata of our society will significantly impact general population health and healthcare costs in the future. Similarly, improving nutrition and thus the health of people living with HIV/AIDS and the incarcerated have ramifications beyond the health status of any one individual as these individuals are all citizens and part of communities. It is particularly important to focus on special populations such as these citizens, as they are often those least likely to have access to or be able to afford healthcare, nutrition education, or healthy foods.

ACRONYMS

AAP	American Academy of Pediatrics
ACA	Affordable Care Act 2010
ACFSA	American Correctional Food Service Association
ADAP	AIDS Drug Assistance Program
AETC	AIDS Education and Training Center
AIDS	Acquired immunodeficiency syndrome
AND	Academy of Nutrition and Dietetics
ANSA	Association of Nutrition Services Agencies
ART	Antiretroviral therapy
AWS	AIDS wasting syndrome
BFHI	Baby-Friendly Hospital Initiative
BMC	Boston Medical Center
BOP	Federal Bureau of Prisons
CDC	Centers for Disease Control and Prevention
DOJ	US Department of Justice
DRI	Dietary reference intake
GI	Gastrointestinal
HAART	Highly active antiretroviral therapy
HHS	Department of Health and Human Services
HIV	Human immunodeficiency virus
IBCLC	International Board-Certified Lactation Consultant
LBM	Lean body mass
LBW	Low birth weight

LDL-C	Low-density lipoprotein cholesterol
MFWI	Mother-Friendly Workplace Initiative
MNT	Medical nutrition therapy
NCCHC	National Commission on Correctional HealthCare
NCHS	National Center for Health Statistics
NEC	Necrotizing enterocolitis
NICU	Neonatal intensive care unit
NIP	National Immunization Program
NIS	National Immunization Survey
OI	Opportunistic infection
PLWH/A	People living with HIV/AIDS
RD	Registered dietitian
RDA	Recommended dietary allowance
RMS	Ross Mothers Survey
RWA	Ryan White HIV/AIDS Treatment Extension Act of 2009
SES	Socioeconomic status
SIDS	Sudden infant death syndrome
UNICEF	United Nations International Children's Emergency Fund
USDA	US Department of Agriculture
WHO	World Health Organization
WIC	Special Supplemental Nutrition Program for Women, Infants, and Children

STUDENT ASSIGNMENTS AND ACTIVITIES DESIGNED TO ENHANCE LEARNING AND STIMULATE CRITICAL THINKING

1. Does a change in state law to explicitly permit public breastfeeding help to increase the rate of breastfeeding by removing or reducing an existing barrier? Suggestion: Compare the changes over time in prevalence of breastfeeding in states with and without breastfeeding legislation.

2. Contact your state's WIC Breastfeeding Coordinator and ask the following questions.
   a. How many WIC infants in your state are exclusively breastfed? Partially breastfed? What are the rates for teenage mothers? First-time mothers?
   b. What are the barriers to breastfeeding?
   c. What percentage of mothers has difficulty breastfeeding?
   d. What are some of the techniques used to convince mothers to breastfeed their infants?
   e. What are the current breastfeeding initiatives being promoted in your state?
   Write a 1–2 page summary of your interview.

3. Search Congress.gov for an update on the most recent activity on the Ryan White Act. Where in the act has nutrition been included?

4. Use healthypeople.gov to list the Healthy People 2020 objectives for breastfeeding and HIV/AIDS. How do these objectives compare to the Healthy People 2010 goals? Given the performance against 2010 goals, are the 2020 goals achievable? Why or why not?

5. Discuss the ethical issues faced by a nutrition professional who is asked to develop a recipe for a food loaf to be used as a reprimand in their detention facility.

6. Contact a correctional facility in your state and ask to speak to the Registered Dietitian. Use the questions listed in the section *Dietary Guidelines and Correctional Menus* to interview the RD. If the 2015 Dietary Guidelines have been published, ask what impact they will have. Summarize the answers and include your assessment of the correctional facility's biggest nutritional challenges. What are your suggestions for addressing these challenges?

7. Are there ramifications to the State of California regulations that require meeting the RDAs and DRIs without reference to the *Dietary Guidelines?* Discuss.

8. What other special populations might have specific nutrition challenges? Answer the following:
   a. Define the special population. What are the characteristics of this population?
   b. What are the particular nutritional needs that this population exhibits?
   c. What programs and/or policies currently exist to meet the nutritional needs of this population?

APPENDIX 6.1 THE INNOCENTI DECLARATION ON THE PROTECTION, PROMOTION, AND SUPPORT OF BREASTFEEDING

The Innocenti Declaration on the protection, promotion, and support of breastfeeding was developed and adopted by participants at the WHO/UNICEF policymakers' meeting on "Breastfeeding in the 1990s: A Global Initiative" cosponsored by the US Agency for International Development (USAID) and the Swedish International Development Authority, held in 1990 at the *Spedale degli Innocenti*, located in Florence, Italy.

The Declaration states:

As a global goal for optimal maternal and child health and nutrition, all women should be enabled to practise exclusive breastfeeding and all infants should be fed exclusively on breast milk from birth to 4–6 months of age. Thereafter, children should continue to be breastfed, while receiving appropriate and adequate complementary foods, for up to two years of age or beyond. This child-feeding ideal is to be achieved by creating an appropriate environment of awareness and support so that women can breastfeed in this manner.

The Declaration set four extremely ambitious operational targets to be met. By 1995, all governments should

- Appoint a national breastfeeding coordinator and establish a multisectoral national breastfeeding committee composed of representatives from relevant government departments, nongovernmental organizations, and health professional associations.
- Ensure that every facility providing maternity services fully practices all of the Ten Steps to Successful Breastfeeding set out in the joint WHO/UNICEF statement "Protecting, promoting and supporting breastfeeding; the special role of maternity services."
- Take action to enforce the principles and aim of all Articles of the International Code of Marketing of Breastmilk Substitutes and subsequent relevant World Health Assembly resolutions. (This goal is regarded as the minimum starting point for effective action.)
- Enact imaginative legislation protecting the breastfeeding rights of working women and establish means for its enforcement.

On the broadest possible scale, international advisory commissions should

- Establish action strategies for protecting, promoting, and supporting breastfeeding, including global monitoring and evaluation of their strategies.
- Support national situation analyses and surveys, and the development of national goals and targets for action.
- Encourage and support national authorities in planning, implementing, monitoring, and evaluating their breastfeeding policies.

Countries have made significant progress in reaching these goals, although they have not been fully achieved. More than 20,000 facilities have been certified and designated as baby friendly in 150 countries.

Source: Innocenti Declaration on the Protection, Promotion, and Support of Breastfeeding. Available at http://www.unicef.org/programme/breastfeeding/innocenti.htm. Accessed January 9, 2015

APPENDIX 6.2 UNITED STATES BREASTFEEDING COMMITTEE

STRATEGIC PLAN: 2009–2013

Goal A: Ensure that quality breastfeeding services are an essential component of healthcare for all families.

Objective 1: Advocate for adoption of evidence-based breastfeeding standards, guidelines, and regulations for accreditation of facilities providing maternity and infant healthcare services.

a. Establish relationships with key organizations, such as the National Quality Forum and The Joint Commission.

b. Advocate for the National Quality Forum and The Joint Commission to adopt measures and standards addressing the Baby-Friendly Hospital Initiative's Ten Steps to Successful Breastfeeding.

c. Advocate for increased funding to support the continuation and expansion of the *Maternity Practices in Infant Nutrition and Care (mPINC)* survey.

d. Develop a toolkit for state coalitions to use to highlight positive mPINC results in their states.

Objective 2: Encourage implementation of core competencies in health professional education.

a. Publish "Core Competencies in Breastfeeding Care for All Health Professionals" on the USBC website.

b. Distribute the Competencies to USBC member organizations and other relevant nonmember organizations.

c. Develop and execute a campaign to promote the Competencies and advocate for their inclusion in health professional education and regulatory programs, including, but not limited to, preservice, postgraduate, continuing education, and competency-assessment programs.

Objective 3: Ensure that healthcare professionals have the knowledge and resources to make evidence-based recommendations and treatment decisions that optimize breastfeeding outcomes.

a. Advocate for the development and dissemination of coordinated education and information to healthcare professionals.

Objective 4: Advocate for quality breastfeeding services in implementation of the ACA and other relevant legislation.

Goal B: Reduce marketing that undermines optimal breastfeeding.

Objective 1: Counteract the negative impact of product marketing.

a. Publish a position statement on marketing of products that impact breastfeeding.

b. Support the publication of a white paper on the economic and environmental impact of formula feeding.

c. Develop and execute a campaign to build public and congressional support for reducing such marketing.

d. Advocate for the elimination of the distribution of formula marketing materials through healthcare professionals and the health system.

e. Advocate for improved monitoring of product marketing claims.

f. Advocate for recognition of the ethical responsibilities of healthcare professionals and organizations related to product marketing.

Goal C: Ensure that women and their families in the workforce are supported in optimal breastfeeding.

Objective 1: Support legislation to provide paid family leave.
   a. Publish a position statement on paid family leave and its impact on breastfeeding.
   b. Approach other stakeholders to support their national campaigns for paid family leave.
   c. Collaborate with state breastfeeding coalitions to support state legislation to provide paid family leave.
Objective 2: Pursue legislation to require or incentivize workplace accommodations for breastfeeding.
   a. Publish a position statement in support of requiring workplace accommodations.
   b. Advocate for passage of federal legislation to require or incentivize workplace accommodations for all employees, and for effective and thorough implementation of such legislation.
   c. Collaborate with state breastfeeding coalitions to pursue state legislation to require or incentivize workplace accommodations, and to facilitate smooth implementation of federal legislation.

Goal D: Ensure that USBC is a sustainable and effective organization, funded, structured, and aligned to do its work.
   a. Secure and maintain funding to support achievement of the strategic goals, and reserves to cushion against the unexpected.
   b. Maintain a staffing structure to support achievement of the strategic goals.
   c. Maintain a strong governance framework, including a committee structure that mobilizes members and volunteers to collaborate to support achievement of the strategic goals, while making the best use of their unique skills and expertise.
   d. Continue to build a multisectoral, diverse membership and cultivate appropriate strategic partnerships.
   e. Maintain a strong partnership with, and provide support for, a network of state, territory, and tribal breastfeeding coalitions.
   f. Serve as an expert voice and a clearinghouse of breastfeeding information.
   g. Coordinate advocacy to ensure that federal legislation and policy protects, promotes, and supports breastfeeding.

Source: United States Breastfeeding Committee. *Strategic Plan: 2009–2013.* Rockville, MD: US Department of Health and Human Services, Health Services and Research Administration, Maternal and Child Health Bureau 2011. Available at http://www.usbreastfeeding.org/Portals/0 /USBC-Strategic-Plan-2009-2013.pdf, accessed January 9, 2015.

APPENDIX 6.3 STATE BREASTFEEDING STATUTES

92% of all states have enacted legislation related to breastfeeding:

- *Forty-six states, the District of Columbia, and the US Virgin Islands allow mothers to breastfeed in any public or private location.* Idaho, Michigan, South Dakota, and Virginia are the exceptions.
- *Twenty-nine states, the District of Columbia, and the US Virgin Islands exempt breastfeeding from public indecency laws.* Alaska, Arizona, Arkansas, Florida, Illinois, Kentucky, Louisiana, Massachusetts, Michigan, Minnesota, Mississippi, Missouri, Montana, Nevada, New Hampshire, New York, North Carolina, North Dakota, Oklahoma, Pennsylvania, Rhode Island, South Carolina, South Dakota, Tennessee, Utah, Virginia, Washington, Wisconsin and Wyoming.
- *Twenty-five states, the District of Columbia, and Puerto Rico have laws related to breastfeeding in the workplace.* Arkansas, California, Colorado, Connecticut, Georgia, Hawaii,

Illinois, Indiana, Louisiana, Maine, Minnesota, Mississippi, Montana, New Mexico, New York, North Dakota, Oklahoma, Oregon, Rhode Island, Tennessee, Texas, Vermont, Virginia, Washington, and Wyoming.

- *Sixteen states and Puerto Rico exempt breastfeeding mothers from jury duty or allow jury duty to be postponed.* California, Connecticut, Idaho, Illinois, Iowa, Kansas, Kentucky, Michigan, Mississippi, Missouri, Montana, Nebraska, Oklahoma, Oregon, South Dakota, and Virginia.
- *Five states and Puerto Rico have implemented or encouraged the development of a breastfeeding awareness education campaign.* California, Illinois, Minnesota, Missouri, and Vermont.

Some unique laws relating to breastfeeding:

- *Virginia* allows women to breastfeed on any land or property owned by the state.
- *Puerto Rico* requires shopping malls, airports, public service government centers, and other select locations to have accessible areas designed for breastfeeding and diaper changing that are not bathrooms.
- *Louisiana* law requires state buildings to provide suitable areas for breastfeeding and lactation, and prohibits any child-care facility from discrimination against breastfed babies.
- *Mississippi* requires licensed child-care facilities to provide breastfeeding mothers with a sanitary place that is not a toilet stall to breastfeed their children or express milk, to provide a refrigerator to store expressed milk, to train staff in the safe and proper storage and handling of human milk, and to display breastfeeding promotion information to the clients of the facility.
- *California* requires the Department of Public Health to develop a training course of hospital policies and recommendations that promote exclusive breastfeeding and specify staff for whom this model training is appropriate. The recommendation is targeted at hospitals with patients who ranked in the lowest 25% of the state for exclusive breastfeeding rates.
- *Maryland* exempts the sale of tangible personal property that is manufactured for the purpose of initiating, supporting, or sustaining breastfeeding from the sales and use tax.
- *California, New York, and Texas* have laws related to the procurement, processing, distribution, or use of human milk.
- *New York* created a Breastfeeding Mothers Bill of Rights, which is required to be posted in maternal healthcare facilities. New York also created a law that allows a child under 1 year of age to accompany the mother to a correctional facility if the mother is breastfeeding at the time she is committed.

Source: National Conference of State Legislatures. 50 State Summary of Breastfeeding Laws (updated June 2014). Available at http://www.ncsl.org/research/health/breastfeeding-state-laws .aspx, accessed January 9, 2015.

REFERENCES

Abrahams SW, Labbok MH. Exploring the impact of the Baby-Friendly Hospital Initiative on trends in exclusive breastfeeding. *Int Breastfeed J.* 2009;4:11. Available at http://www.internationalbreastfeedingjournal .com/content/4/1/11, accessed January 7, 2015.
Academy of Nutrition and Dietetics. Recommendations Summary H/A: Screening and Referral for Medical Nutrition Therapy 2010. Evidence Analysis Library. Printed August 15, 2014. Available at http://www .andeal.org/tmp/pq101.pdf, accessed January 7, 2015.
Academy of Nutrition and Dietetics. Ryan White HIV/AIDS Program Reauthorization. Available at http:// www.eatrightwashington.org/docs/Policy/2013/Issue%20Brief%20Ryan%20White%20PPW%202013 .pdf, accessed February 7, 2015.
Aramark: Correctional Institutions page. Available at http://www.Aramark.com/industries/correctionalinsti tutions, accessed December 26, 2014.

Association of Correctional Food Service Affiliates. About Us. Available at http://www.acfsa.org/about.php, accessed January 9, 2015.

Association of Correctional Food Service Affiliates. Insider. Available at http://www.acfsa.org/insider.php, accessed January 9, 2015.

Aidala A, Yomogida M, the HIV Food & Nutrition Study Team. *Community Health Advisory & Information Network Factsheet: HIV/AIDS, Food & Nutrition Service Needs.* New York: Columbia University Mailman School of Public Health, 2011. New York.

Al Shakir v. Carlson, 605 F. Supp. 374—Dist. Court, MD Pennsylvania, 1984.

Alvarez L. Soy diet is cruel and unusual punishment, Florida inmate claims. *New York Times,* November 11, 2011. Available at http://www.nytimes.com/2011/11/12/us/soy-diet-is-cruel-and-unusual-florida-inmate-claims.html?_r=0, accessed January 9, 2015.

American Academy of Pediatrics Policy Statement. Breastfeeding and the use of human milk. *Pediatrics.* 2012; 129:e827–e841. Available at http://pediatrics.aappublications.org/content/129/3/e827.full, accessed January 7, 2015.

American Dietetic Association. Position of the American Dietetic Association. Promoting and supporting breastfeeding. *J Am Diet Assoc.* 2009;109:1926–1942.

Baby-Friendly USA Designated Facilities as of December 22, 2014. Available at http://www.babyfriendlyusa .org/find-facilities, accessed January 7, 2015.

Baby-Friendly USA. Available at https://www.babyfriendlyusa.org/about-us/baby-friendly-hospital-initiative /the-ten-steps, accessed January 7, 2015.

Baillargeon J, Black SA, Pulvino J, Dunn K. Disease profile of Texas prison inmates. *Ann Epidemiol.* 2000;10(2):74–80. Available at https://www.ncjrs.gov/pdffiles1/nij/grants/194052.pdf.

Ball TM, Wright AL. Healthcare costs of formula-feeding in the first year of life. *Pediatrics.* 1999;103(4 Pt 2):870–876. Available at http://pediatrics.aappublications.org/content/103/Supplement_1/870.full.pdf, accessed January 7, 2015.

Ban the Bags. About. Available at http://banthebags.org/about/, accessed January 7, 2015.

Bartick M, Reinhold A. The burden of suboptimal breastfeeding in the United States: A pediatric cost analysis. *Pediatrics.* 2010;125(5):e1048–e1056. Available at http://pediatrics.aappublications.org/content/125/5 /e1048.full, accessed January 7, 2015.

Binswanger IA, Krueger PM, Steiner JF. Prevalence of chronic medical conditions among jail and prison inmates in the USA compared with the general population. *J Epidemiol Commun Health.* 2009;63(11):912–919.

Binswanger IA, Redmond N, Steiner JF, Hicks LS. Health disparities and the criminal justice system: An agenda for further research and action. *J Urban Health.* 2012;89(1):98–107.

Bondy J, Berman S, Glazner J, Lezotte D. Direct expenditures related to otitis media diagnoses: Extrapolations from a pediatric Medicaid cohort. *Pediatrics.* 2000;105:e72. Available at http://www.pediatrics.org/cgi /content/full/105/6/e72, accessed January 7, 2015.

Bureau of Prisons. Inmate Admission and Orientation Handbook. Updated August 28, 2014. Available at http:// www.bop.gov/locations/institutions/gil/GIL_aohandbook.pdf, accessed January 9, 2015.

Butte NF, King JC. Energy requirements during pregnancy and lactation. *Public Health Nutr.* 2005;8:1010–1027.

Carson EA. Prisoners in 2013. *Bureau of Justice Statistics,* September 30, 2014. Available at http://www.bjs .gov/content/pub/pdf/p13.pdf, accessed January 7, 2015.

Centers for Disease Control and Prevention. Breastfeeding among U.S. Children Born 2001–2011, CDC National Immunization Survey. Available at http://www.cdc.gov/breastfeeding/data/nis_data/, accessed January 7, 2015.

Centers for Disease Control and Prevention. Breastfeeding among U.S. Children Born 2001–2011, CDC National Immunization Survey. Available at http://www.cdc.gov/breastfeeding/data/NIS_data/2007 /state_any.htm, accessed January 7, 2015.

Centers for Disease Control and Prevention. Division of Nutrition, Physical Activity, and Obesity. CDC 2014 Breastfeeding Report Card. Available at http://www.cdc.gov/breastfeeding/pdf/2014breastfeeding reportcard.pdf, accessed January 7, 2015.

Centers for Disease Control and Prevention. HIV Statistics at a Glance. Available at http://www.cdc.gov/hiv /statistics/basics/ataglance.html, accessed January 7, 2015.

Centers for Disease Control and Prevention. HIV/AIDS. Opportunistic Infections. Available at http://www .cdc.gov/hiv/living/opportunisticinfections.html, accessed January 7, 2015.

Centers for Disease Control and Prevention. HIV/AIDS. Prevention Benefits of HIV Treatment. Available at http://www.cdc.gov/hiv/prevention/research/tap/, accessed January 7, 2015.

Centers for Disease Control and Prevention. NIS Survey Methods and Breastfeeding Questions. Available at http://www.cdc.gov/breastfeeding/data/nis_data/survey_methods.htm, accessed January 7, 2015.

Centers for Disease Control and Prevention. PRAMS. Available at http://www.cdc.gov/prams/, accessed February 17, 2015.

Cohen J. Breakthrough of the year. HIV treatment as prevention. *Science.* 2011;334(6063):1628. Available at http://www.sciencemag.org/content/334/6063/1628, accessed January 7, 2015.

Collins SA, Thompson SH. What are we feeding our inmates? *J Correct Health Care.* 2012;18(3):210–218.

Community Servings. History. Available at http://www.servings.org/about/history.cfm, accessed February 7, 2015.

Conklin TJ, Lincoln T, Flanigan TP. A public health model to connect correctional health care with communities. *Am J Public Health.* 1998;88(8):1249–1250.

Controversy over Kosher Meals in Florida Prisons. *CBS,* April 11, 2014. Available at http://miami.cbslocal.com/2014/04/11/controversy-over-kosher-meals-in-florida-prisons/, accessed January 9, 2015.

County of Santa Clara, California. Nutrition Standards 2012 Implementation Guidance. Available at http://www.sccgov.org/sites/planning/PlansPrograms/GeneralPlan/Health/Documents/NUTRITION_STANDARDS_2012.pdf, accessed January 9, 2015.

Curd P, Ohlmann K, Bush H. Effectiveness of a voluntary nutrition education workshop in a state prison. *J Correct Health Care.* 2013;19(2):144–150.

Dietetics in Health Care Communities. Dietary Practice Group of the Academy of Nutrition and Dietetics. Available at http://www.dhccdpg.org, accessed January 9, 2015.

Eat Right. Academy of Nutrition and Dietetics. Nutrition and HIV—AIDS. Available at http://www.eatright.org/Public/content.aspx?id=5546, reviewed April 2014, accessed January 7, 2015.

Elwood MR, Buxton JA, Hislop G, Salmon A, ed. Collaborative community-prison programs for women in BC. Nutrition and exercise program developed by incarcerated women. *BC Med J.* 2012;54(10):509–513. Available at http://www.bcmj.org/articles/collaborative-community-prison-programs-incarcerated-women-bc#a19, accessed January 9, 2015.

Federal Bureau of Prisons. Available at http://www.bop.gov/, accessed January 7, 2015. National Commission on Correctional Health Care. Accreditation and Facility Services. Available at http://www.ncchc.org/accreditation-facility-services, accessed January 9, 2015.

Foundation for Aids Research. HIV and AIDS Facts and Statistics. Available at http://www.amfar.org/About-HIV-and-AIDS/Facts-and-Stats/Statistics—Worldwide, accessed January 7, 2015.

Fox AD, Anderson MR, Bartlett G, Valverde J, Starrels JL, Cunningham CO. Health outcomes and retention in care following release from prison for patients of an urban post-incarceration transitions clinic. *J Health Care Poor Underserved.* 2014;25(3):1139–1152.

Freudenberg N. Jails, prisons, and the health of urban populations: A review of the impact of the correctional system on community health. *J Urban Health.* 2001;78:214–235.

God's Love We Deliver. Our Story. Available at https://www.glwd.org/press/kit.jsp, accessed February 7, 2015.

Golinelli D, Minton TD. US Department of Justice, Bureau of Justice Statistics. Jail Inmates at MidYear 2013 Statistical Tables. Available at http://www.bjs.gov/index.cfm?ty=pbdetail&iid=4988, accessed January 7, 2015.

Granger-Brown A, Buxton JA, Condello L-L, Elwood Martin R, Hislop G, Salmon A. Collaborative community-prison programs for women in BC. Nutrition and exercise program developed by incarcerated women. *BC Med J.* 2012;54(10):509–513. Available at http://www.bcmi.org/articles/collaborative-community-programs-incarcerated-women-bc#a19, accessed January 9, 2015.

Greene J, Pranis K. The Punitiveness Report. Part I. Growth Trends and Recent Research. Institute on Women & Criminal Justice. Available at http://66.29.139.159/institute/hardhit/part1.htm, accessed January 9, 2015.

Greenfeld LA, Snell TL. Women Offenders. US Department of Justice. Office of Justice Programs. Bureau of Justice Statistics. Special Report, December 1999. Available at http://www.bjs.gov/content/pub/pdf/wo.pdf, accessed January 9, 2015.

Hammett TM, Gaiter JL, Crawford C. Reaching seriously at-risk populations: Health interventions in criminal justice settings. *Health Educ Behav.* 1998;25(1):99–120.

Harzke A, Baillargeon J, Pruitt S, Pulvino J, Paar D, Kelley M. Prevalence of chronic medical conditions among inmates in the Texas Prison System. *J Urban Health.* 2010;87(3):486–503.

Health Resources and Services Administration. HIV/AIDS Programs: Ryan White Treatment Modernization Act of 2006, Reauthorization. Available at http://hab.hrsa.gov/abouthab/modernact2006.html, accessed January 7, 2015.

Hellard ME, Aitken CK. HIV in prison: What are the risks and what can be done? *Sex Health.* 2004;1(2):107–113.

Hendricks KM, Dong KR, Gerrior JL, ed. *Nutrition Management of HIV and AIDS.* Chicago: American Dietetic Association, 2009.

Hirschman C, Butler M. Trends and differentials in breast feeding: An update. *Demography.* 1981;18(1):39–54.

HIV/AIDS (2010) Evidence-Based Nutrition Practice Guideline. Available at http://www.andeal.org/tmp/pq100.pdf, accessed January 7, 2015.

Hornung CA, Greifinger RB, Gadre S. *A Projection Model of the Prevalence of Selected Chronic Diseases in the Inmate Population*, Vol. 2. Chicago: NCCHC, 2002, pp. 39–56.

HRSA. Key Provisions of the Affordable Care Act for the Ryan White HIV/AIDS Program. Available at http://hab.hrsa.gov/affordablecareact/keyprovisions.pdf, accessed January 7, 2015.

HRSA. Part B: Aids Drug Assistance Program. http://hab.hrsa.gov/abouthab/partbdrug.html, accessed January 9, 2015.

HRSA. The Ryan White HIV/AIDS Program: 2010 State Profiles. Available at http://hab.hrsa.gov/stateprofiles/index.htm, accessed February 7, 2015.

Innocenti Declaration 2005 on Infant and Young Child Feeding. Available at http://www.unicef-irc.org/publications/435, accessed January 7, 2015.

Innocenti Declaration on the Protection, Promotion, and Support of Breastfeeding. Available at http://www.unicef.org/programme/breastfeeding/innocenti.htm, accessed January 7, 2015.

International Board of Lactation Consultant Examiners homepage. Available at http://www.iblce.org/, accessed January 7, 2015.

James JS. State Prison Expenditures, 2001. US Department of Justice. Office of Justice Programs. Bureau of Justice Statistics. Special Report, June 2004. Available at http://www.bjs.gov/content/pub/pdf/spe01.pdf, accessed January 9, 2015.

Judge David L. Bazelon Center for Mental Health Law. Best Practices: Access to Benefits for Prisoners with Mental Illnesses. A Bazelon Center Issue Brief, 2006.

Kaiser Family Foundation. Updating the Ryan White HIV/AIDS Program for a New Era: Key Issues and Questions for the Future, 2013. Available at http://kaiserfamilyfoundation.files.wordpress.com/2013/04/8431/pdf, accessed January 7, 2015.

Khavjou OA, Clarke J, Hofeldt RM et al. A captive audience: Bringing the WISEWOMAN program to South Dakota prisoners. *Womens Health Issues*. 2007;17:193–201.

Kotz D. All Massachusetts maternity hospitals now ban infant formula gift bags. *Boston Globe*, July 7, 2012. Available at http://www.boston.com/dailydose/2012/07/12/all-massachusetts-maternity-hospitals-now-ban-infant-formula-gift-bags/stcOXl9MRyWbSGLAzXdACO/story.html, accessed January 7, 2015.

Li R, Scanlon KS, Serdula MK. The validity and reliability of maternal recall of breastfeeding practice. *Nutr Rev*. 2005;63:103–110.

Los Angeles County Commission on HIV Health Services. Guidelines for Implementing HIV/AIDS Medical Nutrition Therapy Protocols. Revised December 2002. Available at http://hivcommission-la.info/guidelines_implementing.pdf, accessed January 7, 2015.

Maruschak L. Medical problems of prisoners (NCJ 221740). Washington, DC: Bureau of Justice Statistics, 2008.

Merewood A, Philipp BL. Becoming baby-friendly: Overcoming the issue of accepting free formula. *J Hum Lact*. 2000;16:279–282.

Minton TD. Jail Inmates at Midyear 2012—Statistical Tables. *Bureau of Justice Statistics*, May 2013. Available at http://www.bjs.gov/content/pub/pdf/jim12st.pdf, accessed January 9, 2015.

National Alliance of State and Territorial AIDS Directors "Ryan White Program 2013 Reauthorization." Available at http://www.nastad.org/Docs/095329_NASTAD%20Fact%20Sheet%20on%20Future%20of%20the%20Ryan%20White%20Program.pdf, accessed January 7, 2015.

National Commission on Correctional HealthCare. The Health Status of Soon-to-be-Released Inmates: A Report to Congress, 2002.

National Commission on Correctional Health Care. Guidelines for Disease Management. Available at http://www.ncchc.org/guidelines, accessed January 9, 2015.

National Conference of State Legislatures. Breastfeeding State Laws. Available at http://www.ncsl.org/research/health/breastfeeding-state-laws.aspx, accessed January 5, 2015.

National HIV/AIDS Strategy for the United States, July 2010. Available at http://www.whitehouse.gov/sites/default/files/uploads/NHAS.pdf, accessed January 7, 2015.

Naylor AJ. Baby-Friendly Hospital Initiative. Protecting, promoting, and supporting breastfeeding in the twenty-first century. *Pediatr Clin North Am*. 2001;48:475–483.

Nerad J, Romeyn M, Silverman E, Allen-Reid J, Dieterich D, Merchant J. General nutrition management in patients infected with HIV. *Clin Infect Dis*. 2003;36:552–562.

New Mexico Community Planning and Action Group. Ryan White Program Service Definitions. Available at http://www.nmcpag.org/pdf/ryan_white_program_defs.pdf, accessed January 7, 2015.

Newell v. Asure. United States District Court Middle District of Pennsylvania, December 18, 2014. Available at https://localtvwnep.files.wordpress.com/2015/01/rockne_newell_food_lawsuit.pdf, accessed January 9, 2015.

Parker M, Burnham L, Cook J, Sanchez E, Philipp BL, Merewood A. 10 years after baby-friendly designation: Breastfeeding rates continue to increase in a US neonatal care unit. *J Hum Lact.* 2013;29(3):354–358.

Philipp BL, Merewood A, Miller LW et al. Baby-Friendly Hospital Initiative improves breastfeeding initiation rates in a US hospital setting. *Pediatrics.* 2001;108:677–681.

Picciano MF. Pregnancy and lactation: Physiological adjustments, nutritional requirements and the role of dietary supplements. *J Nutr.* 2003;133:1997S–2002S.

Public Citizen. Successful Initiatives to Limit Formula Marketing in Health Care Facilities: Strategic Approaches and Case Studies. Available at http://www.citizen.org/documents/report-successful-initia tives-formula-marketing.pdf, accessed January 7, 2015.

Rippetoe M, Kilgore L. *Practical Programming for Strength Training.* Wichita Falls, TX: Aasgaard Company. Third Printing, 2008.

Ryan AS. The resurgence of breastfeeding in the United States. *Pediatrics.* 1997;99(4):e12. Available at http:// pediatrics.aappublications.org/content/99/4/e12.short, accessed January 7, 2015.

Ryan AS. The truth about the Ross Mothers Survey. *Pediatrics.* 2004;113:626–267.

Ryan AS, Zhou W. Lower breastfeeding rates persist among the Special Supplemental Nutrition Program for Women, Infants, and Children participants, 1978–2003. *Pediatrics.* 2006;117:1136–1146.

Snell TL. Women in Prison. Survey of State Prison Inmates, 1991. US Department of Justice. Office of Justice Programs. Bureau of Justice Statistics. Special Report, March 1994. Available at http://bjs.gov/content /pub/pdf/WOPRIS.PDF, accessed January 9, 2015.

State of California. California Code of Regulations. Title 15. Crime Prevention and Corrections. Division 3. Rules and Regulations of Adult Institutions, Programs, and Parole. Department of Corrections and Rehabilitation. Updated through January 1, 2014. Article 4. Food Services. Available at http://www .cdcr.ca.gov/Regulations/Adult_Operations/docs/Title15-2014.pdf, accessed January 9, 2015.

Stern M, Greifinger R, Mellow J. Patient safety: Moving the bar in prison healthcare standards. *Am J Public Health.* 2010;100(11):2103–2110.

Steube A. The risks of not breastfeeding for mothers and infants. *Rev Obstet Gynecol.* 2009 Fall;2(4):222–231.

Stoller N. Improving Access to HealthCare for California's Women Prisoners. Executive Summary. A working paper for the California Program on Access to Care, October 2000. Available at http://cpac.berkeley.edu /documents/stollerpaper.pdf, accessed January 6, 2015.

TARGET Center Tools for the Ryan White Community. Health Care and HIV: Nutritional Guide for Providers and Clients. Available at https://careacttarget.org/library/health-care-and-hiv-nutritional-guide-provid ers-and-clients, accessed January 7, 2015.

The Becket Fund for Religious Liberty. Study Group on Religious Dietary Accommodation in Florida's State Prison System, July 26, 2007. Available at http://www.becketfund.org/wp-content/uploads/2012/08 /JDA-Study-Group-Report.pdf, accessed January 9, 2015.

The CDC Guide to Strategies to Support Breastfeeding Mothers and Babies. Atlanta, GA: US Department of Health and Human Services, Centers for Disease Control and Prevention, 2013. Available at http://www .cdc.gov/breastfeeding/pdf/BF-Guide-508.PDF, accessed January 7, 2015.

The Henry J. Kaiser Family Foundation. The HIV/AIDS Epidemic in the United States, April 7, 2014. Available at http://kff.org/hivaids/fact-sheet/the-hivaids-epidemic-in-the-united-states/, accessed January 7, 2015.

United States Breastfeeding Committee. Workplace Support in Federal Law. Available at http://www.usbreast feeding.org/Employment/WorkplaceSupport/WorkplaceSupportinFederalLaw/tabid/175/Default.aspx, accessed January 7, 2015.

United States Department of Agriculture, Food and Nutrition Service, Women, Infants and Children. About WIC—WIC at a Glance. Available at http://www.fns.usda.gov/wic/about-wic-wic-glance, accessed January 9, 2015.

United States Department of Agriculture, Food and Nutrition Service. WIC Breastfeeding Peer Counseling Study Final Implementation Report June 2010. Available at http://www.fns.usda.gov/sites/default/files /wicpeercounseling.PDF, accessed January 7, 2015.

United States Department of Agriculture. Center for Nutrition Policy and Promotion. USDA Food Plans: Cost of Food report for November 2014. Available at http://www.cnpp.usda.gov/sites/default/files/Costof FoodNov2014.pdf, accessed January 9, 2015.

Upton C, Harp S. Cost of Incarcerating Adult Felons. Research Report No. 373. Legislative Research Commission. Available at http://www.lrc.ky.gov/lrcpubs/rr373.pdf, accessed January 9, 2015.

US Department of Agriculture, Food and Nutrition Service, Office of Analysis, Nutrition and Evaluation. *Breastfeeding Intervention Design Study-Final Evaluation Design and Analysis Plan.* Alexandria, VA: McLaughlin JE, Burstein NR, Tao F, Fox MK. Project Officer, McKinney P, 2004.

US Department of Agriculture, Food and Nutrition Service, Office of Analysis, Nutrition and Evaluation. WIC Participant and Program Characteristics 2012, WICPC2012, December 2013. Available at http://www .fns.usda.gov/sites/default/files/WICPC2012_Summary.pdf, accessed January 9, 2015.

US Department of Health and Human Services. *Healthy People 2020.* Washington, DC: US Department of Health and Human Services, Public Health Service, Office of the Assistant Secretary for Health, 2010. Available at http://www.healthypeople.gov/2020/topics-objectives/topic/maternal-infant-and-child-health /objectives, accessed January 7, 2015.

US Department of Health and Human Services, Office of Disease Prevention and Health Promotion. Healthy People 2020. Washington, DC. Available at http://www.healthypeople.gov/2020/topicsobjectives2020 /TechSpecs .aspx?hp2020id=MICH-24. accessed January 5, 2014.

US Department of Justice, Bureau of Justice Statistics. Prevalence of Imprisonment in the U.S. Population, 1974–2001. Available at http://www.bjs.gov/content/pub/pdf/piusp01.pdf, accessed January 7, 2015.

US Government Accountability Office. Women in Prison. Issues and Challenges Confronting the U.S. Correctional Systems, December 1999. Available at http://www.gao.gov/archive/2000/gg00022.pdf, accessed January 9, 2015.

US Government Accountability Office. GAO Highlights. Bureau of Prisons. Eligibility and Capacity Impact Use of Flexibilities to Reduce Inmates' Time in Prison, February 2012. Available at http://www.gao.gov /assets/590/588283.pdf, accessed January 7, 2015.

US Health Resources and Services Administration. Women's Preventive Services Guidelines. Available at http://www.hrsa.gov/womensguidelines, accessed January 7, 2015.

Vanoni J. Menu trends in corrections. *Insider.* Winter 2013. Available at http://www.acfsa.org/Insider /articles/13Winter.pdf, accessed January 9, 2015.

Vitucci N. Facility implements weight loss and nutrition education plan. *Correct Care.* 1999;9.

Wagner P, Sakala L. Mass Incarceration: The Whole Pie. A Prison Policy Initiative Briefing, March 12, 2014. Available at http://www.prisonpolicy.org/reports/pie.html, accessed January 9, 2015.

Wakeen B. Changes in standards and guidelines…. and the impact on correctional menus and diets. *Insider.* Fall 2011. Available at http://www.acfsa.org/Insider/articles/11Fall.pdf, accessed January 9, 2015.

Wakeen B. The non-traditional dietitian's role. *Insider.* Winter 2014. Available at http://www.acfsa.org/Insider /insider2014Winter.pdf, accessed January 9, 2015.

Walensky RP, Paltiel AD, Losina E et al. The survival benefits of AIDS treatment in the United States. *J Infect Dis.* 2006;194:11–19.

Wang EA, Hong CS, Samuels L, Shavit S, Sanders R, Kushel M. Transitions clinic: Creating a community-based model of health care for recently released California prisoners. *Public Health Rep.* 2010;125(2):171–177.

Weimer DR. Summary of State Breastfeeding Laws and Related Issues. Congressional Research Service. The Library of Congress. Order Code RL31633, June 26, 2009. Available at http://maloney.house.gov/sites /maloney.house.gov/files/documents/women/breastfeeding/062609%20CRS%20Summary%20of%20 State%20Breastfeeding%20Laws.pdf, accessed January 5, 2015.

Weimer JP. The Economic Benefits of Breastfeeding: A Review and Analysis. Food and Rural Economics Division, Economic Research Service, US Department of Agriculture. Food Assistance and Nutrition Research Report No. 13. Available at http://www.ers.usda.gov/publications/fanrr-food-assistance-nutri tion-research-program/fanrr13.aspx, accessed January 7, 2015.

Williams BA, McGuire J, Lindsay RG, Baillargeon J, Cenzer IS, Lee SJ, Kushel M. Coming home: Health status and homelessness risk of older pre-release prisoners. *J Gen Intern Med.* 2010;25:1038–1044.

Williams B, Stern M, Mellow J, Safer M, Greifinger R. Aging in correctional custody: Setting a policy agenda for older prisoner healthcare. *Am J Public Health.* 2012;102(8):1475–1481.

Wilper AP, Woolhandler S, Boyd JW, Lasser KE, McCormick D, Bor DH, Himmelstein DU. The health and health care of US prisoners: A nationwide survey. *Am J Public Health.* 2009;99(4):666–672.

World Alliance for Breastfeeding Action (WABA). Women & Work. M.F.W.I. Available at http://www.waba .org.my/whatwedo/womenandwork/mfwi.htm, accessed January 7, 2015.

World Health Organization. Baby Friendly Hospital Initiative. Available at http://www.who.int/nutrition/top ics/bfhi/en/, accessed January 9, 2015.

World Health Organization. *The Optimal Duration of Exclusive Breastfeeding. Report of an Expert Consultation.* Department of Child and Adolescent Health and Development. Geneva, Switzerland: WHO, 2001. Available at http://www.who.int/nutrition/publications/optimal_duration_of_exc_bfeeding_report_eng .pdf, accessed January 7, 2015.

Zell ER, Ezzati-Rice TM, Battaglia MP, Wright RA. National Immunization Survey: The methodology of a vaccination surveillance system. *Public Health Rep.* 2000;115:65–77. Available at http://www.ncbi.nlm .nih.gov/pmc/articles/PMC1308558/, accessed January 7, 2015.

7 Cultural Competency*

> Food and language are the cultural habits humans learn first and the ones they change with the greatest reluctance.
>
> **Gabaccia (1998)**

INTRODUCTION

By 2050, more than 50% of the US population will consist of people from different cultural backgrounds. According to the estimates from the 2011 American Community Survey, roughly 11.7 million, or 29%, of the immigrant population in the United States is from Mexico. Chinese and Indian immigrants make up the second and third largest immigrant groups, with 1.9 million or 5% of the foreign-born population each. As of 2010, India replaced the Philippines as the third largest source country of migration to the United States (Hipsman and Meissner 2013).

The dynamic, growing population shifts in the United States along with the changing health status of various cultural, ethnic, and racial populations invite exciting challenges in the field of health services. There is a plethora of evidence that supports the importance of understanding and applying cultural constructs in care and education (Cynthia and Drago 2009). Cultural competence is vital for public health policy makers and health program planners who are operating in an increasingly multicultural and cross-cultural society. This chapter explores some of the issues pertaining to cultural competence. We discuss cultural competence generally, which includes a discussion on health literacy. We examine the influence of culture competency on healthcare organizations and the role of nutritionists. We conclude with a look at the foodways of some of the major ethnic groups in the United States.

CULTURAL COMPETENCY

Cultural competence is a broad concept that influences a variety of policy-making decisions and shapes interventions to improve accessibility and health outcomes. *Culture* refers to patterns of human behavior that include the language, thoughts, communications, actions, customs, beliefs, values, and institutions of racial, ethnic, religious, or social groups. *Competence* implies functioning effectively (either as an individual or an organization) within the context of the cultural beliefs, behaviors, and needs presented by communities and individuals (Cynthia and Drago 2009).

The need and support for cultural competency dates back to the civil rights movements in the 1960s (Engebretson et al. 2008) and the enactment of the Civil Rights Act of 1964. Title VI of the Civil Rights Act of 1964 mandates that no person in the United States shall, on grounds of race, color, or national origin, be excluded from participation in, be denied the benefits of, or be subjected to discrimination under any program or activity receiving federal financial assistance. Programs or services supported by federal funds must deliver the benefits and services without regard to race, color, or national origin (US Government Publishing Office 1964). "Delivery of services" incorporates the notion that such delivery should be effective, and in turn, effectiveness may be impacted by cultural differences. Over time, the importance of integrating cultural competency into all levels of healthcare has expanded to address health inequities.

---

* Shakiba Muhammadi, MD, MPH, contributed primary research and prepared draft versions of portions of this chapter.

In the 1980s, a range of cultural competency models and frameworks burgeoned, and a variety of terms are used to describe culturally competent healthcare service, such as cultural awareness, cultural sensitivity, and cultural diversity. Many professionals who work in this area have developed their own definitions and explanations. However, the most cited definition of cultural competency is that of Cross et al.: "a set of congruent behaviors, attitudes, and policies that come together in a system, agency, or amongst professionals and enables that system, agency or those professionals to work effectively in cross-cultural situations" (Grant et al. 2013). This is the definition used by the United States Department of Health and Human Services' (HHS's) Health Resources and Services Administration office (US Department of Health and Human Services, http://www.hrsa.gov/culturalcompetence/index.html).

HEALTH DISPARITIES AND THE ROLE OF CULTURAL COMPETENCY

Despite recent progress in overall national health, there are continuing disparities in the incidence of illness and death among populations of racial and ethnic minorities as compared with the US population as a whole, as indicated in *Healthy People 2000* (US Department of Health and Human Services, http://www.cdc.gov/nchs/data/hp2000/hp2k01.pdf), *Healthy People 2010* (US Department of Health and Human Services, http://www.healthypeople.gov/2010/About/goals.htm), and *Healthy People 2020* (US Department of Health and Human Services, https://www.healthypeople.gov/2020/About-Healthy-People).

Healthy People 2000 identified three broad goals, one of which was to reduce health disparities among Americans. Healthy People 2010 identified two overarching goals, one of which was to eliminate health disparities among different segments of the population. Healthy People 2020 (HP 2020) identified four overarching goals, one of which is to achieve health equity, eliminate disparities, and improve the health of all groups. Our nation's health goals are increasingly ambitious.

According to HP 2020, disparity is evident when a health outcome is seen in a greater or lesser extent between populations, and it is important to recognize the impact that social determinants have on health outcomes of specific populations. A *health disparity* is defined by HP 2020 as "a particular type of health difference that is closely linked with social, economic, and/or environmental disadvantage. Health disparities adversely affect groups of people who have systematically experienced greater obstacles to health based on their racial or ethnic group; religion; socioeconomic status; gender; age; mental health; cognitive, sensory, or physical disability; sexual orientation or gender identity; geographic location; or other characteristics historically linked to discrimination or exclusion" (HealthyPeople.gov, http://www.healthypeople.gov/2020/about/foundation-health-measures/Disparities).

Health disparities are found among populations from racial and ethnic minorities, such as African Americans, Latino/Hispanic Americans, and Native Americans, Alaska Natives, and Pacific Islanders. As indicated in Chapter 4, minority groups face a disproportionate burden of disease compared to the nonwhite US population, particularly of chronic diseases. Hypertension, cardiovascular diseases, stroke, diabetes, and anemia (micronutrient deficiencies) are some of the diet-related diseases disproportionately affecting racial and ethnic minorities.

However, health disparities exist among other marginalized populations as well. The need for cultural competence is not limited to just racial and ethnic differences. Healthcare providers may be treating population groups who are ethnically and racially similar to the provider but who are different in other social identities or have differences in healthcare needs. The inclusion of other identities that face discrimination and healthcare disparities into cultural competence policies speaks to a broader concept of diversity competence (US Department of Health and Human Services and Agency for Healthcare Research and Quality 2014).

For policy makers, it is necessary to ensure universal, competent, professional practice. The process of creating competent policies to reduce discrimination of any kind, and thus reduce health inequities, requires an understanding of the interplay between policy, service provision, and the effectiveness of the outcomes on the population in question (Betancourt et al. 2003). Segmented diversity in the workforce may also contribute to the challenge facing public health in meeting the needs of diverse populations, thereby affecting the quality of preventive care and contributing to health disparities.

The National Center for Cultural Competence (NCCC, http://nccc.georgetown.edu/foundations /need.html) has identified reasons for incorporating cultural competence into organizational policy:

- To understand and respond effectively to diverse belief systems related to health and well-being.
- To respond to current and projected demographic changes in the United States.
- To eliminate long-standing disparities in the health and mental health status of diverse racial, ethnic, and cultural groups.
- To improve the quality and accessibility of healthcare services.

Although it is assumed that cultural competence will have a positive effect on health outcomes, research on the effects of cultural competence is still developing. A 2014 literature review of articles published between 2000 and 2012 reviewing cultural competency in health settings found moderate evidence of improvement in healthcare access and utilization but weaker evidence for health outcomes. More rigorous study designs are still needed (Truong et al. 2014).

CULTURAL COMPETENCY INFLUENCERS

Demographic Changes

The makeup of the American population is changing as a result of immigration patterns as well as from significant increases among already extant racially, ethnically, culturally, and linguistically, diverse populations. For example, the growth in the Asian American population has been primarily through immigration, whereas the growth in the Hispanic population in the United States has been primarily due to births (Brown 2014). As another example of a change in immigration patterns, the foreign-born population from Africa in the United States has increased from about 80,000 in 1970 to about 1.6 million in the period from 2008 to 2012 (Box 7.1) (Gambino et al. 2014a).

Another change in immigration pattern concerns destination. The main immigrant destination states have been California, New York, Texas, Florida, Illinois, and New Jersey; however, 10 other states, mostly in the south and west, have experienced over 270% immigrant population growth since 1990. These "new" destination states are North Carolina, Georgia, Tennessee, Arkansas, Nevada, South Carolina, Kentucky, Nebraska, Utah, and Alabama (Hipsman and Meissner 2013).

The 2010 US census reports that whites, African Americans, Hispanics, and Asians all increased in population size between 2000 and 2010; however, over that decade, the Asian population group experienced the fastest rate of population growth, and whites experienced the slowest rate of growth

---

BOX 7.1   FOREIGN-BORN

The US Census Bureau uses the term *foreign-born* to refer to anyone who is not a US citizen at birth. This includes naturalized US citizens, lawful permanent residents (immigrants), temporary migrants (such as foreign students), and humanitarian migrants (such as refugees). The term *foreign-born* also includes those persons who are illegally present in the United States. The terms *native* and *native-born* refer to anyone born in the United States, Puerto Rico, a US island area (e.g., Guam), or abroad of a US citizen parent or parents.

Source: Gambino, C.P. et al., English-Speaking Ability of the Foreign-Born Population in the United States: 2012, American Community Survey Report, June 2014. Available at https://www.census.gov/prod/2014pubs/acs-26.pdf, accessed January 11, 2015.

(Humes et al. 2011a). Based on the 2010 census, the United States is projected to become a majority-minority nation for the first time in 2043, meaning that although the non-Hispanic white population will remain the single largest group, it will not be a majority, and no one group will comprise a majority. By 2060, the total non-Hispanic white population is projected to comprise 43% of the population, while all minorities together will comprise 53% of the population (Box 7.2) (United States Census Bureau 2012).

Hispanics have surpassed African Americans as the country's largest minority group. As of 2013, the Hispanic population of the United States is 54 million people, making the United States second only to Mexico in size of Hispanic population. As of 2012, 38.3 million US residents speak Spanish at home as of 2012, a 121% increase since 1990 (United States Census Bureau 2014); the United States has the fifth largest Spanish-speaking population in the world (Spanish Linguist, http://www.spanishlinguist.com/extra/spanish_speaking_countries_world_figures_and_map.html).

Asian immigration increased by 43% between 2000 and 2010, which is more than any other group. By 2050, Asians will increase from 4.8% as of 2011 to nearly 10% of the US population, 14.7 million (Centers for Disease Control and Prevention, http://www.cdc.gov/minorityhealth/populations/REMP/asian.html).

Hawaiian Native and other Pacific Islander groups, although the smallest, also grew substantially between 2000 and 2010 from 398,835 in 2000 to 540,013 in 2010 (Humes et al. 2011b).

The Pew Research Center estimates that, from 1960 to 2005, immigrants and their descendants accounted for 51% of the increase in the US population. Looking ahead, from 2005 to 2050, immigrants and their descendants are projected to contribute 82% of the total increase in the US population (Pew Research Global Attitudes Project 2014). Healthcare organizations and programs as well as federal, state, and local governments must implement systemic change in order to meet the health needs of this diverse and changing population.

Health Literacy

The Patient Protection and Affordable Care Act of 2010, Title V, defines health literacy as "the degree to which an individual has the capacity to obtain, communicate, process, and understand basic health information and services to make appropriate health decisions." Health literacy is important in making life-changing decisions, which are often made in daily activities, such as grocery shopping, filling prescriptions, and conducting self-monitoring diagnostic tests, such as blood glucose monitoring (Centers for Disease Control and Prevention, http://www.cdc.gov/healthliteracy/Learn/).

This is a broader view of literacy than just an individual's ability to read, the more traditional concept of literacy. As information and technology have increasingly shaped our society, the skills we need to function successfully have gone beyond reading, and literacy has come to include the skills cited in this definition. The Institute of Medicine (IOM) has reported that 90 million US

BOX 7.2 HISPANICS/LATINOS

According to the United States Census Bureau, Hispanics (or Latinos) are those people who classified themselves into one of the specific Spanish, Hispanic, or Latino categories (Mexican, Puerto Rican, or Cuban) in the census 2010 questionnaire, as well as those who indicate that they are "another Hispanic, Latino, or Spanish origin," such as Spain, the Spanish-speaking countries of Central or South America, or the Dominican Republic. People who identify their origin as Spanish, Hispanic, or Latino may be of any race, as origin refers to the heritage, nationality group, lineage, or country of birth.

Source: United States Census Bureau, State & County Quick Facts, Hispanic Origin. Available at http://quickfacts.census.gov/qfd/meta/long_RHI825213.htm, accessed December 10, 2014.

adults "have difficulty locating, matching, and integrating information in written texts with accuracy and consistency" (Consumer Health Informatics Research Resource, http://chirr.nlm.nih.gov /health-literacy.php).

It is essential for every individual to possess the skills to understand information and services and be able to utilize them in order to make healthy decisions. Individuals with low health literacy skills have "less knowledge of disease management and of health-promoting behaviors, report poorer health status, and are less likely to use preventive services" (Consumer Health Informatics Research Resource. Health Literacy, http://chirr.nlm.nih.gov/health-literacy.php).

Culture and language have considerable impact on how patients access and respond to healthcare service, and the level of English proficiency may impact the ability to make healthful decisions as well. Not surprisingly, people who are older or disabled, have a poor education, or come from non–English-speaking homes are more likely to have difficulties with health literacy. In 1995, the Center for Cultural and Linguistic Competency in Health Care was established within the Office of Minority Health (OMH) to serve as a resource center for healthcare professionals to help address the cultural and linguistic barriers to healthcare delivery and increase access to healthcare for people with limited English proficiency (US Department of Health and Human Services, http://minority health.hhs.gov/omh/browse.aspx?lvl=2&lvlid=34).

According to the 2000 census, half of the foreign-born population spoke English less than "very well." This percentage has remained relatively constant at 52% in 2010 and 50% in 2012. The 2012 census also reported that 21% of the foreign-born spoke English "well," 19% spoke English "not well," and 10% spoke English "not at all" (Gambino et al. 2014b).

In 2003, the National Assessment of Adult Literacy (NAAL) survey added a component on health literacy to the survey—the first-ever national assessment specifically aimed at the ability of adults to read and understand health-related information, focusing on one key aspect: the ability of adults to understand and use health-related printed information in daily activities (National Center for Education Statistics, http://nces.ed.gov/naal/fct_hlthliteracy.asp).

Of adults surveyed, 22% were found to have basic health literacy, and 14% had below basic health literacy. Relationships between health literacy and background variables (such as educational attainment, age, race/ethnicity) were also assessed. For example, adults with below basic or basic health literacy were less likely than adults with higher health literacy to get information about health issues from written sources and more likely to get a lot of information about health issues from radio and television. The survey found that white and Asian/Pacific Islander adults had the highest average health literacy and Hispanic adults had the lowest average health literacy compared to adults in other racial and ethnic groups. Adults who spoke only English before starting school had higher average health literacy than those who spoke other languages. Older adults (65+) had lower average health literacy than younger adults. On the average, health literacy increased with educational attainment (Kutner et al. 2006).

Health literacy is emerging as one of the most important cross-cutting issues to affect health service delivery and outcomes in the United States. The HHS recognizes that "culture affects how people communicate, understand and respond to health information." Recognizing that a cultural context may impact health literacy will help public health professionals to provide more effective communication, education, and services (US Department of Health and Human Services, http:// www.health.gov/communication/literacy/quickguide/factsbasic.htm#six).

Nutritionists must also recognize the implications of health literacy challenges. In 2004, the Academy of Nutrition and Dietetics (AND) identified health literacy and nutrition advancement as a public policy priority. Four years later, health and nutrition literacy was identified as a hot topic at AND's 2008 Food and Nutrition Conference and Expo in Chicago, Illinois. However, despite AND's efforts regarding health literacy and growing national interest, discussion of the relevance of diet, food, or nutrition remains lacking in health literacy literature, according to a 2012 literature review. Health literacy measures that focus specifically on nutrition-related outcomes have been developed, however, which have the potential to bolster nutrition-related health literacy research.

In particular, it is important to note that nutrition studies have found that simply equating a low-socioeconomic population to a low-health-literate population (and vice versa) without using a literacy metric can lead to false conclusions about the relationships between health literacy and nutrition outcomes (Carbone and Zoellner 2012).

One of HP 2020's goals is to use health communication strategies and health information technologies to improve health outcomes and healthcare quality, and to achieve health equity. Increasing health literacy is one of the underlying objectives aiming toward this goal. Objective HC/HIT-1 (albeit developmental) is to improve the health literacy of the population and is a new objective for HP 2020. A number of objectives under the health communication strategies and health information technologies goal emphasize skills and techniques associated with culturally competent care (HealthyPeople.gov 2015).

Age

By 2030, 20% of the population of the United States is anticipated to be aged 65 or over, a marked increase compared to 13% in 2010 and 9.8% in 1970. Furthermore, the 65-and-older population is expected to grow faster among minorities than among whites; the 65-and-older nonwhite population is projected to be 39.1% minority in 2050, up from 20.7% in 2012 (Ortman et al. 2014).

Nutrition is one of the major determinants of healthy aging through maintaining optimal physiological functions. In medicine, medical nutrition therapy (MNT) is an effective way to slow disease progression, reduce symptoms of disease, and decrease chronic disease risk. Nutritional support strategies can help maintain health through the years at the end of the life cycle. Registered dietitians (RDs) and dietetic technicians, registered (DTRs) are qualified to provide a broad array of nutritional support within medical settings, including the design of nutritional interventions that incorporate an understanding of cultural practices and environmental and lifestyle factors. Accounting for the language and age group of the target population is a key strategy to increase nutrition program effectiveness and to ensure health equity across all age and population groups.

Sexual Orientation, Gender Identity, and Gender Expression

In HP 2020, lesbian, gay, bisexual, and transgender (LGBT) health and the impact of experienced health disparities among these populations and individuals are recognized for the first time in the Healthy People agenda (The Fenway Institute, http://thefenwayinstitute.org/about/). In 2013, the Centers for Disease Control and Prevention's (CDC's) National Health Survey (NHS) included a section on sexual orientation. As a result, nationally representative data are available for the first time on lesbian, gay, and bisexual Americans. Results from the 2013 NHS survey report that 96.6% of adults identified as "straight," 1.6% identified as gay or lesbian, and .07% identified as bisexual, with the remaining 1.1% answering "something else" or "I don't know the answer," or not answering the question. Significant differences were found in health-related behaviors, health status, healthcare service utilization, and healthcare access among the groups. For the most part, this survey should be able to help track HP 2020 LGBT health objectives (Ward et al. 2014).

However, questions about gender identity and gender expression were not included in the NHS. Research estimations as to gender choices are still tentative, in part due to a lack of agreed-upon definitions and in part due to reluctance by some to answer such questions. One estimate of the transgender population in the United States comes from Gary Gates, a demographer at the Williams Institute, which studies sexual orientation and gender identity law and public policy. Lacking national estimates and extrapolating from state surveys (a 2003 California survey of LGBT tobacco use and Massachusetts surveys in 2007 and 2009), Gates estimates that about 700,000 (0.3%) of US adults are transgender (Box 7.3) (Gates 2011).

Existing research points to a higher prevalence of certain health conditions that disproportionately affect sexual and gender minorities, such as substance abuse, overweight and obesity, and tobacco. Clinicians and public health professionals need to understand the dynamics and expression

---

BOX 7.3 LGBT

GLAAD is self-described as the nation's lesbian, gay, bisexual, and transgender (LGBT) media advocacy organization. GLAAD was formed in 1985 in response to highly defamatory media coverage of AIDS. GLAAD originally stood for *Gay & Lesbian Alliance Against Defamation*, but the full name was formally dropped in 2013 in order to highlight the work inclusive of all members and allies of the LGBT community.

According to GLAAD's "An Ally's Guide to Terminology: Talking About LGBT People & Equality," *transgender* refers to people whose gender identity (the sense of gender that every person feels inside) or gender expression (how a person outwardly expresses his/her gender) is different from the sex that was assigned to them at birth.

Transgender is an adjective, not a noun. A person is not "a transgender," nor is a person "transgendered," which connotes a condition of some kind. Many transgender people do not identify themselves as transgender but, instead, simply male or female.

Always use a transgender person's chosen name. Use pronouns consistent with the person's gender identity or expression. The terms *gender identity* and *gender expression* are not interchangeable.

Transition is the appropriate, accurate term to avoid fixating on surgeries or a person's anatomy. Many transgender people do not or cannot undergo surgery. Terms like *preop* or *postop* should be avoided.

Source: GLAAD, History and Highlights, http://www.glaad.org/about/history, accessed December 14, 2014; GLAAD, Talking About Series. Available at http://www.glaad.org/sites/default/files/allys-guide-to-terminology_1 .pdf, accessed December 14, 2014.

---

of these health issues in LGBT people. To educate a new generation of clinicians, the American College of Physicians has published the first comprehensive text on the care of sexual- and gender-minority patients. In addition to studies finding a high prevalence of mental health disorders, some studies have also found more eating and body image disorders among gay and bisexual men compared with their heterosexual peers. Lesbians are more likely than women of other sexual orientations to be overweight and obese, and are at increased risk for cardiovascular disease, lipid abnormalities, glucose intolerance, and morbidity related to inactivity (Institute of Medicine 2011).

It is critical that population-based surveys and social behavioral research studies continue to expand and improve the measurement of sexual- and gender-minority identity and behavior. Furthermore, public health advocacy for policy changes and supportive programs and services will make a difference in ensuring equity for sexual- and gender-minority patients. The country's views on gender identity and sexual preference have changed dramatically since New York City's Stonewall Uprising of June 28, 1969, which is seen by many as the catalyst for the LGBT movement. As we write this on June 28, 2015, the Supreme Court just ruled that the Fourteenth Amendment (see Chapter 1) does not allow states to discriminate against same-sex couples. The central purpose of the "equal protection" clause of the Amendment is to protect minority groups that have long experienced prejudice and are unable to protect themselves in the democratic process.

CULTURAL COMPETENCY AND HEALTHCARE ORGANIZATIONS

In addition to changes in US demographics and the growing awareness of health disparities, cultural competency within healthcare has been promoted by policy and marketplace factors, such as accreditation, and a move toward patient-centered care. Techniques have been developed to assist healthcare providers in gaining cultural competency. Nutrition education materials need to address health literacy.

POLICY

At the federal level, major policy initiatives have directly addressed cultural competence in a range of rules that cover nearly every healthcare provider in the country (US Department of Health and Human Services, http://www.omhrc.gov/clas/cultural1a.htm). For example, cultural competence is necessary in order for healthcare workers and patients to effectively adhere to the 1998 Consumer Bill of Rights and Responsibilities (President's Advisory Commission 1998), which includes recommendations covering the patient's right to participate in all treatment decisions, the right to respect and nondiscrimination, and a set of responsibilities that all consumers should strive to meet (Box 7.4).

In August 2000, the Health Care Financing Administration (now the Centers for Medicare & Medicaid Services [CMS]) issued guidance regarding interpreter and translation services, emphasizing that federal matching funds are available for states to provide oral interpretation and written translation services for Medicaid beneficiaries. Shortly thereafter, in December of 2000, the HHS OMH promulgated the National Culturally and Linguistically Appropriate Services (CLAS) Standards in Health Care. These standards were updated in 2013 and (now referenced as the enhanced National CLAS Standards) include a collective set of mandates and guidelines that inform, guide, and facilitate both required and recommended culturally competence and linguistically appropriate practices. The 2013 updated standards reflect the growth in knowledge, demographic changes, and new national policies and legislation, such as the Affordable Care Act, and are standards healthcare organizations and providers should follow (US Department of Health and Human Services, http://www.omhrc.gov/omh/programs/2pgprograms/finalreport.pdf). The CMS use these standards as guidance (Box 7.5).

MARKETPLACE FACTORS

To gain a competitive edge in the marketplace, healthcare and promotion programs may leverage culturally competent policies, structures, and practices to provide services for diverse population groups. Additionally, culturally competent policies may decrease the likelihood of liability/malpractice claims, for example, by helping ensure that all treatment is conducted with appropriate informed consent. Also, healthcare organizations and programs face potential claims that their failure to

---

BOX 7.4   THE CONSUMER BILL OF RIGHTS

The 1998 Consumer Bill of Rights and Responsibilities introduced the idea that consumers should assume certain responsibilities that benefit not only individual consumers and their families but also the healthcare system and society as a whole. Some of the responsibilities are listed here:

- Taking responsibility for maximizing healthy habits, such as exercising, not smoking, and eating a healthy diet.
- Becoming involved in specific healthcare decisions.
- Working collaboratively with healthcare providers in developing and carrying out agreed-upon treatment plans.
- Disclosing relevant information and clearly communicating wants and needs.
- Recognizing the reality of risks and limits of the science of medical care and the human fallibility of healthcare professionals.
- Being aware of a healthcare provider's obligation to be reasonably efficient and equitable in providing care to other patients and the community.
- Showing respect for other patients and health workers.

BOX 7.5 THE NATIONAL CULTURALLY AND LINGUISTICALLY APPROPRIATE SERVICES (CLAS) STANDARDS

Principal standard:

- Provide effective, equitable, understandable, and respectful quality care and services that are responsive to diverse cultural health beliefs and practices, preferred languages, health literacy, and other communication needs.

Governance, leadership, and workforce:

- Advance and sustain organizational governance and leadership that promotes CLAS and health equity through policy, practices, and allocated resources.
- Recruit, promote, and support a culturally and linguistically diverse governance, leadership, and workforce that are responsive to the population in the service area.
- Educate and train governance, leadership, and workforce in culturally and linguistically appropriate policies and practices on an ongoing basis.

Communication and language assistance:

- Offer language assistance to individuals who have limited English proficiency and/or other communication needs, at no cost to them, to facilitate timely access to all healthcare and services.
- Inform all individuals of the availability of language assistance services clearly and in their preferred language, verbally and in writing.
- Ensure the competence of individuals providing language assistance, recognizing that the use of untrained individuals and/or minors as interpreters should be avoided.
- Provide easy-to-understand print and multimedia materials and signage in the languages of the populations in the service area.

Engagement, continuous improvement, and accountability:

- Establish culturally and linguistically appropriate goals, policies, and management accountability, and infuse them throughout the organizations' planning and operations.
- Conduct ongoing assessments of the organization's CLAS-related activities and integrate CLAS-related measures into assessment measurement and continuous quality improvement activities.
- Collect and maintain accurate and reliable demographic data to monitor and evaluate the impact of CLAS on health equity and outcomes and to inform service delivery.
- Conduct regular assessments of community health assets and needs and use the results to plan and implement services that respond to the cultural and linguistic diversity of populations in the service area.
- Partner with the community to design, implement, and evaluate policies, practices and services to ensure cultural and linguistic appropriateness.
- Create conflict resolution and grievance resolution processes that are culturally and linguistically appropriate to identify, prevent, and resolve conflicts or complaint.
- Communicate the organization's progress in implementing and sustaining CLAS to all stakeholders, constituents, and the general public.

Source: US Department of Health and Human Services, Public Health Service, The Office of Minority Health, National CLAS Standards. Available at http://minorityhealth.hhs.gov/omh/browse.aspx?lvl=2&lvlid=53, updated December 4, 2014, accessed December 14, 2014.

understand health beliefs, practices, and behavior on the part of providers or patients breaches professional standards of care. In some states, failure to follow instructions because they conflict with values and beliefs may raise a presumption of negligence on the part of the provider.

Accreditation

Watchdog and accrediting organizations have certain minimum requirements regarding cultural competence. For example, the Joint Commission (2014), an independent, not-for-profit organization that accredits and certifies more than 20,500 healthcare organizations and programs in the United States, views the delivery of services in a culturally and linguistically appropriate manner as an important healthcare safety and quality issue Accredited organizations are encouraged to provide equitable care, treatment, and services across diverse populations.

PATIENT-CENTERED CARE

Patient-centered care is a change in focus from disease and its treatments to the patient's engagement in the process with shared decision making. Patient-centered care is achieved by a consistent healthcare team approach that emphasizes effective communication, common language, and the consideration of the best interest of the patient and his or her family.

All individuals have the right and responsibility to fully participate in all decisions related to their healthcare. Those who are unable to fully participate in treatment decisions have the right to be represented by parents, guardians, family members, or other conservators. To ensure the right and ability to participate in treatment decisions, healthcare professionals should provide patients with easily understood information and the opportunity to decide among treatment options consistent with the informed-consent process. Specifically, healthcare professionals should discuss all treatment options with a patient in a culturally competent manner, including the option of no treatment at all; discuss all current treatments a consumer may be undergoing, including those alternative treatments that are self-administered, and discuss all risks, benefits, and consequences to treatment or nontreatment.

All people have the right to considerate, respectful care from all members of the healthcare system at all times and under all circumstances, and must not be discriminated against in the delivery of healthcare services consistent with the benefits covered in their policy or as required by law based on race, ethnicity, national origin, religion, sex, age, mental or physical disability, sexual orientation, genetic information, or source of payment.

Accordingly, it is critical that healthcare providers recognize individual differences and do not participate in *cultural stereotyping*. Because persons of the same cultural group can have very different beliefs and practices, it is important to understand the particular circumstances of the patient or family by obtaining information on place of origin, social and economic background, religion, degree of acculturation, and, most importantly, personal expectations concerning health and medical care.

In sum, although increasing factual knowledge about general cultural beliefs and behaviors is a starting point, effective patient-centered care is really best fully implemented through increasing capacity in skills that can be universally applied, such as communication; medical history-taking techniques that focus on inquiry, reflection, and analysis; and reinforcing attitudes of curiosity, empathy, respect, and humility (Georgetown University 2004). Nutritional professionals and other healthcare providers can use these universally applicable skills to address healthcare biases associated with individual attributes, such as gender orientation or body shape and size (Box 7.6).

The application of patient-centered care and integrating clinical ethics into nutrition practice adds another dimension into healthcare practice. For a nutritionist, patient-centered care requires acquiring the knowledge of religion/spirituality and cultural diversity in order to improve the culture of care and empowerment of the patient and his or her family in the process of healthcare decisions, including those of nutritional support. The ways in which people deal with issues of serious

BOX 7.6   NATIONAL ASSOCIATION TO ADVANCE FAT ACCEPTANCE

Founded in 1969, the National Association to Advance Fat Acceptance (NAAFA) is a human rights organization with the mission of ending size discrimination in all of its forms and supports the concept of Health at Every Size (HAES). NAAFA encourages healthcare organizations to adopt an HAES policy and to include HAES in patients' rights policies (United States Census Bureau 2012). HAES emphasizes overall well-being, instead of focusing on weight as a measurement of health. The general principles of HAES are

- Accepting and respecting the diversity of body shapes and sizes.
- Recognizing that health and well-being are multidimensional and that they include physical, social, spiritual, occupational, emotional, and intellectual aspects.
- Promoting all aspects of health and well-being for people of all sizes.
- Promoting eating in a manner that balances individual nutritional needs, hunger, satiety, appetite, and pleasure.
- Promoting individually appropriate, enjoyable, life-enhancing physical activity, rather than exercise that is focused on a goal of weight loss.

Source: The National Association to Advance Fat Acceptance. Available at http://www.naafaonline.com/dev2/about/index.html, accessed February 9, 2015; The National Association to Advance Fat Acceptance. Available at http://www.naafaonline.com/dev2/education/haes.html, accessed February 9, 2015.

illness are often influenced by their religion/spirituality and culture. Nutritional support is a life-sustaining treatment, and nutrition-support clinicians should be aware of an individual's religion/spirituality and culture, and understand how this context may impact an individual's decisions about health issues. It is important to understand that patients cannot be relegated to a mere diagnosis as they are made up of lifetime events, unique perspective, and distinctive background reflective of family relationships, friends, culture, religion/spirituality, work/profession, and knowledge (Schwartz 2013).

TECHNIQUES AND STRATEGIES FOR ACHIEVING CULTURAL COMPETENCE

To ensure equal access to quality healthcare by diverse populations, Brach and Fraser (2000) identified nine major techniques for achieving cultural competence. The techniques encompass interpreter services, recruitment and retention policies, training, coordination with traditional healers, use of community health workers, culturally competent health promotion (including family/another culture), and administrative and organizational accommodations.

A seminal article by Harris-Davis and Haughton (2000) describes how nutritionists play a role in developing the dietary component of cultural competency training for nonnutritionist staff members. To do this, nutrition professionals should be aware of relevant cultural food and nutrition practices. The overall goal is to use this information to ask questions about "where the client is at" to help inform any needed changes. According to Harris-Davis and Haughton, the nutritionist with multicultural food and nutrition counseling knowledge should (Harris-Davis and Haughton 2000)

- Understand food selection, preparation, and storage within a cultural context.
- Have knowledge of cultural eating patterns and family traditions such as core foods, traditional celebrations, and fasting.
- Become familiar with relevant research and the latest findings regarding food practices and nutrition-related health problems of various ethnic and racial groups.

- Possess specific knowledge of cultural values, health beliefs, and nutrition practices of particular groups served, including culturally different clients.
- Have knowledge about within-group differences and understanding of variations in food practices.
- Apply helping principle of "starting where the client is" by considering changes in eating patterns, such as the addition of American foods or substitution of foods.

An important first step is to be sensitive to patients' cultural beliefs and practices and to convey respect for their cultural values. This may require requesting for help in interpreting behavior, either from a provider who is from the same ethnic group as the patient or from an expert familiar with the group's language, lifestyle, and value preferences. A model for self-assessment of multicultural nutrition counseling competencies may focus on multicultural nutrition counseling skills, multicultural awareness, and knowledge of foods from other cultures (Box 7.7).

The culturally sensitive healthcare provider should also consider these additional suggestions regarding etiquette and communication (Box 7.8):

- Speak slower than usual but not louder.
- Ask questions to increase understanding of the patient's culture as it relates to healthcare practices. For example, ask what types of foods and medicines are administered or avoided

---

BOX 7.7   MULTICULTURAL NUTRITION COUNSELING SKILLS

- Be able to differentiate between individual and universal similarities.
- Be experienced in application of medical nutrition therapy and nutrition-related health promotion/disease prevention strategies that are culturally appropriate.
- Have the ability to use cultural knowledge and sensitivity for appropriate nutrition intervention and materials.
- Take responsibility for collectively working with community leaders or members about unique knowledge or abilities for the benefit of the culturally different client.
- Be able to evaluate new techniques, research, and knowledge as to validity and applicability in working with culturally different populations.

Multicultural awareness

- Be aware of how one's own cultural background and experiences and attitudes, values, and biases influence nutrition counseling.
- Be able to recognize the limits of one's own cultural competencies and abilities.
- Be aware and sensitive to one's own cultural heritage and to valuing and respecting differences.

Multicultural food and nutrition counseling knowledge

- Understand food selection, preparation, and storage with a cultural context.
- Have knowledge of cultural eating patterns and family traditions such as core foods, traditional celebrations, and fasting.
- Familiarize oneself with relevant research and the latest findings regarding food practices and nutrition-related health problems of various ethnic and racial groups.

Source: Reprinted from Harris-Davis, E. and Haughton, B., *J. Am. Diet. Assn.*, 100, 2000. With permission from The American Dietetic Association.

**BOX 7.8   SUGGESTED SCRIPT FOR INTERVIEWING
A CULTURALLY DIVERSE FAMILY**

Be aware of and respect their cultural beliefs:

- Please tell me what languages are spoken in your home and the languages that you understand and speak.
- Please describe your usual diet.
  - Are there certain foods or food combinations that your culture prohibits?
  - Are there times during the year when you change your diet in celebration of religious and other ethnic holidays?
- Are there any other dietary considerations I should know about to serve your health needs?
- Please tell me about your experiences with healthcare providers in your native country. How often each year did you see a healthcare provider before you arrived in the United States? Have you noticed any differences between the type of care you received in your native country and the type you receive here? If yes, could you tell me about those differences?
- Do you use any traditional remedies to improve your health?

Encourage two-way communication:

- Please tell me about beliefs and practices including special events such as birth, marriage, and death that you feel I should know.
- Please tell me if there is anything else I should know. Do you have any questions for me?
- Is there someone, in addition to yourself, with whom you want us to discuss your medical condition?

Source: University of Michigan, Cultural Competence for Clinicians, Enhancing Your Cultural Communication Skills. Available at http://www.med.umich.edu/pteducation/cultcomp.htm, accessed January 20, 2015.

under particular illness conditions or during physiological changes, such as those due to pregnancy. Then ask, "If these are the rules, do you follow them? Why?" Make it clear to your respondents that "no" is a perfectly acceptable response (Pelto et al. 1989).

- Use drawings, models, and gestures to aid communication.
- Use empty packages of food to illustrate.
- Clearly communicate expectations.
- To ascertain understanding, ask the patient to repeat the information provided.
- Where appropriate, formulate treatment plans that take into account cultural beliefs and practices.
- Provide written instructions. Use handouts, if available. Be sure that all written materials are at the appropriate literacy level.

LOW-LITERACY NUTRITION EDUCATION MATERIALS

Until health literacy goals have been accomplished, public and private organizations need to develop appropriate written materials. Nutritionists have access to numerous existing materials, as well as resources providing training about how to create effective, culturally and linguistically appropriate, plain-language health communications.

The National Cancer Institute (NCI) suggests a five-step process for developing publications for people with limited literacy skills: (1) define the target audience, (2) conduct target audience research, (3) develop a concept for the product, (4) develop content and visuals, and (5) pretest and revise draft materials (National Cancer Institute 1994).

Target Audience

The target audience is the group of people the communicator wants to reach with a message. People with limited literacy skills compose a broad target audience, crossing all ethnic and class boundaries. However, there are some common characteristics among low-literate audiences regarding how they interpret and process information:

- Tendency to think in concrete/immediate rather than abstract/futuristic terms.
- Literal interpretation of information.
- Insufficient language fluency to comprehend and apply information from written materials.
- Difficulty with information processing, such as reading a menu, interpreting a bus schedule, following medical instructions, or reading a prescription label.

Conduct Target Audience Research

Learn about the target audience. Look for information on

- Age, sex, ethnicity, income and education levels, places of work, and residence.
- Causative/preventive behaviors related to your topic.
- Related knowledge, attitudes, and practices.
- Patterns of use of related services.
- Cultural habits, preferences, and sensitivities related to your topic.
- Barriers to behavior change.
- Effective motivators (e.g., benefits of change, fear of consequences, incentives, or social support).

Develop a Concept for the Product
- Define the behavioral objective(s) of the material.
- Determine the key information points the reader needs to achieve the behavioral objective(s).
- Select the most appropriate presentation method(s).
- Decide on the reading level for the material if you select a print presentation.
- Organize topics in the order the person will use them.

Develop Content and Visuals

At the end of this step, perform a readability analysis to determine reading level.

Style and Content
- The material is interactive and allows for audience involvement.
- The material presents how-to information.
- Peer language is used whenever appropriate to increase personal identification and improve readability.
- Words are familiar to the audience. Any new words are defined clearly.
- Sentences are simple, specific, direct, and written in the active voice.
- Each idea is clear and logically sequenced (according to audience logic).
- The number of concepts is limited per piece.
- The material uses concrete examples rather than abstract concepts.
- The text highlights and summarizes important points.

Visuals and Layout
- The material uses advance organizers or headers.
- Headers are simple and close to text.
- Layout balances white space with words and illustrations.
- Text uses uppercase and lowercase letters.
- Underlining or bolding rather than all capitals gives emphasis.
- Type style and size of print are easy to read; type is at least 12 point.
- Visuals are relevant to the text, meaningful to the audience, and appropriately located.
- Illustrations and photographs are simple and free from clutter and distraction.
- Visuals use adult rather than childlike images.
- Illustrations show familiar images that reflect cultural context.
- Visuals have captions. Each visual illustrates and is directly related to one message.
- Different styles, such as photographs without background detail, shaded line drawings, or simple line drawings, are pretested with the audience to determine which is understood best.
- Cues, such as circles or arrows, point out key information. Colors used are appealing to the audience (as determined by pretesting).

Pretest and Revise Draft Materials

Pretesting is a qualitative measure of audience response to a product. Pretesting helps ensure that materials are well understood, responsive to audience needs and concerns, and culturally sensitive. Pretest for comprehension, attraction, and acceptability.

Comprehension
- Does the respondent understand what the material is recommending and how and when to do it? Is anything unclear, confusing, or hard to believe?
- Suitability of the words used: "What does this mean when it says to eat balanced meals? How do you do that?"
- Distinguishing key details: "Which vegetables have lots of fiber?"
- Meaning or relationship of visuals to text: "Looking at this picture, how will you cut down on fat in your soups or stocks when cooking?"

Attraction
- What kind of feelings does the material generate? Enthusiasm, just OK, or a "turnoff"?
- Questions you may ask: "Are the people in the material attractive to you? Is there anything you don't like about the people (or pictures) in this material? How about the color and the layout of the material?"

Acceptability
- Is the material compatible with the target audience? Is it realistic? Would it offend people in any way? Are the hairstyles, clothing, etc., appropriate? Is it supportive of ethnic practices? Does it invoke personal involvement?
- Questions you may ask: "Can you see yourself carrying out the actions called for in the materials? Do you think your friends and neighbors would be willing to cook their foods this way?"

FOODWAYS OF SOME ETHNIC/RACIAL GROUPS IN THE UNITED STATES

This section contains generalizations about ethnic and cultural food practices of some ethnic/racial groups in the United States. Unless otherwise indicated, the information is based on information gathered by the Ohio State University Extension Department (OSU). OSU developed a series of fact sheets developed to address cultural diversity in American eating and stresses that the fact sheets are designed as an awareness tool for a novice working with a cultural group previously unknown to him or her. The goal is to assist novice educators in addressing any cultural barriers that may impact educational effectiveness (Ohio State University, http://ohioline.osu.edu/lines/food.html#FOODF).

It is important not to assume that the characteristics cited here apply to all individuals of a single cultural group. Not all people of a particular group have the same quality of diets, level of concern about their health, or understanding about the relationship of diet to health, or practice the same cooking techniques. Other variations exist in cultural groups, such as socio-economic status, religion, age, education, length of time in the United States, and location of origin; thus, caution needs to be taken not to generalize or imply that these characteristics apply to all individuals.

Additional research into specific cultural groups and assessment of individuals you may work with is not only recommended but also necessary. In particular, for nutrition educators working with women and children, asking about both traditional and individual practices of maternal nutrition while pregnant and child breastfeeding and weaning practices (and reasons behind such practices) is essential.

AFRICAN AMERICANS

More than 35 million Americans claim African ancestry. Unlike other immigrants to the United States prior to the 1860s, most Africans came to North America against their will. The centuries-long battle African Americans waged for freedom, dignity, and full participation in American society utterly transformed and shaped the nation. The present-day African American population, like many other ethnic groups, is several generations removed from their original land and culture. Thus, many practices and habits have been lost, dropped, simulated, or modified. For many among this population group of African American families, the greatest influence is the lifestyle of their parents or grandparents who lived in the southern United States.

The popular term for African American cooking with southern roots is *soul food.* Many soul food dishes are rich in nutrients, as found in collard greens and other leafy green and yellow vegetables, legumes, beans, rice, and potatoes. Other parts of the diet, however, are low in fiber, calcium, and potassium, and high in fat; food preparation traditionally emphasizes frying, barbecuing, and serving foods with gravy and sauces.

However, immigration to the United States also includes more recent, voluntary migration, from Africa, the Caribbean, and the West Indies. Some describe a difference between the population groups as "black Americans versus African immigrants." The foodways of voluntary, more recent African immigrants will naturally reflect closer connections to homeland and culture, with variations in tastes and content. An Ethiopian vegetable stew is often served with a sour-raised spongy flatbread known as *injera,* whereas a Ghanese stew would likely be served atop rice or yams.

The US Census Bureau defines blacks or African Americans as people having origins in any of the black racial groups of Africa. When the census reports statistics regarding the black or African American population, it includes people who marked their race(s) as "Black, African Am., or Negro" or who reported entries such as African American; Sub-Saharan African (e.g., Kenyan and Nigerian); or Afro-Caribbean, such as Haitian and Jamaican. As of 2012, the population of African Americans including those of more than one race was estimated at 44.5 million, making up 14.2% of the total US population, and those who identified only as African American made up 13.1% of the US population—over 39 million people. By 2060, the African American population (including those of more than one race) is projected to be 77.4 million people, making up 18.4% of the total US population (Centers for Disease Control and Prevention 2014).

As of 2010, the top four leading causes of death for African Americans are heart disease, cancer, stroke, and diabetes. Health disparities are rampant. In 2009, African Americans had the largest death rates from heart disease and stroke compared with other racial and ethnic populations; obesity prevalence among African American adults was the largest compared to other race ethnicity groups from 2007 to 2010, and as of 2010, the prevalence of diabetes among African American adults was nearly twice as large as that for white adults. Infants of African American women in 2008 had the largest death rate, which was more than twice as large as infants of white women. African Americans had the largest incidence and death rates from colorectal cancer in 2008 of all racial and ethnic populations despite similar colorectal screening rates in white adults.

Nutrients of interest for the African American population include vitamin D, as the CDC reports that non-Hispanic blacks (31%) were more likely to be vitamin D deficient compared to non-Hispanic whites (3%), yet conversely, clinical data show that non-Hispanic blacks have better bone health—greater bone density and fewer fractures—than other races/ethnic groups (Centers for Disease Control and Prevention 2012).

Milk with added vitamin D provides a convenient source of the vitamin, but many African Americans may be lactose intolerant (US National Library of Medicine, http://ghr.nlm.nih.gov /condition/lactose-intolerance).

Lactose intolerance is due to the gradually decreasing activity (expression) of the *LCT* gene after infancy. Adults who can still digest lactose are considered lactase persistent (Wiley 2004). Fortified nondairy alternatives may be good options for increasing vitamin D intake for lactose-intolerant individuals. The rate of calcium absorption from fortified soy beverages is lower than the rate of calcium absorption from cow's milk; thus, soy beverages are often fortified with extra calcium. One cup of soy milk fortified to 500 mg of calcium yields approximately the same amount of absorbable calcium as does one cup of cow's milk (Zhao et al. 2005).

Many African Americans are Protestant and have no specific food restrictions. However, many may be members of religious groups that may have some restrictions or dietary preference such as Seventh-day Adventists or Jehovah's Witnesses, or may be Jewish or Muslim.

Taboos about child rearing and nursing more likely may be present if older grandparents are heads of households. Although as of 2012, the rate of teenage pregnancy is continuing to decline in general, the rate of teenage pregnancy is still higher in African Americans, with 43.9 births per 1000 females aged 15–19 years (compared with 20.5 for whites) (Centers for Disease Control and Prevention 2014).

Besides the formal and traditional American occasions and holidays, a large number of African Americans observe and celebrate Kwanzaa, an African American cultural holiday born out of the whirlwind of social and political changes of the 1960s, an era rich in expressions of freedom and self-identity. Kwanzaa was created in 1966 by Maulana Karenga, PhD (chairperson from 1991 to 2002 (Clark 2002) of the Department of Black Studies at California State University in Long Beach), to provide an opportunity for the African American community to celebrate their heritage and reinforce positive community values through the principles of unity, self-determination, collective work and responsibility, cooperative economics, purpose, creativity, and faith (The Official Kwanzaa Web site, http://www.officialkwanzaawebsite.org/index.html).

Kwanzaa is observed for 7 days, starting December 26; December 31 is celebrated with ceremonies, a buffet, and festive attire.

Teaching Implications

Nutrition educators should focus on the methods of food preparation, encouraging families to explore modifying the sodium, fat, and sugar content of traditional foods and using herbs and spices to replace high-sodium seasonings or high-fat meat such as fatback and ham hocks when cooking dandelion, turnip, and collard greens. Greens that take less time to cook (and thus also may require less fat to prepare), such as Swiss chard, might be of interest. As noted above, sampling alternatives for dairy beverages may also be of interest. Recommendations that are generally applicable to improving the typical diet of any American are also appropriate, such as substituting fresh fruits for fruit drinks and fruit juice, increasing the amount of fresh vegetables consumed and decreasing the amount of meat consumed, removing the fat and skin from meat, and eating less of high-fat processed meat products such as bologna and sausage (Burke and Raia 1995).

HISPANICS

According to the 2010 census, 50.5 million (16%) people residing in the United States were of Hispanic (or Latino) origin. Among US residents, 31.8 million were of Mexican origin, by far the largest group, comprising 63% of the total Hispanic population. The next largest group (4.6 million) was those of Puerto Rican origin, comprising 9% of the total Hispanic population. Although the census adds the next largest group, those of Cuban origin, to the Mexican and Puerto Rican group to describe the total as "about three-quarters of the Hispanic population in the United States," the Cuban group is just 1.8 million, and the next largest group, Salvadoran, is not much farther behind at 1.6 million (Ennis et al. 2011).

The US Census Bureau created and tested the term *Hispanic* in 1970 for use as an ethnic category based on "Spanish origin or descent"; the term does not denote race or color. The term became officially used in 1973 by the Department of Health, Education, and Welfare (HEW); the Office of Education, for data-gathering purposes; and the US census from 1980 to date (Ennis et al. 2011). The term *Hispanic* encompasses Mexican, Puerto Rican, Central American, South American, Caribbean, and Spanish peoples who share some common cultural values. Hispanics may be of any race, may have a multicultural ethnic identity, and may not speak Spanish. The term *Latino* may be preferred over the term *Hispanic* by many members of this population (US Census Bureau, http://www.census.gov/eeo/special_emphasis_programs/hispanic_heritage.html).

The diversity among this population is extensive due to differing patterns of Spanish settlement, interactions with indigenous populations, and slaves brought from Africa. Mexico, Puerto Rico, and other Latin American countries have hundreds of years of separate history, as well as entirely different native populations present when the Spaniards arrived. Such diversity also brings variations in food composition, names, recipes and traditions even among similar foods and diet patterns. For example, individuals in some, but not all, Hispanic cultures may have a "hot–cold" classification of foods, which may be determined through characteristics of the foods such as method of preparation, rather than temperature. Balancing a meal between hot and cold ingredients is considered to be health promoting, and the treatment for diseases considered to have one classification (i.e., hot) may include meals emphasizing the other classification (i.e., cold). Although the number of individuals who practice such hot–cold dietary balancing may be small, one study has reported that Latinos in general are more likely than non-Latinos to consider certain foods as herbal medicines (Kittler et al. 2012).

Studies of the impact of acculturation and length of residence in the United States report that Hispanics residing in the United States for a longer time tend to have macronutrient profiles more similar to those of non-Hispanic whites. More acculturated Hispanics consume fewer ethnic foods and more foods related to the non-Hispanic white eating patterns than those less acculturated (Bermúdez et al. 2000).

The following section examines some Hispanic subpopulation groups in more detail: Mexican Americans, Puerto Ricans, Cuban Americans, and Dominican Americans.

MEXICAN AMERICANS

Millions of people in the United States today identify themselves as Mexican immigrants or Mexican Americans. It is important to realize that the Mexican American population of the United States has some of the oldest inhabitants of the nation, as some Mexicans were already living in the southern and western regions of the North American continent centuries before the United States existed. Mexican immigrants and their descendants now make up a significant portion of the US population, particularly in California, Texas, Arizona, New Mexico, and Colorado.

The cultural inheritance of Mexican Americans is rich and complex, reflecting the influences of Spain, Mexico, indigenous cultures, and years of survival and adaptation. Immigration law and public opinion on Mexican immigration has swung back and forth throughout the nation's history, at times welcoming immigrants and at other times slamming the door shut on them (Library of Congress, http://www.loc.gov/teachers/classroommaterials/presentationsandactivities /presentations/immigration/mexican.html), this tension most recently visible in arguments over President Obama's Deferred Action for Childhood Arrivals (DACA) program, which was announced in June 2012, and President Obama's executive actions regarding immigration in late 2014.

The family unit is the single most important social unit in the life of Hispanics. Family responsibilities come before all others. Gender differentiation and male dominance are issues to consider while working with Hispanic families. Traditionally, the father is the leader of the family, and the mother runs the household and shops and prepares the food. If the family is religious, it is important to acknowledge such beliefs, as the church community may play a significant role in daily family life. A majority of Mexicans are Roman Catholic, but Evangelical Protestantism is a fast-growing religion, especially among immigrants.

The Mexican diet of today is rich in a variety of foods and dishes that represent a blend of pre-Columbian, Spanish, French, and, more recently, American culture. The typical Mexican diet is rich in complex carbohydrates, provided mainly by corn (including tortillas), beans, rice, and breads, and contains an adequate amount of protein in the forms of beans, eggs, fish and shellfish, and a variety of meats. Traditional cooking methods emphasize frying and the use of lard.

The daily meal pattern in the typical Mexican American home varies according to the availability of traditional foods and the degree of assimilation into American society.

With emigration to the United States, major changes occur in the diet of many Mexican Americans. A 2011 study reported that Mexican American families often acculturate completely within one generation in the United States. One marked change observed was a significantly lower consumption of corn tortillas. Additionally, the number of Mexicans who drink fruit juice nearly triples when Mexicans migrate to the United States, and consumption of sugar-sweetened sodas nearly doubles. Saturated fat intake also increases, along with typical American dishes such as salty snacks, pizza, and French fries. Conversely, healthy changes include a higher intake of lower-fat milk, meat and fish, and high-fiber bread. An increase in vegetable consumption postmigration has been observed, perhaps due to the adoption of American-style salads and vegetable side dishes as compared to traditional Mexican dishes, in which vegetables are mainly used as pickled condiments or ingredients in soup, rice, pasta, or meat entrée preparation. The study authors acknowledge that the dietary intake reference for the Mexican diet is based on the most recently available Mexican national dietary intake information, which was gathered in 1999, and recognize this weakness. As any culture's typical diet will change over time due to external social and environmental influences, the typical level of corn tortilla consumption in the Mexican diet may be less remarkably different today from the level of corn tortilla consumption by Mexican Americans (Batis et al. 2011).

Nutrients of concern for the Mexican American population include vitamin D and iron. According to a 2012 report from the CDC and data from National Health and Nutrition Examination Survey (NHANES) 2003–2006 reports, Mexican Americans (12%) were more likely to be vitamin D deficient compared to non-Hispanic whites (3%), and the prevalence of iron deficiency, as based on a low-body-iron (<0 mg/kg) analysis method, was higher in Mexican American children compared to non-Hispanic black and non-Hispanic white children, and was also higher in Mexican American and non-Hispanic black women aged 12–49 years compared to non-Hispanic white women (Centers for Disease Control and Prevention 2012).

Teaching Implications

Healthcare providers need to understand Hispanic culture, beliefs, norms, food practices, and terminology to best assist clients. Providers need to (1) support and stimulate the preservation of healthy cultural food practices among Mexican American clientele; (2) when appropriate, suggest modifications of traditional dishes that are high in sodium, fat, and sugar; (3) increase clients' knowledge of healthy food selections from typical American fare, and (4) gain support from clients' families to enhance their acceptance of the diet.

The diets of pregnant Mexican American women of marginal social and economic standing are deficient in dietary iron, vitamin A, and calcium. Providers should encourage the consumption of low-fat cheeses, lean red meat, fresh fruits, and vegetables, as well as monitor beverage intake, since carbonated soft drinks and presweetened drinks are widely consumed.

Efforts to promote better diets among the Hispanic elderly need to focus on maintenance or adoption of healthful dietary patterns based on ethnic and modern foods that will satisfy the biological, emotional, and social needs of the diverse Hispanic groups in the United States. Continuing efforts to teach diverse groups of older adults about meeting current recommendations for macronutrient intake should consider the effects of acculturation and how migration factors may positively influence the use of certain foods and, perhaps, negatively affect others (Bermudez et al. 2000).

The healthcare provider may intervene with Hispanic clients and communities in culturally sensitive ways, which includes viewing culture as an enabler rather than a resistant force. For example, incorporating cultural beliefs into the plans of care may include respecting the culture of familialism (prioritizing the needs of the family as a unit, rather than as individuals) and taking time for pleasant conversation.

PUERTO RICANS

Puerto Rico has been a possession of the United States since 1898 but has never been a state. Its people have been US citizens since 1917, but they have no vote in Congress. As citizens, the people of Puerto Rico can move throughout the 50 states just as any other American can. This is considered internal migration, not immigration. However, in moving to the mainland, Puerto Ricans leave a homeland with its own distinct identity and culture, and the transition has involved many of the same cultural conflicts and emotional adjustments that most immigrants face. For example, Puerto Ricans of African heritage may find greater overt discrimination in the United States than experienced in the homeland (Kittler et al. 2012).

At first, only very few Puerto Ricans came to the continental United States. Although the United States tried to promote Puerto Rico as a glamorous tourist destination, in the early twentieth century the island suffered a severe economic depression. Poverty was rife, and few of the island's residents could afford the long boat journey to the mainland. In 1910, there were fewer than 2000 Puerto Ricans in the continental United States, mostly in small enclaves in New York City. By the 1930s, there were only 40,000 more. After the end of World War II, however, Puerto Rican migration exploded. Although there were 13,000 Puerto Ricans in New York City in 1945, by 1946, there were more than 50,000. Over the next decade, more than 25,000 Puerto Ricans would come to the continental United States each year, peaking in 1953, when more than 69,000 arrived. By 1955, nearly 700,000 Puerto Ricans had migrated to the United States, and by the mid-1960s, more than a million had. There were a number of reasons for this sudden influx. The continuing depression in Puerto Rico made many Puerto Ricans eager for a fresh start, and US factory owners and employment agencies had begun recruiting heavily on the island. In addition, the postwar years saw the return home of thousands of Puerto Rican war veterans, whose service in the US military had shown them the world. But perhaps the most significant cause was the sudden availability of affordable air travel. After centuries of immigration by boat, the Puerto Rican migration became the first great airborne migration in US history (Library of Congress 2004). As of 2012, close to 5 million residents from Puerto Rico make up just over 9% of the total Hispanic population of the United States (Pew Research Center 2012).

Most of the food available on the island is imported from the United States, and common American foods—pizza, hot dogs, canned soups—are also common Puerto Rican foods. As Puerto

Ricans are American citizens, and migration is fluid and circular, the food culture of Puerto Ricans living on the mainland is similar to those of their relatives on the island. Typically, a light breakfast of strong coffee (with milk) and bread may be followed by a light lunch of rice and beans (*arroz con gandules*) or a starchy vegetable such as potatoes or plantains with or without dried salt cod (*bacalao*). Americanized Puerto Ricans may substitute a sandwich and soft drink for the more traditional noonday meal. A late-day dinner may consist of foods from the more traditional lunch. Salad consumption is erratic; snacking on low-nutrient-density foods is common (Kittler and Sucher 2004). Generally, increasing calcium intake and varieties of vegetables may be helpful dietary adjustments.

Heart disease and diabetes mellitus (nutrition-related chronic diseases) are two of the three leading causes of mortality in Puerto Rico. Earlier reports indicated that Puerto Rican Americans had the highest death rates from hypertension-related mortality among Hispanic subpopulations, perhaps from the greater prevalence of classic risk factors (diabetes mellitus, obesity, physical inactivity) (Centers for Disease Control and Prevention 2006), but the death rate from heart disease has declined in the last decade. Overweight and obesity are also of concern for the population (Departmento De Salud 2012).

A 2010 longitudinal cohort study on Puerto Ricans living in Boston supports observations that Puerto Ricans in the United States experience considerable health disparities. Some of these health disparities exceed those reported in other Hispanic subgroups, including Mexican Americans. The cohort study found a higher prevalence of physical and cognitive disability, type 2 diabetes, obesity, depressive symptomatology, hypertension, and self-reported heart disease compared to published reports for similarly aged Mexican Americans, and of even more concern, the high prevalence of these conditions was observed even for those in the younger age category (Tucker et al. 2010).

The Puerto Rican culture places an emphasis on families; women are usually the decision makers and purchasers of food and preparation, and meals are traditionally family events.

Teaching Implications

Nutrition education that challenges cultural beliefs that complications of diabetes are unavoidable may be critical for this population (Kittler et al. 2012). Teachers may benefit from involving trusting older female members of the community and engaging learners on a personal level. Even if extensive one-to-one engagement is not feasible, individual contact can be made in a manner such as handing papers to each person rather than passing the papers down the row. As Puerto Ricans typically like to touch and feel close (both physically and emotionally) to those around them, you may also be asked personal questions.

Due to the high prevalence of obesity and overweight in the population, nutritional education should involve methods of maintaining an ideal body weight; encouraging low-fat dairy products, unsweetened fruit juices and beverages, and creative food preparation that uses less fat and oil would all be helpful to this end. Ethnic heritage and identity may be strongly maintained (Kittler et al. 2012); thus, asking about how foods contribute to ethnic identity may be helpful. If adapting the preparation of cultural recipes is challenging, the introduction of specific healthy food alternatives for consumption outside of particularly meaningful dishes may be helpful. And, as with any American diet, encouraging the consumption of a variety of vegetables and discouraging sugar use would also be helpful.

Cuban Americans

Cuban immigration occurred in very distinct waves, creating differing populations of Cuban Americans. At the beginning of the twentieth century, between 50,000 and 100,000 Cubans moved between Havana and Florida every year, following the sugar, coffee, and tobacco industries. At this time, some Cubans were already arriving as political refugees, and in the 1950s, the ranks of refugees swelled under the regime of Fulgenico Batista. The subsequent 1959 Cuban Revolution and the transformation of Cuba economically and politically created a new impetus for people to leave—now the refugees were the wealthiest elite and members of Batista's regime. The first wave of migrants numbered over 200,000, until air flights were suspended between the countries in 1962. When a few air flights were allowed between 1965 and 1973, another 300,000 flew out. Not only were these migrants typically white Cubans of higher socioeconomic background; they also were perceived as refugees from a dictatorial regime and thus welcomed with offers of assistance and, by a 1966 act of Congress, permanent residency for those who lived in the United States for a year. The next wave of immigrants was of a much different composition. In 1980, the Cuban government opened a port city for those Cubans who wanted to leave, and in response, Cuban Americans organized a flotilla of private yachts, commercial ships, and boats to ferry Cubans to the United States. More than 125,000 migrants left during the 6 months the port was open; however, this wave was far less affluent than the first migrants, and as a few thousand had been in prison in Cuba, they were less warmly received. After this, Cubans took to the seas to cross the 90 mi. at their own peril, many in homemade rafts. Hundreds died during these journeys, and by the end of the 1990s, the countries reached an agreement that the United States would return boats to Cuba (Library of Congress, http://www.loc.gov/teachers/classroommaterials/presentationsandactivities/presentations /immigration/cuban5.html). On December 17, 2014, President Obama announced a change in policies toward normalizing relations with Cuba; the effect of this on migration remains to be seen (The White House 2014).

Cuban cuisine has been influenced by Spanish, French, African, Arabic, Chinese, and Portuguese cultures (University of Miami, http://www.education.miami.edu/ep/littlehavana/Cuban_Food/Cuban _Cuisine/cuban_cuisine.html).

Mainstays of the Cuban diet are bananas and other tropical fruits, rice and black beans (*moros y cristianos*), pork, fried plantains, and strong, sweet coffee. Traditional Cuban cooking is primarily peasant cuisine that has little concern with measurements, order, and timing. Most of the food is sautéed or slow-cooked over a low flame. Very little is deep-fried, and there are no heavy or creamy sauces.

Most Cuban cooking relies on a few basic spices, such as garlic, cumin, oregano, and bay laurel leaves. Many dishes use a *sofrito* as their basis. The sofrito consists of onion, green pepper, garlic, oregano, and ground pepper quick-fried in olive oil. The sofrito, which gives the food its flavor, is used when cooking black beans, stews, many meat dishes, and tomato-based sauces. Meats and poultry are usually marinated in citrus juices, such as lime or sour orange juices, and then roasted over low heat until the meat is tender and literally falling off the bone. Another common staple of the Cuban diet is root vegetables such as *yucca*, *malanga*, and *boniato*, which are found in most Latin markets. These vegetables are flavored with a marinade, called *mojo*, which includes hot olive oil, lemon juice, sliced raw onions, garlic, cumin, and a little water.

A 1995 study comparing the diet of Mexican Americans, Puerto Ricans, and Cuban Americans noted the distinguishing characteristics of the Cuban American population at the time as being older and having attained higher levels of education and economic status than Mexican Americans and the mainland Puerto Rican population. The study also found differences in macronutrient intakes amongst these populations and concluded that dietary research, recommendations, and interventions should be targeted individually to each group (Loria et al. 1995).

However, updated general information on Cuban American diet and health concerns is difficult to find, as Cuban Americans are the least studied of the three largest Hispanic subgroups (Exebio et al. 2011), perhaps in part because of the demographic changes in the population due to the various restrictions on immigration. For example, recent health information from the CDC (2014) about HIV in the Hispanic American population states that behavioral risk factors for HIV infections differ by country of birth and provides one such example, but does not break out summary details for all subpopulations. The 2012 CDC National Report on Biochemical Indicators of Diet and Nutrition in the US Population provides details only for the following races/ethnic groups: Mexican American, non-Hispanic black, and non-Hispanic white.

As with other Hispanic populations, Cuban Americans are at a higher risk for diabetes. The most recent CDC (2014) statistics available report that among Hispanic adults, the age-adjusted rate of diagnosed diabetes was 8.5% for Central and South Americans, 9.3% for Cubans, 13.9% for Mexican Americans, and 14.8% for Puerto Ricans, compared to 7.6% for non-Hispanic whites.

Teaching Implications

Although current research on Cuban American diet and nutrition status is limited, awareness of some Cuban American values may assist nutrition educators and program planners. The following suggestions, which may be used as a starting point, are derived from a monograph introducing the Cuban culture to rehabilitation service providers (Brice, http://cirrie.buffalo.edu/culture/monographs/cuba/).

Earlier-wave Cuban Americans may be more reliant on extended family, while later arrivals, familiar with the social support of the Cuban communist government, may seek a group or community-level system of support. Cuban American males may display machismo or very traditional-role types of interaction. Traditionally, they may perceive their role in the household as one of provider and disciplinarian.

In general, social relationships are important. Attendance at Cuban social events and the use of the Spanish language are important social identifiers. Success in building personal relationships may facilitate nutrition education, as may the use of humor and puns. Building in immediate reinforcement to diet objectives may help for those who are more present oriented.

An individual assessment may be made regarding nutrients of concern, but in general, nutrition education can focus on diabetes and heart-healthy diet patterns.

Dominican Americans

According to the 2010 census, more than 1,410,000 Dominicans live in the United States. Immigration increased dramatically from the early 1960s (when just over 90,000 Dominicans were admitted to the United States) through the mid-1990s and began to decline thereafter. From 1988 to 1998, over 400,000 Dominicans migrated to the United States. Two-thirds settled in New York and northern New Jersey; the remainder live primarily in Miami, Los Angeles, Boston, Houston, Chicago, Philadelphia, and Portland (Castro and Boswell 2002). In general, Dominican-born residents in the United States suffer from low levels of education, income, and occupational status. Almost half are high school dropouts, and less than 10% are college graduates. On the other hand, only 8.8% of Dominican Americans born in the United States fail to complete high school, and 21.7% are college graduates (Motel and Patten 2012). Dominicans have higher levels of education than the Hispanic population overall. Some 15% of Dominicans ages 25 and older—compared with 13% of all US Hispanics—have obtained at least a bachelor's degree (Brown and Patten 2013).

Green plantains, boiled and fried, mashed with olive oil, and served with onions and avocado, is a staple food, traditionally served for breakfast, which can include a variety of additions such as fried eggs, peppers, fried white cheese, and pork. Lunch is traditionally the main meal in the Dominican Republic over which the family gathers, but for Dominican American families in which both parents were out working, dinner has become the more substantial meal. The main meal of the day can include meat; rice; beans; fritters (plantains, yucca, sweet potato); salad (numerous vegetables, seasoned with olive oil and vinegar); dessert; and coffee (Gray 2001).

As a Hispanic subgroup, the Dominican population reflects the influence of significant mixing of European, Hispanic, and African people and culture. The health concerns associated with the Hispanic population in general, such as diabetes, are present in the Dominican American population, but with variations. Some health disparities are not as marked; for example, a 2010 cross-sectional study of women found that prevalence of metabolic syndrome was lowest among Dominican women, for whom prevalence was one-third to one-half that among other Hispanic groups, which supported similar results observed in another study previously (Derby et al. 2010).

Conversely, another study reports that some specific cardiovascular risk factors may be of greater prevalence among Dominican Americans than other Hispanic groups and furthermore notes that hypertension is highly prevalent, recommending that blood pressure surveillance and control be especially aggressive in Dominican Americans. The significant admixture of African ancestry could be one possible reason for this significantly higher prevalence of hypertension among Dominican Americans in comparison with Mexican, Puerto Rican, and other Hispanic Americans (Allison et al. 2008).

Past immigrant experience in the United States has led to social expectations of cultural and linguistic assimilation within two to three generations. With the fluidity and ease of modern travel, immigration from regions closer in distance to the United States, and greater access of greater communication, the immigrant experience today can be of a more transnational nature for many. Connections to the homeland may be maintained, even after the second generation is born on US soil. The Dominican American community of Washington Heights, NY, is representative of this new immigrant paradigm (Dicker, https://www.hostos.cuny.edu/OAA/eng/pdf/Dicker.pdf).

Teaching Implications

Dominican Americans may divide their time to a significant extent between the United States and the Dominican Republic, which may also mean difficulties in scheduling classes or follow-up sessions. The strength of transnationalism includes language; it has been reported that 93% of Dominican Americans speak Spanish at home, and over half (54%) are not proficient in English. Thus, the ability to speak Spanish may be a critical requirement for the educator, but even a fluent Spanish speaker of a different background may need to learn more about cultural and environmental differences in order to achieve the best efficacy of nutrition education. Traditionally, mild health concerns were treated through an informal system of older women (Kittler et al. 2012); nutritional education that involves dietary changes for children might be most effective if involving trusting older female members of the community, who may act as babysitters or consultants for younger working mothers. Respecting transnationalism may include seeking ideas on how to adapt dishes to work in both the United States and the homeland.

ASIAN AMERICANS

The US Government's Office of Management and Budget defines *Asians* as people having origins in any of the original peoples of the Far East, Southeast Asia, or the Indian subcontinent, including, for example, Cambodia, China, India, Japan, Korea, Malaysia, Pakistan, the Philippine Islands, Thailand, and Vietnam. According to the United States Census Bureau, the 2010 census statistics on the Asian population includes people who indicated their race(s) as "Asian"; reported entries such as "Asian Indian," "Chinese," "Filipino," "Korean," "Japanese," and "Vietnamese"; or provided other detailed Asian responses. More than 56 ethnic groups from Asia and the Pacific Islands (speaking over 100 languages) live in the United States (Centers for Disease Control and Prevention 2014).

As of 2011, the Asian American population in the United States is estimated to be 18.2 million people, with the three largest groups being Chinese (4 million; except Taiwanese descent), Filipinos (3.4 million), and Asian Indians (3.2 million). The next largest population groups are Vietnamese (1.9 million), Koreans (1.7 million), and Japanese (1.3 million) (Centers for Disease Control and Prevention, http://www.cdc.gov/minorityhealth/populations/REMP/asian.html). According to the Census Bureau, for Asian American population groups numbering 1 million or more, the highest proportion of each group lived in California as of 2010 (Hoeffel et al. 2012).

The Census Bureau estimates that by the year 2050, there will be 40.6 million Asians living in the United States, comprising 9.2% of the total US population (Centers for Disease Control and Prevention, http://www.cdc.gov/minorityhealth/populations/REMP/asian.html).

The immigration history, pattern, and experience of Asian Americans is wide ranging and far beyond the scope of this text; nutrition educators should inform themselves as to relevant history and cultural influences when working with populations. Asian Americans also practice a number of religions, including Confucianism, Buddhism, Taoism, and Shintoism (Japanese only). A large number of native Filipinos are Roman Catholic.

However, two key elements draw the diverse cultures of the Asian region together when it comes to food: the composition of meals (emphasis on vegetables and rice, with relatively little meat) and cooking techniques. Most Asians living in the United States adhere to a traditional Asian diet interspersed with American foods, particularly breads and cereals. Dairy products are not consumed in large amounts, except for ice cream. Calcium is consumed through tofu, green vegetables (such as bok choy), and small fish (bones eaten). Fish, pork, and poultry comprise the main proteins. Significant amounts of nuts and dried beans are also eaten. Vegetables and fruits make up a large part of their food intake. Rice is the mainstay of the diet and is commonly eaten at every meal. Asian food preparation techniques include stir-frying, barbecuing, deep-frying, boiling, and steaming. All ingredients are carefully prepared (chopped, sliced, and so on) prior to starting the cooking process. A typical day's menu might include hot cereal, bread, fruit juice, soy milk, fruit, nuts, and rice for breakfast; rice or bread with vegetables or fruits for lunch; and rice and vegetable soup mixed with tofu, vegetables, fish, or meat for dinner.

Although the composition of Asian meals may be relatively similar, the tastes can be wide ranging. For example, Thai food is generally spicy, hot, and high in sodium, and hot peppers are used daily. Conversely, garlic and hot peppers are not common ingredients in Japanese cuisine. Fish sauce is indispensable for a Vietnamese table. Koreans eat kimchee with every meal. Kimchee is cabbage marinated in salt water, layered with peppers and spices in crockery, and left to ferment through November and December.

The California Department of Health Care Services has developed some general nutrition recommendations that might be applicable to Asian Americans, which include encouraging the following (Nguyen 2006): breastfeeding; the maintenance of traditional, nutrient-rich diets; changing grain consumption to whole grains (brown rice, whole-wheat noodles); consuming lactose-free dairy products or alternative sources of calcium and lean meats without skin; the reduction of oil and fats used in cooking; steaming/boiling; and reducing reliance on salty condiments and cooking sauces.

The following sections examine two Asian American subpopulation groups in more detail: Vietnamese and Hmong.

VIETNAMESE

The Vietnamese come from both remote agricultural and fast-paced urban areas of Southeast Asia. Most Vietnamese practice Buddhism, but some practice Confucianism or Taoism. Vietnamese Americans are one of the fastest-growing American Asian Pacific Islander (AAPI) groups in the United States. From 1990 to 2000, the Vietnamese population in the United States grew by 83% (614,547 to 1,122,528) (Barnes and Bennett 2002), and from 2000 to 2010, by 42% to 1,737,433 (including individuals reporting more than one race). As of 2010, 37% of Vietnamese immigrants settled in California, with the next largest state population in Texas, at 13.1% (Hoeffel et al. 2012).

The basic food in Vietnam is rice or rice noodles supplemented with vegetables, eggs, and small amounts of meat and fish. French-style bread and wheat noodles are also consumed. Although similar to Chinese cooking, Vietnamese cooking uses little fat or oil for frying. *Nuoc mam* fish sauce is a principal ingredient in almost every Vietnamese dish. Fruits such as bananas, mangos, papayas, oranges, watermelon, and pineapple are popular. Vietnamese eat a wide variety of vegetables. Soybeans, mung beans, and peanuts are used extensively, and lettuce, bean sprouts, and herbs are often served raw as accompaniments to meals. Traditionally, the consumption of dairy products is not emphasized; these are mainly consumed as ice cream, sweetened condensed milk, and shelf-stable processed cheese products. Many Vietnamese have varying degrees of lactose intolerance. Hot green tea and coffee are frequently drunk without adding sugar, milk, or lemon. Milk consumption, already low in adults, remains low or nonexistent in pregnant or lactating women; some pregnant Vietnamese immigrants may have diets low in calcium, vitamin E, and thiamin.

Vietnamese eat three meals a day with some snacking on fruits and soups. A light breakfast may consist of soup (*pho*), rice, or rice noodles; thin slices of beef, chicken, or pork; bean sprouts; greens; green tea or green coffee; boiled eggs; and crusty bread. Lunch and dinner are similar in content—rice, fish or meat, a vegetable dish with *nuoc mam* or fish sauce, plus tea or coffee. Smaller portions are served at dinner.

Vietnamese migration started as a refugee flow and, over time, became oriented toward family reunification. The immigrant Vietnamese population has encountered significant social challenges in the United States. An intervention conducted by the University of California, Berkeley, Department of Nutritional Sciences and Toxicology from 2002 to 2005 aimed at developing a culturally sensitive and relevant nutrition education program describes some of the challenges the population faced at that time as compared with other Asian American/Pacific Islander groups, namely, lower socioeconomic status, greater likelihood of difficulties with the English language, social isolation, and low reading levels. Additionally, as many Vietnamese may rely on traditional beliefs about health and medicine, the limited access to culturally appropriate and literacy-appropriate education materials may contribute to a poor dietary intake when faced with limited access to familiar foods (University of California Berkeley, http://nature.berkeley.edu/departments /nut/extension/vietnamese.health/).

Vietnamese Americans are at risk for hypertension, and consequently, strokes. Heart disease is the second leading cause of death among Vietnamese. Studies from 1978 to 1985 and from 1991 found that Vietnamese American women had the highest rates of hypertension among all Asian American groups. A 1996 National Institute of Health publication reported that cervical cancer is the most common cancer among Vietnamese women, with a rate five times higher than that of Caucasian women (Nguyen 2006).

Teaching Implications

Education is extremely important to the Vietnamese. Their learning system traditionally emphasized memorization and repetition, not critical study. Vietnamese show great respect to elders, superiors, and strangers. They clasp both hands against their chests in welcome. Shaking hands is seldom done; a smile and nod would suffice. Beckoning with a finger is a sign of contempt used toward an animal or inferior.

Vietnamese people tend to be polite and delicate. Because frankness and outspokenness are usually considered rude, true feelings are often veiled. Vietnamese people may just smile and nod when they do not understand you. Keep in mind that this means, "Yes, I hear you," or, "Yes, I see what you mean even though I don't truly understand it!" Vietnamese are typically friendly and giving people, and hospitality and food are related. A Vietnamese person might not ask, "How are you?" but rather, "Have you eaten yet?"

Respect for parents and for ancestors is a key virtue in Vietnamese families. The oldest male in the family is the head of the household and the most important family member. His oldest son is the second leader of the family. Sometimes, related families live together in a big house and help each other.

Even though Vietnamese immigrants range from farmers to urban dwellers, their move to the United States is still one of enormous cultural change. They are a people of tradition yet are open to try new American ways. Unfamiliarity with most US grocery items may require a total introduction to American food culture. In their home country, Vietnamese either grow food or purchase it daily and traditionally lack refrigeration. Education about how to store perishable foods may be helpful for those Vietnamese adapting to the more common American rhythm of purchasing food on a less frequent basis. Education and health providers can also encourage home and community gardening as a source of native vegetables. When access to familiar foods is limited, introducing unfamiliar vegetables, fruits, and legumes will be helpful.

Hmong

The Hmong are a highly developed people with a rich culture who lived in northeast China under the leadership of the Hmong king Chiyou. They were invaded over 5000 years ago and forced to migrate to southern China, some eventually arriving in Southeast Asia, principally the rural mountain areas of Laos. In 1975, when Laos was taken over by communists, the Hmong began to disperse to many parts of the world, including the United States. In 2010, there were 260,073 Hmong in the United States, an increase of over 39% from 2000 (Barnes and Bennett 2002; Hoeffel et al. 2012), 64,000 of whom live in the Minneapolis–St. Paul metropolitan area (Hoeffel et al. 2012).

Although some Hmong have converted to Christianity or other religions, traditionally, the Hmong follow an animist religion, believing in spirits in all places and every aspect of life. They also have close family and clan relationships and are divided into clans or tribes that share the same paternal ancestry. Each clan has a leader who oversees all relations. Clans will move to the same area in the United States to maintain their closeness. Each clan has a shaman (wise man/medicine man) who deals with spiritual and physical problems, similar to the functions of a minister, psychologist, and doctor. As the clan leader and the shaman are important to the Hmong family members, it is important for the healthcare worker to gain their respect. The book *A Spirit Catches You and You Fall Down* is an excellent starting point for learning about Hmong culture and, in particular, the potential depth of cultural differences about how we think about health, medicine, and healthcare. The extreme cultural clash presented in the book is gripping and evocative; the reader, however, must take care to step back and reflect that cultural clashes may be far less obvious than the ones described.

The Hmong staple food is white rice. Their diet is enhanced by a variety of vegetables, fish, meat, and traditional spices. They eat three meals a day; snacking is not part of their native culture. A typical day's menu might include light soup with rice, pumpkin, vegetables, chicken, or pork (eaten very early, for breakfast) and nonglutinous rice, fried or steamed meat, pork, chicken, or beef (eaten at noon or before for lunch and eaten late in the evening for dinner).

Most of a Hmong's daily calories are from the carbohydrates/grain group, but vegetables are also consumed in large amounts. The Hmong diet could be enhanced with the addition of a variety of inexpensive, available vegetables. Meats and fish are used in small amounts as enhancements. The amounts are sufficient, however, to provide ample protein. Popular fruits are bananas, mangos, pineapples, coconuts, lichees, and jackfruit. As with vegetables, additional varieties of fruit could enhance the Hmong diet. In particular, citrus fruits should be emphasized for their vitamin C content.

Fresh milk and cheese are typically unavailable to Hmong in their native country. This, along with lactose intolerance, discourages the consumption of dairy products. Overall fat content in the diet is low. Relatively few households in Laos eat sweets. A steamed rice cake may be eaten occasionally. Hmong food is usually homegrown. Meats are usually fresh, home butchered, and shared among clan members to keep storage time short. Meals are served in a communal style. Food is placed (and replenished) in the middle of the table, and each person eats from the center with a spoon or fork. Using fingers to eat is impolite. Cooking methods include stir-frying, boiling, steaming, and roasting over an open fire. Vegetable oils and pork fat are the principal fats used in cooking. Food is usually chopped in uniform pieces before cooking. Seasonings are an essential aspect of Hmong cooking. Fish sauce and soy sauce, both of which are high in sodium, replace table salt. Hot peppers, ginger, garlic, coriander, coconut, and lemongrass contribute to the robust flavor (Nguyen 2006).

During pregnancy and lactation, many women do not include milk in their diet, instead following traditional dietary patterns during pregnancy and after birth. The book *A Spirit Catches You and*

You Fall Down is an excellent starting point for further exploration of Hmong dietary patterns and culture. More critically, many Hmong women do not sufficiently increase their caloric intake during pregnancy or postpartum.

Work done during the 1990s found that riboflavin, calcium, iron, magnesium, and zinc consumption were found to be less than 80% of the Recommended Dietary Allowance (RDA) in Hmong adults at that time, and that major health concerns include increased risk of heart disease and diabetes, and increased incidence of obesity.

Teaching Implications

The Hmong do not feel comfortable with direct eye contact. As Hmong education is traditionally oral, many of the elders do not read; children of immigrant families may play a significant role in helping the family navigate a new culture and language. Nonetheless, the Hmong are a willing and hospitable group of learners. Many times in teaching situations, they will nod and say, "Yes," which means, "Yes, I am listening to you," not, "Yes, I understand."

The Hmong people have experienced an enormous cultural change in their move to the United States. The Hmong mother is caught between her husband, who wants homeland cooking, and her children, who are becoming Americanized and expect her to cook American meals. The cultural generation gap caused as younger members acculturate (a phenomenon also experienced in particular by other Southeast Asian immigrant groups) can be of significant impact.

CONCLUSION

Working within a rapidly diversifying society requires the health professional to seek cultural competency. Practicing in a culturally competent manner is a difficult, time-consuming, ongoing process. Our discussion on culture and foodways is limited in scope and is offered not as facts to learn but as a guide toward the questions a nutrition health educator may need to ask in order to positively affect communication and improve health status.

There are inherent challenges in attempting to untangle social factors (e.g., socioeconomic status, environmental impacts, the binding necessities of daily life that may conflict with ideal values) from cultural factors as both may variably influence any given individual who might identify as part of a larger population. Accordingly, understanding and addressing social context and influencers has emerged as a critical component of cultural competence. As an example, a 2015 report on a tobacco intervention notes expanding cultural competency to "include the context of community history, group norms, and other dynamics related to resisting or facilitating factors informing the planning of solution strategies" (Douglas et al. 2015).

A need exists to develop a more comprehensive approach to devising and implementing cultural competence in nutrition care at different levels and perspectives, including efforts at addressing health literacy. The assessment of cross-cultural relations, knowledge, awareness about the dynamics that result from cultural differences, and adaptation of services helps to design policies, guidelines, and strategies that meet cultural needs and national goals. Culturally competent healthcare systems incorporate the HP 2020 goals of increasing health equity, eliminating disparities, and improving the health of all groups, at all levels of care (Betancourt et al. 2003).

ACRONYMS

AND	Academy of Nutrition and Dietetics
CCLCH	Center for Cultural and Linguistic Competency in Health Care
CDC	Centers for Disease Control and Prevention
CLAS	Culturally and Linguistically Appropriate Services
CMS	Centers for Medicare & Medicaid Services

DTR	Dietetic technician, registered
HAES	Health at Every Size
HEW	Department of Health, Education, and Welfare
HHS	US Department of Health and Human Services
HIV	Human immunodeficiency virus
HRSA	Health Resources and Services Administration
IOM	Institute of Medicine
LGBT	Lesbian, gay, bisexual, and transgender
MHI	Minority Health Initiative
MNT	Medical nutrition therapy
NAAFA	National Association to Advance Fat Acceptance
NAAL	National Assessment of Adult Literacy
NCCC	National Center for Cultural Competence
NCI	National Cancer Institute
NCMHD	National Center on Minority Health and Health Disparities
NHS	National Health Survey
NIH	National Institutes of Health
OMH	Office of Minority Health
RD	Registered dietitian

STUDENT ASSIGNMENTS AND ACTIVITIES DESIGNED TO ENHANCE LEARNING AND STIMULATE CRITICAL THINKING

1. Use the Internet to research community health workers (CHW) and answer the following questions:
    a. What is the definition of a CHW?
    b. What are some job titles that CHWs may have?
    c. What services do CHWs provide? In what types of settings do CHWs serve?
    d. Is there a standardized training and credentialing program for CHWs? If yes, describe the program. If no, what might be the reasons that such a program does not exist?
    e. What are the benefits of utilizing CHWs? What are the drawbacks?
2. What is your favorite meal cooked by an older relative? Is it prepared in the most healthful manner? If not, what steps could be taken to improve the healthfulness of the dish? If someone else (personally unknown to you) told you or your relative that the dish needed to be changed, would you listen to them and make the change? What would convince you?
3. You have been asked to teach a nutrition in-service to a group of low-literacy adults. Develop a 10- to 15-minute lesson plan, one teaching material (visual aid), and one handout to teach one of the following topics:
    • Portion size education.
    • Increasing fruit and vegetable consumption.
    • How to read a food label.
    • Monitoring and modifying sodium intake (labels and cooking).
4. Read the excerpt from Anne Fadiman's book, *The Spirit Catches You and You Fall Down* (http://www.spiritcatchesyou.com/bookexcerpt.htm). Answer the following questions:
    a. How do traditional Hmong and American birth practices differ?
    b. Describe the role of food in the traditional Hmong birth experiences. How does this differ from American practices/beliefs?
    c. As a nutritionist working in clinical care, what questions would you ask a Hmong woman that was referred to you by her ob-gyn?

    d. As a nutritionist working in clinical care, what questions would you ask a woman from your own culture that was referred to you by her ob-gyn? How would you characterize or discern her as a cultural peer?

5. This chapter briefly touches on the need to be culturally sensitive to gender identity and expression. Search the Internet and do a literature review regarding nutritional needs for transgender persons. What did you find? What questions should you ask of any clients or patients who are transgender persons? Are there questions you should not ask?

6. Make a list of foods listed in this chapter that you are not familiar with. Pick three and research them. Describe what they are, how they are usually prepared, and what nutrients they provide. Be sure to state the cultural group(s) that typically consumes these foods. Include any additional information you think is important or interesting. Use the following questions to help you:

- Where is the food from?
- What is the best time/season to purchase this food?
- How long does it take this food to grow?
- Can this food be eaten raw? If not, how can one cook this food?
- How long can this food be stored?
- How should this food be stored?
- What other foods are typically eaten with this one?

REFERENCES

Allison MA, Budoff MJ, Wong ND, Blumenthal RS, Schreiner PJ, Criqui MH. Prevalence of risk factors for subclinical cardiovascular disease in selected US Hispanic Ethnic Groups. The multi-ethnic study of atherosclerosis. *Am J Epidemiol*. 2008;167(8):962–969.

Barnes JS, Bennett CE. Census Brief 2000. The Asian Population 2000, February 2002. Available at http://www.census.gov/prod/2002pubs/c2kbr01-16.pdf, accessed January 24, 2015.

Batis C, Hernandez-Barrera L, Barquera S, Rivera JA, Popkin BM. Food acculturation drives dietary differences among Mexicans, Mexican Americans, and Non-Hispanic Whites. *J Nutr*. 2011;141(10):1898–1906.

Bermúdez OI, Falcón LM, Tucker KL. Intake and food sources of macronutrients among older Hispanic adults: Association with ethnicity, acculturation, and length of residence in the United States. *J Am Diet Assoc*. 2000;100(6):665–673.

Betancourt JR, Green AR, Carrillo JE, Ananeh-Firempong O, 2nd. Defining cultural competence: A practical framework for addressing racial/ethnic disparities in health and health care. *Public Health Rep*. 2003;118(4):293–302.

Brach C, Fraser I. Can cultural competency reduce racial and ethnic health disparities? A review and conceptual model. *Med Care Res Rev*. 2000;57(Suppl 1):181–217.

Brice A. Introduction to Cuban Culture for Rehabilitation Service Providers. Available at http://cirrie.buffalo.edu/culture/monographs/cuba/, accessed December 23, 2014.

Brown A. U.S. Hispanic and Asian Populations Growing, but for Different Reasons. PEW Research Center, June 26, 2014. Available at http://www.pewresearch.org/fact-tank/2014/06/26/u-s-hispanic-and-asian-populations-growing-but-for-different-reasons/, accessed December 10, 2014.

Brown A, Patten E. Hispanics of Dominican Origin in the United States, 2011, June 19, 2013. Available at http://www.pewhispanic.org/2013/06/19/hispanics-of-dominican-origin-in-the-united-states-2011/, accessed December 23, 2014.

Burke CB, Raia SP. *Ethnic and Regional Food Practices. A Series. Soul and Traditional Southern Food Practices and Customs*. Chicago: The American Dietetic Association, 1995.

Carbone ET, Zoellner JM. Nutrition and health literacy: A systematic review to inform nutrition research and practice. *J Acad Nutr Diet*. 2012;112(2):254–265.

Castro MJ, Boswell TD. The Dominican Diaspora Revisited: Dominicans and Dominican-Americans in a New Century. Dante B. Fascell North-South Agenda Paper No. 53, January 2002.

Centers for Disease Control and Prevention. Asian American Populations. Available at http://www.cdc.gov/minorityhealth/populations/REMP/asian.html, accessed January 10, 2015.

Centers for Disease Control and Prevention. Asian American Populations. Available at http://www.cdc.gov/minorityhealth/populations/REMP/asian.html, accessed January 20, 2014.

Centers for Disease Control and Prevention. Asian American Populations. Available at http://www.cdc.gov/minorityhealth/populations/REMP/asian.html, accessed June 10, 2014.

Centers for Disease Control and Prevention. Health Literacy. Learn about Health Literacy. Available at http://www.cdc.gov/healthliteracy/Learn/, accessed December 14, 2014.

Centers for Disease Control and Prevention. Teen Pregnancy. Last updated June 9, 2014. Available at http://www.cdc.gov/teenpregnancy/longdescriptors.htm, accessed December 14, 2014.

Centers for Disease Control and Prevention. 2nd National Report on Biochemical Indicators of Diet and Nutrition in the U.S. Population, 2012. Available at http://www.cdc.gov/nutritionreport/pdf/ExeSummary_Web_032612.pdf, accessed December 22, 2014.

Centers for Disease Control and Prevention. Black or African American Populations. Updated February 10, 2014. Available at http://www.cdc.gov/minorityhealth/populations/REMP/black.html, accessed December 23, 2014.

Centers for Disease Control and Prevention. HIV among Latinos. Fact Sheet. Updated December 8, 2014. Available at http://www.cdc.gov/hiv/risk/racialethnic/hispaniclatinos/facts/index.html, accessed December 23, 2014.

Centers for Disease Control and Prevention. Hypertension-related mortality among Hispanic United States, 1995–2002. *MMWR*. 2006;55(7):177–180. Available at http://www.cdc.gov/mmwr/preview/mmwrhtml/mm5507a3.htm, accessed December 23, 2014.

Centers for Disease Control and Prevention. 2014 National Diabetes Statistics Report. Available at http://www.cdc.gov/diabetes/pubs/statsreport14/national-diabetes-report-web.pdf, accessed December 23, 2014.

Centers for Disease Control and Prevention. Observances—May Asian American & Pacific Islander Heritage Month. Updated May 9, 2014. Available at http://www.cdc.gov/minorityhealth/observances/AAPI.html, accessed December 23, 2014.

Civil Rights Act of 1964, Pub. L. 88-352, 78 Stat. 241, enacted July 2, 1964. Available at http://www.gpo.gov/fdsys/pkg/STATUTE-78/pdf/STATUTE-78-Pg241.pdf, accessed December 14, 2014.

Clark ML. Vision marks black studies chairman's legacy. *On-Line 49er*. 2002;10(20). Available at http://www.csulb.edu/~d49er/archives/2002/fall/news/v10n20-vis.shtml, accessed February 7, 2015.

Consumer Health Informatics Research Resource. Health Literacy. Available at http://chirr.nlm.nih.gov/health-literacy.php, accessed June 20, 2014.

Cynthia MG, Drago L. Using cultural competence constructs to understand food practices and provide diabetes care and education. *Diabetes Spectr*. 2009;22(1):43–47.

Departmento De Salud, Gobierno De Puerto Rico. Puerto Rico Community Health Assessment: Secondary Data Profile, September 28, 2012. Available at http://www.salud.gov.pr/Datos/EstadisticasVitales/Estudio%20de%20Necesidades/PRCHA_Secondary%20data%20analysis_final_2012.pdf, accessed December 23, 2014.

Derby C, Wildman RP, McGinn AP et al. Cardiovascular risk factor variation within a Hispanic cohort: SWAN, the Study of Women's Health Across the Nation. *Ethn Dis*. 2010 Autumn;20(4):396–402.

Dicker S. Dominican Americans in Washington Heights, New York: Language and Culture in a Transnational Community. Available at https://www.hostos.cuny.edu/OAA/eng/pdf/Dicker.pdf, accessed December 23, 2014.

Douglas MR, Carter SR, Wilson AP, Chan A. A neo-strategic planning approach to enhance local tobacco control programs. *Am J Prev Med*. 2015;48(1):S13–S20.

Engebretson J, Mahoney J, Carlson ED. Cultural competence in the era of evidence-based practice. *J Prof Nurs*. 2008;24(3):172–178.

Ennis SR, Rio-Vargas M, Albert NG. The Hispanic Population: 2010. 2010 Census Briefs. United States Census Bureau, May, 2011. Available at http://www.census.gov/prod/cen2010/briefs/c2010br-04.pdf, accessed December 14, 2014.

Exebio JC, Zarini CG, Exebio C, Huffman FG. Healthy Eating Index scores associated with symptoms of depression in Cuban-Americans with and without type 2 diabetes: A cross sectional study. *Nutr J*. 2011;10:135. Available at http://www.nutritionj.com/content/10/1/135, accessed December 23, 2014.

The Fenway Institute. Available at http://thefenwayinstitute.org/about/, accessed December 14, 2014.

Gabaccia DR. *We Are What We Eat*. Cambridge, MA: Harvard University Press, 1998.

Gambino CP, Trevelyan EN, Fitzwater JT. The Foreign-Born Population from Africa: 2008–2012. American Community Survey Briefs, October 2014a. Available at http://www.census.gov/content/dam/Census/library/publications/2014/acs/acsbr12-16.pdf, accessed December 10, 2014.

Gambino CP, Acosta YD, Grieco EM. English-Speaking Ability of the Foreign-Born Population in the United States: 2012. American Community Survey Report, June 2014b. Available at https://www.census.gov/prod/2014pubs/acs-26.pdf, accessed June 11, 2014.

Gates GJ. How Many People are Lesbian, Gay, Bisexual, and Transgender? The Williams Institute, April 2011. Available at https://escholarship.org/uc/item/09h684x2, accessed December 14, 2014.

Georgetown University. Health Policy Institute. Cultural Competence in Health Care: Is It Important for People with Chronic Conditions? Issue Brief No. 5, February 2004. Available at https://hpi.georgetown.edu /agingsociety/pubhtml/cultural/cultural.html, accessed December 14, 2014.

Grant J, Parry Y, Guerin P. An investigation of culturally competent terminology in healthcare policy finds ambiguity and lack of definition. *Aust N Z J Public Health*. 2013;37(3):250–256.

Gray DM. *High Literacy and Ethnic Identity: Dominican American Schooling in Transition*. Lanham, MD: Rowman and Littlefield, 2001.

Harris-Davis E, Haughton B. Model for multicultural nutrition counseling competencies. *J Am Diet Assoc*. 2000;100(10):1178–1185.

HealthyPeople.gov. Healthy People 2020 Topics & Objectives. Health Communication and Information Technology. Updated January 2, 2015. Available at https://www.healthypeople.gov/2020/topics-objectives /topic/health-communication-and-health-information-technology, accessed January 2, 2015.

HealthyPeople.gov. HealthyPeople 2020. Foundation Health Measures. Disparities. Available at http://www .healthypeople.gov/2020/about/foundation-health-measures/Disparities, accessed December 14, 2014.

Hipsman F, Meissner D. Immigration in the United States: New Economic, Social, Political Landscapes with Legislative Reform on the Horizon. Migration Policy Institute, April 16, 2013. Available at http:// www.migrationpolicy.org/article/immigration-united-states-new-economic-social-political-landscapes -legislative-reform, accessed December 23, 2014.

Hoeffel E, Rastogi S, Kim MO, Shahid H. 2010 Census Briefs. *The Asian Population: 2010*, March 2012. Available at http://www.census.gov/prod/cen2010/briefs/c2010br-11.pdf, accessed December 23, 2014.

Humes K, Jones NA, Ramirez RR. Overview of Race and Hispanic Origin: 2010. 2010 Census Briefs, March 2011. Available at http://www.census.gov/prod/cen2010/briefs/c2010br-02.pdf, accessed December 10, 2014.

Immigration. Library of Congress. Available at http://www.loc.gov/teachers/classroommaterials/presentation sandactivities/presentations/immigration/mexican.html, accessed January 22, 2015.

Immigration ... Puerto Rican/Cuban. The Library of Congress. Available at http://www.loc.gov/teachers /classroommaterials/presentationsandactivities/presentations/immigration/cuban5.html, accessed December 23, 2014.

Institute of Medicine (US) Committee on Lesbian, Gay, Bisexual, and Transgender Health Issues and Research Gaps and Opportunities. *The Health of Lesbian, Gay, Bisexual, and Transgender People Building a Foundation for Better Understanding*. Washington, DC: National Academies Press, 2011.

Joint Commission. Advancing Effective Communication, Cultural Competence, and Patient-and-Family -Centered Care. Available at http://www.jointcommission.org/Advancing_Effective_Communication, updated November 24, 2014, accessed December 14, 2014.

Kittler PM, Sucher KP. Caribbean Islanders and South Americans. *Food and Culture*, 4th ed. Belmont, CA: Thomson/Wadsworth, 2004, chap. 10.

Kittler PG, Sucher K, Nelms M. *Food and Culture*, 6th ed. Belmont, CA: Wadsworth, 2012.

Kutner M, Greenberg E, Jin Y, Paulsen C. The Health Literacy of America's Adults. Results from the 2003 National Assessment of Adult Literacy, September 2006. Available at http://nces.ed.gov/pubs2006 /2006483.pdf, accessed December 14, 2014.

Library of Congress. Immigration...Puerto Rico/Cuba. American Memory, 2004. Available at http://memory .loc.gov/learn/features/immig/cuban3.html, accessed June 22, 2014.

List of Spanish Speaking Countries by Population. Available at http://www.spanishlinguist.com/extra/spanish _speaking_countries_world_figures_and_map.html, accessed December 10, 2014.

Loria CM, Bush TL, Carroll MD, Looker AC, McDowell MA, Johnson CL, Sempos CT. Macronutrient intakes among adult Hispanics: A comparison of Mexican Americans, Cuban Americans, and mainland Puerto Ricans. *Am J Public Health*. 1995;85(5):684–689.

Motel S, Patten E. Hispanics of Dominican Origin in the United States, 2010, June 27, 2012. Available at http://www.pewhispanic.org/2012/06/27/hispanics-of-dominican-origin-in-the-united-states-2010, accessed December 23, 2014.

National Cancer Institute. Clear & Simple: Developing Effective Print Materials for Low-Literate Readers. Pub. No. NIH 95-3594, December 1994.

National Center for Cultural Competence. The Compelling Need for Cultural and Linguistic Competence. Available at http://nccc.georgetown.edu/foundations/need.html, accessed December 10, 2014.

National Center for Education Statistics. National Assessment of Adult Literacy (NAAL). Available at http:// nces.ed.gov/naal/fct_hlthliteracy.asp, accessed December 14, 2014.

Nguyen KP. Chapter 18: Health and Dietary Issues Affecting Asians. *California Food Guide: Fulfilling the Dietary Guidelines for Americans*, March 9, 2006. Available at http://www.dhcs.ca.gov/formsandpubs/publications/CaliforniaFoodGuide/18HealthandDietaryIssuesAffectingAsians.pdf, accessed December 23, 2014.

The Official Kwanzaa Web site. Available at http://www.officialkwanzaaweb site.org/index.html, accessed January 22, 2015.

Ohio State University Extension Fact Sheets. Food, Home & Family Series. HYG-5000. Available at http://ohioline.osu.edu/lines/food.html#FOODF, accessed December 14, 2014.

Ortman JM, Velkoff VA, Hogan H. An Aging Nation: The Older Population in the United States. Population Estimates and Projections. Current Population Reports, May 2014. Available at http://www.census.gov/prod/2014pubs/p25-1140.pdf, accessed December 10, 2014.

Pelto GH, Pelto PJ, Messer E. Symbolic, folkloric and medicinal factors, Appendix C in *Research Methods in Nutritional Anthropology*. Toyko: The United Nations University, 1989.

Pew Research Global Attitudes Project. Attitudes about Aging: A Global Perspective, January 30, 2014. Available at http://www.pewglobal.org/2014/01/30/chapter-2-aging-in-the-u-s-and-other-countries-2010-to-2050/#fn-29179-5, accessed December 10, 2014.

President's Advisory Commission on Consumer Protection and Quality in the HealthCare Industry. Quality First: Better HealthCare for All Americans, 1998. Available at http://www.hcqualitycommission.gov/final/, accessed January 20, 2015.

Promoting Good Health through Diet & Lifestyle. Available at http://nature.berkeley.edu/departments/nut/extension/vietnamese.health/, accessed December 23, 2014.

Quick Guide to Health Literacy. Health Literacy Basics. US Department of Health and Human Services. Available at http://www.health.gov/communication/literacy/quickguide/factsbasic.htm#six, accessed January 11, 2015.

Rosario D. Cuban Cuisine. Available at http://www.education.miami.edu/ep/littlehavana/Cuban_Food/Cuban_Cuisine/cuban_cuisine.html, accessed January 20, 2015.

Schwartz DB. Integrating patient-centered care and clinical ethics into nutrition practice. *Nutr Clin Pract.* 2013;28(5):543–555.

Statistical Portrait of Hispanics in the United States, 2012, Detailed Hispanic Origin: 2012. Available at http://www.pewhispanic.org/2014/04/29/statistical-portrait-of-hispanics-in-the-united-states-2012/#hispanic-population-by-nativity-2000-and-2012, accessed December 22, 2014.

Truong M, Paradies Y, Priest N. Interventions to improve cultural competency in healthcare: A systemic review of reviews. *BMC Health Serv Res.* 2014;14:99.

Tucker KL, Mattei J, Noel SE et al. The Boston Puerto Rican Health Study, a longitudinal cohort study on health disparities in Puerto Rican adults, challenges and opportunities. *BMC Public Health.* 2010;10:107.

United States Census Bureau. Hispanic Heritage Month. Available at http://www.census.gov/eeo/special_emphasis_programs/hispanic_heritage.html, accessed December 14, 2014.

US Department of Health and Human Services. Public Health Service. The Office of Minority Health. Assuring Cultural Competence in HealthCare: Recommendations for National Standards and an Outcomes-Focused Research Agenda. Recommendations for National Standards and a National Public Comment Process. Available at http://www.omhrc.gov/clas/cultural1a.htm, accessed June 20, 2014.

US Department of Health and Human Services. Office for Minority Health. Final CLAS Report: National Standards for Culturally and Linguistically Appropriate Services in HealthCare. Available at http://www.omhrc.gov/omh/programs/2pgprograms/finalreport.pdf, accessed June 20, 2014.

US National Library of Medicine, Genetics Home Reference. Available at http://ghr.nlm.nih.gov/condition/lactose-intolerance, accessed October 20, 2014.

US Department of Health and Human Services. *Healthy People 2000*. Final Review. Available at http://www.cdc.gov/nchs/data/hp2000/hp2k01.pdf, accessed December 10, 2014.

US Department of Health and Human Services. *Healthy People 2010*. About Healthy People. (archive site). Available at http://www.healthypeople.gov/2010/About/goals.htm, accessed December 10, 2014.

US Department of Health and Human Services. *Healthy People 2020*. About Healthy People. Available at https://www.healthypeople.gov/2020/About-Healthy-People, accessed December 10, 2014.

US Department of Health and Human Services. Health Resources and Services Administration. Culture, Language and Health Literacy. Available at http://www.hrsa.gov/culturalcompetence/index.html, accessed December 14, 2014.

US Department of Health and Human Services, Agency for Healthcare Research and Quality. Improving Cultural Competence to Reduce Health Disparities for Priority Populations. Research Protocol, July 18, 2014. Available at http://effectivehealthcare.ahrq.gov/ehc/products/573/1934/cultural-competence-protocol-140709.pdf, accessed December 23, 2014.

US Department of Health and Human Services. Center for Linguistic and Cultural Competency in Health Care. Available at http://minorityhealth.hhs.gov/omh/browse.aspx?lvl=2&lvlid=34, accessed February 9, 2015.

United States Census Bureau. U.S. Census Bureau Projections Show a Slower Growing, Older, More Diverse Nation a Half Century From Now. Wednesday, December 12, 2012. Available at https://www.census.gov/newsroom/releases/archives/population/cb12-243.html, accessed December 10, 2014.

United States Census Bureau. Facts for Features: Hispanic Heritage Month 2014: Sept. 15–Oct. 15. September 8, 2014. Available at http://www.census.gov/newsroom/facts-for-features/2014/cb14-ff22.html, accessed December 10, 2014.

Ward BW, Dahlhamer JM, Galinksy AM, Joestl SS. Sexual Orientation and Health Among U.S. Adults: National Health Interview Survey, 2013. *National Health Statistics Report.* No. 77, July 15, 2014. Available at http://www.cdc.gov/nchs/data/nhsr/nhsr077.pdf, accessed December 14, 2014.

The White House. Office of the Press Secretary. Statement by the President on Cuba Policy Changes, December 17, 2014. Available at http://www.whitehouse.gov/the-press-office/2014/12/17/statement-president-cuba-policy-changes, accessed December 23, 2014.

Wiley AS. "Drink milk for fitness": The cultural politics of human biological variation and milk consumption in the United States. *Am Anthropol.* 2004;106(3):506–517.

Zhao Y, Martin BR, Weaver CM. Calcium bioavailability of calcium carbonate fortified soymilk is equivalent to cow's milk in young women. *J Nutr.* 2005;135:2379–2382.

8 Food and Nutrition Policies*

I think it is important to realize that nutrition as such is not a science. Rather, nutrition is an agenda for action based on a number of sciences: physiology, organic chemistry, biochemistry, epidemiology, psychology, sociology, and economics, as well as a number of other fields like agriculture, food technology, political science, and human relations. While the scientific basis is indispensable if nutritionists are going to be authoritative in what they do, the science by itself does not constitute nutrition unless and until a program of action is incorporated as part of the discipline.

Jean Mayer
President of Tufts University, 1989 (Mayer 1989)

Politics is who gets what, when and how.

Harold Lasswell
Politics: Who Gets What, When and How, 1936 (Lasswell 1936)

INTRODUCTION

US food policy affects the safety, integrity, nutritional quality, and accessibility of the nation's food supply as well as the nutritional guidance given to the American population. Food and nutrition policy makers advocate for policies, regulations, and programs designed to protect and advance the health and nutritional status of the American public. National nutrition policy includes such disparate programs as the nation's food and nutrition guidelines issued jointly by the US Department of Agriculture (USDA) and the Department of Health and Human Services (HHS), labeling, and micronutrient fortification. It is not surprising, then, that federal nutrition policies exert considerable influence on state and local decision makers, stakeholders, and consumers.

After defining policy and reviewing types of food and nutrition policy, we use a case study to illustrate how national nutrition policy is made. We then highlight nutrition and health policies and actions that encompass physical activity as well as nutrition, with special attention to efforts in schools. We then look at micronutrient fortification and labeling policies for additional examples of nutrition policy. We touch on the intersection of US policies concerning hunger, agriculture, and public health. Finally, this chapter concludes with an example of nutrition policy advocacy. After all that, we must leave the detailed discussion of federal food and nutrition policy embodied in the *Dietary Guidelines for Americans* and the USDA's MyPlate food guidance system for Chapter 9.

MAKING POLICY

DEFINITIONS

Polis is the Greek word for city-state. In classical Greece, a polis was a unit of governmental and social organization through which Greek citizens identified themselves by means of their common language, customs, history, religion, and a nearby city center or metro*polis*. Derived from the Greek word *polis* are the English words *politics* and *policy* (and also *polite*).

Politics may be thought of as the activity through which people make, preserve, and amend the rules under which they live. Although politics usually refers to government, it is observed in all human group interactions, including corporate, academic, and religious. Institutions arrive at decisions through their politics. As the method of making decisions for groups, politics is the process by which rules for group

---

* Kate O'Connor and Megan Trusdell contributed primary research and prepared draft versions of portions of this chapter.

behavior are established, competition for positions of leadership is regulated, the disruptive effects of disputes are minimized, a community's decisions are made, and policies are established.

Policy, on the other hand, may be regarded as a principle (basic generalization that is accepted as true) or rule (formal regulation that has the force of law) to guide decision making; statements, plans, practices, principles, or rules adopted by a government or other organization for the purpose of guiding or controlling institutional and community behavior; or an established plan or course of action adopted to address specific issues or achieve particular goals.

In the context of government and public service, a *regulation* (as a process) is the control of something by rules. A *rule* is a principle or condition that customarily governs behavior ("it was his rule to take a walk before breakfast"; "short haircuts were the regulation"). And a *ruling* is an interpretation of a regulation (an authoritative rule).

TYPES OF FOOD AND NUTRITION POLICY

Policy and environmental changes can affect large segments of the population simultaneously. People are more likely to adopt healthy behaviors when supportive community norms and health policies are in place, such as safe walking and cycling trails; incentives to schools to increase physical education; low-fat/high-fruit-and-vegetable menu selections in restaurants, schools, and employee cafeterias; and menu labeling in chain restaurants.

Food and nutrition policy may take the form of a guiding policy statement, a set of goals, an initiative that works to achieve specific goals, a law, a rule or regulation (interpreting law), or even a practice. Examples of the various types of policy are as follows:

- *Policy statement*: *Dietary Guidelines for Americans.*
- *Comprehensive goals*: *Healthy People 2020.*
- *Initiative*: *Let's Move!*
- *Law*: Patient Protection and Affordable Care Act of 2010 (PPACA).
- *Regulation*: The US Food and Drug Administration (FDA) promulgates Final Rules on Calories Labeling of Articles of Food in Vending Machines, as required by PPACA.
- *Practice*: A workplace installs vending machines; removes vending machines; selects vendors to supply the contents; and sets criteria (or the lack thereof) for the contents. These practices manifest underlying (even if not articulated) food policies of the workplace.

INFORMING POLICY: AN ECOLOGICAL APPROACH

Behavior change is more likely to endure when a person's environment also changes in a manner that supports the behavior change, requiring public health practitioners to move beyond a strictly educational approach to broader efforts that produce environmental change. Interventions should address not only the intentions and skills of individuals but also their physical and social environments, including social norms and habits of friends and family (White House Task Force on Childhood Obesity 2010). The *spectrum of prevention* is a paradigm that promotes a multifaceted range of activities for effective prevention. It consists of six levels of increasing scope, beginning with a focus on the individual and family, community norms, institutional practices, and, finally laws. The specific activity levels included in the spectrum are

- Strengthening individual knowledge and skills.
- Promoting community education.
- Educating providers.
- Fostering coalitions and networks.
- Changing organizational practices.
- Influencing policy and legislation.

The levels are complementary and, when used together, result in greater effectiveness than would be possible by implementing just any single activity. The spectrum assists practitioners and community-based organizations in developing comprehensive, multifaceted prevention initiatives that result in environmental and norms change (Cohen and Swift 1999). This ecological approach provides the basis for many public health efforts, such as Let's Move! (White House Task Force on Childhood Obesity 2010) and Healthy People 2020 (US Department of Health and Human Services, http://www.healthypeople.gov/2020/about/foundation-health-measures/Determinants-of-Health).

INITIATING POLICY

Suggesting a new policy or revisions to an existing policy is initiated by a politician, political party, professional or professional organization, special interest groups, or other stakeholders that have enlisted political support. Very briefly, the process of introducing a policy includes these activities (Chapman 1990; Chapman and Edmonds 2007):

1. Documenting needs through assessments, surveillance, monitoring, literature review, and so on.
2. Drafting a preliminary statement that refers to past and existing policies.
3. Seeking support from stakeholders, as well as key legislators and policy makers.
4. Mobilizing a grassroots constituency. Policy is made, in part, through the visibility and organization of public interest constituencies. (President Franklin Delano Roosevelt once told a group of businessmen who had come to lobby him: "I agree with everything you say. Now go out there and *make* me do it!")
5. Securing public and professional comments and input.
6. Implementing the policy.
7. Monitoring the policy, once it has been implemented.
8. Evaluating the policy. To what extent does it produce the desired results? When it is no longer serving its purpose, return to step 1.

CASE STUDY: GENESIS OF A NATIONAL NUTRITION POLICY

This case study examines the process of developing a national nutrition policy for the labeling of foods eaten away from home (Lichtenstein et al. 2006; The Keystone Forum on Away-From-Home Foods 2006; US Department of Health and Human Services 2001; Center for Food Safety and Applied Nutrition 2004).

In 2002, Americans spent about 46% of their total food budget on food eaten away from home, an increase from 27% in 1962. Foods eaten in chain restaurants tend to be less nutritious and higher in calories than foods prepared at home (Guthrie et al. 2002; Lin et al. 1999). Nutrition labeling law at the time exempted much of the food-away-from-home sector from mandatory labeling regulations. Because consumers are less likely to be aware of the ingredients and nutrient content of away-from-home food than of foods prepared at home, public health advocates have called for mandatory nutrition labeling for major sources of food eaten away from home, such as fast-food and chain restaurants (Center for Science in the Public Interest 2003).

A USDA Economic Research Service (ERS) assessment of a food-away-from-home nutrition labeling policy indicates that even if a labeling policy has no direct effect on consumer intake, it could still benefit consumers through producer-initiated reformulation of products. If a labeling policy required disclosure of nutritionally negative attributes such as calories, fat, and sodium content, companies selling products with high amounts of energy and these nutrients may choose to reformulate their products rather than risk losing sales. Thus, product reformulation may benefit all consumers who use the products, not just those who read the label. In fact, healthier restaurant fare resulting from reformulation may prove to be the largest benefit of menu labeling (Variyam 2005).

In 2002, the surgeon general recommended that nutrition information be available to customers at restaurants. In 2004, the FDA's Obesity Working Group released a comprehensive report entitled *Calories Count* (US Food and Drug Administration and Center for Food Safety and Applied Nutrition 2004), outlining a series of key recommendations for ways the FDA can help stem the rising tide of obesity in areas within its authority. A major set of recommendations in the report calls on the FDA to encourage the restaurant industry to provide nutrition information. As a result, the FDA urged the restaurant industry to launch a nationwide, voluntary, point-of-sale nutrition information campaign for customers that includes information on calories.

The report also calls on the FDA to work with a third-party facilitator to begin a national policy dialogue to seek consensus-based solutions to specific aspects of the obesity problem involving foods consumed away from home. To implement this recommendation, the FDA hired a nonprofit organization that assists diverse participants achieve consensus on pressing public policy issues to convene a forum on away-from-home foods. This forum, consisting of a broad range of key stakeholders, met to consider what could be done to support consumers' ability to manage their energy intake, within the scope of away-from-home foods, to prevent undue weight gain and obesity. The final report was delivered to the FDA on June 2, 2006. Recommendation 4.1 of the report states that "away-from-home food establishments should provide consumers with calorie information in a standard format that is easily accessible and easy to use" (The Keystone Forum on Away-From-Home Foods 2006).

Not coincidentally, on June 6, 2006, Senator Tom Harkin (D-Iowa) reintroduced in the Senate the Menu Education and Labeling Act (MEAL Act, S 3484) "to amend the Federal Food, Drug, and Cosmetic Act to extend the food labeling requirements of the Nutrition Labeling and Education Act (NLEA) of 1990 to enable customers to make informed choices about the nutritional content of standard menu items in large chain restaurants." The purpose of the MEAL Act was to close a loophole created by the NLEA, which requires most retail food packages to provide nutrition information but exempts restaurant food from these requirements. The MEAL Act would have required chain restaurants with 20 or more business locations to provide consumers with information about calories, sodium, fat, and *trans* fat on standard menu items. Just two weeks after the MEAL Act was introduced, the American Heart Association (AHA) gave menu labeling a tacit endorsement in their diet and lifestyle recommendations for cardiovascular disease risk reduction: "When you eat food that is prepared outside of the home, follow the AHA 2006 Diet and Lifestyle Recommendations" (Lichtenstein et al. 2006). One would need to know what is in the food in order to follow the AHA recommendations; the only way to know that would be through nutrient disclosure. The MEAL Act died in committee and was later reintroduced by Senator Harkin on March 13, 2008 (S 2784). This attempt also failed.

However, on March 23, 2010, President Barack Obama signed the PPACA (P.L. 111-148). Section 4205 of the PPACA requires that calories be posted on menus and menu boards (including drive-through menu boards) at restaurants and similar retail food establishments with 20 or more outlets nationwide. The law also requires vending machine operators who own or operate 20 or more vending machines to disclose calorie content for certain items. Additional nutrient information—such as fat, saturated fat, cholesterol, sodium, and sugar—must be made available in writing upon request. Any individual restaurant, chain, or vending operator that is not covered by this law may voluntarily elect to comply with the requirements and register with the FDA. The FDA issued final regulations about the requirements for restaurants, similar retail food establishments, and vending machines on December 1, 2014 (Food and Drug Administration 2014).

NUTRITION AND HEALTH POLICIES

DIETARY GUIDELINES FOR AMERICANS

The Dietary Guidelines are literally a set of guidelines that form the basis for federal food and nutritional education programs. These guidelines encourage Americans to focus on eating a healthful diet—one that focuses on foods and beverages that help achieve and maintain a healthy weight,

---

BOX 8.1   *DIETARY GUIDELINES FOR AMERICANS*

P.L. 101-445, Section 301 (7 U.S.C. 5341) directs the Secretaries of the US Departments of Agriculture (USDA) and Health and Human Services (HHS) to issue at least every 5 years a joint report entitled *Dietary Guidelines for Americans*. The law instructs that this publication contain nutritional and dietary information and guidelines for the general public, be based on the preponderance of scientific and medical knowledge current at the time of publication, and be promoted by each federal agency in carrying out any federal food, nutrition, or health program. Issued voluntarily by USDA and HHS in 1980, 1985, and 1990, the 1995 edition was the first statutorily mandated report.

Source: US Department of Agriculture, *Dietary Guidelines for Americans, 2015*, Overview. Available at http://www.health.gov/dietaryguidelines/2015.asp, accessed January 26, 2015.

TABLE 8.1
Development of the 2015 Dietary Guidelines—A Chronology

Fall 2012/winter 2013	The US Department of Health and Human Services (HHS) and the US Department of Agriculture (USDA) solicited nominations for the Dietary Guidelines Advisory Committee (DGAC).
Spring/summer 2013	DGAC members were appointed, and request for public comments was initiated. Work groups were established to identify topic areas.
June 2013	DGAC held its first public meeting.
Fall 2013/winter 2014	Subcommittees were established to begin reviews on current scientific evidence.
January 2014	DGAC held its second public meeting, which included public oral testimony.
March 2014	DGAC held its third public meeting.
Spring/summer/fall 2014	DGAC to hold subsequent public meetings and review current scientific evidence.
Fall 2014/winter 2015	DGAC to issue report to the secretaries of HHS and USDA. DGAC report to be published and made available to public for comment.
Winter/spring/summer 2015	HHS and USDA to consider DGAC's scientific recommendations and public agency comments. Departments to prepare the *Dietary Guidelines for Americans* policy document.
Fall 2015	HHS and USDA to jointly publish and release the eighth edition of the *Dietary Guidelines for Americans*.

Source: US Department of Health and Human Services and US Department of Agriculture, *2015 Dietary Guidelines for Americans. Timeline.* Available at http://www.health.gov/dietaryguidelines/2015-dga-timeline.pdf, accessed February 11, 2015.

---

promote health, and prevent disease (US Department of Agriculture 2015). The seventh edition of the guidelines was released in 2010 and is the current federal policy (US Department of Agriculture and US Department of Health and Human Services 2010).* Whereas the *Dietary Guidelines* are not themselves a law but, rather, a statement of the nation's nutrition policy, P.L. 101-445, Title III, 7 U.S.C. 5301 *et seq.* require that a panel of experts be chosen every 5 years to review them (Box 8.1).

This panel examines the scientific literature that has been published since the last review and, if necessary, recommends updates to the guidelines. The law also requires the secretaries of the USDA and HHS to review all federal dietary guidance-related publications for the general public. Table 8.1 provides a chronology for the development of the 2015 *Dietary Guidelines* (US Department of Health and Human Services and US Department of Agriculture 2014).

---

* PowerPoint slides regarding the 2015 edition of the *Dietary Guidelines for Americans* are available for textbook adopters. Current information is also available at the *Dietary Guidelines* home page: http://health.gov/dietaryguidelines/.

BOX 8.2   FUNDING COORDINATION

One way a government indicates its policies is through its funding priorities. For example, in 2011, several one-time federal funding opportunities were available to community-based organizations and state and territorial governments for projects addressing Healthy People 2020 overarching goals, topic areas, and objectives. In addition, Healthy People 2020 serves as a foundational resource for the four strategic directions and seven strategic priorities outlined in the National Prevention Council's *National Prevention Strategy*. The National Prevention Council—made up of the surgeon general (council chair) and representatives from 17 federal departments, agencies, and offices—provides coordination and leadership at the federal level and identifies ways that agencies can work both individually and together (including through funding coordination) to improve the health of the nation.

Source: National Prevention Council, *National Prevention Strategy*, US Department of Health and Human Services, Office of the Surgeon General, Washington, DC, 2011. Available at http://www.surgeongeneral.gov/initiatives/pre vention/strategy/report.pdf, accessed January 27, 2015.

The *Dietary Guidelines* are intended primarily for use by policy makers, healthcare providers, nutritionists, and nutrition educators. In particular, the information in the guidelines is useful for developing educational materials, aiding policy makers in designing and implementing nutrition-related programs, and improving the regulation of food by providing guidance for the inclusion of health claims and nutrient content claims on food labels.

HEALTHY PEOPLE

Since 1979, HHS has supported nationwide efforts to formulate and monitor national disease prevention and health promotion objectives. Healthy People, a comprehensive set of 10-year national goals and objectives for improving the health of all Americans, is at the forefront of this agenda (HealthyPeople.gov, 2015). The most current edition, *Healthy People 2020*, was released in 2010 to provide guidance during the second decade of the twenty-first century (Box 8.2) (HealthyPeople.gov, http://www.healthypeople.gov/2020/LHI/default.aspx).

Origins of Healthy People: 1979–1990

Healthy People began in 1979 with *Healthy People: The Surgeon General's Report on Health Promotion and Disease Prevention* (Public Health Service 1979). The report contained general goals for reducing preventable death and injury in different age groups by the year 1990. Healthy People was a landmark in the history of public health, as it presented for the first time a national public health agenda developed as a consensus among the health community. In 1980, a companion piece—*Promoting Health/Preventing Disease: Objectives for the Nation* (Public Health Service 1980)—set forth 226 measurable health objectives organized into 15 strategic areas. These objectives, referred to as "the 1990 health objectives," called for improvements in health status, risk reduction, public and professional awareness, health services and protective measures, and surveillance and evaluation. These companion reports served as the blueprint for future decennial health priorities.

Healthy People 2000

In 1990, HHS published Healthy People 2000 (Centers for Disease Control and Prevention 2009), which established three overarching goals and grew to 319 objectives in 22 priority areas. The Healthy People 2000 goals were to (1) increase the span of healthy life, (2) reduce health disparities, and (3) provide access to preventive health services.

Healthy People 2010

Building on the experiences of the first two decades of objectives, on public hearings, and on a public comment process that generated more than 11,000 public comments, in January 2000, HHS issued Healthy People 2010, the third generation of 10-year disease prevention and health promotion objectives for the nation. Healthy People 2010 was a comprehensive set of national health objectives, based on scientific evidence, for the first decade of the twenty-first century. It identified two overarching goals—to increase the quality and years of healthy life, and to eliminate health disparities—exemplified by 467 objectives in 28 specific focus areas (US Department of Health and Human Services 2000) (Centers for Disease Control and Prevention 2011).

Healthy People 2020

In the past decade, great strides have been made since the previous set of objectives, Healthy People 2010. For example, life expectancy at birth has increased, while rates of death from coronary heart disease and stroke have decreased. However, public health challenges, such as obesity, adolescent cigarette smoking, adult binge drinking, and suicide, persist (Centers for Disease Control and Prevention 2011). As a result, Healthy People 2020 has set an agenda with four overarching goals: (1) attaining high-quality, longer lives free of preventable disease, disability, injury, and premature death; (2) achieving health equity, eliminating disparities, and improving the health of all groups; (3) creating social and physical environments that promote good health for all; and (4) promoting quality of life, healthy development, and healthy behaviors across all life stages (US Department of Agriculture and US Department of Health and Human Services 2010).

To meet these goals, Healthy People 2020 offers an estimated 1200 objectives organized into 42 topic areas. Table 8.2 lists the Healthy People 2020 objectives for the Nutrition and Weight Status topic area. Many of these objectives measure the nation's progress in implementing the recommendations of the *Dietary Guidelines for Americans*. Table 8.3 contains diet- and nutrition-related objectives from five additional topic areas: adolescent health, diabetes, educational and community-based programs, food safety, and heart disease and stroke.

DATA2020 is the interactive data system used to track all 1200 Healthy People objectives. For each objective, DATA2020 provides the baseline status, desired target, target-setting method, data source(s), and links for additional information. For some objectives, data are also available by demographic population groups, such as race, ethnicity, sex, educational attainment, and income. Data are searchable by topic area and data source, and DATA2020 is updated as new data become available (US Department of Health and Human Services, http://www.healthypeople.gov/2020/Data/default.aspx).

Each decennial edition of Healthy People is subject to a midcourse review to assess the status of the objectives. Through this review, HHS, other federal agencies, and subject matter experts assess the data trends during the first half of the decade, consider new science and available data, and make changes to ensure that Healthy People remains current, accurate, and relevant, while simultaneously assessing emerging public health priorities (US Department of Health and Human Services 2005). At the time of this writing, the midcourse review for Healthy People 2020 was not yet published.

FEDERAL ACTION STEPS

The USDA's Food and Nutrition Service (FNS) works with other federal agencies to coordinate the federal government's efforts in promoting healthy eating and active lifestyles. The following are various examples of memoranda of understanding (MOUs) signed by two or more federal agencies:

- *Information sharing related to food safety, public health, and other food-associated activities (2011).* The USDA and the FDA of the HHS are working together to enhance the exchange of information related to food safety, public health, and associated regulatory, marketing, trade, and research activities that substantially affect public health (US Department of Agriculture and US Department of Health and Human Services 2011).

TABLE 8.2

Healthy People 2020, **Nutrition and Weight Status Objectives**

Objective	Description	Baseline (Year)	2020 Target	Data Source
	Healthier Food Access			
NWS-1	Increase the number of states with nutrition standards for foods and beverages provided to preschool-aged children in child care	24 states (2006)	34 states and District of Columbia	NRC, state child care licensing websites
NWS-2.1	Increase the proportion of schools that do not sell or offer calorically sweetened beverages to students	9.3% of schools (2006)	21.3% of schools	SHPPS, CDC/NCHHSTP
NWS-2.2	Increase the proportion of school districts that require schools to make fruits or vegetables available whenever other food is offered or sold	6.6% of schools (2006)	18.6%	SHPPS, CDC/NCHHSTP
NWS-3	Increase the number of states that have state-level policies that incentivize food retail outlets to provide foods that are encouraged by the *Dietary Guidelines for Americans*	8 states (2009)	18 states and District of Columbia	State Indicator Report on Fruits and Vegetables, CDC
NWS-4	(Developmental) Increase the proportion of Americans who have access to a food retail outlet that sells a variety of foods that are encouraged by the *Dietary Guidelines for Americans*	N/A	N/A	TBD
	Healthcare and Work Site Settings			
NWS-5.1	Increase the proportion of primary care physicians who regularly assess body mass index (BMI) of their adult patients	48.7% (2009)	53.6%	National Survey of Energy Balance Related Care among Primary Care Physicians, FDA, NIH/NCI
NWS-5.2	Increase the proportion of primary care physicians who regularly assess BMI for age and sex of their child or adolescent patients	49.7% (2008)	54.7%	National Survey of Energy Balance Related Care among Primary Care Physicians, FDA, NIH/NCI/ARP
NWS-6.1	Increase the proportion of physician office visits made by patients with a diagnosis of cardiovascular disease, diabetes, or hyperlipidemia that include counseling or education related to diet or nutrition	20.8% (2007)	22.9%	NAMCS, CDC/NCHS
NWS-6.2	Increase the proportion of physician office visits made by adult patients who are obese that include counseling or education related to weight reduction, nutrition, or physical activity	28.9% (2007)	31.8%	NAMCS, CDC/NCHS
NWS-6.3	Increase the proportion of physician visits made by all child or adult patients that include counseling about nutrition or diet	12.2% (2007)	15.2%	NAMCS, CDC/NCHS
NWS-7	(Developmental) Increase the proportion of work sites that offer nutrition or weight management classes or counseling	N/A	N/A	Follow-up to the 2004 National Worksite Health Promotion Survey, AWHP, ODPHP

(Continued)

TABLE 8.2 (CONTINUED)

Healthy People 2020, **Nutrition and Weight Status Objectives**

Objective	Description	Baseline (Year)	2020 Target	Data Source
	Weight Status			
NWS-8	Increase the proportion of adults who are at a healthy weight	30.8% (2005–2008)	33.9%	NHANES, CDC/NCHS
NWS-9	Reduce the proportion of adults who are obese	33.9% (2005–2008)	30.5%	NHANES, CDC/NCHS
NWS-10.1	Reduce the proportion of children aged 2–5 years who are considered obese	10.7% (2005–2008)	9.6%	NHANES, CDC/NCHS
NWS-10.2	Reduce the proportion of children aged 6–11 years who are considered obese	17.4% (2005–2008)	15.7%	NHANES, CDC/NCHS
NWS-10.3	Reduce the proportion of children aged 12–19 years who are considered obese	17.9% (2005–2008)	16.1%	NHANES, CDC/NCHS
NWS-10.4	Reduce the proportion of children aged 2–19 years who are considered obese	16.1% (2005–2008)	14.5%	NHANES, CDC/NCHS
NWS-11	(Developmental) Prevent inappropriate weight gain in youth and adults	N/A	N/A	NHANES, CDC/NCHS
	Food Insecurity			
NWS-12	Eliminate very low food security among children	1.3% (2008)	0.2%	CPS, census, DOL/BLS
NWS-13	Reduce household food insecurity and, in doing so, reduce hunger	14.6% (2008)	6.0%	CPS, census, DOL/BLS
	Food and Nutrient Consumption			
NWS-14	Increase the contribution of fruits to the diets of the population aged 2 years or older	0.5 cup (2001–2004)	0.9 cup	NHANES, CDC/NCHS
NWS-15.1	Increase the contribution of total vegetables to the diets of the population aged 2 years or older	0.8 cup (2001–2004)	1.1 cup	NHANES, CDC/NCHS
NWS-15.2	Increase the contribution of dark green vegetables, orange vegetables, and legumes to the diets of the population aged 2 years or older	0.1 cup (2001–2004)	0.3 cup	NHANES, CDC/NCHS
NWS-16	Increase the contribution of whole grains to the diets of the population aged 2 years or older	0.3 oz. (2001–2004)	0.6 oz.	NHANES, CDC/NCHS
NWS-17.1	Reduce consumption of calories from solid fats	18.9% (2001–2004)	16.7%	NHANES, CDC/NCHS
NWS-17.2	Reduce consumption of calories from added sugars	15.7% (2001–2004)	10.8%	NHANES, CDC/NCHS
NWS-17.3	Reduce consumption of calories from solid fats and added sugars in the population aged 2 years or older	34.6% (2001–2004)	29.8%	NHANES, CDC/NCHS
NWS-18	Reduce consumption of saturated fat in the population aged 2 years or older	11.3% (2003–2006)	9.5%	NHANES, CDC/NCHS
NWS-19	Reduce consumption of sodium in the population aged 2 years or older	3641 mg (2003–2006)	2300 mg	NHANES, CDC/NCHS
NWS-20	Increase consumption of calcium in the population aged 2 years or older	1118 mg (2003–2006)	1300 mg	NHANES, CDC/NCHS

(*Continued*)

TABLE 8.2 (CONTINUED)
Healthy People 2020, **Nutrition and Weight Status Objectives**

Objective	Description	Baseline (Year)	2020 Target	Data Source
	Iron Deficiency and Anemia			
NWS-21.1	Reduce iron deficiency among young children aged 1–2 years	15.9% (2005–2008)	14.3%	NHANES, CDC/ NCHS
NWS-21.2	Reduce iron deficiency among young children aged 3–4 years	5.3% (2005–2008)	4.3%	NHANES, CDC/ NCHS
NWS-21.3	Reduce iron deficiency among females aged 12–49 years	10.4% (2005–2008)	9.4%	NHANES, CDC/ NCHS
NWS-22	Reduce iron deficiency among pregnant females	16.1% (2005–2008)	14.5%	NHANES, CDC/ NCHS

Source: US Department of Health and Human Services, Healthy People 2020: Nutrition and Weight Status Objectives. Available at http://www.healthypeople.gov/2020/topicsobjectives2020/objectiveslist.aspx?topicId=29, accessed February 11, 2015.

Note: *Abbreviations:* ARP, Annual Research Program; AWHP, Association for Worksite Health Promotion; BLS, Bureau of Labor Statistics; CDC, Centers for Disease Control and Prevention; CPS, Current Population Survey; DOL, Department of Labor; FDA, US Food and Drug Administration; NAMCS, National Ambulatory Medical Care Survey; NCHHSTP, National Center for HIV/AIDS, Viral Hepatitis, STD, and TB Prevention; NCHS, National Center for Health Statistics; NCI, National Cancer Institute; NHANES, National Health and Nutrition Examination Survey; NIH, National Institutes of Health; NRC, National Resource Center for Health and Safety in Child Care and Early Education; ODPHP, Office of Disease Prevention and Health Promotion; SHPPS, School Health Policies and Practices Study; TBD, to be determined.

- *Information sharing related to regulatory oversight over genetically engineered (GE) plants and the foods derived from such plants (2011).* The Environmental Protection Agency, FDA, and USDA have agreed to share with each other information about GE plants and the foods derived from such plants, including nonpublic information exempt from public disclosure (known as *trade secrets* or *confidential business information*) (US Department of Health and Human Services et al. 2011).
- *Promoting public health and recreation (2008).* The Department of the Interior, Army, Department of Transportation, USDA, and HHS work in concert to promote healthy lifestyles through sound nutrition, physical activity, and recreation in America's great outdoors (US Department of Health and Human Services et al. 2008).

Let's Move!

Launched by First Lady Michelle Obama in 2010, Let's Move! is a comprehensive, nationwide initiative dedicated to solving the challenge of childhood obesity "within a generation" by providing parents with helpful information and fostering environments that support healthy choices (Let's Move! 2010). As part of this effort, President Barack Obama established the first-ever Task Force on Childhood Obesity to help coordinate strategies, identify key benchmarks, and outline an action plan to end the issue of childhood obesity. The goal of this action plan is to reduce the childhood obesity rate to just 5% by 2030, which reflects the obesity rate in the 1970s. In total, the report presents a series of 70 specific recommendations focusing on five areas: early childhood; empowering parents and caregivers; healthy foods in schools; access to healthy, affordable food; and increasing physical activity (Let's Move! 2011).

In addition, the Partnership for a Healthier America (http://ahealthieramerica.org/about/about -the-partnership/)—a nonpartisan nonprofit that brings together public, private, and nonprofit

TABLE 8.3

Healthy People 2020, **Food- and Nutrition-Related Objectives in the Areas of Adolescent Health, Diabetes, Educational and Community-Based Programs, Food Safety, and Heart Disease and Stroke**

Objective	Description	Baseline (Year)	Target 2020	Data Source
	Adolescent Health			
Goal: Improve the healthy development, health, safety, and well-being of adolescents and young adults				
AH-6	Increase the proportion of schools with a school breakfast program	68.6% (2006)	75.5%	SHPPS, CDC/NCHHSTP
	Diabetes			
Goal: Reduce the disease and economic burden of diabetes mellitus (DM) and improve the quality of life for all persons who have, or are at risk for, DM				
D-16.2	Increase the proportion of persons at high risk for diabetes with prediabetes who report trying to lose weight	50.0% (2005–2008)	55.0%	NHANES, CDC/NCHS
D-16.3	Increase the proportion of persons at high risk for diabetes with prediabetes who report reducing the amount of fat or calories in their diet	48.5% (2005–2008)	53.4%	NHANES, CDC/NCHS
	Educational and Community-Based Programs			
Goal: Increase the quality, availability, and effectiveness of educational and community-based programs designed to prevent disease and injury, improve health, and enhance quality of life				
ECBP-10.8	Increase the number of community-based organizations (including local health departments, tribal health services, nongovernmental organizations, and state agencies) providing population-based primary prevention services nutrition	86.1% (2008)	94.7%	NPLHD, NACCHO
	Food Safety			
Goal: Improve food safety and reduce foodborne illnesses				
FS-4	Reduce severe allergic reactions to food among adults with a food allergy diagnosis	29.3% (2006)	21.0%	Food Safety Survey, FDA
	Heart Disease and Stroke			
Goal: Improve cardiovascular health and quality of life through prevention, detection, and treatment of risk factors for heart attack and stroke; early identification and treatment of heart attacks and strokes; and prevention of repeat cardiovascular events				
HDS-9.1	(Developmental) Increase the proportion of adults with prehypertension who meet the recommended guidelines for body mass index (BMI)	N/A	N/A	NHANES, CDC/NCHS
HDS-9.2	(Developmental) Increase the proportion of adults with prehypertension who meet the recommended guidelines for saturated fat consumption	N/A	N/A	NHANES, CDC/NCHS
HDS-9.3	(Developmental) Increase the proportion of adults with prehypertension who meet the recommended guidelines for sodium intake	N/A	N/A	NHANES, CDC/NCHS
HDS-9.5	(Developmental) Increase the proportion of adults with prehypertension who meet the recommended guidelines for moderate alcohol consumption	N/A	N/A	NHANES, CDC/NCHS

(Continued)

TABLE 8.3 (CONTINUED)

Healthy People 2020, Food- and Nutrition-Related Objectives in the Areas of Adolescent Health, Diabetes, Educational and Community-Based Programs, Food Safety, and Heart Disease and Stroke

Objective	Description	Baseline (Year)	Target 2020	Data Source
	Heart Disease and Stroke			
HDS-10.1	(Developmental) Increase the proportion of adults with hypertension who meet the recommended guidelines for BMI	N/A	N/A	NHANES, CDC/NCHS
HDS-10.2	(Developmental) Increase the proportion of adults with hypertension who meet the recommended guidelines for saturated fat consumption	N/A	N/A	NHANES, CDC/NCHS
HDS-10.3	(Developmental) Increase the proportion of adults with hypertension who meet the recommended guidelines for sodium intake	N/A	N/A	NHANES, CDC/NCHS
HDS-10.5	(Developmental) Increase the proportion of adults with hypertension who meet the recommended guidelines for physical activity	N/A	N/A	NHANES, CDC/NCHS
HDS-13.1	(Developmental) Increase the proportion of adults with elevated low-density lipoprotein (LDL) cholesterol who have been advised by a healthcare provider regarding a cholesterol-lowering diet	N/A	N/A	NHANES, CDC/NCHS
HDS-13.3	(Developmental) Increase the proportion of adults with elevated LDL cholesterol who have been advised by a healthcare provider regarding cholesterol-lowering weight control	N/A	N/A	NHANES, CDC/NCHS
HDS-14.1	(Developmental) Increase the proportion of adults with elevated LDL cholesterol who adhere to the prescribed cholesterol-lowering diet	N/A	N/A	NHANES, CDC/NCHS
HDS-14.3	(Developmental) Increase the proportion of adults with elevated LDL cholesterol who adhere to the prescribed cholesterol-lowering weight control	N/A	N/A	NHANES, CDC/NCHS

Source: US Department of Health and Human Services, Healthy People 2020: Diet & Nutrition-Related Objectives. Available at http://www.healthypeople.gov/2020/data-search/Search-the-Data, accessed February 11, 2015.

Note: Abbreviations: CDC, Center for Disease Control and Prevention; FDA, US Food and Drug Administration; NACCHO, National Association of County and City Health Officials; NCHHSTP, National Center for HIV/AIDS, Viral Hepatitis, STD, and TB Prevention; NCHS, National Center for Health and Statistics; NHANES, National Health and Nutrition Examination Survey; NPLHD, National Profile of Local Health Departments; SHPPS, School Health Policies and Practices Study.

leaders to build meaningful commitments and develop strategies to end childhood obesity—also supports the First Lady's cause by encouraging, tracking, and communicating commitments to healthier lifestyles from partner organizations. In collaboration with Let's Move! (http://www .letsmove.gov/partnership-healthier-america), the Partnership will work alongside the federal government to build solutions to fight obesity that can be measured and tracked. As a result, Let's Move! initiatives include all levels of government, the private sector, healthcare professionals, community organizations, parents, and schools, as illustrated in Tables 8.4 and 8.5.

Although this comprehensive initiative sets long-term goals, the temporality of these activities remains in question. Prior executive-level efforts to improve the nation's food and physical activity

TABLE 8.4
Selected Let's Move! Initiatives

Initiative	Description
Let's Move! Cities, Towns and Counties	• Supports local elected officials who are working to build healthier communities. • Local elected officials who sign up must be willing to commit to five goals that are designed to promote the health of local constituents.
Chefs Move to Schools	• Pairs chefs with schools and school districts to help schools improve children's health and nutrition.
Let's Move! Faith and Communities	• Helps faith-based and neighborhood organizations promote healthy living for children and communities. • Children learn many lessons about healthy living and well-being in faith- and community-based settings that set the foundation for their lifestyles as adults.
Let's Move Outside!	• Created to help kids and their families take advantage of being outdoors. • Web page provides ideas on what to do, what to bring, and where to go outside.
Let's Move! Museums and Gardens	• National initiative to provide opportunities for millions of museum and garden visitors to learn about healthy food choices and physical activity through interactive exhibits, children's after-school and summer programs, and healthy food service.
Let's Move! in Indian Country	• Seeks to improve the health of American Indian and Alaska Native children who are affected by childhood obesity. • Tribal governments, urban Indian centers, private businesses, youth leaders, and the nonprofit sector are each asked to play a key role by working together to raise the next generation of healthy children.
Let's Move! Child Care	• A voluntary initiative to empower child care and early education providers. • Helping children get off to a healthy start in child care and early education programs is critical to solving the problem of childhood obesity within a generation.
Let's Move! in the Clinic	• Seeks to engage healthcare professionals through clinical efforts and actions to work with patients to address childhood obesity.
Let's Move! Salad Bars 2 Schools	• An initiative of the Food Family Farming Foundation, National Fruit and Vegetable Alliance, United Fresh Produce Association Foundation, and Whole Foods Market to support salad bars in schools.

Source: Let's Move!, About Let's Move: Initiatives. Available at http://www.letsmove.gov/initiatives, accessed February 11, 2015.

habits, such as HealthierUS initiated in 2002 under President George W. Bush, were retained only in part by the Obama administration. For an example of one sustained activity, see the section on the HealthierUS School Challenge (HUSSC) later in this chapter.

State and Local Action Steps

On the local level, a goal of Let's Move! is to expand community efforts and effective strategies to mobilize public and private sector resources in supporting families to lead healthier lives. From the standpoint of public health nutrition, three of the initiative's most important goals are

1. To help parents make healthy family choices around food and nutrition
2. To serve healthier food in schools
3. To improve access to healthy, affordable food (First Lady Michelle Obama Launches Let's Move 2010)

Promoting wellness at work, in schools, and in community-based settings is an important step in helping people to help themselves. Education and social support can induce people to take charge

TABLE 8.5
Selected Accomplishments of Three Let's Move! Initiatives

Let's Move! Faith and Communities	• Bread for the City is the largest food pantry in Washington, DC. The organization serves 31,609 low-income District of Columbia residents through its medical and legal clinics, as well as its social services program. The organization is well aware that its food pantry may be the only source of healthy foods for the over 9000 people per month who rely on its offerings. • Through grants, this organization is also able to provide a rooftop garden and seasonal free farmers' market that distributes thousands of pounds of free product and helps eligible clients apply for SNAP and WIC benefits.[a]
Let's Move! Museums and Gardens	• The Atlanta Botanical Garden (Georgia) opened an edible garden that includes a green wall made from herbs and an on-site outdoor kitchen, featuring "Grow It and Eat It" cooking demonstrations. • The Detroit Science Center (Michigan) features the "Good Health Can't Weight" exhibit collection. • The Oregon Museum of Science and Industry (Portland, Oregon) touring exhibit "Every Body Eats" explores healthy food choices. • The Children's Museum of Manhattan (New York) is adapting the National Institute of Health's "We Can!" materials to communicate to parents of young children messages about healthy eating habits, balancing food intake, and increasing physical activity.[b]
Let's Move Salad Bars 2 Schools	• In January 2012, Kiana School in Alaska implemented a salad bar in their cafeteria because the cold weather and lack of sunlight limit the fruits and vegetables grown there. Fruits and vegetables are flown in from Anchorage to the coastal town of Kotzebue and then take off again in small aircraft to reach Kiana.[c]

Source: [a]Data from US Department of Health and Human Services, Communities on the Move! Let's Move! Faith & Communities: Resources and Success Stories. Available at http://www.hhs.gov/partnerships/letsmove/communities _on_the_move/, accessed February 11, 2015. [b]Data from Institute of Museum and Library Services, Let's Move! Museums and Gardens. Available at http://www.imls.gov/about/lets_move_projects.aspx, accessed February 11, 2015. [c]Data from Let's Move! Blog, Kiana School in Alaska Gets a Salad Bar, June 18, 2012. Available at http:// www.letsmove.gov/blog/2012/06/18/kiana-school-alaska-gets-salad-bar, accessed February 11, 2015.

of their health. Examples of such initiatives include physical activity strategies such as motivational signs and reminders placed near elevators and escalators encouraging the use of stairs for health benefits or weight loss (Andersen et al. 1998); school health programs that provide environments and instruction that promote healthy eating and daily physical activity, such as the HUSSC (US Department of Agriculture, http://www.fns.usda.gov/hussc/healthierus-school-challenge); and community-based programs that bring together health advisors, nurses, nutritionists, and representatives of faith-based organizations to support, encourage, and help people obtain the information they need for health promotion, and primary and secondary disease prevention.

HealthierUS School Challenge

In 2004, Secretary of Agriculture Tom Vilsack launched the HUSSC. This federal-level, voluntary certification program provides incentives to schools enrolled in Team Nutrition that have created healthier school environments to help address the problems of childhood overweight and obesity. As its name implies, the HUSSC is an extension of HealthierUS, an initiative preceding Let's Move! that encouraged all Americans to eat a nutritious diet and become physically active each day (HealthierUS. gov, http://webarchive.library.unt.edu/eot2008/20080916003723/http:/healthierus.gov/). The HUSSC strives to improve the health of the nation's children by promoting healthier school environments, nutrition, and physical activity in schools. To help meet this goal, the FNS of the USDA (2014) identifies those schools that have made changes to improve the quality of the foods served, provide students with nutrition and physical education, and offer opportunities for physical activity.

The HUSSC program was designed to build upon USDA's Team Nutrition program. To be recognized by the program, K-12 schools must enroll in Team Nutrition and meet higher standards than those required by the National School Lunch Program (NSLP) and School Breakfast Program (SBP), among other criteria (Box 8.3).

Examples of nutrition-related HUSSC criteria are provided in Table 8.6. As part of the criteria, local wellness policies must also be consistent with the Healthy, Hunger-Free Kids Act of 2010 (HHFKA, P.L. 111-296) (US Department of Agriculture 2014). Schools apply for the HUSSC by submitting an application in hard copy to their state child nutrition agency or electronically to the USDA, and those receiving a HUSSC award commit to meeting the criteria throughout their 4-year certification period (US Department of Agriculture 2015). As of January 21, 2015, HUSSC awards have been given to schools in 50 states and the District of Columbia, with 7022 schools certified (4773 Bronze, 1315 Silver, 577 Gold, and 357 Gold Awards of Distinction) (US Department of Agriculture 2015).

BOX 8.3   TEAM NUTRITION SCHOOLS

Team Nutrition is an initiative that supports the Child Nutrition Programs through training and technical assistance for food service, nutrition education for children and their caregivers, and school and community support for healthy eating and physical activity.[1] To be designated as a Team Nutrition school, individual schools must submit an enrollment form and agree to the following eight statements:

- Support USDA's Team Nutrition goal and values.
- Demonstrate a commitment to help students meet the *Dietary Guidelines for Americans*.
- Designate a Team Nutrition school leader who will establish a school team.
- Distribute Team Nutrition materials to teachers, students, and parents.
- Involve teachers, students, parents, food service personnel, and the community in interactive and entertaining nutrition education activities.
- Participate in the NSLP/SBP.
- Demonstrate a well-run Child Nutrition Program.
- Share successful strategies and programs with other schools.[2]

Becoming a Team Nutrition school will help schools focus attention on the important role that nutritious school meals, nutrition education, and a health-promoting school environment play in helping students learn to enjoy healthy eating and physical activity. This is achieved through demonstrating a commitment to empower students to make food and physical activity choices that reflect the *Dietary Guidelines for Americans*; making sure school meals that meet these guidelines taste good and appeal to children; building programs on science, education, communication, and technical resources; involving schools and communities; providing age-appropriate messages in the language they speak and the media they use; and focusing on positive messages regarding food and physical activity.[3]

Source:
[1]Data from Food and Nutrition Service, US Department of Agriculture, Team Nutrition, updated February 2, 2015. Available at http://www.fns.usda.gov/tn/team-nutrition, accessed February 10, 2015.
[2]Data from Food and Nutrition Service, US Department of Agriculture, Team Nutrition School Enrollment Form. Available at http://www.fns.usda.gov/sites/default/files/enrollmentform.pdf, accessed February 10, 2015.
[3]Data from Food and Nutrition Service, US Department of Agriculture, Team Nutrition—Join the Team, updated December 16, 2014. Available at http://www.fns.usda.gov/tn/join-team, accessed February 10, 2015.

TABLE 8.6
Examples of 2012 HealthierUS School Challenge Criteria

Food Group	Bronze	Silver	Gold	Gold Award of Distinction
Breakfast Criteria				
Fruits				
# fresh fruit per week	At least 1	At least 1	At least 2	At least 2
Dried fruit must have no added sweetener	X	X	X	X
Grains				
% grains offered weekly that are whole-grain rich	50%	50%	70%	100%
Lunch Criteria				
Vegetables				
# additional 1/2 cup vegetable offering per week from any of three vegetable subgroups	1	1	2	2
Fruits				
# fresh fruit per week	1	2	3	4
Additional Criteria				
Nutrition Education				
(Elementary school) Provided to all full-day students in all grades	X	X	X	X
(Middle school) Offered in at least one grade during the school year	X	X		
(Middle school) Offered in at least two grades during the school year			X	X
(High school) Offered in two courses required for graduation	X	X	X	X
Physical Education				
(Elementary school) Minimum time weekly	45 minutes	45 minutes	90 minutes	150 minutes
(Middle and high school) Offered to at least two grades	X	X	X	X

Source: Food and Nutrition Service, US Department of Agriculture, HealthierUS School Challenge—Recognizing Excellence in Nutrition and Physical Activity. Available at http://www.fns.usda.gov/sites/default/files/2012criteria _chart.pdf, accessed February 11, 2015.

Local Wellness Policies in Schools

The Child Nutrition and WIC Reauthorization Act of 2004 (P.L. 108-205, Sec. 204) requires that each local educational agency participating in a federal school food program develop and implement a local wellness policy as of 2006. In 2010, the Robert Wood Johnson Foundation published a report that summarizes the progress of local wellness policies across the country between school years 2006–2007 and 2010–2011 (Chriqui et al. 2013). The major findings of this report identify areas where progress has been made in adopting and strengthening the written policies, as well as opportunities for improvement. The overall progress shows that in 2010–2011, nearly all (99%) students nationwide were enrolled in a school district with a wellness policy. However, only 46% of these students were in a district that required all five of the wellness policy elements—nutrition education, school meals, physical activity, implementation and evaluation, and competitive foods—and this number had dropped significantly from 56% in 2009–2010. As a result, there continues to be a wide gap in compliance among mandatory policy provisions, mostly in terms of competitive foods and beverages guidelines. However, between 2009–2010 and 2010–2011, the majority of schools complied with the guidelines for nutrition education (95%), school meals (91%), and physical activity goals (90%) (Chriqui et al. 2013).

In 2010, Congress passed the HHFKA (P.L. 111-296, Sec. 204) (US Government Publishing Office 2010), which added new provisions for local school wellness policies related to implementation, evaluation, and progress reporting. Overall, local wellness policies continue to encourage schools to promote student health and nutrition, including preventing obesity and combating problems associated with poor nutrition and physical inactivity (Chriqui et al. 2013). The HHFKA further strengthens these policies so that they may become useful tools in establishing, evaluating, and maintaining healthy school environments (Box 8.4) (US Department of Agriculture 2014).

BOX 8.4   COMPONENTS OF A LOCAL WELLNESS POLICY

At a minimum, local wellness policies must include the following components. Italicized items are new provisions required by the Healthy, Hunger-Free Kids Act of 2010 (P.L. 111-296, Sec. 204).

- Goals for *nutrition promotion* and education, physical activity, and other school-based activities that promote student wellness.
- All foods available on each school campus under the jurisdiction of the local educational agency during the school day must promote student health and reduce childhood obesity.
- The local educational agency permits parents, students, representatives of the school food authority, *teachers of physical education, school health professionals*, the school board, school administrators, and the general public to participate in the development, implementation, and periodic review and update of the local school wellness policy.
- *A requirement that the local educational agency inform and update the public (including parents, students, and others in the community) about the wellness policy's content and implementation.*
- A requirement that the local educational agency periodically measure and *make available to the public an assessment on the implementation*, including (1) the extent to which schools are in compliance with the local school wellness policy, (2) extent to which the local school wellness policy compares with the model local wellness policies, and (3) a description of the progress made in attaining the goals of the local wellness policy.

Source: Healthy, Hunger-Free Kids Act of 2010, Pub. L. no. 111-296, 124 Stat. 3183 (2010), online. Available at http://www.gpo.gov/fdsys/pkg/PLAW-111publ296/pdf/PLAW-111publ296.pdf, accessed January 26, 2015; United States Department of Agriculture Food and Nutrition Service, Comparison Chart of 2004 vs. 2010 Requirements, Local School Wellness Policies, updated June 17, 2013. Available at http://www.fns.usda.gov/sites/default/files/lwpcomparisonchart.pdf, accessed January 15, 2015.

   The USDA was allotted $3 million for fiscal year (FY) 2011 to assist schools in establishing healthy school nutrition environments, reducing childhood obesity, and preventing diet-related chronic diseases. The HHFKA states that the secretary of agriculture shall provide technical assistance that includes (1) resources and training on designing, implementing, promoting, disseminating, and evaluating local wellness policies; (2) modeling of local wellness policies and best practices recommended by nongovernmental organizations and federal and state agencies; and (3) technical assistance as required to promote sound nutrition and establish healthy school nutrition environments (US Government Publishing Office 2010). This assistance, to be provided by the Department of Education (ED), FNS (USDA), as well as HHS and the Centers for Disease Control and Prevention (CDC), includes relevant and applicable examples of schools and local educational agencies that have taken steps to offer healthy options for foods sold or served in schools. Team Nutrition provides resources for establishing and evaluating local wellness and healthy school nutrition environments at http://healthymeals.nal.usda.gov/local-wellness -policy-resources/school-nutrition-environment-and-wellness-resources-0. Additional resources—in the form of a series of seven briefs—are available from the CDC and Robert Wood Johnson Foundation's Bridging the Gap program at http://www.cdc.gov/healthyyouth/npao/wellness.htm (Box 8.5).

BOX 8.5   TEAM NUTRITION LOCAL WELLNESS POLICY RESOURCES

- *Fact Sheets for Healthier School Meals*: fact sheets describing how schools can implement the major recommendations from the *2010 Dietary Guidelines for Americans* within the school meal pattern requirements and nutrition standards.[1]
- *Serving Up MyPlate—A Yummy Curriculum*: a collection of classroom materials that help elementary school teachers integrate nutrition education into math, science, English, language arts, and health to introduce the importance of eating from all five food groups using the MyPlate icon and a variety of hands-on activities.[2]
- *Healthier Middle Schools—Everyone Can Help*: a series of communication tools designed to help engage teachers, principals, parents, food service managers, and students in school wellness efforts.[3]
- *Making It Happen—School Nutrition Success Stories*: a compilation of successful and innovative K-12 schools across the United States that improved their school nutrition environments and the nutritional quality of foods and beverages offered and sold on school campuses.[4]
- *Recipes for Healthy Kids: Cookbooks for Homes, Child Care Centers and Schools*: 30 delicious, kid-approved recipes developed by teams of school nutrition professionals, chefs, students, parents, and other community members.[5]

Source:
[1]Data from United States Department of Agriculture, Food and Nutrition Service, Fact Sheets for Healthier School Meals, published August 21, 2012. Available at http://www.fns.usda.gov/tn/factsheets-healthier-school-meals, accessed February 11, 2015.
[2]Data from United States Department of Agriculture, Food and Nutrition Service, Serving Up MyPlate: A Yummy Curriculum, published October 3, 2012. Available at http://www.fns.usda.gov/tn/serving-myplate-yummy -curriculum, accessed February 11, 2015.
[3]Data from United States Department of Agriculture, Food and Nutrition Service, Resource Library—Healthier Middle Schools, Team Nutrition, published January 29, 2014. Available at http://www.fns.usda.gov/tn/resource -library-healthier-middle-schools, accessed February 11, 2015.
[4]Data from United States Department of Agriculture, Food and Nutrition Service, Making It Happen! School Nutrition Success Stories, updated February 12, 2014. Available at http://www.fns.usda.gov/tn/making-it-happen -school-nutrition-success-stories, accessed February 11, 2015.
[5]Data from United States Department of Agriculture, Food and Nutrition Service, Recipes for Healthy Kids: Cookbook for Homes, published January 17, 2014. Available at http://www.fns.usda.gov/tn/recipes-healthy-kids -cookbook-homes, accessed February 11, 2015.

MICRONUTRIENT FORTIFICATION AND LABELING

Fortification of the food supply has long been used as a tool to help meet people's nutrient needs (Gerrior et al. 2004). In addition to the calorie menu labeling policy described in the beginning of this chapter, there are a number of other current and proposed labeling policies at the federal and state levels.

MICRONUTRIENT FORTIFICATION: BACKGROUND

Examples include the micronutrient fortification of salt, milk, and water, and the enrichment of grain products. *Enrichment*, in the United States, usually refers to a food product that has nutrients added to replace those lost in processing, such as those added to refined flour, whereas *fortified* refers to the addition of vitamins not originally found in the food, such as vitamin D added to milk or soy beverages, but the terms *fortified* and *fortification* are often used to generally cover both situations. Food fortification and enrichment are governed by FDA rules (standards of identity) but remain voluntary in the sense that manufacturers are not required to produce enriched or fortified food products. However, if a manufacturer chooses to produce and market food as enriched or fortified, they must follow FDA regulations.

Iodization of Salt

Fortification in the United States began in 1924 when iodized salt was introduced in Michigan, resulting in a decrease from 38.6% to 9% in the prevalence of goiter in that state. The success of these efforts made the Michigan experience with iodized salt one of the most noteworthy food fortification programs in applied public health in the twentieth century. Between 1924 and 1928, the use of iodized salt spread rapidly throughout the country. Salt manufacturers were eager to produce the iodized product because, from a marketing perspective, it made sense to offer the (literally) new and improved salt. Doing so was an assurance the salt producers would not lag behind the competition (Bishai and Nalubola 2002). Table salt continues to be available without iodide as well as in the iodized form.

Fortification of Milk with Vitamins D and A

In 1921, it was estimated that 75% of infants in New York City were afflicted with rickets. By the 1930s, rickets was recognized as a major public health problem in the United States, particularly in the northeastern states. Accordingly, the practice of supplementing cow's milk with chemically synthesized vitamin D was initiated, given the high consumption of milk within the population. Fortified milk has nearly eliminated this disorder in the United States.

The concentration of vitamin D in cow's milk has been estimated to be between 5 and 40 international units (IU) per liter (Reeve et al. 1982), rather low from the perspective of the 400–800 IU per day (depending on age) recommended by the Food and Nutrition Board of the Institute of Medicine (IOM):

- Birth–1 year: 400 IU (10 µg, Adequate Intake [AI]).
- 1–70 years: 600 IU (15 µg, Recommended Dietary Allowance [RDA]).
- >70 years: 800 IU (20 µg, RDA) (Institute of Medicine and Food and Nutrition Board 2011).

In the United States, nearly all milk is now voluntarily fortified with 400 IU vitamin D per quart (385 IU/L) (Institute of Medicine and Food and Nutrition Board 2011). Most fat-free milk and dried nonfat milk solids sold in the United States are also fortified with vitamin A (a fat-soluble vitamin) to replace the amount lost when the fat is removed from the whole milk.

Enrichment and Fortification of Grain Products

In 1941, President Franklin D. Roosevelt convened the National Nutrition Conference for Defense, which led to the first recommended dietary allowances of nutrients and resulted in the issuance of

War Order Number 1, a program to enrich wheat flour with vitamins and iron (Achievements in public health 1999). With the end of World War II, the FDA established formal standards of identity specifying the nutrients to be added to food items marketed as enriched: pasta (1946), white bread (1952), cornmeal and grits (1955), and white rice (1958) (Backstrand 2002).

Folic acid was added to the "enrichment formula" for cereal and other grain products in order to prevent neural tube defects. In 1996, the FDA introduced mandatory fortification of all enriched cereal-grain products with folic acid at a dose of 140 µg/100 g of cereal-grain (about double what was originally intended) (US Department of Health and Human Services and US Food and Drug Administration 1996). The prevalence of low serum folate in the population has decreased from a range of 16–22% prior to the fortification program to 0.5–1.7% subsequent to fortification (Pfeiffer et al. 2005).

How long will the fortification of grains with folic acid continue? Vitamin B_{12} deficiency is common in older people, with prevalence increasing from about 5% at 65 years of age to 20% at the age of 80. Clinicians have voiced concern about the safety of elevated intakes of folate in older people who have low vitamin B_{12} status. Such people appear to have a more rapid deterioration of cognitive function in the presence of a high folate intake. This concern has delayed the introduction of mandatory folic acid fortification in the United Kingdom (Clarke 2006).

Fluoridation of Water

Fluoridation of community drinking water, begun in 1945, is a major contributor to the decline in dental caries (tooth decay) during the second half of the twentieth century. The history of water fluoridation is a classic example of clinical observation leading to epidemiologic investigation and community-based public health intervention. Although other fluoride-containing products are available (such as toothpastes, gels, mouth rinses, tablets, and drops), water fluoridation remains the most equitable and cost-effective method of delivering fluoride to most members of most communities regardless of age, educational attainment, or income level. Water fluoridation is especially beneficial for communities of low socioeconomic status, which have a disproportionate burden of dental caries and have less access than higher-income communities to dental-care services and other sources of fluoride. Water fluoridation may help reduce such dental health disparities.

Slightly more than two-thirds of the people in the United States (67% or 211 million) were receiving fluoridated water in 2012, including 11 million people served by over 6000 public water systems that have natural fluoride levels greater than or equal to 0.7 ppm. However, approximately 103 million Americans do not have access to fluoridated water, including nearly 89% of Hawaii residents, 85% of New Jersey residents, and 77% of Oregon residents (Centers for Disease Control and Prevention 2012). There is no universal consensus on the desirability of fluoridating the water supply; concomitant with the decline in dental caries prevalence and incidence in developed countries has been an increase in the prevalence of dental fluorosis (Warren and Levy 2003). Still, Healthy People 2020 calls for about 80% of the population served by community water systems to receive optimally fluoridated water by 2020 (US Department of Health and Human Services, http://www.healthypeople.gov/2020/topicsobjectives2020/objectiveslist.aspx?topicId=32).

Since the early days of community water fluoridation, the prevalence of dental caries has declined in communities both with and without fluoridated water in the United States. This trend has been attributed largely to the diffusion of fluoridated water to areas without fluoridated water through bottling and processing of foods and beverages in areas with fluoridated water as well as the widespread use of fluoride toothpaste (Centers for Disease Control and Prevention 1999). On the other hand, the increased consumption of bottled water, with its variable fluoride content, can lead to a decreased exposure to fluoride among some segments of the population. Solely drinking bottled water may not provide sufficient fluoride to maintain optimal dental health (Bartels et al. 2000; Johnson and DeBaise 2003; Lalumandier and Ayers 2000). FDA requires that fluoride be listed on the label of bottled waters only if the bottler adds fluoride during processing; the concentration of fluoride is regulated but does not have to be stated on the label. Few bottled water brands have labels listing the fluoride concentration (Centers for Disease Control and Prevention 2001).

FOOD ALLERGEN LABELING

Food allergy is an immunologic disease responsible for substantial morbidity and some mortality in the US population. It occurs in 5% of infants and young children and 2% of adults. Approximately 30,000 anaphylactic episodes and 150 deaths per year are due to food allergy (US Food and Drug Administration 2014). Published reports document the increasing prevalence of food allergy and food-induced anaphylaxis, but the reasons for these increases are poorly understood. (See Chapter 13 for additional information on food allergies and labeling.)

Eight foods (milk, eggs, fish, crustacean shellfish, tree nuts, peanuts, wheat, and soybeans) cause over 90% of all allergic reactions to foods (US Food and Drug Administration 2014). The most effective strategy to prevent an allergic episode is strict food avoidance. Since its founding, the Food Allergy and Anaphylaxis Network (FAAN) has advocated for simple, clear, and accurate food labels that would allow allergic people to make informed choices about the foods they eat. In 2012, FAAN merged with the Food Allergy Initiative—a group of concerned parents and grandparents committed to advancing food allergy research—to form Food Allergy Research & Education (FARE, http://www.foodallergy.org/about/history), the nation's leading organization dedicated to food allergy research, education, advocacy, and awareness (Box 8.6).

BOX 8.6   FOOD ALLERGY RESEARCH & EDUCATION (FARE)

Formed in 2012, FARE is the world's largest private source of funding for food allergy research and the leading national organization working on behalf of the millions of Americans with food allergies. FARE is the result of a merger between two long-standing organizations, the Food Allergy and Anaphylaxis Network (FAAN) and the Food Allergy Initiative (FAI):

- Founded in 1991 by Anne Muñoz-Furlong, FAAN designed and offered educational programs, resources, and training tools to individuals and families, educators, health professionals, camp personnel, restaurant staff, food manufacturers, and others. FAAN's accomplishments included involvement in the Food Allergen Labeling and Consumer Protection Act of 2004 (FALCPA), the creation of Food Allergy Awareness Week, and educational programs taught in schools across the country. FAAN played a major role in raising public awareness of the seriousness of food allergies.
- FAI was founded in 1998 by a group of concerned parents and grandparents committed to advance food allergy research, a field that received little federal or private support at the time. FAI invested in clinical trials of new therapies, basic research, and epidemiological studies in the United States and abroad. Many FAI-funded projects were conducted in partnership with federal agencies, including the National Institutes of Health (NIH). FAI's advocacy was critical in increasing the federal investment in food allergy research, from $4 million in 2004 to $31 million in 2014.

FARE's website (http://www.foodallergy.org) provides a number of resources searchable by audience, as well as tips for managing food allergies at home, work, school, college, and camp; while traveling; and when dining out.

Source: Food Allergy Research & Education. Available at http://www.foodallergy.org/, accessed February 10, 2015.

Due in part to FAAN's advocacy, the Food Allergen Labeling and Consumer Protection Act of 2004 (FALCPA) was passed in 2004 (US Government Publishing Office 2004). The law, effective January 1, 2006, requires the labeling of any food containing a protein derived from one or more of the following: milk; eggs; fish (e.g., bass, flounder, cod); crustacean shellfish (e.g., crab, lobster, shrimp); tree nuts (e.g., almonds, pecans, walnuts); peanuts; wheat; and soybeans.

Gluten-Free Labeling

In the United States, an estimated 3 million Americans suffer from celiac disease. Celiac disease is a chronic inflammatory autoimmune disorder, whereby the consumption of gluten triggers the production of antibodies that attack and damage the lining of the small intestine. Such damage limits an individual's ability to absorb nutrients, increasing the risk of nutritional deficiencies, osteoporosis, growth retardation, infertility, miscarriages, short stature, and intestinal cancers.

There is no cure for celiac disease. Therefore, the only way to manage this disease is to avoid eating gluten-containing foods. Gluten is a protein that occurs naturally in wheat, rye, barley, and crossbreeds of these grains, and is typically found in breads, cakes, cereals, pastas, and many other foods (US Food and Drug Administration 2015). Unless food products are properly labeled, consumers may not know whether a food contains gluten, which could cause serious health complications for those with celiac disease.

As a result, the FALCPA directed HHS to define the term *gluten-free* for use in food labels. In 2007, the FDA published a proposed rule that defined the term *gluten-free* as food that does not contain any of the following: (1) an ingredient that is any type of wheat, rye, barley, or crossbreed of these grains; (2) an ingredient that is derived from these grains and that has not been processed to remove gluten; or (3) an ingredient that is derived from these grains and that has been processed to remove gluten, if it results in the food containing 20 or more ppm gluten. More than 6 years after the FDA (2014) published its proposed rule in 2007, the final rule was published on August 5, 2013 with full compliance required by August 5, 2014.

The final rule was issued under the authority of FALCPA and establishes requirements for the use of gluten-free claims. Manufacturers can voluntarily use the gluten-free claim to clearly inform consumers about which of their foods meet FDA's gluten-free requirements (US Food and Drug Administration 2014). As of August 5, 2014, manufacturers must be in compliance with the rule, meaning that if a food label bears the claim "gluten-free," "free of gluten," "without gluten," or "no gluten" but fails to meet the requirements as listed above, the food would be considered misbranded and subject to regulatory enforcement action by FDA.

Labeling of Genetically Modified Organisms

Altering genetic material in a way that does not occur naturally results in a GE or genetically modified organism (GMO). In other words, these plants or animals have been genetically manipulated with genetic material from bacteria, viruses, or other plants and animals (Non-GMO Project, http://www.nongmoproject.org/learn-more/what-is-gmo).

Although many characteristics of food products are required to be identified on the label, as of the end of 2014, the fact that a food product is genetically modified is not one of those characteristics. (See Chapter 13 for more on GMOs.)

GMOs are in 80% of processed foods and also account for varying amounts of nonprocessed foods (Non-GMO Project, http://www.nongmoproject.org/learn-more/). In the United States, circa 2010–2011, about 95% of the sugar beet crop, 94% of the soy crop, 90% of the canola crop, 88% of corn (including sweet corn), and most of the Hawaii crop of papaya are genetically modified. Other crops include cotton, alfalfa (first planted in 2011), and zucchini and yellow summer squash (Non-GMO Project, http://www.nongmoproject.org/learn-more/what-is-gmo).

The purpose of genetically altering foods is to increase the quantity, nutritional content, and/or disease-resistance qualities in order to efficiently feed an ever-growing population. Some argue that GMOs can mitigate world hunger or provide critically needed nutrients for countries whose main dietary staple is rice. For example, golden rice (rice that has been genetically engineered to produce and accumulate beta-carotene) has been in development since the 1980s (Golden Rice Project, http://www.goldenrice.org).

In the United States, GMOs were first approved by the FDA in 1982 and were introduced to grocery stores 12 years later. Yet questions around consumer and environmental safety have grown in recent years. Many food activists highlight evidence that GE foods are unsafe, pointing to studies with animals such as rats, chickens, cows, and pigs. For example, in one experiment, pigs that were fed GE corn and soy experienced higher stomach inflammation than those that ate conventional food (Carman et al. 2013). But according to the World Health Organization (WHO, http://www.who.int/foodsafety/publications/biotech/20questions/en/), GM foods on the international market that "have passed risk assessments are not likely to present risks for human health." These safety assessments evaluate GMOs based on six criteria: toxicity, allergenicity, specific components thought to have toxic or nutritional properties, stability of the inserted gene, nutritional effects, and unintended effects (Non-GMO Project, http://www.nongmoproject.org/learn-more/what-is-gmo).

In addition to the potential impact on human health, concerns have been raised about the environmental effects of GMOs. More than 80% of GMOs grown worldwide are engineered for herbicide tolerance (Non-GMO Project, http://www.nongmoproject.org/learn-more/what-is-gmo), which is a plant's ability to resist the toxic effects of certain chemicals used to eliminate weeds. As a result, crops can continue to grow and thrive even in the presence of the applied chemical (UC Davis Seed Biotechnology Center, http://sbc.ucdavis.edu/files/191418.pdf). Other issues of concern include the loss of biodiversity and the increased use of chemicals in agriculture.

Recently, consumers have expressed growing interest in knowing whether their foods are produced using genetic engineering. Yet genetic modification is not something that can be determined through sight, taste, or smell. This has led to national and international calls for GMO labeling. As of January 2015, 64 countries require the labeling of GMO foods, including 15 nations in the European Union, as well as Japan, Australia, Russia, New Zealand, and China, though the GMO labeling policies vary from country to country (Just Label It, http://justlabelit.org/right-to-know/labeling-around-the-world/).

In the United States, GMO labeling is not mandatory; however, in 2013–2014 alone, over half of the states attempted to pass laws surrounding different facets of the GMO debate (Kucinich 2014). Table 8.7 provides a selection of enacted and pending GMO-related bills. Some of the common themes incorporated in potential legislation have included GE food labeling, food misbranding, use of GE seeds or plants to grow agriculture, and the opposition of GE plants and salmon. For example, Alaska enacted a joint resolution (HJR 5) on March 25, 2013, that opposes the FDA's preliminary finding that genetically modified salmon would not significantly impact the environment and requests further examination of the consequences of releasing GE fish into US waters. The resolution also states that, if the FDA approves GE salmon, product labeling requirements should include the words "genetically modified" prominently displayed on the front of the package. Hawaii also passed a resolution (SR 85) on April 3, 2014, that requests the state's congressional delegation to introduce legislation in the US Congress to clarify food labeling requirements for GMO foods. Connecticut enacted a law (Act 13-183) on June 25, 2013, that requires labeling of GE foods and seed with the phrase "produced with genetic engineering." Maine enacted a law (Chapter 436 of the Public Laws of the 126th Maine Legislature) on January 12, 2014, that requires disclosure of genetic engineering of any food at the point of retail sale. Lastly, Vermont passed a GE labeling law (Act 120) on May 8, 2014, requiring that food offered for sale in Vermont after July 1, 2016, be labeled as produced entirely or in part from genetic engineering using the phrase "produced with genetic engineering."

TABLE 8.7

Selection of Enacted and Pending GMO-Related Bills (as of May 28, 2014)

State	Bill	Year	Status	Summary
Alaska	HJR 5	2013	Enacted	Opposes FDA's finding that GE salmon would not significantly impact the environment Urges further examination of GE salmon Requests that GE salmon, if approved for use, be labeled as genetically modified
Connecticut	H 6527	2013	Enacted	Requires labeling of GE food
California	S 1381	2014	Pending	Requires labeling of GE food
Georgia	H 1152	2014	Pending	Requires labeling of GE food
Hawaii	SR 85	2014	Enacted	Requests the state's congressional delegation to introduce legislation in US Congress to clarify food labeling requirements of GMO foods
Hawaii	S 2454	2014	Pending	Establishes a GMO task force to determine whether the state should regulate the agricultural use of GMOs
Maine	H 490	2014	Enacted	Requires labeling of GE food
Massachusetts	H 3996	2014	Pending	Requires labeling of GE food
Missouri	S 533, H 1396	2014	Pending	Requires labeling of GE food
New Hampshire	S 411	2014	Pending	Requires labeling of GE food
New Jersey	S 91, A 1359	2014	Pending	Requires labeling of GE food
New York	A 3525	2014	Pending	Requires labeling of GE food
Vermont	S 89	2014	Enacted	Requires labeling of GE food

Source: National Conference of State Legislatures, Agriculture and Rural Development Legislation Database, updated March 25, 2014. Available at http://www.ncsl.org/research/agriculture-and-rural-development/agriculture-and-rural-development-legislation-data.aspx, accessed February 11, 2015.

One of the main challenges in GMO labeling in the United States is the vast number of concerned stakeholders, ranging from the FDA and food manufacturers to consumers. Both supporters and opponents of GMO labeling use a variety of arguments to justify their position. Supporters of mandatory labeling, primarily consumers, argue for their right to know what is in the food they are purchasing (Raab and Grobe 2003). Those opposed to mandatory labeling, such as food processors and retailers, argue that the FDA already requires labels on foods that pose a potential health risk (e.g., nuts) and that the FDA has not found conclusive evidence of any such risk with GE foods. In addition, food processors forecast an increased cost for both consumers and the food industry (Carter and Gruere 2003). Aside from the cost of changing the actual label, food producers predict a loss of sales stemming from a negative reaction to a GMO designation. Overall, the possible change in any government policy inevitably comes with arguments from opponents and proponents, and the issue of GMO labeling continues to ignite a fierce debate.

NUTRITION LABELING

Until the late 1960s, information on the nutrient content of foods was rarely available to consumers on food labels, mainly because most meals were prepared at home from basic ingredients and there was little demand for nutritional information. However, as the number of processed foods on the market increased, consumers requested information that would help them understand the products they were purchasing. In response, the 1969 White House Conference on Food, Nutrition, and Health recommended that the FDA consider developing a system for identifying the nutritional content of food. In 1972, the FDA proposed regulations outlining a specific format to provide nutrition information on packaged food labels; however, the inclusion of this information was voluntary (except when nutrition claims were made on the label, in labeling, or in advertising, or when nutrients were added to the food). Nutrition labels, when used, were to include the number of calories; grams of protein, carbohydrate, and fat; and RDA of protein, vitamins A and C, thiamin, riboflavin, niacin, calcium, and iron. Sodium, saturated fat, and polyunsaturated fat could also be added at the manufacturer's discretion. All nutrient information was to be reported on the basis of an average or usual serving size (Institute of Medicine 2010).

As new knowledge about the relationship between diet and disease grew, consumers demanded more information on food labels, leading to an increase in food manufacturers' use of new and undefined (and at times misleading) health claims on product labels. During the late 1980s and early 1990s, several changes were made to standardize nutrition claims and require uniform nutrition labeling. Most significantly, the NLEA of 1990 granted the FDA explicit authority to require nutrition labeling on most food packages and specified the nutrients to be listed on the nutrition label. It also required that nutrients be presented in the context of the daily diet; required that serving sizes represent a typical amount consumed and are expressed in a common and appropriate household measure; and provided for a voluntary nutrition labeling program for raw fruits, vegetables, and fish. The USDA, which oversees meat and poultry, adopted the NLEA requirements for meat and poultry product labels for consistency (Institute of Medicine 2010).

Final regulations mandating nutrition labeling in the form of a Nutrition Facts panel on most packaged foods for both agencies were published in 1993. Nutrients required to be listed on nutrition labels include calories, calories from fat, total fat, saturated fat, cholesterol, sodium, total carbohydrate, dietary fiber, sugars, protein, vitamins A and C, calcium, and iron. The regulations established the Daily Reference Values (DRVs) to be used in reporting values of total fat, saturated fat, cholesterol, total carbohydrate, dietary fiber, protein, sodium, and potassium (all other required nutrients had RDAs established at the time). Regulations also established general principles for the use of nutrient content claims and health claims (Institute of Medicine 2010). Figure 8.1 shows the Nutrition Facts label as required by the 1993 federal policy.

Since 1993, minor changes to the label policy have been made, including the addition of trans fatty acids to nutrition labels and amendment of regulations pertaining to sodium levels in foods that use the term "healthy" on product labels (Institute of Medicine 2010). Despite the availability of nutrition information on food products, Americans are eating larger serving sizes, and rates of obesity, heart disease, and diabetes remain high. As such, in 2005, the FDA began seeking comments on amending the nutrition label. In March 2014, the FDA published a proposed rule to update the list of nutrients that are required or permitted to be declared on the label; provide updated DRVs and Reference Daily Intake values based on current dietary recommendations; amend requirements for foods meant for children under 4 years old and pregnant and lactating women and establish nutrient reference values for these subgroups; and revise the format and appearance of the Nutrition Facts label (US Food and Drug Administration 2014). Specific proposed changes are shown in Figure 8.2 (Box 8.7).

Following the publication of the proposed rule on March 3, 2014, a 90-day comment period ensued to solicit the public's feedback and suggestions, both positive and negative. Based on comments received, the FDA may make modifications before publishing the final rule. Once the final rule is published, it will become effective 60 days afterward, and businesses will be expected to comply with the new rules within 2 years of the effective date (US Food and Drug Administration 2014). As of January 2015, the FDA's final rule remains pending.

Nutrition Facts

Serving Size 1 cup (228g)
Servings Per Container 2

Amount Per Serving	
Calories 260	Calories from Fat 120

	% Daily Value*
Total Fat 13g	**20%**
Saturated Fat 5g	**25%**
Trans Fat 2g	
Cholesterol 30mg	**10%**
Sodium 660mg	**28%**
Total Carbohydrate 31g	**10%**
Dietary Fiber 0g	**0%**
Sugars 5g	
Protein 5g	

Vitamin A 4%	•	Vitamin C 2%	
Calcium 15%	•	Iron 4%	

*Percent Daily Values are based on a 2,000 calorie diet.
Your Daily Values may be higher or lower depending on
your calorie needs:

	Calories:	2,000	2,500
Total Fat	Less than	65g	80g
Sat Fat	Less than	20g	25g
Cholesterol	Less than	300mg	300mg
Sodium	Less than	2,400mg	2,400mg
Total Carbohydrate		300g	375g
Dietary Fiber		25g	30g

Calories per gram:

Fat 9	•	Carbohydrate 4	•	Protein 4

FIGURE 8.1   Nutrition Facts label. (Original file available at http://ecfr.gpoaccess.gov/graphics/pdfs/er11jy03 .001.pdf.) (From 21 CFR 101.9(d)(12).)

HUNGER, AGRICULTURE, AND PUBLIC HEALTH

POLICY REGARDING DOMESTIC HUNGER

The federal government initially responded to hunger among the low-income US population during the Depression. Interest waned during the Second World War and the Korean War. In the 1960s, the federal government was again forced to acknowledge hunger's presence in the United States by a study entitled *Hunger, USA* and a documentary called *Hunger in America* (Nestle and Guttmacher 1992). The ensuing social pressure resulted in a "nutrition safety net," comprised of programs such as WIC.

The face of hunger has changed during the past century, from that of the rail-thin Appalachian farmer to that of the overweight, minority urbanite. During this time, the concept of food insecurity and the contradiction of food deprivation and obesity, rather than frank malnutrition, have become the dominant issues facing victims of domestic hunger.

First Half of the Twentieth Century

At the beginning of the twentieth century, matters pertaining to the well-being of poor citizens in the United States were left to local charities rather than the federal government. With the advent of the Depression in the 1930s, the conditions of the poor, particularly widespread hunger, became a

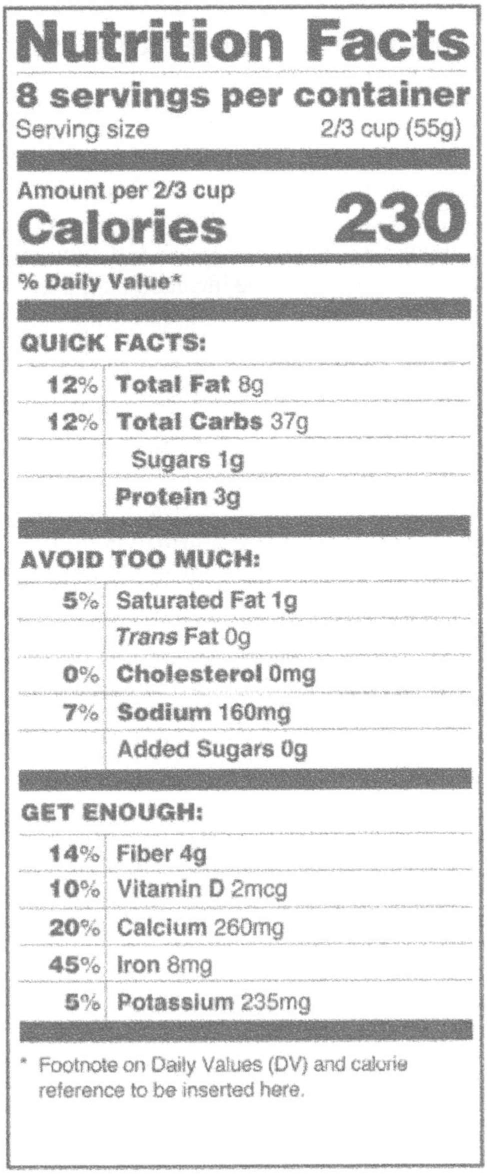

Nutrition Facts

8 servings per container

Serving size · 2/3 cup (55g)

Amount per 2/3 cup

Calories · **230**

% Daily Value*

QUICK FACTS:

12%	**Total Fat** 8g	
12%	**Total Carbs** 37g	
	Sugars 1g	
	Protein 3g	

AVOID TOO MUCH:

5%	Saturated Fat 1g
	Trans Fat 0g
0%	**Cholesterol** 0mg
7%	**Sodium** 160mg
	Added Sugars 0g

GET ENOUGH:

14%	Fiber 4g
10%	Vitamin D 2mcg
20%	Calcium 260mg
45%	Iron 8mg
5%	Potassium 235mg

* Footnote on Daily Values (DV) and calorie reference to be inserted here.

FIGURE 8.2 Proposed Nutrition Facts label. (Original file available at https://s3.amazonaws.com/images .federalregister.gov/ep03mr14.002/original.png.) (From US Food and Drug Administration, *Federal Register*, 79, 2014.)

national concern. In response, President Franklin D. Roosevelt launched the New Deal, a suite of federal programs designed to alleviate the widespread unemployment and suffering caused by the prevailing economy conditions. Major initiatives to deal with hunger introduced by way of the New Deal involved the purchase and distribution of surplus agricultural products, which were given to needy families, and Aid to Dependent Children (ADC), which provided cash assistance (welfare) for the care of widows and orphaned children.

Scant attention was paid to the lives and living conditions of Americans in local communities while the government was preoccupied with the external threats occasioned by the Second World War and throughout the 1940s while the United States helped to rebuild war-torn Europe and Japan.

BOX 8.7   PROPOSED CHANGES TO THE NUTRITION FACTS LABEL

- Require information about "added sugars" because Americans are consuming too much.
- Update daily values for sodium, dietary fiber, and vitamin D.
- Require the amount of potassium and vitamin D to be on the label because they are new "nutrients of public health significance." Calcium and iron would remain required, while vitamins A and C could be included on the label voluntarily.
- Remove "calories from fat" because research shows that the type of fat is more important than the amount.
- Change the serving size requirements to reflect how people are currently eating and drinking according to recent food consumption data. By law, serving sizes must be based on the amounts people actually eat, rather than on the amounts they "should" be eating.
- Require packaged foods and drinks that are typically consumed in one sitting to be labeled as a single serving, and nutritional information to be declared for the entire package. For larger packages, manufacturers would have to provide a dual-column label to indicate both "per serving" and "per package" nutritional information.
- Make calories and serving sizes more prominent, given public health concerns over obesity, diabetes, and cardiovascular disease.
- Move the % Daily Value to the left of the label, so it comes first.
- Change the footnote to more clearly explain the meaning of the % Daily Value.

Source: US Food and Drug Administration, Proposed Changes to the Nutrition Facts Label, updated August 1, 2014. Available at http://www.fda.gov/food/guidanceregulation/guidancedocumentsregulatoryinformation/labelingnutrition /ucm385663.htm#Summary, accessed February 11, 2015.

As the nation made the transition from World War II into the Korean War, communism became the dominant interest of political leaders in the mid- to late 1950s. However, with the resumption of economic prosperity and the demise of perceived external threats in the late 1950s to early 1960s, the federal government refocused its attention on internal conditions (Brown 2003).

Second Half of the Twentieth Century

The road to the US national nutrition policy in the 1970s was paved by media coverage of hunger in America during the raised-consciousness era of the civil rights movement and the War on Poverty. In the late 1960s, the nation was stunned to learn of chronic hunger and malnutrition in the South (Galer-Unti 1995). In 1968, the Citizens' Board of Inquiry into Hunger and Malnutrition issued a study, *Hunger, USA* (1968), reporting that millions of citizens suffered from hunger, even extreme malnutrition like that experienced by people in the Third World. Also in 1968, the award-winning documentary *Hunger in America* was televised, which showed the faults of the Food Stamp Program (FSP) in combating hunger in the Mississippi Delta, on Indian reservations, in migrant camps, and in inner cities. Existing food programs were either insufficient or not reaching people who needed them most and, as a result, hunger was widespread (Eisinger 1998). By the end of the decade, the government's failure to adequately address hunger in America was being heavily criticized (Kotz 1969).

Within this climate, President Nixon convened the 1969 White House Conference on Food, Nutri-tion, and Health (National Nutrition Summit 2000, http://www.nns.nih.gov/1969/conference.htm).

The conference, a seminal event that focused public attention on the importance of nutrition in the life and well-being of the US population, led to an action-oriented agenda that helped shape the nutrition safety net. For example, the conference proposed a specific recommendation of food supplementation for high-risk pregnant women and their infants, one of the major factors leading to the creation of what is now known as WIC. Initiatives for food labeling and a feeding program for the elderly were also developed at the conference.

While considerable progress had been made since 1969 in solving the problem of hunger in the United States, there remained serious concerns about household food security in some segments of the population, and there has been a troubling rise in the prevalence of overweight and obesity. Thus, a National Nutrition Summit (http://www.nns.nih.gov/2000/background/background.htm) was convened in 2000 to develop a human nutrition policy for the twenty-first century. The summit identified continuing challenges and emerging opportunities for the United States, focusing on nutrition and lifestyle issues across the life span, particularly those relevant to overweight and obesity. A number of overarching themes emerged from the National Nutrition Summit, as described in Table 8.8, which paved the way for current national nutrition policy regarding nutrition assistance programs and the obesity crisis. Chapter 11 contains an in-depth discussion of the various programs that comprise the nation's nutrition safety net, and Chapter 5 examines programs developed in response to escalating rates of obesity.

US Farm Policy and Health

Beginning in the era of the Great Depression, the USDA created, and continues to support, farm policies that encourage the overproduction of a select few multiple-use agricultural products (bulk agricultural commodities) in an effort to help the American farmer gain economic stability and drive down the price of food. Grains, meats, soybeans, and dairy are current examples of these commodity products. Farmers receive economic subsidies from the USDA's Farm Services Agency to offset the cost of producing these agricultural commodities.

Background

The first American agricultural assistance programs addressed the increased yield patterns these farmers had developed in support of the World War I effort. At the end of the war, farmers continued to grow crops at a record pace, resulting in an oversupply, followed by plummeting prices. The severe economic problems faced by this large segment of society, where about 25% of the US population then resided, needed mitigation. Relief came in the form of the first Agricultural Adjustment Act (AAA) in 1933, which helped stabilize the agricultural sector through guaranteed minimum farm prices and other supply management techniques. This system helped to ensure an abundant supply of food at artificially reduced prices. In effect, the government was encouraging continued increased production by buying the surplus. Since then, farm price and income support programs have formed the core of agricultural policy in the United States.

A common topic in the debate over US farm programs is that current policies were tailored for a time in American agriculture that no longer exists. The United States is no longer a nation of farmers. Furthermore, the change in the structure of farms over the last century raises questions about the efficacy of policies with roots in an agriculturally based economy (Dimitri et al. 2005).

As indicated in Table 8.9, at the beginning of the twentieth century, most of the nation's approximately 6 million farms were small and diversified. Today they are confined to fewer, larger, and more specialized operations. In 1900, 41% of the workforce was employed in agriculture; over a century later, that percentage has dropped to less than 1%. Over the same period, both the US farm population and rural population dwindled as a share of the nation's overall population.

Farming continues to move toward fewer, larger operations producing the bulk of farm commodities, complemented by a growing number of smaller farms. In 2007, 37% of very large family farms ($500,000 or more in annual sales) and 13% of nonfamily farms had gross sales of at least

TABLE 8.8

National Nutrition Summit 2000: General Overarching Themes and Themes Regarding Obesity

Area	General Recommendations[a]	Obesity Recommendations[b]
Federal agency coordination	Improve federal agency coordination and increase partnerships among and between public and private interests to create more visibility for healthy lifestyle behaviors. Draw on the strengths of communities and build partnerships at all levels (e.g., federal, state, local, public, private) to eliminate hunger, improve nutrition, encourage physical activity, and enhance the community food environment.	Better federal agency coordination is needed along with more partnerships of public and private interests at the federal, state, and local levels.
Targeted national campaigns aimed at behavior change in high-risk groups	Based on the research outcomes, identify cost-effective and exemplary health promotion practices and programs; promote national campaigns that target specific behavioral changes (e.g., obesity prevention and treatment, dietary and physical activity habits, behavioral change barriers) among high-risk groups (e.g., elderly citizens, reproductive-aged women, physically inactive adolescents, and children); and employ multichannel and culturally relevant methodologies. Piggyback campaigns on existing national media and education campaigns involving the healthcare system, schools, work sites, and communities.	National campaigns are needed that target specific behavioral change. Interventions should use multichannel and culturally relevant approaches to target high-risk groups such as inactive children and youth who consume diets rich in fat and added sugar.
Education	Educate the public about the various nutrition and physical activity requirements for different populations (e.g., infants, children, reproductive-aged women, and elderly) to facilitate the appropriate implementation of prevention and intervention strategies.	Interventions should use multichannel and culturally relevant approaches to target high-risk groups such as inactive children and youth who consume diets rich in fat and added sugar.
Supportive environments	Supportive environments to promote and practice healthy behaviors are needed.	Prevent overweight and obesity among US citizens through creation of a supportive environment for promoting healthy lifestyles and encouraging people to practice appropriate nutrition and activity behaviors, including changes in the physical environment, health policy, and social norms.
Diet and exercise as primary prevention	Encourage and support healthy dietary and physical activity behaviors across all levels of society to improve health status.	Interventions should use multichannel and culturally relevant approaches to target high-risk groups such as inactive children and youth who consume diets rich in fat and added sugar.

(Continued)

TABLE 8.8 (CONTINUED)
National Nutrition Summit 2000: General Overarching Themes and Themes Regarding Obesity

Area	General Recommendations[a]	Obesity Recommendations[b]
Awareness	Deliver more expertly effective communication of nutrition and health messages intended to raise awareness that hunger continues to exist. Deliver more expertly effective communication of nutrition and health messages intended to raise recognition that poor dietary practices, overweight, and lack of physical activity contribute to poor health.	Prevention and treatment of obesity must become a healthcare priority if the obesity epidemic is to be reversed.
Economics	Conduct economic analyses of the ramifications of poor nutrition and physical inactivity. Food insecurity and the epidemic of obesity may increase the burden on our healthcare system because of comorbidity and related losses in production. Conduct this analytic research through federal agencies and the use of grant programs as a broader base of issues come forward. Examples of economic analyses include the increment in healthcare cost related to obesity, the impact on productivity of workers due to comorbidities, the impact that recruiting physically unfit soldiers places on the military, the impact on Medicare, and the role of food assistance in making the transition from poverty.	Prevention and treatment of obesity must become a healthcare priority if the obesity epidemic is to be reversed.
Research	Conduct applied and behavioral research to identify cost-effective and exemplary health promotion practices and programs. Conduct basic and clinical research to determine how dietary constituents and physical activity influence pathways to health and to identify those who will benefit from dietary change and increased physical activity. Conduct research in the areas of behavioral change, cost-effectiveness of interventions, and identification of exemplary practices and programs to change population behaviors. Conduct research to understand which factors act as barriers to behavioral change and identify the changes that can be made to facilitate positive behavioral change. Conduct research and evaluation to determine how to best communicate these messages to individuals and specific populations.	
Food security	Publicize the message that food security is the foundation of a healthy lifestyle by raising awareness of the links among poverty, hunger, and health to better engage the public in the fight against hunger and poor nutrition. Maintain and strengthen federal nutrition assistance programs as an integral part of every community's nutrition safety net.	

Source: [a]Picciano MF, Coates PM, Cohen BE. The National Nutrition Summit: History and continued commitment to the nutritional health of the US population. *J Nutr.* 2003; 133(6):1942–1952. [b]Stockmyer C, Kuester S, Ramsey D, Dietz WH. National Nutrition Summit, May 30, 2000: Results of the Obesity Discussion Groups. *Obes Res.* 2001;9:41S–52S.

TABLE 8.9

A Century of Structural Changes in US Agriculture

	1900[a]	1930[a]	2000/2002[a]	2009/2012
US rural population as a share of the nation's overall population	60%	48%	28%	17%[b]
US farm population as a share of the overall US population	39%	28%	1%	N/A
Percentage of workforce employed in agriculture	41%	21.5%	1.9%	0.7%[c]
Average size of farms (in acres)	146	151	441	434[d]
Number of farms (in millions)	5.7	6.3	2.13	2.11[d]
Average number of commodities produced per farm	5	4.5	1	N/A

Source: [a]Data from Dimitri, C. et al., The 20th Century Transformation of US Agriculture and Farm Policy, *ERS Electronic Information Bulletin* number 3, June 2005. Available at http://www.ers.usda.gov/publications/eib-economic-information-bulletin/eib3.aspx#.U6yBsqhFyPM, accessed February 11, 2015. [b]Data from The World Bank, Rural Population (% of Total Population), 2012. Available at http://data.worldbank.org/indicator/SP.RUR.TOTL.ZS, accessed February 11, 2015. [c]Data from Central Intelligence Agency, The World Factbook: United States. Available at https://www.cia.gov/library/publications/the-world-factbook/geos/us.html, accessed February 11, 2015. [d]Data from 2012 Census of Agriculture, volume 1, chapter 1: US National Level Data, Table 1, Historical Highlights: 2012 and Earlier Census Years. Available at http://www.agcensus.usda.gov/Publications/2012/Full_Report/Volume_1_Chapter_1_US/st99_1_001_001.pdf, accessed February 11, 2015.

$1 million. These "million-dollar farms" make up about 2% of all US farms, but they account for 53% of the value of production. In fact, million-dollar farms dominate the production of five major farm products: high-value crops (fruits, vegetables, tree nuts, and nursery and greenhouse products); hogs; dairy; poultry; and beef (Hoppe and Banker 2010).

The current larger farms are more productive than were the agricultural operations in the middle of the twentieth century. Advances in plant and animal breeding have facilitated mechanization and increased yields, enhanced by the rapid development of inexpensive chemical fertilizers and pesticides since 1945. As a result, the level of US farm output more than doubled between 1948 and 2011, growing at an average annual rate of 1.49% (US Department of Agriculture 2014).

Despite these changes, the government has continued supporting American farming (albeit through crop insurance programs instead of direct payments), particularly in commodity crop production. Government support, in conjunction with the efficiencies of modern production, drives down the price of the commodities, making vast quantities available to the food industry at low costs. In particular, the low cost of corn, wheat, and soybeans results in the low prices of their by-products, which include high-fructose corn syrup (HFCS), hydrogenated fats, and corn-fed meats (Box 8.8) (Schoonover and Muller 2006).

Health Implications of Current US Farm Policy

Because corn sweeteners and soy- and corn-based fats are inexpensive to produce and procure, the food industry has an incentive to use these inexpensive ingredients in the processed foods they create (Box 8.9). The result is a food supply that contains a large and ever-increasing number of relatively inexpensive, highly caloric food products (Box 8.10).

These foods fall into the very dietary categories that have been linked to obesity. In 2010, of 21,528 new food and beverage products introduced into the market, about three-quarters were candies, beverages, condiments, processed meats, baked goods, breakfast cereals, and desserts—all foods high in added sugars and fats (US Department of Agriculture 2014). Such products taste good, have a long shelf life, provide participation in social trends and the pleasure of trying new

BOX 8.8 CORN AND ITS DERIVATIVES

Corn is one example of an inexpensive bulk agricultural commodity crop that can be developed into many other products.[1,2,3] Corn on the cob is sold in its unprocessed state or is minimally processed to produce corn products such as flours and meals used as an ingredient in home cooking and in mass production of cereals, breads, and other starchy foods. But corn in itself is not a high-value commodity until it is transformed into other items, such as high-fructose corn syrup (HFCS) or animal feed, which, due to the cheap price of the raw ingredients, becomes a valuable way to increase the opportunity for profit in food production.

HFCS has become a food industry staple used as a sweetener to replace sugar in many products. In the 1970s, the price of sugar increased, which led the food industry to explore other options for food sweeteners. Food scientists learned that corn could be converted into a sweetener that is six times sweeter than regular sucrose at a fraction of the cost. HFCS also gives food a longer shelf life, helps avoid freezer burn in frozen foods, gives items a more "natural and fresh" look, and most importantly, is inexpensive to produce. This discovery led the food industry to begin replacing sugar with HFCS in many processed foods, including bread and canned vegetables, over the past 40 years because of its economic benefits. Today, HFCS has replaced sugar as the sweetener in most sweetened carbonated beverages sold in the United States.

Corn can also be manufactured into inexpensive animal feed that allows varying livestock industries to lower their production costs. By using an inexpensive feed to raise livestock, the varying industries are able to sell their product, such as chicken and beef, at a lower price to the food industry. This, in turn, allows fast-food restaurants to sell hamburgers and chicken nuggets on their dollar menu.

Source:
[1] Data from Haddad, L., *Dev. Policy Rev.*, 21, 2003.
[2] Data from Critser, G., *Fat Land: How Americans Became the Fattest People in the World*, Houghton Mifflin Company, New York, 2003.
[3] Data from Tillotson, J., *Annu. Rev. Nutr.*, 24, 2004.

things, and on a per-caloric basis, cost much less than fruits and vegetables. Low-income people find these foods particularly attractive because they are often more available and more affordable than healthier choices (Drewnowski and Darmon 2005).

A dichotomy, therefore, exists between

US nutrition policies that attempt to guide food consumption in the interests of human health, such as the *Dietary Guidelines for Americans*	and	US farm policies that encourage increased food production and food industry objectives that promote increased food consumption.

BOX 8.9 CORN PRODUCTS

Corn products are not fresh food. To make them, you're using corn as an industrial raw material ... I avoid foods with more than five ingredients on the label, and I eat as few processed foods as I can—in particular, anything made with high-fructose corn syrup. It's not evil, but it's a marker of a highly processed food.

Michael Pollan

Source: Q & A Michael Pollan. Think Global, Eat Local, *Washington Post*, June 28, 2006, p. F01.

BOX 8.10   FOOD SUPPLY CALORIES

From 1970 to 2010, *per capita* calories from the US food supply increased from 2109 to 2568 (adjusted for spoilage and waste).

Source: US Department of Agriculture, Economic Research Service, Average Daily per Capita Calories from the US Food Availability, Adjusted for Spoilage and Other Waste. Available at http://www.ers.usda.gov/data-products /food-availability-%28per-capita%29-data-system/.aspx#.U620GajR3jY, accessed February 11, 2015.

Obesity is one marker of how the conflict is proceeding (Tillotson 2003). As a result of this tension, contemporary critics of the system, such as Dr. Marion Nestle and journalist Michael Pollan, argue that US farm policy is one (though not the only) cause of the obesity epidemic.

Corn and Soy

The ability of fast-food restaurants to sell hamburgers inexpensively (for example, the dollar menu) can be linked to cheap commodities. Corn and soybeans are also used to produce low-cost animal feed for the animals that become fried chicken and hamburger patties. Animal feed in the form of soy meal also produces soy oil as a by-product. It therefore contributes not only to the burger but also to the side orders of fried potatoes and fried onion rings. Thus, in the short run, US farm policy makes poor eating habits an economically sensible choice (Schoonover and Muller 2006).

Produce

As discussed, a number of USDA farm policies function as disincentives for American farmers to grow healthier foods (Box 8.11). For example, more subsidies focus on bulk commodities, whereas few have been instituted to encourage the production of fruits and vegetables. High-value produce crops receive a lower level of government economic support and risk management insurance, resulting in more farmers focusing on high-bulk agricultural commodities rather than produce. Although a farmer might generate a higher return in the market for high-value produce, the lack of support makes growing fruits and vegetables a riskier proposition for the farmer. Thus, the subsidized production of agricultural commodities contributes to an artificially depressed production of fruits and vegetables. In the United States, the cost of fresh fruits and vegetables has increased by 40% over the past 20 years, while that of food with dubious nutritional value (junk food) has decreased by 25% when taking inflation into consideration (Box 8.11) (Tillotson 2004).

Social Implications of Current US Farm Policy

Bulk commodity subsidies also discourage farmers from focusing on diverse crops for local consumption. Many rural farm communities are unable to sustain themselves because they concentrate on one bulk commodity. Rural areas now depend on food imports in order to have a diverse food supply in their community. For example, in an agricultural region of southeastern Minnesota, only $2 million of the total $500 million that local residents spent on food went directly to local farmers. This situation has become the norm in many American agricultural communities as a consequence

---

BOX 8.11   COMMODITY SUBSIDIZATION

The government does not subsidize fruit and vegetable production the way it supports corn, soybeans, sugar cane, and sugar beets.

Marion Nestle

Source: Nestle, M., *What to Eat*, North Point Press, New York, 2006.

BOX 8.12   SUSTAINABLE FOOD SYSTEMS

We will not have sustainable food systems merely by working to improve the environment or even by keeping local farmers in business with a two-tiered system: healthy, fresh, local food for the well-off and cheap industrialized food for the poor. Truly sustainable food systems will be those that provide good jobs for all of those working with food and good food for everyone who eats.

Joan Gussow

Source: Gussow, J.D. and Clancy, K.L., *J. Nutr. Educ.,* 18, 1986.

---

of farm policies that reward bulk agricultural commodity products that are, for the most part, not for direct consumption or are distributed out of the community, rather than diverse crops to feed local communities (Waltner-Toews and Lang 2000).

AGRICULTURAL POLICY CHANGES

As we have seen, current policies that encourage overproduction and provide subsidies for bulk agricultural commodities leave farmers of fresh produce at an economic disadvantage (Schoonover and Muller 2006). The challenge to economists, public health experts, and the USDA is to institute changes that will help reverse the effects of current US agricultural policy and provide the general public with a healthier food supply that remains affordable. To succeed, any new farm policies must consider both the health and well-being of the population as well as the economic exigencies of the agricultural and food industry sectors (Box 8.12).

Economic subsidies to encourage farmers to produce healthy foods that are, in turn, economically affordable for the American public could lead to higher consumption of fruits and vegetables and place US farm policy in line with the current dietary guidelines. Creating economic subsidies for high-value produce would also drive down the price of high-value crops, making purchase and production of healthier foods an economically sensible choice for the food industry. For example, the USDA could help improve public health by creating a retail-based mechanism to provide participants in its Supplemental Nutrition Assistance Program (SNAP) with significant monetary incentives to purchase health-promoting foods, such as minimally processed fruits, vegetables, and whole-grain products. This incentive program could be underwritten by redirecting some of the funds currently allocated to annual commodity support payments. The redirected funds could be used to reimburse retailers and wholesaler–distributors for lost revenues and to provide growers and processors with direct payments.

US FARM BILL

The federal omnibus farm policy, popularly known as the "farm bill," serves as the major US agricultural legislation that outlines provisions on commodity programs, trade, conservation, credit, agricultural research, nutrition assistance programs, and marketing. The farm bill is usually renewed every 5 years and is often subject to great debate, as it includes price supports for farmers; environmental, food safety, and trade provisions; and social welfare program allotments, most notably SNAP. SNAP is the nation's largest food and nutrition assistance program (Box 8.13).

The most recent farm bill—the $956 billion Agricultural Act of 2014—was signed into law by President Obama after 4 years of contentious, partisan arguments over farming subsidies and efforts to reduce financing for SNAP. The bill trimmed $8 billion from SNAP over the next decade and eliminated $5 billion in direct subsidies to farmers for their crops, whether they grow them or not. Instead, the federally subsidized crop insurance program was expanded by $7 billion over the next 10 years. Farmers pay for insurance each year and receive payments in the years they take a loss. Eighteen

BOX 8.13   SELECTED HIGHLIGHTS OF FARM BILLS, 1996–2014

Federal Agriculture Improvement and Reform Act of 1996

- Removed link between payments to farmers from the US government and farm commodity prices.
- Replaced adjustable payments with seven annual declining fixed payments independent of farm commodity prices.
- Eliminated programs that paid farmers to idle acreages of land and gave farmers the freedom to plant any crop on contract acres, with limitations on fruits and vegetables.
- Required farmers receiving payments to sign contracts that obligated them to comply with conservation plans, wetland provisions, and planting flexibility stipulations, as well as to continue the agricultural use of the land.
- Dropped requirement for farmers to purchase crop insurance in order to be eligible for payments, so long as the farmer waived eligibility for emergency crop loss assistance.
- Extended the authority of the Food for Progress Program to provide assistance in the administration, sale, and monitoring of food assistance programs to strengthen private-sector agriculture in recipient countries through 2002.
- Amended the Agricultural Act of 1980 to establish a Food Security Commodity Reserve, authorizing a 4-million-ton reserve of corn, grain sorghum, rice, and wheat.
- Reauthorized the Food Stamp Program (FSP) for 2 years, with additional criteria for disqualification of food stores and wholesale food concerns from program violations.
- Reauthorized food distribution and assistance programs, including the Commodity Supplemental Food Program (CSFP), the Soup Kitchen and Food Bank Program, and The Emergency Food Assistance Program (TEFAP).
- Reauthorized appropriations over 2 years for federal agricultural research, extension, and education programs administered by the Agricultural Research Service and the Cooperative State Research, Education, and Extension Service.[1]

Farm Security and Rural Investment Act of 2002

- Continued direct payments for eligible producers of wheat, corn, barley, grain sorghum, oats, upland cotton, and rice; direct payments newly available to producers of soybeans, other oilseeds, and peanuts.
- Required that at least $200 million be spent by the USDA to purchase fruits, vegetables, and other specialty crops, of which $50 million is allotted for fresh fruits and vegetables for schools through the Department of Defense's Fresh program.
- Dedicated $17.1 billion over 10 years in conservation to preserve farmland, save wetlands, and improve water quality and soil conservation on farms.
- Reauthorized Food for Peace program through FY 2007 to help combat hunger and encourage development overseas, and authorized the president to establish the McGovern–Dole International Food for Education and Child Nutrition Program providing US agricultural commodities and financial and technical assistance for foreign preschool and school feeding programs and for pregnant and nursing women and young children.
- Required that, in 2 years, retailers must provide country-of-origin information to consumers for perishable fruits and vegetables, peanuts, fresh beef, lamb, pork, and farm-raised and wild fish/shellfish.

- Reauthorized the FSP with expanded eligibility for noncitizens, increased benefits for larger households, extensive state options to conform food stamp rules to other assistance programs, "transitional" benefits for those leaving cash welfare, a new "quality control" system with eased penalties on states, and a new system of high-performance bonuses to states.
- Reauthorized and added funding to TEFAP and nutrition assistance for Puerto Rico and American Samoa.
- Reauthorized the CSFP and nutrition assistance on Indian reservations.
- Reauthorized university research and state cooperative extension programs at such sums as may be necessary through FY 2007.
- Authorized farmers' market promotion program.
- Created national organic certification cost-share program.
- Created a new USDA assistant secretary for civil rights.[2,3]

Food, Conservation, and Energy Act of 2008

- Continued direct payments, a system that paid producers regardless of whether they incurred losses, but set new standards for farm commodity and disaster program benefit eligibility.
- Established a new disaster assistance program.
- Included a pilot program funded at $60 million over 4 years to evaluate the effectiveness of local or regional procurement of food for humanitarian assistance.
- Renamed the FSP to the Supplemental Nutrition Assistance Program (SNAP) and invested $5.4 billion to the program.
- Increased the minimum SNAP benefit to $14 and indexed the level to future inflation.
- Expanded the Fresh Fruit and Vegetable Program, which provides free fresh fruits and vegetables to low-income children in schools, by investing $1 billion over the next decade.
- Nearly doubled the funding available to food banks for commodity purchases to $1.256 billion.
- Expanded the Senior Farmers' Market Nutrition Program by $50 million.
- Provided $50 million for competitive grants for community food projects, such as school gardens.
- Created the National Institute of Food and Agriculture within the USDA.
- Provided $78 million in mandatory funds for the Organic Research and Extension Initiative and $230 million for the Specialty Crop Research Initiative.
- Funded the Beginning Farmers and Ranchers Development Program with $75 million for FY 2009 to FY 2012.
- Provided $33 million to develop and expand farmers' markets across the country.
- Allotted $377 million over the next decade for a new pest and disease program.
- Required retailers to label the country of origin of meat, fish, fruits and vegetables, ginseng, peanuts, pecans, and macadamia nuts by September 30, 2008.[4]

Agricultural Act of 2014

- Eliminates direct payments and expanded crop insurance.
- Reduces crop insurance premiums during the first 5 years of farming.
- Restores livestock disaster assistance, which expired in FY 2011.

- Provides $200 million for job training and $100 million to increase fruit and vegetable purchases through SNAP.
- Provides $250 million in additional funding for TEFAP.
- Authorizes $125 million for the Healthy Food Financing Initiative to make nutritious food more accessible.
- Provides $100 million for the Beginning Farmers and Ranchers Development Program.
- Renames *FMPP* to *Farmers Market and Local Food Promotion Program* and increases funding to $30 million annually.
- Increases funding for the Specialty Crop Block Grant Program to $72.5 million annually to promote fruit and vegetable production.
- Funds the Organic Cost Share program at $11.5 million annually—a new resource for organic farmers.
- Increases funding for pest and disease management and disaster prevention to $62.5 million per year, and $75 million in FY 2018 and beyond.[5]

Source:
[1]Data from Economic Research Service, US Department of Agriculture, 1996 FAIR Act Frames Farm Policy for 7 Years, Agricultural Outlook Supplement, April 1996. Available at http://webarchives.cdlib.org/sw1vh5dg3r/http:/ers .usda.gov/publications/agoutlook/aosupp.pdf, accessed February 11, 2015.
[2]Data from Becker, G.S., CRS Report for Congress: The 2002 Farm Law at a Glance, Report no. RS21233, June 7, 2002, Congressional Research Service, The Library of Congress. Available at http://digital.library.unt.edu /ark:/67531/metacrs2127/m1/1/high_res_d/RS21233_2002Jun07.pdf, accessed February 11, 2015.
[3]Data from Becker, G.S. and Womach, J., The 2002 Farm Bill: Selected Highlights, updated November 14, 2003, Congressional Research Service. Available at http://www.cnie.org/nle/crsreports/briefingbooks/Agriculture /The%202002%20Farm%20Bill%20Selected%20Highlights.htm, accessed February 11, 2015.
[4]Data from US Senate Agriculture, Nutrition and Forest Committee, Farm Bill: Investments for the Future, The Food, Conservation and Energy Act of 2008, May 8, 2008. Available at http://www.ag.senate.gov/issues/2008 -farm-bill, accessed February 11, 2015.
[5]Data from US Department of Agriculture, 2014 Farm Bill Highlights. Available at http://www.usda.gov/documents /usda-2014-farm-bill-highlights.pdf, accessed February 11, 2015.

companies administer the insurance program and are paid $1.4 billion a year to sell policies to farmers (Nixon 2014). The crop insurance was well appreciated by farmers during the historic droughts of 2012, which impacted more than 80% of the country (US House Committee on Agriculture 2014).

While money for SNAP was reduced, a greater emphasis was placed on increasing the consumption of fruits and vegetables and improving the availability of health food in neighborhoods that have few grocery stores. The current farm bill pays special attention to produce over traditional commodity crops like soybeans and sorghum, as well as organically grown products. These shifts stem from a perceived growing market in addition to profound changes in nutrition policy and eating habits across the country. Policy revisions have come about in efforts to combat childhood obesity and diabetes, as well as in response to highly publicized health campaigns, such as the farm-to-table movement promoted by First Lady Michelle Obama and other national figures (Steinhauer 2014). Funding for fruits and vegetables and organic programs will increase by more than 50% over the next decade, while traditional commodities' subsidies were cut by more than 30% to $23 million. Money to help growers transition from conventional to organic farming rose to $57.5 million from $22 million, and funds for oversight of the nation's organic food program nearly doubled to $75 million over 5 years (Steinhauer 2014).

Proposals for the Next US Farm Bill

Each new federal farm bill provides an opportunity to influence the overall direction of US farm policy. Because the farm bill contains hundreds of programs and provisions that impact the US food system, it provides a unique opportunity to institute policies that foster systemic changes that could lead to a healthier food supply. The Food and Agriculture Policy Collaborative, a partnership of national and local organizations including the Food Research and Action Center (FRAC) and the National Sustainable Agriculture Coalition, recommends the following policy goals:

- Protect and strengthen SNAP, which reduces food poverty, improves nutrition and child health, and increases household food security.
- Expand the Healthy Food Finance Initiative, which supports efforts to improve access to nutritious food at affordable prices, provides flexible one-time grants and loans to fresh food retailers, and creates public–private partnerships to bring economically sustainable businesses providing access to healthy food to underserved areas.
- Create and expand healthy food incentives programs that provide families participating in SNAP with supplemental benefits to purchase locally grown fruits and vegetables at farmers' markets. The programs increase families' access to affordable, nutritious fresh food and increase markets for small and midsized farmers.
- Build a sustainable local and regional food system through policy reform that expands farming and marketing opportunities for new and existing family farmers. Such a system spurs economic growth, expands access to "good food," and helps socially disadvantaged farmers and ranchers have opportunities to acquire, own, operate, and retain farms and ranches (Food and Agriculture Policy Collaborative, http://frac.org/pdf/food_ag_policy _collaborative_hfhe.pdf).

The American Farm Bureau Federation, an independent organization of farm and ranch families, also has a list of grassroots campaigns and priority issues, including the following:

- Securing a reliable and competent workforce for the nation's farms and ranches.
- Protecting proprietary data collected from farming and agricultural operations, as farmers are using technology to better match varieties of seeds with field characteristics.
- Replacing the current federal income tax with a fair and equitable tax system that encourages success, savings, investment, and entrepreneurship.
- Opposing mandatory labeling at the state and federal levels. "Mandatory labels would mislead consumers about the safety of biotechnology, erode the credibility of FDA, and discourage consumer acceptance of new, beneficial technologies."
- Supporting US government involvement in the development of international standards for biotechnology (American Farm Bureau Federation, http://www.fb.org/index.php ?action=issues.home).

In sum, overproduction and the consequent reduction in the cost of some foods is an environmental force favoring the occurrence of obesity. US farm policy, specifically crop subsidies and incentives for bulk agricultural commodities, promotes obesity by creating a relatively inexpensive, high-calorie food source for the food industry to use in the production of low-cost foods replete with added fats and sugars. This creates an environment that conflicts with the Dietary Guidelines' suggestion to limit the amount of sugars and fats in one's diet and makes eating unhealthy foods less expensive in the short term. To improve the food environment in which we live, economists, health experts, and policy makers must promote new farm policies that result in a healthier food supply while not undermining economic prosperity for both the food industry and the American farmer.

TAKING ACTION

Food and nutrition advocates focus on the particular needs of vulnerable segments of the population: low-income children and families; populations with special needs due to age or physiologic status; ethnic, linguistic, and racial minorities; immigrants; and groups at risk due to malnutrition, obesity, disability, and other conditions. Food and nutrition advocates also aim to protect the environment by encouraging the consumption of locally produced, minimally processed food.

Advocacy Goals

Goals of food and nutrition advocacy include

- Education and training.
- Monitoring and modifying food and nutrition policy.
- Developing intervention models.
- Field application of methods.
- Identifying the most successful approaches to alleviating problems of food insecurity and hunger, and to improving the nutritional health of the American population.
- Monitoring and evaluating programs.
- Communicating food and nutrition advice to nutrition and health professionals, policy makers in government and in the private sector, and the American public.
- Advocacy for policy, regulation, and programs designed to advance the health and nutritional status of the American public.
- Advocacy for policy and regulations to protect the environment.

Different approaches are available to affect nutrition policy. Activists can propose new policies, as well as support policies they believe in that have been introduced by others. As an example, the following case study describes the steps taken by the Center for Science in the Public Interest (CSPI) to promote passage of a bill designed to improve school food. CSPI followed the steps necessary for making policy that are outlined at the beginning of this chapter.

Case Study: Promoting the Child Nutrition Promotion and School Lunch Protection Act

1995
- S 1074, the Healthy Lifestyles and Prevention America Act (HeLP America), is introduced in the Senate by Tom Harkin (D-Iowa) on May 18. The legislation was designed as a comprehensive bill to improve the health of Americans and reduce healthcare costs by reorienting the nation's healthcare system toward prevention, wellness, and self-care. Section 102, entitled Child Nutrition Promotion and School Lunch Protection, would require the USDA to apply the same standards for competitive foods as for school lunches, and to apply those standards to all foods sold on campus throughout the school day. The bill was sent to the Committee on Finance, where it remained because it received no congressional support in the form of cosponsors.
- In anticipation of Section 102 being resubmitted as a separate bill entitled the Child Nutrition Promotion and School Lunch Protection Act, CSPI called on nutrition activists to support the legislation. Through the National Alliance for Nutrition and Activity (NANA) and the Internet, CSPI signed on more than 80 national, state, and local organizations to support the bill (see http://www.cspinet.org/new/pdf/nana_coalition.pdf for the list of supporters).

2006
- In April, bipartisan S 2592/HR 5167 was introduced in the Senate and the House.
- In June, CSPI released a compendium of state policies regarding competitive foods. The report demonstrates that most state nutrition policies fail to keep nutrition-poor foods and sugary drinks out of schools. The report, School Foods Report Card, is posted on the CSPI website: http://cspinet.org/new/pdf/school_foods_report_card.pdf.

BOX 8.14   LETTER OF SUPPORT

Dear:

As your constituent, I urge you to cosponsor the bipartisan Child Nutrition Promotion and School Lunch Protection Act (S 2592/HR 5167).

The bill would require the USDA to bring its nutrition standards for foods sold out of vending machines, school stores, and a la carte in line with current nutrition science, and to apply those standards to all foods sold on campus throughout the school day.

In a state-by-state review of school food and beverage policies published in June 2006 (http://cspinet.org/new/pdf/school_foods_report_card.pdf), the Center for Science in the Public Interest found that most states allow far too much junk food to be sold in schools through vending machines and school stores, and on a la carte lines. With junk foods tempting children at nearly every other public place in America, school should be one locale where parents do not need to worry about what their children are eating. Just as Congress has enacted strong nutrition standards for school lunch and breakfast programs, it should take similar steps to assure that all school foods are healthy.

Children's poor diets and rising rates of pediatric obesity are national problems that need a national response. Please let me know if I can count on you to cosponsor S 2592 and HR 5167.

Sincerely,
Name, professional credentials
Contact information

Note: The Center for Science in the Public Interest generously made their materials available for inclusion in this chapter.

- Also in June, CSPI mounted a letter-writing campaign to Congress. Activists on CSPI's e-mail lists were asked to encourage their legislators to cosponsor (support) the bill. CSPI provided a model letter (Box 8.14).

2010–2013

- Fifteen years after the HeLP America Act was introduced, the NANA coalition led the effort to pass the HHFKA. HHFKA authorizes the USDA to update national nutrition standards for all foods sold on the school campus throughout the school day. These standards apply to competitive foods sold through vending machines, a la carte lines, school stores, and fundraisers on campus during the school day.
- Following the release of the USDA's proposed Smart Snacks in School nutrition standards in 2013, NANA continued to advocate for healthier foods in schools with a series of fact sheets, including a comparison of competitive food standards, information on sports drinks, and healthy fundraising ideas (available at http://www.cspinet.org/nutritionpolicy /priority_nutritionprogram.html). The Smart Snacks in School nutrition standards took effect on July 1, 2014.

CONCLUSION

What people choose to eat is affected by far more than personal selection. The foods available through our food system are determined by agricultural and economic policies. US farm policies and nutrition policies often lack coherence and are not necessarily designed specifically to improve the health of US consumers. When our agricultural policies encourage overproduction of energy-dense, low-nutrient foods, these policies are in direct conflict with federal nutritional guidelines, which advocate nutrient-dense, low-energy foods.

Although the focus of the nation's nutritional guidelines and support has shifted from malnutrition in the 1930s to overnutrition presently, the low-income segment of our population remains most negatively affected. Federal and state efforts have already shown success with policies around fortification, labeling, and school food environments. Legislation such as the farm bill as well as local wellness policies can be an effective tool for encouraging production and consumption of fresh fruits and vegetables rather than processed foods dense with added fats and sugars, and in turn, encouraging health.

ACRONYMS

AAA	Agricultural Adjustment Act
ADC	Aid to Dependent Children
AHA	American Heart Association
AI	Adequate intake
CDC	Centers for Disease Control and Prevention
CSFP	Commodity Supplemental Food Program
CSPI	Center for Science in the Public Interest
DRV	Daily Reference Value
ED	US Department of Education
ERS	Economic Research Service
FAAN	Food Allergy and Anaphylaxis Network
FAI	Food Allergy Initiative
FALCPA	Food Allergen Labeling and Consumer Protection Act of 2004
FARE	Food Allergy Research & Education
FDA	US Food and Drug Administration
FNS	Food and Nutrition Service (USDA)
FRAC	Food Research and Action Center
FSP	Food Stamp Program
GE	Genetically engineered
GMO	Genetically modified organism
HeLP America	Healthy Lifestyles and Prevention America Act
HFCS	High-fructose corn syrup
HHFKA	Healthy, Hunger-Free Kids Act of 2010
HHS	US Department of Health and Human Services
HUSSC	HealthierUS School Challenge
IOM	Institute of Medicine
IU	International units
MEAL Act	Menu Education and Labeling Act
MOUs	Memoranda of understanding
NANA	National Alliance for Nutrition and Activity (at CSPI)
NLEA	Nutrition Labeling and Education Act
NSLP	National School Lunch Program
PPACA	Patient Protection and Affordable Care Act
RDA	Recommended Dietary Allowance
SBP	School Breakfast Program
SNAP	Supplemental Nutrition Assistance Program
TEFAP	The Emergency Food Assistance Program
USDA	US Department of Agriculture
WHO	World Health Organization
WIC	Special Supplemental Nutrition Program for Women, Infants, and Children

**STUDENT ASSIGNMENTS AND ACTIVITIES DESIGNED TO ENHANCE
LEARNING AND STIMULATE CRITICAL THINKING**

1. Find a nutrition-related bill that has been introduced recently to Congress (http://www
   .congress.gov). Search the Internet to find out if any organizations are in support or opposition of the bill. Then, write a letter to your legislators in support of or in opposition to the bill.
2. Discuss three guidelines that you think should be added or changed in the development of
   the next set of Dietary Guidelines, and your reasoning for these changes.
3. Read the Healthy People 2020 Midcourse Review. How is the nation progressing in the
   Nutrition and Weight Status Objectives, as listed in Table 8.2? Describe areas where
   improvement is needed, and identify programs and policies that may help the nation meet
   each of these objectives.
4. Obtain the local wellness policy for the school district where you live, work, or attend
   school. Does this policy meet all of the required elements? If not, what is missing?
   Using the resources available through Team Nutrition (http://healthymeals.nal.usda.gov
   /local-wellness-policy-resources/school-nutrition-environment-and-wellness-resources-0)
   and the Centers for Disease Control and Prevention (http://www.cdc.gov/healthyyouth
   /npao/wellness.htm), how could this local wellness policy be strengthened to further
   improve student health?
5. Since the passing of the Healthy, Hunger-Free Kids Act of 2010 (HHFKA), US schools
   have been working hard to meet the updated nutrition standards for school meals. However,
   several groups, including some food companies, Republican politicians, and the School
   Nutrition Association, have been working hard to change legislation so that schools may
   be granted waivers from the requirements if they are losing money. In fact, during the
   2013–2014 legislative session, more than five bills were introduced in Congress to weaken
   or delay the nutrition standards. Using http://www.congress.gov and the Internet, answer
   the following questions:
   • Describe three of the bills introduced in Congress to weaken or delay the nutrition
     standards. What do they propose? How far did each bill progress in the legislative
     process? How many legislative sponsors did each bill have by the end of the 2013–2014
     legislative session?
   • Why is the School Nutrition Association advocating for waivers and relaxed nutrition
     standards, when they helped pass the HHFKA in 2010?
   • Why does improving the health of school food garner so much debate?
6. The Agriculture Act of 2014 (2014 farm bill) cut $8.6 billion in SNAP benefits. Briefly
   discuss the implications of such a large cut in funding.
   Then, read the February 5, 2014, *Washington Post* article by Niraj Chokshi, Why the
   Food Cuts in the Farm Bill Affect Only a Third of States (http://www.washingtonpost
   .com/blogs/govbcat/wp/2014/02/05/why-the-food-stamp-cuts-in-the-farm-bill-affect
   -only-a-third-of-states/), as well as the following materials:
   • FRAC fact sheet: SNAP Cuts = Cuts in Meals for Americans Struggling to Heat and
     Eat (http://frac.org/pdf/snap_cuts_and_heat_and_eat.pdf).
   • CBPP's Greenstein on the cuts: Commentary: Nutrition Title of Farm Bill Agreement
     Drops Draconian Cuts and Represents Reasonable Compromise (http://www.cbpp.org
     /cms/index.cfm?fa=view&id=4081).
   • Feeding America fact sheet: SNAP (Food Stamps): Facts, Myths, and Realities (http://
     feedingamerica.org/how-we-fight-hunger/programs-and-services/public-assistance
     -programs/supplemental-nutrition-assistance-program/snap-myths-realities.aspx#).
   • Senate Agriculture Committee Chairwoman Debbie Stabenow's fact sheet: 2014 Farm
     Bill: Addressing Misuse, Protecting Food Assistance (http://www.ag.senate.gov/newsroom
     /press/release/2014-farm-bill-addressing-misuse-protecting-food-assistance).

Who will be affected by the $8.6 billion in SNAP cuts, and why? What is the issue around "Heat and Eat?" What are the pros and cons of these cuts?

7. Read the following article:

Close, R.S. and Schoeller, D.A., The financial reality of overeating, *J. Am. Col. Nutr.*, 25:203–209, 2996 (http://graphics8.nytimes.com/packages/pdf/business/20061202money3.pdf).

Discuss whether a poor family can afford to pass up "supersizing" a meal at a fast-food restaurant.

8. Numerous comments were received by the FDA in regard to the proposed changes to the Nutrition Facts label. Review 15 of the public comments, available at http://www.regulations .gov/#!docketDetail;D=FDA-2012-N-1210. Choose comments from a variety of stakeholder groups, including consumers, health professionals, food companies, politicians, researchers, etc. What are the arguments for and against the proposed changes? Which groups support these positions, and why? Assuming that the rule has been finalized, how do these comments compare to the final, revised label?

9. Define the term *junk food*. What foods are included and excluded from your definition? Why? Who would support and oppose your definition, and why? Several public health professionals have proposed a "junk food" tax. Based on your definition, do you think this is feasible and appropriate? Explain your answer.

REFERENCES

1969 White House Conference on Food, Nutrition, and Health. Available at http://www.nns.nih.gov/1969 /conference.htm, accessed February 11, 2015.

American Farm Bureau Federation. Farm Bureau Priority Issues. Available at http://www.fb.org/index .php?action=issues.home, accessed January 27, 2015.

Andersen RE, Franckowiak SC, Snyder J, Bartlett SJ, Fontaine KR. Can inexpensive signs encourage the use of stairs? Results from a community intervention. *Ann Intern Med*. 1998;129(5):363–369.

Backstrand JR. The history and future of food fortification in the United States: A public health perspective. *Nut Rev*. 2002;60(1):15–26.

Bartels D, Haney K, Khajotia SS. Fluoride concentrations in bottled water. *J Okla Dent Assoc*. 2000;91(1):18–22.

Bishai D, Nalubola R. The history of food fortification in the United States: Its relevance for current fortification efforts in developing countries. *Econ Dev Cult Change*. 2002;51(1):37–53.

Carman JA, Vlieger HR, Ver Steeg LJ et al. A long-term toxicology study on pigs fed a combined genetically modified (GM) soy and GM maize diet. *J Org Syst*. 2013;8(1):38–54.

Carter C, Gruere G. Mandatory labeling of genetically modified foods: Does it really provide consumer choice? *The Journal of Agrobiotechnology Management and Economics*. 2003;6(1–2):68–70. Available at http://www.agbioforum.org/v6n12/v6n12a13-carter.htm, accessed February 11, 2015.

Center for Science in the Public Interest. *Anyone's Guess: The Need for Nutrition Labeling at Fast-Food and Other Chain Restaurants*. Washington, DC: Center for Science in the Public Interest, November 2003. Available at http://www.cspinet.org/restaurantreport.pdf, accessed January 16, 2015.

Centers for Disease Control and Prevention. Achievements in public health, 1900–1999: Safer and healthier foods. *MMWR*. 1999;48(40):905–913.

Centers for Disease Control and Prevention. Achievements in public health, 1900–1999: Fluoridation of drinking water to prevent dental caries. *MMWR*. 1999;48(41):933–940. Available at http://www.cdc.gov /mmwr/preview/mmwrhtml/mm4841a1.htm, accessed January 25, 2015.

Centers for Disease Control and Prevention. Recommendations for using fluoride to prevent and control dental caries in the United States. *MMWR*. 2001;50(RR14):1–42. Available at http://www.cdc.gov/MMWr /preview/mmwrhtml/rr5014a1.htm, accessed January 25, 2015.

Centers for Disease Control and Prevention. *Healthy People 2000*. Updated October 14, 2009. Available at http://www.cdc.gov/nchs/healthy_people/hp2000.htm, accessed January 20, 2015.

Centers for Disease Control and Prevention. *Healthy People 2010*. Updated November 8, 2011. Available at http://www.cdc.gov/nchs/healthy_people/hp2010.htm, accessed January 10, 2015.

Centers for Disease Control and Prevention. *Healthy People 2020*. Updated October 14, 2011. Available at http://www.cdc.gov/nchs/healthy_people/hp2020.htm, accessed January 7, 2015.

Centers for Disease Control and Prevention. 2012 Water Fluoridation Statistics. Available at http://www.cdc.gov /fluoridation/statistics/2012stats.htm, accessed January 25, 2015.

Citizen's Board of Inquiry into Hunger and Malnutrition in the United States. *Hunger, USA*. Boston: Beacon Press, 1968.

Chapman N. Developing agency, community, and state policies. In Kaufman M, eds. *Nutrition in Public Health: A Handbook for Developing Programs and Services*. Rockville, MD: Aspen Publishers, 1990, Chap. 5.

Chapman N, Edmonds MT. Develop agency, community, and state nutrition policies. In Kaufman M, ed. *Nutrition in Promoting the Public's Health: Strategies, Principles, and Practice*. Sudbury, MA: Jones and Barlett Publisher, 2007, Chap. 5.

Chriqui JF, Resnick EA, Schneider L, Schermbeck R, Adcock T, Carrion V, Chaloupka FJ. *School District Wellness Policies: Evaluating Progress and Potential for Improving Children's Health Five Years after the Federal Mandate. School Years 2006–2007 through 2010–2011*, Vol. 3. Chicago: Bridging the Gap Program, Health Policy Center, Institute for Health Research and Policy, University of Illinois at Chicago, 2013. Available at http://www.bridgingthegapresearch.org/_asset/13s2jm/WP_2013_report .pdf, accessed February 10, 2015.

Clarke R. Vitamin B12, folic acid, and the prevention of dementia. *N Engl J Med*. 2006;354(26):2817–2819.

Cohen L, Swift S. The spectrum of prevention: Developing a comprehensive approach to injury prevention. *Injury Prev*. 1999;5(3):203–207.

Dimitri C, Effland A, Conklin N. The 20th Century Transformation of US Agriculture and Farm Policy. ERS Electronic Information Bulletin Number 3, June 2005. Available at http://www.ers.usda.gov/publications /eib-economic-information-bulletin/eib3.aspx#.U6yBsqhFyPM, accessed January 27, 2015.

Drewnowski A, Darmon N. The economics of obesity: Dietary energy density and energy cost. *Am J Clin Nutr*. 2005;82(Suppl):265S–273S.

Eisinger PK. *Toward an End to Hunger in America*. Washington, DC: The Brookings Institution Press, 1998.

First Lady Michelle Obama Launches Let's Move: America's Move to Raise a Healthier Generation of Kids [Press Release]. Washington, DC: The White House Briefing Room, February 9, 2010. Available at http://www.whitehouse.gov/the-press-office/first-lady-michelle-obama-launches-lets-move-americas -move-raise-a-healthier-genera, accessed January 26, 2015.

Food and Drug Administration. Final Rule. Food Labeling; Calorie Labeling of Articles of Food in Vending Machines, December 1, 2014. Available at https://www.federalregister.gov/articles/2014/12/01/2014 -27834/food-labeling-calorie-labeling-of-articles-of-food-in-vending-machines, accessed February 11, 2015.

Food Allergy Research & Education. History. Available at http://www.foodallergy.org/about/history, accessed February 10, 2015.

Food Allergen Labeling and Consumer Protection Act of 2004, Pub. L. no. 108–282, Title II, 118 Stat. 905 (2004). Available at http://www.gpo.gov/fdsys/pkg/PLAW-108publ282/pdf/PLAW-108publ282.pdf, accessed January 26, 2015.

Food and Nutrition Service. US Department of Agriculture. HealthierUS School Challenge. Available at http://www.fns.usda.gov/hussc/healthierus-school-challenge, accessed January 26, 2015.

Food and Nutrition Service. US Department of Agriculture. HealthierUS School Challenge—Vision. Updated August 22, 2014. Available at http://www.fns.usda.gov/hussc/vision, accessed January 20, 2015.

Food and Nutrition Service. US Department of Agriculture. Application Criteria. Updated February 25, 2014. Available at http://www.fns.usda.gov/hussc/healthierus-school-challenge-criteria-application-criteria, accessed January 20, 2015.

Food and Nutrition Service. US Department of Agriculture. Recognizing Excellence in Nutrition and Physical Activity. Updated February 2, 2015. Available at http://www.fns.usda.gov/hussc/healthierus -school-challenge, accessed February 10, 2015.

Food and Agriculture Policy Collaborative. Healthy Food, Healthy Economies. Available at http://frac.org/pdf /food_ag_policy_collaborative_hfhe.pdf, accessed January 27, 2015.

Galer-Unti R. *Hunger and Food Assistance Policy in the United States*. New York: Garland Publishing, 1995.

Gerrior S, Bente L, Hiza H. Nutrient Content of the US Food Supply, 1909–2000. Home Economics Research Report No. 56. US Department of Agriculture, Center for Nutrition Policy and Promotion, 2004. Available at http://www.cnpp.usda.gov/sites/default/files/nutrient_content_of_the_us_food_supply/Food Supply1909-2000.pdf, accessed February 10, 2015.

Golden Rice Project. Available at http://www.goldenrice.org, accessed February 11, 2015.

Guthrie JF, Lin B-H, Frazao E. Role of food prepared away from home in the American diet, 1977–1978 versus 1994–1996: Changes and consequences. *J Nutr Educ Behav*. 2002;34(3):140–150.

HealthyPeople.gov. History and Development. Healthy People. Updated February 9, 2015. Available at http://www.healthypeople.gov/2020/about/history.aspx, accessed February 10, 2015.

HealthyPeople.gov. Leading Health Indicators. Healthy People 2020. Available at http://www.healthypeople.gov/2020/LHI/default.aspx, accessed February 10, 2015.

HealthierUS.gov. Available at http://webarchive.library.unt.edu/eot2008/20080916003723/http:/healthierus.gov/, accessed January 20, 2015.

Healthy, Hunger-Free Kids Act of 2010, Pub. L. no. 111–296, 124 Stat. 3183 (2010). Available at http://www.gpo.gov/fdsys/pkg/PLAW-111publ296/pdf/PLAW-111publ296.pdf, accessed February 10, 2015.

Hoppe RA, Banker DE. *Structure and Finances of US Farms: Family Farm Report, 2010 Edition*. EIB-66. US Department of Agriculture, Economic Research Service, July 2010. Available at http://www.ers.usda.gov/publications/eib-economic-information-bulletin/eib66.aspx#.U62nWqjR3jY, accessed January 27, 2015.

Institute of Medicine. *Examination of Front-of-Package Nutrition Rating Systems and Symbols: Phase I Report*. Washington, DC: The National Academies Press, 2010.

Institute of Medicine, Food and Nutrition Board. *Dietary Reference Intakes for Calcium and Vitamin D*. Washington, DC: National Academy Press, 2011.

Johnson SA, DeBaise C. Concentration levels of fluoride in bottled drinking water. *J Dent Hyg*. 2003;77(3): 161–167.

Just Label It. Right to Know, Labeling around the World. Available at http://justlabelit.org/right-to-know/labeling-around-the-world/, accessed February 11, 2015.

Kotz N. *Let Them Eat Promises: The Politics of Hunger in America*. Englewood Cliffs, NJ: Prentice-Hall, 1969.

Kucinich E. Members of Congress, Farmers and Businesses Call on Obama to Fulfill Campaign Promise on GMO Labeling. *The Huffington Post*. Last updated March 18, 2014. Available at http://www.huffingtonpost.com/elizabeth kucinich/post_6676_b_4612219.html, accessed February 11, 2015.

Lalumandier JA, Ayers LW. Fluoride and bacterial content of bottled water vs. tap water. *Arch Fam Med*. 2000;9(3):246–250.

Lasswell HD. *Politics: Who Gets What, When and How*. New York: McGraw-Hill, 1936.

Let's Move! Learn the Facts, February 9, 2010. Available at http://www.letsmove.gov/learn-facts/epidemic-childhood-obesity, accessed January 22, 2015.

Let's Move! White House Task Force on Childhood Obesity Report to the President, February 2011. Available at http://www.letsmove.gov/white-house-task-force-childhood-obesity-report-president, accessed January 22, 2015.

Let's Move! The Partnership for a Healthy America. Available at http://www.letsmove.gov/partnership-healthier-america, accessed January 22, 2015.

Lichtenstein H, Appel LJ, Brands M et al. Diet and lifestyle recommendations revision 2006. A scientific statement from the American Heart Association Nutrition Committee. *Circulation*. 2006;114(1):82–96.

Lin B-H, Frazao E, Guthrie J. Away-From-Home Foods Increasingly Important to Quality of American Diet. Agriculture Information Bulletin No. 749. US Department of Agriculture, Economic Research Service, January 1999. Available at http://www.ers.usda.gov/publications/aib-agricultural-information-bulletin/aib749.aspx#.U58eA6iW8zw, accessed January 16, 2015.

Mayer J. National and International Issues in Food Policy. Lowell Lecture, May 15, 1989.

National Nutrition Summit 2000. Available at http://www.nns.nih.gov/2000/background/background.htm, accessed February 11, 2015.

Nestle M, Guttmacher S. Hunger in the United States: Rationale, methods, and policy implications of state hunger surveys. *J Nutr Educ*. 1992;24(1 Suppl):18S–22S.

Nixon R. Senate passes long-stalled farm bill, with clear winners and losers. *NY Times*, February 5, 2014, p. A15.

Partnership for a Healthier America. About the Partnership. Available at http://ahealthieramerica.org/about/about-the-partnership/, accessed January 22, 2015.

Pfeiffer CM, Caudill SP, Gunter EW, Osterloh J, Sampson EJ. Biochemical indicators of B vitamin status in the US population after folic acid fortification: Results from the National Health and Nutrition Examination Survey 1999–2000. *Am J Clin Nutr*. 2005;82(2):442–450.

Public Health Service. *Healthy People: The Surgeon General's Report on Health Promotion and Disease Prevention*. Washington, DC: US Department of Health, Education, and Welfare, Public Health Service. DHEW Publication No. PHS 79-55071, 1979. Available at http://profiles.nlm.nih.gov/ps/access/NNBBGK.pdf, accessed January 20, 2015.

Public Health Service. *Promoting Health/Preventing Disease: Objectives for the Nation*. Washington, DC: US Department of Health and Human Services, Public Health Service, 1980. Available at http://legacy.library.ucsf.edu/tid/xsi52f00/pdf;jsessionid=43F27DB72EE8FE592C9547B909F4120D.tobacco03, accessed January 20, 2015.

Raab C, Grobe D. Labeling genetically engineered food: The consumer's right to know. *AgBioForum*. 2003; 6(4): 155–161. Available at http://www.agbioforum.org/v6n4/v6n4a02-raab.htm, accessed February 11, 2015.

Reeve LE, Jorgensen NA, DeLuca HF. Vitamin D compounds in cows' milk. *J Nutr*. 1982;112(4):667–672.

Schoonover H, Muller M. *Food without Thought: How US Farm Policy Contributes to Obesity*. Minneapolis, MN: The Institute for Agricultural and Trade Policy, 2006. Available at http://www.iatp.org/files /421_2_80627.pdf, accessed January 27, 2015.

Steinhauer J. Farm bill reflects shifting American menu and a senator's persistent tilling. *NY Times*, March 9, 2014, p. A16.

The Keystone Forum on Away-From-Home Foods: Opportunities for Preventing Weight Gain and Obesity. Final Report, May 2006. Available at https://keystone.org/images/keystone-center/spp-documents /2011/Forum_on_Away-From-Home_Foods/forum_report_final_5-30-06.pdf, accessed January 16, 2015.

The Non-GMO Project RSS. What is GMO? Available at http://www.nongmoproject.org/learn-more/what-is -gmo, accessed February 11, 2015.

The Non-GMO Project RSS. GMO Facts. Available at http://www.nongmoproject.org/learn-more/, accessed February 11, 2015.

The Non-GMO Project RSS. What is GMO? Available at http://www.nongmoproject.org/learn-more/what-is -gmo, accessed February 11, 2015.

Tillotson JE. Pandemic obesity: Unintended policy consequences. *Nutr Today*. 2003;38(4):116–119.

Tillotson J. America's obesity: Conflicting public policies, industrial economic development, and unintended consequences. *Ann Rev Nutr*. 2004;24:617–643.

UC Davis Seed Biotechnology Center. What Is Herbicide Tolerance? Biotechnology for Sustainability. Available at http://sbc.ucdavis.edu/files/191418.pdf, accessed February 11, 2015.

US Department of Agriculture Food and Nutrition Service. Local Wellness Policy—Background. Team Nutrition. Updated July 21, 2014. Available at http://www.fns.usda.gov/tn/local-school-wellness-policy, accessed February 10, 2015.

US Department of Agriculture, Economic Research Service. Agricultural Productivity in the US Updated October 31, 2014. Available at http://www.ers.usda.gov/data-products/agricultural-productivity-in-the-us.aspx#.U62spKjR3jZ, accessed January 27, 2015.

US Department of Agriculture, Economic Research Service. Processing & Marketing: New Products. Updated October 30, 2014. Available at http://ers.usda.gov/topics/food-markets-prices/processing-marketing/new -products.aspx#.U62wuajR3jZ, accessed January 27, 2015.

US Department of Agriculture. *Dietary Guidelines for Americans*, 2015. Available at http://www.health.gov /dietaryguidelines/2015.asp, accessed January 26, 2015.

US Department of Agriculture, US Department of Health and Human Services. *Dietary Guidelines for Americans, 2010*, 7th ed. Washington, DC: US Government Printing Office, December 2010. Available at http://www.health.gov/dietaryguidelines/dga2010/DietaryGuidelines2010.pdf, accessed January 26, 2015.

US Department of Agriculture, US Department of Health and Human Services. Memorandum of Understanding Concerning Information Sharing Related to Food Safety, Public Health, and Other Food-Associated Activities. MOU 225012-0007, 2011. Available at http://www.fda.gov/AboutFDA /PartnershipsCollaborations/MemorandaofUnderstandingMOUs/DomesticMOUs/ucm294512.htm, accessed February 11, 2015.

US Department of Health and Human Services. *Healthy People 2010: Understanding and Improving Health*, 2nd ed. Washington, DC, November 2000. Available at http://www.healthypeople.gov/2010/Document /pdf/uih/2010uih.pdf, accessed January 20, 2015.

US Department of Health and Human Services. *The Surgeon General's Call to Action to Prevent and Decrease Overweight and Obesity*. Rockville, MD: US Department of Health and Human Services, Public Health Service, Office of the Surgeon General, 2001. Available at http://www.ncbi.nlm.nih.gov /books/NBK44206/pdf/TOC.pdf, accessed January 16, 2015.

US Department of Health and Human Services. Solicitation for written comments on the proposed changes to *Healthy People 2010* through the Midcourse Review. *Fed Reg*. 2005;70:47206–47207.

US Department of Health and Human Services. Healthy People 2020: Oral Health Objectives. Available at http://www.healthypeople.gov/2020/topicsobjectives2020/objectiveslist.aspx?topicId=32, accessed January 25, 2015.

US Department of Health and Human Services. *Healthy People 2020: How to Use DATA2020*. Available at http://www.healthypeople.gov/2020/Data/default.aspx, accessed January 25, 2015.

US Department of Health and Human Services. Healthy People 2020: Determinants of Health. Available at http://www.healthypeople.gov/2020/about/foundation-health-measures/Determinants-of-Health, accessed January 26, 2015.

US Department of Health and Human Services, US Food and Drug Administration. Food standards: Amendment of standards of identity for enriched grain products to require addition of folic acid. *Fed Reg.* 1996;61:8781–8797. Available at http://www.gpo.gov/fdsys/pkg/FR-1996-03-05/pdf/96-5014 .pdf#page=1, accessed January 25, 2015.

US Department of Health and Human Services, US Department of Agriculture. *2015 Dietary Guidelines for Americans. Timeline*, 2014. Available at http://www.health.gov/dietaryguidelines/2015-dga-timeline.pdf, accessed January 26, 2015.

US Department of Health and Human Services, US Department of Agriculture, US Department of the Interior, US Department of the Army, US Department of Transportation. Memorandum of Understanding to Promote Public Health and Recreation, 2008. Available at http://www.fhwa.dot.gov/environment /recreational_trails/overview/mou_pubhealth08.pdf, accessed January 20, 2015.

US Department of Health and Human Services, US Department of Agriculture, Environmental Protection Agency. Memorandum of Understanding Concerning Information Sharing in the Regulatory Oversight over Genetically-Engineered Plants and the Foods Derived from Such Plants. 10-2000-0058-MU. 225-11-0001, 2011. Available at http://www.epa.gov/oppbppd1/biopesticides/pips/biotech-mou.pdf, accessed January 20, 2015.

US Food and Drug Administration. Food Allergen Labeling and Consumer Protection Act of 2004: Questions and Answers. Updated December 16, 2014. Available at http://www.fda.gov/food/guidanceregulation /guidancedocumentsregulatoryinformation/allergens/ucm106890.htm, accessed February 10, 2015.

US Food and Drug Administration. Food Facts. Gluten and Food Labeling: FDA's Regulation of "Gluten-Free" Claims. Updated January 29, 2015. Available at http://www.fda.gov/Food/ResourcesForYou /Consumers/ucm367654.htm, accessed February 10, 2015.

US Food and Drug Administration. Questions and Answers: Gluten-Free Food Labeling Final Rule. Updated August 5, 2014. Available at http://www.fda.gov/Food/GuidanceRegulation/GuidanceDocuments RegulatoryInformation/Allergens/ucm362880.htm, accessed February 11, 2015.

US Food and Drug Administration. Food Labeling: Revision of the Nutrition and Supplement Facts Label. Proposed Rule. *Fed Reg.* 2014;79:11879–11987. Available at https://www.federalregister.gov/articles /2014/03/03/2014-04387/food-labeling-revision-of-the-nutrition-and-supplement-facts-labels, accessed February 11, 2015.

US Food and Drug Administration, Center for Food Safety and Applied Nutrition. Calories Count: Report on the Working Group on Obesity, March 12, 2004. Available at http://www.fda.gov/Food/FoodScienceResearch /ConsumerBehaviorResearch/ucm081696.htm, accessed January 16, 2015.

US House Committee on Agriculture. House-Senate Negotiators Announce Bipartisan Agreement on Final Farm Bill [Press Release], January 27, 2014. Available at http://agriculture.house.gov/press-release /house-senate-negotiators-announce-bipartisan-agreement-final-farm-bill, accessed February 11, 2015.

Variyam JN. Nutrition Labeling in the Food-Away-From-Home Sector: An Economic Assessment. US Department of Agriculture, Economic Research Service. Economic Research Report No. ERR-4, April 2005. Available at http://www.ers.usda.gov/publications/err-economic-research-report/err4.aspx# .U58ihaiW8zw, accessed January 16, 2015.

Waltner-Toews D, Lang TA. A new conceptual base for food and agricultural policy: The emerging model of links between agriculture, food, health, environment, and society. *Glob Change Hum Health.* 2000;1(2):116–130.

Warren JJ, Levy SM. Current and future role of fluoride in nutrition. *Dent Clin North Am.* 2003;47(2):225–243.

White House Task Force on Childhood Obesity. Report to the President. Solving the Problem of Childhood Obesity Within a Generation, May 2010. Available at http://www.letsmove.gov/sites/letsmove.gov/files /TaskForce_on_Childhood_Obesity_May2010_FullReport.pdf, accessed January 26, 2015.

World Health Organization. 20 Questions on Genetically Modified Foods. Available at http://www.who.int /foodsafety/publications/biotech/20questions/en/, accessed February 11, 2015.

9 Food and Nutrition Guidance

Eat food. Not too much. Mostly plants.

Michael Pollan (2007)

INTRODUCTION

Everyone, it seems, offers advice about what we should eat. Diet books are perennial best sellers, with the eating plans they espouse providing the basis for endless articles in women's consumer magazines and fitness and health magazines, and are the subject for television talk shows and newspaper columns. Perhaps less well known is the more credible advice issued by the US Department of Agriculture (USDA) and the Department of Health and Human Services (HHS), and from voluntary health organizations such as the American Heart Association (AHA) and the American Cancer Society (ACS). This chapter examines federal food and nutrition guidance aimed at health promotion and guidelines from voluntary as well as federal health associations for the primary and secondary prevention of cardiovascular diseases (CVDs), cancer, and diabetes. In this chapter, we review the early twentieth century food guidance from the USDA focusing on avoiding dietary deficiencies. We then examine the growth in population-based health promotion dietary recommendations from the federal government in the 1970s and the transition to a joint effort by the USDA and HHS to provide complementary messages to the public. Next we discuss how we measure diet as "healthy" and illustrate the difference between food-group–based guidance and nutrient-based guidance. Finally, we turn to current federal dietary guidance and discuss disease prevention guidance from federal and voluntary health organizations.

USDA FOOD GUIDANCE, 1900s–1970: EATING TO PREVENT DEFICIENCIES

The USDA has been issuing food and nutrition recommendations for more than 100 years.* USDA food scientist W.O. Atwater's research on food composition and nutritional needs ushered in the USDA's long history of food guides. By emphasizing variety, proportionality, and moderation in food intake in 1902, he set the stage for all future work in the field of dietary recommendations (Box 9.1).

A food guide translates nutrient intake recommendations into food intake recommendations and provides a conceptual framework for selecting the kinds and amounts of foods needed for a nutritionally sound diet. The USDA's first food guide, published in 1916, categorized foods into five groups: milk and meat, cereals, vegetables and fruits, fats and fatty foods, and sugars and sugary foods. That guide was followed in 1917 by dietary recommendations that were based on these five food groups. The concept of categorizing food into groups has remained a constant theme in USDA dietary guidance to date, as illustrated in Table 9.1.

---

* This discussion about the history of food guidance is adapted from these two USDA sources: Davis C, Saltos E. Dietary recommendations and how they have changed over time. In Frazao E, ed. *America's Eating Habits: Changes and Consequences.* Washington, DC: Economic Research Service. US Department of Agriculture. Agriculture Information Bulletin No. 750, 1999, pp. 33–50. Available at http://www.ers.usda.gov/publications/aib-agricultural-information-bulletin/aib750.aspx#.UgENZ1OISUc, accessed February 2, 2015; Welsh SO, Davis C, Shaw A. *USDA's Food Guide: Background and Development.* US Department of Agriculture. Human Nutrition Information Service. Nutrition Education Division. Miscellaneous Publication No. 1514, September 1993. Available at http://www.cnpp.usda.gov/sites/default/files/archived_projects/FGPBackgroundAndDevelopment.pdf, accessed February 2, 2015.

BOX 9.1   A WARNING MORE THAN 100 YEARS OLD

Unless care is exercised in selecting food, a diet may result which is one-sided or badly balanced, that is, one in which either protein or fuel ingredients (carbohydrate and fat) are provided in excess ... The evils of overeating may not be felt at once, but sooner or later they are sure to appear, perhaps in an excessive amount of fatty tissue, perhaps in general debility, perhaps in actual disease.

W.O. Atwater, 1902

Source: Davis, C. and Saltos, E., Dietary recommendations and how they have changed over time, in Frazao, E., ed., *America's Eating Habits: Changes and Consequences*, Economic Research Service, US Department of Agriculture, Washington, DC, Agriculture Information Bulletin no. 750, 1999, 33–50. Available at http://www .ers.usda.gov/publications/aib-agricultural-information-bulletin/aib750.aspx#.UgENZ1OISUc, accessed February 2, 2015.

In the 1920s, guides were released using these same five food groups to suggest amounts of foods to purchase each week for families of varying sizes. During the Depression, economic constraints influenced dietary guidance. In 1933, the USDA developed its first food plans at four cost levels to help people with food shopping. The plans were organized into 12 major food groups to buy and use within a week to meet nutritional needs. Research to provide guidance on selecting a healthful diet at different cost levels continues at the USDA (Box 9.2).

At the beginning of the US entry into World War II, President Franklin D. Roosevelt convened the National Nutrition Conference for Defense, a meeting notable to the nutrition community for at least two reasons. For one, the conference resulted in the development in 1941 of the first Recommended Dietary Allowances (RDAs), published in 1943 by the Food and Nutrition Board of the National Academy of Sciences (NAS). The first edition of the RDAs listed specific recommended intakes for calories and nine essential nutrients: protein, iron, calcium, vitamin A, vitamin C, vitamin D, thiamine, riboflavin, and niacin. The National Nutrition Conference for Defense also addressed the need for public nutrition education and provided suggestions for an effective nutrition education program (Box 9.3).

As part of national defense efforts, the USDA released the Basic 7 food guide in 1943 in the form of a leaflet entitled *National Wartime Nutrition Guide*. This was revised in 1946 as the *National Food Guide*. This guide specified a foundation diet that would provide a major share of the RDAs for nutrients but only a portion of caloric needs. It was assumed that people would include more foods than the guide recommended to meet their energy and nutrient requirements. In those days, little guidance was provided on the use of fats and sugars. The wartime version of the Basic 7 was intended to help people cope with limited supplies of certain foods.

The 1946 version suggested numbers of servings within each food group and was widely used for over a decade. However, its complexity and lack of specifics regarding serving sizes necessitated modification. In 1956, the USDA released what became known as its Basic 4 Food Groups (dairy, grains, meat and alternates, and fruits and vegetables). Used for the next two decades, the focus of this foundation diet was on getting adequate nutrients (Box 9.4).

USDA AND HHS DIETARY GUIDANCE, 1970s TO 2010: HEALTH PROMOTION

By the end of the 1970s, research had implicated the role of diet (namely, the overconsumption of fat, saturated fat, cholesterol, and sodium) in the development of some chronic diseases, drawing attention to the need for new guidance on diet and health. Dietary advice began a new direction that shifted the focus of recommendations from obtaining enough nutrients to recommendations

TABLE 9.1

Principal USDA Food Groups, 1916 through 2015

Year	Type of Food Guide	Title	Food Groups
1916	Buying guides	*Food for Young Children,* developed by Caroline Hunt	1. Meat and other protein-rich foods, including milk 2. Cereals and other starchy foods 3. Vegetables and fruit 4. Fatty food 5. Sugars
1930s	Buying guides	Food plans at four cost levels, developed by Hazel K. Stiebeling	1. Milk 2. Lean meat/poultry/fish 3. Dry mature beans, peas, nuts 4. Eggs 5. Flours and cereals 6. Leafy green and yellow vegetables 7. Potatoes and sweet potatoes 8. Other vegetables and fruits 9. Tomatoes and citrus 10. Butter 11. Other facts 12. Sugars
1940s	Foundation diet	Basic 7	1. Milk and milk products 2. Meat, poultry, fish, eggs, dried beans, peas, nuts 3. Bread, flour, and cereals 4. Leafy green and yellow vegetables 5. Potatoes and other fruits and vegetables 6. Citrus, tomato, cabbage, salad greens 7. Butter, fortified margarine
1956–1970s	Foundation diet	Basic 4	1. Milk group 2. Meat group 3. Bread and cereal group 4. Vegetable and fruit group
1979	Foundation diet	*Hassle-Free Food Guide*	1. Milk–cheese group 2. Meat, poultry, fish, and beans group 3. Breads, cereal, rice, pasta 4. Vegetable–fruit group 5. Fats, sweets, alcohol
1984–2005	Total diet	*Food Guide Pyramid*	1. Milk, yogurt, cheese 2. Meat, poultry, fish, eggs, dry beans, nuts 3. Breads, cereals, rice, pasta 4. Vegetables: dark green/deep yellow, starchy legumes, other 5. Fruit: citrus and others 6. Fats, oils, sweets
2005–2011	Total diet	*MyPyramid*	1. Milk group 2. Meat and beans group, including eggs, fish, poultry, dry beans, nuts and seeds, and peanut butter 3. Grain group 4. Vegetable group, including dark green and orange vegetables, starchy vegetables, other vegetables, and legumes 5. Fruit group 6. Oils 7. Discretionary calorie allowance

(Continued)

TABLE 9.1 (CONTINUED)
Principal USDA Food Groups, 1916 through 2015

Year	Type of Food Guide	Title	Food Groups
2011– present	Total diet	*MyPlate*	1. Dairy group, including milk, cheese, and yogurt 2. Protein group, including meats, poultry, eggs, beans and peas, processed soy products, nuts and seeds, and seafood 3. Grain group 4. Vegetable group, including dark green, red, and orange vegetables; starchy vegetables; other vegetables; and beans and peas 5. Fruit group 6. Oils

Source: Davis, C. and Saltos, E., Dietary recommendations and how they have changed over time, in Frazao, E., ed., *America's Eating Habits: Changes and Consequences*, Economic Research Service, Washington, DC, US Department of Agriculture, Agriculture Information Bulletin no. 750, 1999, 33–50. Available at http://www.ers.usda .gov/publications/aib-agricultural-information-bulletin/aib750.aspx#.UgENZ1OISUc, accessed February 2, 2015; US Department of Agriculture, MyPyramid Food Intake Patterns, April 2005. Available at http://www.choosemyplate .gov/food-groups/downloads/MyPyramid_Food_Intake_Patterns.pdf, accessed February 2, 2015; US Department of Agriculture, MyPlate Food Groups. Available at http://www.choosemyplate.gov/food-groups/, accessed February 2, 2015.

BOX 9.2   IMAGES OF HISTORICAL DIETARY GUIDANCE

Illustrations of historical food guides are available in the various links that trace the USDA's food guides from the 1890s to the present: http://fnic.nal.usda.gov/dietary-guidance /dietary-guidelines/historical-dietary-guidance.

BOX 9.3   SUGGESTIONS FOR EFFECTIVE NUTRITION EDUCATION

The suggestions provided in 1941 by the National Nutrition Conference for Defense reflect essential program characteristics that remain applicable today. Effective nutrition education must

- Reach the whole population—all groups, all races, both sexes, all creeds, all ages.
- Recognize motives for action and include suggestions on what to do and how to do it.
- Develop qualified leadership.
- Drive home the same ideas many times and in many ways.
- Employ every suitable education tool available.
- Adapt those tools to the many and varied groups to be reached and use them with intelligence and skill.
- Consider all phases of individual, family, and group situations that have a bearing upon the ability to produce, buy, prepare, conserve, and consume food.
- Afford opportunity for participation in making, putting into effect, and evaluating local nutrition programs.
- Enlist the fullest participation of all citizens and work through every possible channel to reach the people.
- Be adequately financed.

BOX 9.4   BASIC 4 FOUNDATION DIET (RELEASED IN 1956 BY THE USDA)

Milk group: 2 cups or more

Meat group: Two or more 2–3 oz. servings

Bread, cereal: Four or more (1 oz. dry cereal, 1 slice bread, 1/2–3/4 cup cooked cereal)

Vegetable, fruit: Four or more (includes dark green/yellow vegetables frequently and
citrus daily, 1/2 cup or average-size piece)

BOX 9.5   NUTRIENT-BASED GUIDANCE

By the 1970s, it was generally recognized that dietary guidance should not only target adequacy but also provide guidance related to moderation of those dietary components being consumed in excess. This paved the way for nutrient-based dietary guidance, which focuses primarily on nutrients and other food factors, such as cholesterol, saturated fats, and *trans* fats. A food-based approach presents recommendations in terms of number of servings or amounts of food to be consumed from each of the food groups. In contrast, nutrient-based guidance presents recommendations for single food factors, stated in terms of either the weight (in grams) or percentage of calories that should be provided by one or more of the energy nutrients (carbohydrate, protein, fat). Nutrient-based recommendations also specify the amounts to be consumed of fiber (grams) and vitamins and minerals (milligrams and micrograms).

---

of decreasing intakes of food components associated with heart disease, stroke, and some forms of cancer.

The USDA began addressing the role of fats, sugars, and sodium in risks for chronic diseases in its 1979 *Hassle-Free Guide to a Better Diet*, a modified Basic 4 plan that added and highlighted a fifth food group—fats, sweets, and alcoholic beverages—targeted for moderation. Additionally, we see the beginning of a consistent voice from the federal government on diet and health, as food guidance from the USDA begins following population health dietary guidelines jointly published by the USDA and HHS (Box 9.5).

DIETARY GOALS FOR THE UNITED STATES, 1977

In 1968, the US Senate formed the Committee on Nutrition and Human Needs (meant to address hunger and malnutrition), but cooperation of Congress on dietary goals remained elusive. However, with the developing research on CVD, the Committee on Nutrition and Human Needs found a foothold in addressing diet and health—a reported eight US senators died in office of heart disease in the 1960s and 1970s (Aubrey 2014).

Eight years later, in February 1977, led by Senator George McGovern (D-South Dakota), the committee released the *Dietary Goals for the United States* (US Congress 1977a), which recommended that Americans:

- Increase carbohydrate intake to 55–60% of calories.
- Decrease dietary fat intake to no more than 30% of calories, with a reduction in intake of saturated fat and approximately equivalent distributions among saturated, polyunsaturated, and monounsaturated fats to meet the 30% target.
- Decrease cholesterol intake to 300 mg per day.
- Decrease sugar intake to 15% of calories.
- Decrease salt intake to 3 g per day.

These goals were the focus of so much controversy among some nutritionists, industry groups, the scientific community, and others concerned with food, nutrition, and health that the committee released Supplemental Views to the report in November 1977 (US Congress 1977b) and a second edition in December 1977 (US Congress 1977c). Table 9.2 summarizes the goals of the first and second editions. Although the first and second editions were released in the same calendar year, it is instructive to note the differences in the recommendations of the two reports. Developing dietary guidelines and the political processes involved can never be completely separated, because the outputs are not simply scientific statements. Dietary recommendations have economic consequences for many different groups (Dwyer 2001).

When the average US diet as of 1977 and the quantitative recommendations of the *Dietary Goals* are represented in side-by-side bar graphs, as in Figure 9.1, it is evident that the *Dietary Goals* advocate a more plant-based diet.

Key to this interpretation is the recommended protein distribution. To decrease consumption of total fats, one needs to consume less vegetable oil and fat derived from animal sources. For example, the dietary modification to decrease fats would require using less oil in cooking and salad dressings, switching from high-fat to lower-fat meat and poultry products, and replacing the reduction in calories with an increased intake of foods rich in complex carbohydrates and naturally occurring sugars such as grain products, fruits, and vegetables. To maintain the proportion of calories derived from protein, as illustrated in the bar graph, the source of protein calories should switch from animal to plant products.

TABLE 9.2

Dietary Goals for the United States, 1977

Dietary Goals for the United States, 1st Edition, February 1977	*Dietary Goals for the United States,* 2nd Edition, December 1977
	To avoid overweight, consume only as much energy (calories) as is expended; if overweight, decrease energy intake and increase energy expenditure
Increase carbohydrate intake to 55–60% of calories	Increase the consumption of complex carbohydrates and "naturally occurring" sugars from about 28% to about 48% of energy intake
Decrease sugar intake to 15% of calories	Reduce the consumption of refined and processed sugars by about 45% to account for about 10% of total energy intake
Decrease dietary fat intake to no more than 30% of calories, with a reduction in intake of saturated fat, and recommended approximately equivalent distributions among saturated, polyunsaturated, and monounsaturated fats to meet the 30% target	Reduce overall fat consumption from approximately 40% to about 30% of energy intake
	Reduce saturated fat consumption to account for about 10% of total energy intake, and balance that with polyunsaturated and monounsaturated fats, which should account for about 10% of energy intake each
Decrease cholesterol intake to 300 mg per day	Reduce cholesterol consumption to about 300 mg per day
Decrease salt intake to 3 g per day	Limit the intake of sodium by reducing the intake of salt to about 5 g per day

Source: US Congress, Senate Select Committee on Nutrition and Human Needs, *Dietary Goals for the United States*, 1st ed., US Government Printing Office, Washington, DC, 1977; US Congress, Senate Select Committee on Nutrition and Human Needs, *Dietary Goals for the United States*, 2nd ed., US Government Printing Office, Washington, DC, 1977.

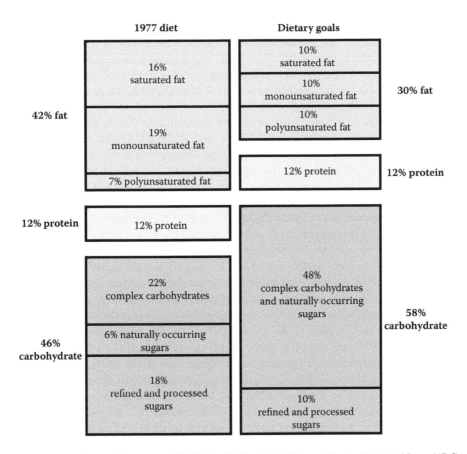

FIGURE 9.1 Comparison of the average US diet in 1977 and the *Dietary Goals*. (Adapted from US Congress, Senate Select Committee on Nutrition and Human Needs, *Dietary Goals for the United States*, 1st ed., US Government Printing Office, Washington, DC, 1977.)

In essence, the 1977 *Dietary Goals* recommended replacing some higher-biological-value protein (from animal products) with lower-biological-value protein (from plants). Similarly, the recommendation to decrease cholesterol derived exclusively from animal products—principally from egg yolks—would be achieved by decreasing intake of whole eggs and/or meat. In other words, the dietary goals advocated a diet that approached vegetarianism. The message to reduce consumption of meat and eggs would result in negative economic consequences for producers and marketers of these products, arousing their opposition to the recommendations.

DIETARY GUIDELINES FOR AMERICANS, 1980–

Perhaps in part due to the opposition from food producers, the USDA did not adopt the *Dietary Goals* directly but instead, in conjunction with the Department of Health, Education, and Welfare (now the HHS), conducted a supporting investigation of the underlying science, resulting in the first issuance of the *Dietary Guidelines for Americans* in 1980 (Dietary Guidelines Advisory Committee 2010), a consumer-facing brochure titled *Nutrition and Your Health: Dietary Guidelines for Americans* (US Department of Agriculture 1980).

With the release of the first edition of the *Dietary Guidelines for Americans*, the USDA began work on developing a new food guide, *A Pattern for Daily Food Choices*, designed to help consumers implement the *Dietary Guidelines* in their daily food choices. Focusing on the total diet rather than the foundation diet described by earlier guides, the new food guide emphasized making food selections both to meet nutrient objectives and to moderate intake of those components related to the risk of chronic diseases. It suggested numbers of servings from each of five major food groups (bread, cereal, rice, and pasta; vegetables; fruit; milk, yogurt, and cheese; and meat, poultry, fish, dry beans, eggs, and nuts) and recommended sparing use of a sixth food group—fats, oils, and sweets. The food guide was initially presented as a food wheel graphic but also appeared as a table in several USDA publications published in the 1980s.

The *Dietary Guidelines for Americans* generated considerable discussion by nutrition scientists, consumer groups, the food industry, and others, such that the US Senate directed that a committee be established to review scientific evidence and recommend revisions to the guidelines.* In 1983, a federal advisory committee of nine nutrition scientists selected from outside the federal government was convened to review and make recommendations about the first edition of the *Dietary Guidelines*. Based on the committee's recommendations, HHS and USDA jointly issued a second edition of the guidelines in 1985 (US Department of Agriculture 1985). Although nearly identical to the first edition, some changes were made for clarity; others reflected advances in scientific knowledge of the associations between diet and a range of chronic diseases. The second edition received wide acceptance and was used as a framework for consumer education messages.

In 1989, USDA and HHS established a second advisory committee that considered whether the 1985 *Dietary Guidelines* needed revision and then proceeded to make recommendations for revision in a report to the secretaries. *The Surgeon General's Report on Nutrition and Health* (1988) and the National Research Council's (NRC's) report *Diet and Health: Implications for Reducing Chronic Disease Risk* (1989) were key resources used by this committee.

The 1990 *Dietary Guidelines* (US Department of Agriculture, HHS 1990) contained additional refinements to reflect increased understanding of the science of nutrition and how best to communicate this to consumers. The language of the new *Dietary Guidelines for Americans* was more positive, was oriented toward the total diet, and provided more specific information regarding food selection. For the first time, numerical recommendations were made for intakes of total dietary fat and of saturated fat.

In 1990, with the passage of P.L.101-445 (US Government Publishing Office 1990), Congress formally instructed USDA and HHS to issue the dietary guidelines at least every 5 years. The legislation directed that the guidelines must (1) contain nutritional and dietary information and guidelines for the general public; (2) be based on the preponderance of current scientific and medical knowledge; and (3) be promoted by each federal agency in carrying out any federal food, nutrition, or health program. In other words, the act made the report official federal policy on nutrition guidance. Thus, while the USDA and HHS voluntarily issued the *Dietary Guidelines* in 1980, 1985, and 1990, the subsequent editions were statutorily mandated.

Food Guide Pyramid, 1992–2005

In 1992, the USDA's *Food Guide Pyramid* (US Department of Agriculture 1992) was released with the objective of translating the *Dietary Guidelines* into food choices. The pyramid recommended that choices come primarily from the grains, vegetables, and fruit groups (plant foods), with less from the meat and dairy groups (animal foods) and even less from fats, oils, and sweets. Within the pyramid, food groups were arranged to indicate proportionality of servings, with accompanying text that provided the recommended number of servings from each group. For more than a decade (1992–2005), the Food Guide Pyramid was widely used by nutrition and health professionals, educators, media, and the food industry, and helped to disseminate the nutritional messages of the *Dietary Guidelines* (Davis and Saltos 1999).

---

* The discussion about the history of the *Dietary Guidelines* is adapted from: 2005 *Dietary Guidelines* Advisory Committee. Report of the *Dietary Guidelines* Advisory Committee on the *Dietary Guidelines for Americans, 2005*, August 19, 2004. Available at http://www.health.gov/dietaryguidelines/dga2005/report/, accessed February 2, 2015.

The philosophical goals (Welsh et al. 1993) that guided the process of developing the Food Guide Pyramid continue to be relevant today. The principles of designing a food guide ensure that it

- Promotes overall health and well-being (rather than prevents a particular disease).
- Is based on up-to-date research.
- Focuses on the total diet, not a core or foundation diet.
- Is useful to the target audience, builds on previous food guides, and contains recognizable food groups based on a conceptual framework.
- Meets its nutritional goals in a realistic manner, based on the incorporation in the diet of commonly used foods.
- Permits maximum flexibility, allowing consumers to eat in a manner that suits their tastes.
- Presents practical ways to meet nutritional needs, which might mean using different plans for different activity and age levels; however, because families generally eat the same foods, members should be able to meet their needs by choosing different serving sizes from each of the food groups.

The 1990 *Dietary Guidelines* and the Food Guide Pyramid reflect the key concepts of variety, proportionality, and moderation introduced by Atwater a century ago. Table 9.3 illustrates how the Food Guide Pyramid serves as a mechanism for translating the key concepts of the *Dietary Guidelines*.

The 1995 edition of the *Dietary Guidelines for Americans* (US Department of Agriculture, HHS 1995) continued to support the concepts elucidated in earlier editions. New information included the Food Guide Pyramid, Nutrition Facts labels, and boxes highlighting good food sources of key nutrients. Starting with the second edition of the *Dietary Goals* and continuing through the first four editions of the *Dietary Guidelines*, recommendations have been presented as seven individual guidelines. The 2000 edition (US Department of Agriculture, HHS 2000) expanded to 10 guidelines, created by separating physical activity from the weight guideline, splitting the grains from fruits and vegetables for greater emphasis, and introducing a new guideline about safe food handling. The progression from 7 to 10 guidelines is illustrated in the guidelines summary (1980 through 2000) in Figure 9.2.

TABLE 9.3

The Food Guide Pyramid as a Mechanism for Translating the Key Concepts of the *Dietary Guidelines for Americans*, 1990

Dietary Guidelines for Americans, 1990	Key Concepts of the USDA Food Guide Pyramid, 1992			
	Variety	Proportionality	Moderation	Usability
Eat a variety of foods	✓	✓		
Choose a diet with plenty of vegetables, fruits, and grain products	✓	✓		
Maintain a healthy weight		✓	✓	
Choose a diet low in fat, saturated fat, and cholesterol			✓	
Use sugars only in moderation			✓	
Use salt and sodium only in moderation			✓	
If you drink alcoholic beverages, do so in moderation			✓	

Source: Welsh S.O. et al., *USDA's Food Guide: Background and Development*, US Department of Agriculture, Human Nutrition Information Service, Nutrition Education Division, Miscellaneous publication no, 1514. September 1993. Available at http://www.cnpp.usda.gov/sites/default/files/archived_projects/FGPBackgroundAndDevelopment.pdf, accessed February 2, 2015.

1980	1985	1990	1995	2000	
7 Guidelines	7 Guidelines	7 Guidelines	7 Guidelines	10 Guidelines, clustered into 3 groups	
Eat a variety of foods	Eat a variety of foods	Eat a variety of foods	Eat a variety of foods		
Maintain ideal weight	Maintain desirable weight	Maintain healthy weight	Balance the food you eat with physical activity—maintain or improve your weight	Aim for a healthy weight	Aim for fitness
				Be physically active each day	
Avoid too much fat, saturated fat, and cholesterol	Avoid too much fat, saturated fat, and cholesterol	Choose a diet low in fat, saturated fat, and cholesterol		Let the Pyramid guide your food choices	Build a healthy base
Eat foods with adequate starch and fiber	Eat foods with adequate starch and fiber	Choose a diet with plenty of vegetables, fruits, and grain products	Choose a diet with plenty of grain products, vegetables, and fruits	Choose a variety of grains daily, especially whole grains	
				Choose a variety of fruits and vegetables daily	
				Keep food safe to eat	
			Choose a diet low in fat, saturated fat, and cholesterol	Choose a diet that is low in saturated fat and cholesterol and moderate in total fat	Choose sensibly
Avoid too much sugar	Avoid too much sugar	Use sugars only in moderation	Choose a diet moderate in sugars	Choose beverages and foods to moderate your intake of sugars	
Avoid too much sodium	Avoid too much sodium	Use salt and sodium only in moderation	Choose a diet moderate in salt and sodium	Choose and prepare foods with less salt	
If you drink alcohol, do so in moderation	If you drink alcoholic beverages, do so in moderation	If you drink alcoholic beverages, do so in moderation	If you drink alcoholic beverages, do so in moderation	If you drink alcoholic beverages, do so in moderation	

Shading indicates how the order in which the guidelines are presented has changed over time.

FIGURE 9.2 *Dietary Guidelines for Americans,* 1980–2000. (From US Department of Agriculture, Center for Nutrition Policy and Promotion, *Dietary Guidelines for Americans,* 1980 to 2000, May 30, 2000. Available at http://www.health.gov/dietaryguidelines/1980_2000_chart.pdf, accessed February 2, 2015.)

The sixth edition (US Department of Agriculture, HHS 2005a) of the *Dietary Guidelines* was released in January 2005 and identifies 41 key recommendations grouped into nine general topics:

- Adequate nutrients within calorie needs.
- Weight management.
- Physical activity.
- Food groups to encourage.
- Fats.
- Carbohydrates.
- Sodium and potassium.
- Alcoholic beverages.
- Food safety.

The key recommendations are based on a preponderance of the scientific evidence regarding nutritional factors important for lowering the risk of chronic disease and promoting health. Of the 41 key recommendations, 23 are considered to be applicable to everybody, and 18 are focused on the 10 special population groups listed in Box 9.6. The 23 recommendations applicable to the general population are listed in Table 9.4.

The integrated messages comprising the guidelines are meant to be implemented as a whole. When taken together, they encourage most Americans to eat fewer calories, be more active, and make wiser food choices.

BOX 9.6   SPECIAL POPULATIONS

Slightly more than half of the 2005 *Dietary Guidelines* recommendations address the general public; the rest target special populations:

- Children and adolescents.
- Women of childbearing age who may become pregnant.
- Pregnant women, including women in the first trimester of pregnancy.
- Breastfeeding women.
- Middle-aged adults, people over age 50, and older adults.
- Blacks and people with dark skin.
- People exposed to insufficient ultraviolet band radiation (i.e., sunlight).
- Those who need to lose weight, including overweight children, overweight adults, and overweight children with chronic diseases and/or on medication.
- Individuals with hypertension.
- Those who are immunocompromised.

DISSENSION AND CONTROVERSY

The process of guideline development should be transparent and iterative. The pursuit of consensus is driven by an evidence-based review based on the science, coupled with discussion, formulation, and evaluation of guidelines (Box 9.7).

During the process and, indeed, in the final report, failure to achieve unanimous agreement is inevitable. Not all parties will agree when issues of emerging science are being considered and when one segment or another of the food industry is threatened. These points are illustrated when one reviews the comments received by the *Dietary Guidelines* Advisory Committee.

Public comments were solicited five times during the development of the 2005 *Dietary Guidelines*. For the final solicitation, the public was asked to provide oral or written comments on the *Report of the Dietary Guidelines Advisory Committee on the Dietary Guidelines for Americans, 2005 to the Secretaries of Health and Human Services and Agriculture*. In all, more than 400 responses were received.

In the past, the *Dietary Guidelines* settled for minor tweaks. The "avoid too much sugar" guideline in 1980 and 1985 evolved into "use sugars only in moderation" in 1990, "choose a diet moderate in sugars" in 1995, and "choose beverages and foods to moderate your intake of sugars" in 2000. In the 2005 revision, however, Americans are urged to "choose food and beverages low in added sugars. Added sugars contribute calories with few, if any, nutrients." Despite the impassioned and lengthy, 1700-word statement submitted by the Sugar Association, Inc., to the 2005 *Dietary Guidelines* Advisory Committee, the 2005 *Dietary Guidelines* take a harder line on sugars than ever before (Box 9.8).

On the other hand, the 2005 *Dietary Guidelines* recommendation to increase dairy intake from 2 to 3 cups per day has been met with skepticism by some who believe that the recommendation is the result of intense lobbying by the National Dairy Council (Kuehn 2005). The chairman of the Nutrition Department at the Harvard University School of Public Health argues that "dairy products shouldn't occupy the prominent place they do in [US dietary guidance], nor should they be the centerpiece of the national strategy to prevent osteoporosis" (Willett 2001). Other sources of calcium are available such as collards, tofu, spinach, calcium-fortified orange juice, and calcium supplements (Box 9.9).

The evidence, some of the milk critics say, is scant to support nutrition guidelines focused specifically on increasing intake of milk or other dairy products for bone health (Lanou et al. 2005). Other

TABLE 9.4

Dietary Guidelines for Americans, 2005: Topic Areas, Goals, and Key Recommendations for the General Population

Topic Area	Goal	Key Recommendations for the General Population (Objectives)
Adequate nutrients within calorie needs	Consume a variety of foods within and among the basic food groups while staying within energy needs	• Consume a variety of nutrient-dense foods and beverages within and among the basic food groups while choosing foods that limit the intake of saturated and *trans* fats, cholesterol, added sugars, salt, and alcohol. • Meet recommended intakes within energy needs by adopting a balanced eating pattern, such as the US Department of Agriculture (USDA) Food Guide or the Dietary Approaches to Stop Hypertension (DASH) eating plan.
Weight management	Control calorie intake to manage body weight	• To maintain body weight in a healthy range, balance calories from foods and beverages with calories expended. • To prevent gradual weight gain over time, make small decreases in food and beverage calories and increase physical activity.
Physical activity	Be physically active every day	• Engage in regular physical activity and reduce sedentary activities to promote health, psychological well-being, and a healthy body weight. • To reduce the risk of chronic disease in adulthood, engage in at least 30 minutes of moderate-intensity physical activity, beyond usual activity at work or home on most days of the week. • For most people, greater health benefits can be obtained by engaging in physical activity of more vigorous intensity or longer duration. • To help manage body weight and prevent gradual, unhealthy body weight gain in adulthood: engage in approximately 60 minutes of moderate- to vigorous-intensity activity on most days of the week while not exceeding caloric intake requirements. • To sustain weight loss in adulthood, participate in at least 60–90 minutes of moderate-intensity physical activity daily while not exceeding caloric intake requirements. Some people may need to consult with a healthcare provider before participating in this level of activity. • Achieve physical fitness by including cardiovascular conditioning, stretching exercises for flexibility, and resistance exercises or calisthenics for muscle strength and endurance.
Food groups to encourage	Increase daily intake of fruits and vegetables, whole grains, and nonfat or low-fat milk and milk products	• Consume a sufficient amount of fruits and vegetables while staying within energy needs. Two cups of fruit and 2 1/2 cups of vegetables per day are recommended for a reference 2000-calorie intake, with higher or lower amounts depending on the calorie level. • Choose a variety of fruits and vegetables each day. In particular, select from all five vegetable subgroups (dark green, orange, legumes, starchy vegetables, and other vegetables) several times a week. • Consume three or more 1 oz. equivalents of whole-grain products per day, with the rest of the recommended grains coming from enriched or whole-grain products. In general, at least half the grains should come from whole grains. • Consume 3 cups per day of fat-free or low-fat milk or equivalent milk products.

(Continued)

TABLE 9.4 (CONTINUED)
Dietary Guidelines for Americans, **2005: Topic Areas, Goals, and Key Recommendations for the General Population**

Topic Area	Goal	Key Recommendations for the General Population (Objectives)
Fats	Choose fats wisely for good health	• Consume less than 10% of calories from saturated fatty acids and less than 300 mg per day of cholesterol, and keep *trans* fatty acid consumption as low as possible. • Keep total fat intake between 20% and 35% of calories, with most fats coming from sources of polyunsaturated and monounsaturated fatty acids, such as fish, nuts, and vegetable oils. • When selecting and preparing meat, poultry, dry beans, and milk or milk products, make choices that are lean, low fat, or fat free. • Limit intake of fats and oils high in saturated and/or *trans* fatty acids, and choose products low in such fats and oils.
Carbohydrates	Choose carbohydrates wisely for good health	• Choose fiber-rich fruits, vegetables, and whole grains often. • Choose and prepare foods and beverages with little added sugars or caloric sweeteners. Aim for amounts suggested by the USDA Food Guide and the DASH eating plan. • Reduce the incidence of dental caries by practicing good oral hygiene and consuming sugar- and starch-containing foods and beverages less frequently.
Sodium and potassium	Choose and prepare foods with little salt	• Consume less than 2300 mg of sodium (approximately 1 tsp. of salt) per day. • Choose and prepare foods with little salt. At the same time, consume potassium-rich foods, such as fruits and vegetables.
Alcoholic beverages	If you drink alcoholic beverages, do so in moderation	• Those who choose to drink alcoholic beverages should do so sensibly and in moderation—defined as the consumption of up to one drink per day for women and up to two drinks per day for men. • Alcoholic beverages should not be consumed by some individuals, including those who cannot restrict their alcohol intake, women of childbearing age who may become pregnant, pregnant and lactating women, children and adolescents, individuals taking medications that can interact with alcohol, and those with specific medical conditions. • Alcoholic beverages should be avoided by individuals engaging in activities that require attention, skill, or coordination, such as driving or operating machinery.

Food safety	Keep food safe to eat	• To avoid microbial foodborne illness:
		  • Clean hands, food contact surfaces, and fruits and vegetables. Meat and poultry should not be washed or rinsed.
		  • Separate raw, cooked, and ready-to-eat foods while shopping, preparing, or storing foods.
		  • Cook foods to a safe temperature to kill microorganisms.
		  • Chill (refrigerate) perishable food promptly and defrost foods properly.
		  • Avoid raw (unpasteurized) milk or any products made from unpasteurized milk, raw or partially cooked eggs or foods containing raw eggs, raw or undercooked meat and poultry, unpasteurized juices, and raw sprouts.

Source: US Department of Agriculture, US Department of Health and Human Services, *Dietary Guidelines for Americans, 2005,* 6th ed., HHS publication no.: HHS-ODPHP-2005-01-DGA-A, USDA publication no.: Home and Garden Bulletin no. 232. January 2005. Available at http://www.health.gov/dietaryguidelines/dga2005/document/default.htm, accessed February 2, 2015.

BOX 9.7   ITERATION

Iteration is the repetition of a process. It describes a procedure that repeats until some condition is satisfied. Successive approximations, each based on the preceding approximations, are processed in such a way as to arrive at the desired solution. Iteration describes the systematic process used for development of the *Dietary Guidelines*. The previous guidelines are reviewed and critiqued by nutrition specialists along with healthcare professionals, industry, consumers, and other stakeholders. The resulting revised guidelines are reviewed again by stakeholders, and revised again before being reviewed by USDA and HHS and released to the public.

BOX 9.8   2005 DIETARY GUIDELINES COMMENTARY
FROM THE SUGAR ASSOCIATION, INC.

In August 2004, the HSS and USDA announced that public comments were being accepted on the *Report of the Dietary Guidelines Advisory Committee on the Dietary Guidelines for Americans, 2005 to the Secretaries of Health and Human Services and Agriculture*. Individuals and organizations were encouraged to provide written comments within the month. The committee received 42 comments regarding carbohydrates and sugars.

These statements were extracted from the comments submitted by The Sugar Association.

... There is no validated body of irrefutable evidence that corroborates the popular theory that added sugars reduce the nutrient adequacy of the American diet ...

Terminology—sugar-sweetened drinks. The Food and Drug Administration has defined sugar to mean sucrose for the purpose of ingredient labeling, 21 C.F.R. 101.4(b)(20). For the purposes of ingredient labeling, the term *sugar* shall refer to sucrose, which is obtained from sugar cane and sugar beets, in accordance with the provisions of 184.1854. The term *sugars* (plural) is used to designate all mono- and disaccharides. Therefore, The Association (i.e., The Sugar Association, Inc.) takes strong issue with the use of the term *"sugar-sweetened drinks"* to denote caloric beverages throughout the committee's final recommendations and asks that the Agencies not allow this terminology in the messages developed to communicate dietary guidance to the American public.

Very few beverages, and all major soft drinks, have not contained sugar since the mid-1980s. High fructose corn syrup is the major sweetener in nearly all caloric beverages and to use the term "sugar-sweetened drinks" is not only inaccurate but misleads the consuming public ... the sucrose share of the US caloric sweetener market has fallen from nearly 86% in 1970 to 43% in 2003.

Source: Comments of the Sugar Association, Inc, September 27, 2004, previously found at http://www.health.gov /dietaryguidelines/dga2005/comments/readComments.htm, no longer available.

BOX 9.9   USDA NATIONAL NUTRIENT DATABASE: CALCIUM CONTENT

An extensive list of the calcium content of foods is available online from the USDA National Nutrient Database for Standard Reference, Release 27, at http://ndb.nal.usda.gov. The USDA's Nutrient Database is used in food policy, research, and nutrition monitoring; is the foundation of most food and nutrition databases in the United States; and is maintained by the Nutrient Data Laboratory (NDL).

stakeholders that weighed in heavily during the 2005 *Dietary Guidelines* revision process were the United Fresh Fruit and Vegetable Association, Soft Drink Association, American Meat Institute, National Cattlemen's Beef Association, and Wheat Foods Council (Nestle 2002). Understandably, various other interest groups such as vegetarians representing varying levels of strictness and supporters of organic or pesticide-free agriculture also want their principles represented in the guidelines. Not all points are included.

As the government should deliver state-of-the-art nutrition advice unfettered by special interests, one former Washington insider suggested that the responsibility for developing nutrition guidance be moved solely to the HHS as their policy makers do not represent agricultural interests and are therefore less likely than USDA employees to be influenced by pressures from food lobbies (Light 2004).

MYPYRAMID, 2005–2010

In 2005, *MyPyramid* (US Department of Agriculture 2005b) replaced the Food Guide Pyramid. The two-page graphic, available at http://www.choosemyplate.gov/food-groups/downloads/MiniPoster .pdf, was developed by the USDA's Center for Nutrition Policy and Promotion (CNPP). MyPyramid is both a symbol and an interactive food guidance system designed to assist Americans in identifying healthier lifestyle choices to improve their overall health. MyPyramid is also an educational tool intended to translate recommendations from the 2005 *Dietary Guidelines* into concrete recommendations concerning the kinds and amounts of food to eat. In addition, MyPyramid's design was intended to make consumers aware of the health benefits of simple, modest improvements in nutrition, physical activity, and lifestyle behavior. The central message of MyPyramid is "Steps to a Healthier You," consistent with the former *HealthierUS* initiative that emphasized nutrition combined with physical activity, prevention, and a healthier lifestyle (HealthierUS.gov, http://webarchive .library.unt.edu/cot2008/20080916003723/http:/healthierus.gov/).

While MyPyramid retained the pyramid concept of its predecessor in food guidance, it simplified the illustration in order to describe several key concepts:

- *Variety*, symbolized by the six different colored stripes representing the five food groups and the oils and fats group that should be consumed each day. Orange represents grains; green, vegetables; red, fruits; blue, dairy and calcium-rich foods; purple, nondairy, protein-rich foods (such as meat, poultry, fish, eggs, and dried beans and legumes); and yellow, fats and oils. *Recommendation*: Eat foods from all food groups and subgroups.
- *Moderation*, represented by the narrowing of each food group from bottom to top. The wider base stands for foods with little or no solid fats, added sugars, or caloric sweeteners, which should be selected more often to obtain the most nutritionally dense diet. *Recommendation*: Choose forms of foods that limit intake of saturated and *trans* fats, added sugars, cholesterol, salt, and alcohol.
- *Proportionality*, suggested by the varied widths of the stripes. *Recommendation*: Eat more of some foods (fruits, vegetables, whole grains, fat-free or low-fat milk products) and less of others (foods high in saturated or *trans* fats, added sugars, cholesterol, salt, and alcohol).
- *Physical activity*, represented by the steps and the person climbing them, as a reminder of the importance of daily physical activity. *Recommendation*: Be physically active every day.
- *Personalization*, operationalized by the MyPyramid website, which is accessible to consumers who want to obtain more in-depth information about food choices that match their own needs. Consumers could also use the MyPyramid Tracker to maintain a log of daily food intake and check improvement over time.
- *Gradual improvement*, encouraged by the slogan "Steps to a Healthier You," which suggests that small steps can lead to improved diet and lifestyle.

DEFINING AND MEASURING HEALTHY DIETS

HEALTHY EATING INDEX

To assess and monitor the dietary status of Americans, in 1995, the USDA's CNPP developed the Healthy Eating Index (HEI). Designed to measure compliance with the 1990 edition of the *Dietary Guidelines*, the HEI gauges relative intake of the key dietary components identified in the guidelines. The 1995 index comprises 10 components, each representing different aspects of a healthful diet. Components 1–5 measure the degree to which a person's diet conforms to serving recommendations for the five major food groups of the 1992 Food Guide Pyramid (grains, vegetables, fruits, milk, and meat). Components 6–9 conform to recommendations in the 1995 *Dietary Guidelines* for total fat and saturated fat consumption as a percentage of total food energy intake and total cholesterol and sodium intake. Lastly, component 10 measures variety in a person's diet. Scores for each component are given equal weight; the maximum combined score for the 10 components is 100. An HEI score above 80 implies a good diet; a score between 51 and 80 suggests that the diet needs to be improved; and a score below 51 indicates a poor diet (Basiotis et al. 2002; Kennedy et al. 1995).

The HEI has been used for developing nutrition education, evaluating interventions, and monitoring diet quality. For example, as indicated in Table 9.5, the USDA used the HEI to evaluate children's diets. According to the statistics in the table, the average child across all age groups has a diet that needs improvement. As children get older, their diet quality declines. In particular, the lower-quality diets of older children are linked to declines in their fruit and sodium scores (Box 9.10).

The HEI was revised to reflect the 2005 *Dietary Guidelines for Americans* and is based on nutrient density of the diet (density standards per 1000 calories) (Zelman and Kennedy 2005). In the HEI-2005, the recommendation to limit discretionary calories is addressed by crediting the absence of solid fats, alcohol, and added sugars (SoFAAS) in the diet. This category accounts for

TABLE 9.5
Original Healthy Eating Index—Overall and Component Mean Scores for Children, 1989–2000

	1989–1990			1994–1996			1998–2000		
				Ages					
Component	2–6	7–12	13–18	2–6	7–12	13–18	2–6	7–12	13–18
HEI Score									
Overall	70.2	66.6	59.2	69.4	64.6	59.9	70.3	64.1	61.0
1. Grains	7.6	7.0	6.3	7.7	7.5	6.9	8.0	7.5	6.8
2. Vegetables	5.2	5.0	5.6	5.3	5.2	5.9	5.6	4.8	5.3
3. Fruits	6.2	4.6	3.1	6.0	4.1	3.2	5.8	3.7	3.1
4. Milk	8.6	8.3	6.7	7.3	7.1	5.3	7.3	6.9	7.5
5. Meat	6.6	7.0	7.1	5.7	5.7	6.3	5.4	5.5	6.0
6. Total fat	6.7	6.9	6.1	7.3	7.1	7.0	7.3	7.2	7.1
7. Saturated fat	3.7	4.2	4.0	5.5	5.7	6.2	5.8	6.2	6.2
8. Cholesterol	9.4	8.7	8.1	9.0	8.6	7.6	9.0	8.6	8.1
9. Sodium	9.1	7.3	5.8	8.4	6.6	5.6	8.0	6.4	5.7
10. Variety	7.2	7.7	6.5	7.3	7.1	6.0	8.1	7.5	7.2

Source: Federal Interagency Forum on Child and Family Statistics, Table ECON4.D *Healthy Eating Index: Overall and Component Mean Scores and Percentages for Children Ages 2–18, 1989–90, 1994–96, and 1999–2000,* in America's Children: Key National Indicators of Well-Being, 2005, US Government Printing Office, Washington, DC, 2005: 129. Available at http://www.childstats.gov/pdf/ac2005/ac_05 .pdf, accessed February 2, 2015.

20 out of the total 100 possible points. The recommendation to consume a variety of vegetables is addressed by crediting consumption of dark green and orange vegetables and legumes, as well as total vegetables.

RECOMMENDED DIETARY ALLOWANCES AND DIETARY REFERENCE INTAKES

Until 1997, the RDAs served as a benchmark for nutritional adequacy. They were designed to suggest the levels of nutrients adequate to meet the nutrient needs of the majority of healthy people. Subsequently, the Dietary Reference Intakes (DRIs) reflect a shift in emphasis from preventing deficiency to decreasing the risk of chronic disease.

History of the Recommended Dietary Allowances

During World War II, the NRC determined that a set of dietary standards was needed in the event that food would have to be rationed. These standards would be used to make nutrition recommendations for the armed forces, civilians, and the overseas population who might need food relief. All available data concerning nutrient needs was surveyed to create a tentative set of allowances, which was then reviewed by experts before being accepted in 1941. The allowances were meant to provide superior nutrition for civilians and military personnel; therefore, they included a margin of safety. The first edition, published in 1943, was intended to provide "standards to serve as a goal for good nutrition." The RDAs were revised 9 times; the 10th and last edition was published in 1989.

Dietary Reference Intakes

In 1997, at the suggestion of the Institute of Medicine (IOM) of the NAS, the RDAs were incorporated into a broader set of dietary guidelines called the DRIs, which are used by both the US and Canada. The DRIs are a set of nutrient-based reference values that have replaced the 1989 RDAs in the US and the Recommended Nutrient Intakes (RNIs) in Canada. The DRI tables can be found online at http://fnic.nal.usda.gov/dietary-guidance/dietary-reference-intakes/dri-tables. In addition, the USDA provides an interactive tool to determine DRI values for individuals based on sex, age, height, weight, and activity level (http://fnic.nal.usda.gov/fnic/interactiveDRI/).

This set of nutrient reference values, collectively referred to as the DRIs, includes the RDA, Estimated Average Requirement (EAR), Adequate Intake (AI), and Tolerable Upper Intake Level (UL). The RDAs represent the average daily dietary nutrient intake level sufficient to meet the nutrient requirements of almost all healthy individuals (97.5%) in a particular life stage and gender group. AI is used when a definitive RDA cannot be determined from the scientific data. The UL is the maximum amount of a nutrient at which no adverse effects have been observed. The DRIs differ from the 1989 RDAs in at least two respects: First, DRIs are concerned with a reduction in the risk of chronic disease, rather than merely the absence of signs of deficiency. Second, when data are available, ULs are established to avoid the risk of adverse effects from excess consumption (Box 9.11) (National Research Council 2006).

BOX 9.11   THE FOUR COMPONENTS
OF THE DIETARY REFERENCE INTAKES

- *Estimated Average Requirement (EAR)*: The average daily nutrient intake level estimated to meet the requirements of half the healthy individuals in a particular life stage and gender group. It is used to plan and assess dietary adequacies for population groups.
- *Recommended Dietary Allowance (RDA)*: The usual daily dietary nutrient intake level sufficient to meet the nutrient requirements of nearly all (97.5%) healthy individuals in a particular life stage and gender group. It is derived from the EAR: if the distribution of requirements in the group is assumed to be normal, the RDA can be derived as the EAR plus 2 standard deviations of requirements.
- *Adequate Intake (AI)*: The recommended average daily intake level based on observed or experimentally determined approximations or estimates of nutrient intake assumed to be adequate for a group (or groups) of apparently healthy people. It is used when an RDA and EAR cannot be determined.
- *Tolerable Upper Intake Level (UL)*: The highest average daily nutrient intake level that is likely to pose no risk of adverse health effects for almost all individuals in the general population. As intake increases above the UL, the potential risk of adverse health effects may increase.

Source: National Research Council, *Dietary Reference Intakes: The Essential Guide to Nutrient Requirements*, The National Academies Press, Washington, DC, 2006.

TABLE 9.6
Dietary Reference Intake: Acceptable Macronutrient Distribution Ranges (as Percentage of Total Energy)

Macronutrient	Children, 1–3 years	Children, 4–18 years	Adults
Fat	30–40	25–35	20–35
Carbohydrate	45–65	45–65	45–65
Protein	5–20	10–30	10–35

Additional Macronutrient Recommendations

Macronutrient	Recommendation
Dietary cholesterol	As low as possible while consuming a nutritionally adequate diet
Trans fatty acids	As low as possible while consuming a nutritionally adequate diet
Saturated fatty acids	As low as possible while consuming a nutritionally adequate diet
Added sugars	Limit to a maximal intake of no more than 25% total energy[a]

Source: National Research Council, *Dietary Reference Intakes: The Essential Guide to Nutrient Requirements*, The National Academies Press, Washington, DC, 2006.

[a]   It is easy to misinterpret the meaning of limit sugar to no more than 25% of calories. The NRC is trying to say that it would be difficult to obtain all the nutrients one needs on a diet that derives one-quarter of its energy from added sugar.

BOX 9.12   DRIs FOR ENERGY, NUTRIENTS, AND FIBER

Energy	EER
Carbohydrate	EAR, RDA, AMDR
Fiber	AI
Fat	AMDR
Protein	EAR, RDA, AMDR
Vitamins and minerals	EAR, RDA, AI, UL

In addition to the set of four nutrient reference values, two other references are provided: the Estimated Energy Requirement (EER) and the Acceptable Micronutrient Distribution Ranges (AMDRs). The EER is the average dietary energy intake that is predicted to maintain energy balance in a healthy adult of a specific age, gender, weight, height, and physical activity level consistent with good health. AMDRs reflect our interest in nutrition-related chronic disease risks and recommend percentage ranges of calories for daily macronutrients (protein, fat, carbohydrate). Table 9.6 provides the recommended AMDRs for children and adults; as an example, for adults, the acceptable range for carbohydrates is 45–65% of calories; for fat, 20–35% of calories; and for protein, 10–35% of calories (Box 9.12) (National Research Council 2006).

Micronutrients

The DRIs for micronutrients (vitamins and minerals) include the EAR, RDA, AI, and UL. When sufficient information is available on the distribution of nutrient requirements, a nutrient will have both an EAR and an RDA. When information is not sufficient to determine an EAR (and, thus, an RDA), an AI is set for the nutrient. In addition, many nutrients have a UL. For some nutrients, however, data are insufficient to estimate the UL reliably. The absence of a UL indicates that the current evidence does not permit its estimation, which is not the same as saying that there is no point at which adverse effects may occur due to overconsumption of that nutrient.

Energy, Fiber, and the Macronutrients

A different set of DRIs has been developed for energy, fiber, and the macronutrients (carbohydrate, protein, and fat) (National Research Council 2006).

Energy

The food energy (calorie) requirement is expressed in terms of EER. An adult EER is the dietary energy intake needed to maintain energy balance in a healthy adult of a given age, gender, weight, height, and level of physical activity. For children and pregnant and lactating women, the EER accounts for the needs associated with growth, deposition of tissues, and the secretion of milk at rates that are consistent with good health.

Fiber

For fiber, the DRI is expressed as an AI. The fiber AI increases from 19 g per day for children through the age of 3 years to 25 g per day for females and 38 g per day for males aged 19–50 years, as illustrated in Table 9.7. For adults, this is the equivalent of 14 g per 1000 calories intake. Many legumes such as baked beans, black beans, kidney beans, navy beans, and pinto beans deliver about 6–8 g of fiber per 1/2-cup serving. Other legumes such as garbanzo beans, great northern beans, lentils, lima beans, and split peas provide slightly less fiber, at 5 g for a 1/2-cup serving. The USDA National Nutrient Database for Standard Reference, Release 27, at http://ndb.nal.usda.gov, is a convenient tool for looking up the micronutrient and macronutrient value of foods, including fiber content.

TABLE 9.7
**Dietary Reference Intake: Adequate Intake
for Total Fiber (g per day)**

Age	Female	Male
0–6 months	ND	ND
7–12 months	ND	ND
1–3 years	19	19
4–8 years	25	25
9–13 years	26	31
14–18 years	26	38
19–50 years	25	38
Pregnancy, 14–50 years	28	–
Lactation, 14–50 years	29	–
>50 years	21	30

Source: National Research Council, *Dietary Reference Intakes:
The Essential Guide to Nutrient Requirements*, The
National Academies Press, Washington, DC, 2006.
Note: ND, not determined.

Macronutrients

For intake of fat, protein, and carbohydrate, the DRIs include AMDRs, expressed as a percentage of energy intakes. EARs and RDAs are also available for carbohydrate and protein.

Additional Recommendations

Saturated fatty acids, *trans* fatty acids, and dietary cholesterol have no known protective role in preventing chronic disease and are not required at any level in the diet, although many of the foods containing these fats do provide other valuable nutrients. Animal products, bakery items, and full-fat dairy products are the primary sources of these fats. As there is no intake level of saturated fatty acids, *trans* fatty acids, or dietary cholesterol at which there is no adverse effect, no UL is set for them. Instead, the DRI calls for intakes of dietary cholesterol, *trans* fatty acids, and saturated fatty acids "as low as possible while consuming a nutritionally adequate diet" (Box 9.13, Table 9.6).

Added Sugar

Whereas the acceptable range for carbohydrates is 45–65% of total calories, almost inexplicably, the DRI also recommends that added sugars be limited to 25% or less of total energy intake (Table 9.6). It is difficult to consume a nutritionally adequate diet when added sugar provides one-fourth or more of daily energy intake. In contrast, the World Health Organization (WHO) recommends that 10% or less of total calories come from added sugars (Report of a Joint WHO/FAO Expert Consultation 2003). As early as 1977, reducing the consumption of refined and processed sugars to about 10% of energy intake was one of the *Dietary Goals* for the US (Table 9.2).

USES OF THE DIETARY REFERENCE INTAKES

The introduction of the DRIs, especially the EAR and the UL, provided better tools for use in dietary assessment and planning for individuals and for groups than did the RDAs published through 1989 (the "old" RDAs). The DRIs were developed anticipating a variety of uses, such as assessment of diets of individuals and groups, design and evaluation of diets in a variety of institutions, creation of nutrition guidelines and education programs, and development of regulations around the nutritional

BOX 9.13 *TRANS* FATTY ACIDS AND THE LAW OF UNINTENDED CONSEQUENCES

Trans fatty acids (also known as *trans* fats) are chemically classified as unsaturated fatty acids; however, once in the body, they behave more like saturated fatty acids. Both *trans* and saturated fatty acids increase the risk of heart disease in vulnerable people by raising low-density lipoprotein cholesterol levels. The magnitude of this effect may be greater for *trans* fatty acids than for saturated fats.

Trans fats are found in partially hydrogenated vegetable oils, such as margarine and shortening, with lower levels found in meats and dairy products. For the food industry, partially hydrogenated vegetable oils are attractive because of their long shelf life, their stability during deep-frying, and their semisolidity, which can be customized to enhance the palatability of baked goods and sweets.[1]

Fatty acids are the chemical compounds that comprise fats. They are chains of carbon atoms with attached hydrogen atoms. A *saturated* fatty acid has the maximum possible number of hydrogen atoms attached to every carbon atom, and is therefore described as saturated with hydrogen atoms. Conversely, sometimes, a pair of hydrogen atoms in the middle of a chain is missing, creating a gap that leaves two carbon atoms connected by a double bond, rather than a single bond. The missing hydrogen atoms cause the chain to be described as *unsaturated*. A fatty acid that has one double bond is said to be *monounsaturated*. Fatty acids having more than one double bond are called *polyunsaturated*. When the hydrogen atoms at a double bond are positioned on the same side of the carbon chain, it is described as a *cis* (meaning "same" in Latin) configuration. In nutrition labeling, all monounsaturated and polyunsaturated fatty acids are in the *cis* configuration.

Trans fatty acids are produced from vegetable oils through a manufacturing process known as *partial hydrogenation*. Hydrogen atoms are added to unsaturated sites on fatty acids, eliminating double bonds and resulting in a more solid fat with a longer shelf life. Some double bonds and hydrogen atoms end up on opposite sides of the carbon chain. This type of configuration is called *trans* (meaning "across" in Latin). The structures of saturated and unsaturated fatty acids are depicted below.

Portion of a **saturated fatty acid**	Portion of a ***cis*-unsaturated fatty acid**	Portion of a ***trans*-unsaturated fatty acid**
H H | | ...– C – C –... | | H H	H H | | ...– C = C –...	H | ...– C = C –... | H

The same molecule, containing the same number of atoms, with a double bond in the same location, can be either a *trans* or a *cis* fatty acid, depending on the conformation of the double bond. In most naturally occurring unsaturated fatty acids, the hydrogen atoms are on the same side of the double bonds of the carbon chain (*cis* configuration—meaning "on the same side" in Latin). However, partial hydrogenation reconfigures most of the double bonds that do not become chemically saturated, twisting them so that the hydrogen atoms end up on different sides of the chain. This type of configuration is called *trans*, which means "across" in Latin (White 2009).

At the time the Food and Drug Administration (FDA) ruled that effective 2006, *trans* fatty acids be declared in the nutrition label of conventional foods and dietary supplements, the average consumption of industrially produced *trans* fatty acids in the US was 2–3% of total calories consumed.[2,3] In response, many food companies have removed *trans* fat from their products and replaced it with palm oil, a saturated fat that was taken out of many products in the late 1980s after an effective campaign waged in part by the American Soybean Association and the Center for Science in the Public Interest helped turn Americans away from all forms of tropical oils.[4] If the increased consumption of palm oil results in a negative health outcome (or a negative social outcome due to deforestation), this would be considered an example of the law of unintended consequences.

Source:
[1] Data from Mozaffarian, D. et al., *N. Engl. J. Med.*, 354, 2006.
[2] Data from Allison, D.B. et al., *J. Am. Diet. Assoc.*, 99, 1999.
[3] Data from US Department of Health and Human Services, US Food and Drug Administration, Center for Food Safety and Applied Nutrition, Food Labeling: Trans Fatty Acids in Nutrition Labeling, Nutrient Content Claims, and Health Claims, August 2003. Available at http://www.fda.gov/Food/GuidanceRegulation/GuidanceDocuments RegulatoryInformation/LabelingNutrition/ucm053479.htm, accessed February 2, 2015.
[4] Data from Severson, K. and Warner, M., Fat Substitute Is Pushed Out of the Kitchen, *New York Times*, February 13, 2005. Available at http://www.nytimes.com/2005/02/13/business/13transfat.html?_r=0, accessed February 2, 2015.

quality of the food supply. Indeed, separate IOM reports have been published addressing the role of the DRIs in dietary assessment (National Research Council 2000) and planning (National Research Council 2003a), as well as labeling and fortification (National Research Council 2003b).

Between 1997 and 2011, 14 DRI reports have been published: 8 nutrient-specific reports, 2 reports explaining appropriate uses of the DRIs, and 4 related or derivative reports. As of 2015, no further DRI reports have been published (Box 9.14).

CURRENT FEDERAL FOOD, NUTRITION, AND LIFESTYLE GUIDANCE (2010–2015)

Since 1980, the *Dietary Guidelines for Americans* have been updated every 5 years. A *Dietary Guidelines* Advisory Committee was established to assist in the preparations of the 1995, 2000, 2005, 2010, and 2015 editions of the guidelines (US Department of Health and Human Services 2013). (The 2015 *Dietary Guidelines for Americans* was still under development as of the writing of this book.)

Although the guidelines have remained consistent, there have been changes through the years that reflect emerging science. The guidelines have evolved into a document that attempts to reflect scientific consensus and provides the statutory basis of federal nutrition education efforts.

DIETARY GUIDELINES FOR AMERICANS, 2010

The seventh edition of the *Dietary Guidelines* was released in January 2011 (US Department of Agriculture 2010) and is the current policy as of the time of writing this book. The policy document is available online at http://www.cnpp.usda.gov/DGAs2010-PolicyDocument.htm. An abbreviated Executive Summary with recommendations appears in Tables 9.8 and 9.9.

The *Dietary Guidelines* provide dietary advice for Americans ages 2 years and over. The recommendations are based on current scientific knowledge about the relationship between dietary intake and health promotion and reduction of risk for major chronic diseases. The document forms the basis for federal nutrition policy, sets standards for nutrition assistance programs, and guides nutrition

**BOX 9.14   DIETARY REFERENCE INTAKE REPORTS ISSUED
BY THE INSTITUTE OF MEDICINE, 1997–2011**

1. Dietary Reference Intakes for Vitamin D and Calcium (2011)
2. Dietary Reference Intakes Research Synthesis Workshop Summary (2006)
3. Dietary Reference Intakes for Water, Potassium, Sodium, Chloride, and Sulfate (2005)
4. Dietary Reference Intakes for Energy, Carbohydrate, Fiber, Fat, Fatty Acids, Cholesterol, Protein, and Amino Acids (Macronutrients) (2005)
5. Dietary Reference Intakes: Guiding Principles for Nutrition Labeling and Fortification (2003)
6. Dietary Reference Intakes: Applications in Dietary Planning (2003)
7. Dietary Reference Intakes: Proposed Definition of Dietary Fiber (2001)
8. Dietary Reference Intakes for Vitamin A, Vitamin K, Arsenic, Boron, Chromium, Copper, Iodine, Iron, Manganese, Molybdenum, Nickel, Silicon, Vanadium, and Zinc (2001)
9. Dietary Reference Intakes for Vitamin C, Vitamin E, Selenium, and Carotenoids (2000)
10. Dietary Reference Intakes: Applications in Dietary Assessment (2000)
11. Dietary Reference Intakes: Proposed Definition and Plan for Review of Dietary Antioxidants and Related Compounds (1998)
12. Dietary Reference Intakes for Thiamin, Riboflavin, Niacin, Vitamin B_6, Folate, Vitamin B_{12}, Pantothenic Acid, Biotin, and Choline (1998)
13. Dietary Reference Intakes: A Risk Assessment Model for Establishing Upper Intake Levels for Nutrients (1998)
14. Dietary Reference Intakes for Calcium, Phosphorus, Magnesium, Vitamin D, and Fluoride (1997)

Source: US Department of Agriculture, National Agricultural Library, DRI Reports. Available at http://fnic.nal.usda.gov/dietary-guidance/dietary-reference-intakes/dri-reports, accessed February 2, 2015.

education programs. In particular, the guidelines are the source of the information contained in the USDA's food guidance system, *MyPlate*. Following the release of the 2010 *Dietary Guidelines*, MyPlate, a more individualized and interactive food guidance tool, replaced MyPyramid.

The guidelines provide the rationale for food and nutrition legislation and play a role in developing policies aimed at preventing disease and promoting optimal health as well as in assessing the impact of prevention policies on population behavior and health outcomes (Schneeman and Mendelson 2002). Federal nutrition assistance programs such as the USDA's National School Lunch and School Breakfast Programs (NSLP/SBP), Supplemental Nutrition Assistance Program (SNAP), and Special Supplemental Nutrition Program for Women, Infants, and Children (WIC) use the principles in the *Dietary Guidelines* as the scientific underpinning for designing nutrition assistance benefit structures.

All federal dietary guidance for the public must be consistent with the *Dietary Guidelines*. The CNPP chairs the USDA Dietary Guidance Working Group, which reviews the USDA and dietary guidance materials to ensure consistency with the *Dietary Guidelines*. In sum, the guidelines enable the federal government to speak with one voice on nutrition issues for the health of the American public.

Dietary Advice

The purpose of the *Dietary Guidelines* is to summarize and synthesize the current knowledge about foods and food components into an interrelated set of recommendations for healthy eating that can be adopted by the public. To optimize the beneficial impact of these recommendations on

TABLE 9.8

Dietary Guidelines for Americans, 2010: Topic Areas and Key Recommendations for the General Population

Topic Area	Key Recommendations for the General Population
Balancing calories to manage weight	• Prevent and/or reduce overweight and obesity through improved eating and physical activity behaviors. • Control total calorie intake to manage body weight. For people who are overweight or obese, this will mean consuming fewer calories from foods and beverages. • Increase physical activity and reduce time spent in sedentary behaviors. • Maintain appropriate calorie balance during each stage of life—childhood, adolescence, adulthood, pregnancy and breastfeeding, and older age.
Foods and food components to reduce	• Reduce daily sodium intake to less than 2300 mg, and further reduce intake to 1500 mg among people who are 51 or older and those of any age who are African American or have hypertension, diabetes, or chronic kidney disease. The 1500 mg recommendation applies to about half of the US population, including children, and the majority of adults. • Consume less than 10% of calories from saturated fatty acids by replacing them with monounsaturated and polyunsaturated fatty acids. • Consume less than 300 mg per day of dietary cholesterol. • Keep trans fatty acid consumption as low as possible by limiting foods that contain synthetic sources of trans fat, such as partially hydrogenated oils, and by limiting other solid fats. • Reduce the intake of calories from solid fats and added sugars. • Limit the consumption of foods that contain refined grains, especially refined grain foods that contain solid fats, added sugars, and sodium. • If alcohol is consumed, it should be consumed in moderation—up to one drink per day for women and two drinks per day for men—and only by adults of legal drinking age.
Foods and nutrients to increase	Individuals should meet the following recommendations as part of a healthy eating pattern while staying within their calorie needs: • Increase vegetable and fruit intake. • Eat a variety of vegetables, especially dark green, red, and orange vegetables and beans and peas. • Consume at least half of all grains as whole grains. Increase whole-grain intake by replacing refined grains with whole grains. • Increase intake of fat-free or low-fat milk and milk products, such as milk, yogurt, cheese, or fortified soy beverages. • Choose a variety of protein foods, which include seafood, lean meat and poultry, eggs, beans and peas, soy products, and unsalted nuts and seeds. • Increase the amount and variety of seafood consumed by choosing seafood in place of some meat and poultry. • Replace protein foods that are higher in solid fats with choices that are lower in solid fats and calories and/or are sources of oils. • Use oils to replace solid fats where possible. • Choose foods that provide more potassium, dietary fiber, calcium, and vitamin D, which are nutrients of concern in American diets. These foods include vegetables, fruits, whole grains, and milk and milk products.
Building healthy eating patterns	• Select an eating pattern that meets nutrient needs over time at an appropriate calorie level. • Account for all foods and beverages consumed and assess how they fit within a total healthy eating pattern. • Follow food safety recommendations when preparing and eating foods to reduce the risk of foodborne illness.

Source: US Department of Agriculture, US Department of Health and Human Services, *Dietary Guidelines for Americans, 2010,* 7th ed., US Government Printing Office, Washington, DC, December 2010.

TABLE 9.9

Dietary Guidelines for Americans, **2010: Key Recommendations for Specific Population Groups**

Population Group	Key Recommendations
Women capable of becoming pregnant	• Choose foods that supply heme iron, which is more readily absorbed by the body; additional iron sources; and enhancers of iron absorption such as vitamin C-rich foods. • Consume 400 µg per day of synthetic folic acid (from fortified foods and/or supplements) in addition to food forms of folate from a varied diet.
Women who are pregnant or breastfeeding	• Consume 8–12 oz. of seafood per week from a variety of seafood types. • Due to its high methyl mercury content, limit white (albacore) tuna to 6 oz. per week, and do not eat the following four types of fish: tilefish, shark, swordfish, and king mackerel. • If pregnant, take an iron supplement, as recommended by an obstetrician or other healthcare provider.
Individuals ages 50 years and older	• Consume foods fortified with vitamin B_{12}, such as fortified cereals, or dietary supplements.

Source: US Department of Agriculture, US Department of Health and Human Services, *Dietary Guidelines for Americans, 2010,* 7th ed., US Government Printing Office, Washington, DC, December 2010.

health, the guidelines should be implemented in their entirety. The 2010 *Dietary Guidelines* recommendations are grouped into four general topic areas as described in Table 9.8 and encompass two main concepts: (1) maintain calorie balance over time to achieve and sustain a healthy weight, and (2) focus on consuming nutrient-dense foods and beverages.

Maintain Calorie Balance

Those individuals most successful at achieving and maintaining a healthy weight do so through continued attention to caloric balance: consuming only enough calories to meet their needs while engaging in regular physical activity. In order to halt and reverse obesity and improve health, many Americans must decrease their consumption of calories and increase calorie expenditure through physical activity.

Although the *Dietary Guidelines* are aimed at changing individual behaviors, the document does acknowledge that individuals make food and physical activity choices within an environmental context that promotes overconsumption of calories and discourages physical activity (US Department of Agriculture 2010). This environmental context (and the ensuing behavioral choices made by individuals) have contributed to the dramatic increases in obesity and weight-related conditions, such as CVD, type 2 diabetes, and some types of cancer. To reverse these trends, a coordinated, system-wide approach is needed. As such, several strategies are described that can be implemented by various sectors of influence (e.g., educators, communities and organizations, health professionals, small and large businesses, and policy makers) to support individuals and families in achieving the dietary intake recommendations, as highlighted in Table 9.10.

Nutrient Density

Like its predecessor, the 2010 *Dietary Guidelines* recommend consuming a variety of nutrient-dense foods and beverages within and among the basic food groups. Nutrient-dense foods provide more nutrients and generally fewer calories per unit volume than energy-dense, nutrient-poor foods. Foods low in nutrient density often supply too much sodium and too many calories from solid fats, added sugars, and refined grains, but relatively small amounts of micronutrients, sometimes none at all.

The greater the consumption of foods or beverages low in nutrient density, the more difficult it is to consume enough nutrients without gaining weight, especially for sedentary individuals. Selecting low-fat forms of foods in each group and foods free of added sugars—in other words, nutrient-dense versions of foods—allows an individual to meet his or her nutrient needs without overconsuming

TABLE 9.10

Dietary Guidelines for Americans, 2010: Multisectoral Strategies for Helping Americans Make Healthy Choices

Guiding Principle	Strategies
Ensure that all Americans have access to nutritious foods and opportunities for physical activity	• Create local-, state-, and national-level strategic plans to achieve *Dietary Guidelines* and *Physical Activity Guidelines* recommendations among individuals, families, and communities. • Recognize health disparities among subpopulations and ensure equitable access to safe and affordable healthy foods and opportunities for physical activity for all people. • Expand access to grocery stores, farmers' markets, and other outlets for healthy foods. • Develop and expand safe, effective, and sustainable agriculture and aquaculture practices to ensure availability of recommended amounts of healthy foods to all segments of the population. • Increase food security among at-risk populations by promoting nutrition assistance programs. • Facilitate attainment of the nutrition, food safety, and physical activity objectives outlined in Healthy People 2020.
Facilitate individual behavior change through environmental strategies	• Empower individuals and families with improved nutrition literacy and gardening and cooking skills to heighten enjoyment of preparing and consuming healthy foods. • Initiate partnerships with food producers, suppliers, and retailers to promote the development and availability of appropriate portions of affordable, nutritious food products (including, but not limited to, those lower in sodium, solid fats, and added sugars) in food retail and food service establishments. • Develop legislation, policies, and systems in key sectors such as public health, healthcare, retail, school food service, recreation/fitness, transportation, and nonprofit/volunteer to prevent and reduce obesity. • Support future research that will further examine the individual, community, and system factors that contribute to the adoption of healthy eating and physical activity behaviors; identify best practices and facilitate adoption of those practices. • Implement the US National Physical Activity Plan to increase physical activity and reduce sedentary behavior.
Set the stage for lifelong health eating, physical activity, and weight management behaviors	• Ensure that all meals and snacks sold and served in schools and child-care and early childhood settings are consistent with the *Dietary Guidelines*. • Provide comprehensive health, nutrition, and physical education programs in educational settings, and place special emphasis on food preparation skills, food safety, and lifelong physical activity. • Identify approaches for assessing and tracking children's body mass index (or other valid measures) for use by health professionals to identify overweight and obesity and implement appropriate interventions. • Encourage physical activity in school, child-care, and early childhood settings through physical education programs, recess, and support for active transportation initiatives (e.g., walk-to-school programs). • Reduce children's screen (television and computer) time. • Develop and support effective policies to limit food and beverage marketing to children. • Support children's programs that promote healthy nutrition and physical activity throughout the year, including summer.

Source: US Department of Agriculture, US Department of Health and Human Services, *Dietary Guidelines for Americans, 2010,* 7th ed., US Government Printing Office, Washington, DC, December 2010.

calories. However, the US food supply is replete with foods not in their most nutrient-dense form, such as potatoes deep-fried into chips, popcorn popped in oil and drizzled with butter, chicken breaded and deep-fat-fried, and whole milk-based sugar-sweetened drinks. Most people will exceed calorie recommendations if they consistently choose higher-fat foods within the food groups.

Based on data from the Third National Health and Nutrition Examination Survey (NHANES III), adults who consumed energy-dense, nutrient-poor foods were likely to have a high energy intake, marginal micronutrient intake, poor compliance with dietary guidance related to nutrients and food groups, and low serum concentrations of vitamins and carotenoids (the precursors to vitamin A) (Kant 2000). Similarly, in children, a high intake of low-nutrient-density foods is related to an overall higher energy intake and a lower intake of the major food groups and micronutrients. Nearly one-third of the daily energy intake of American children and adolescents comes from relatively energy-dense, low-nutritional-value foods (Kant 2003).

REVISED HEALTHY EATING INDEX

Publication of the 2010 *Dietary Guidelines* prompted the update of the HEI-2005. The HEI-2010 retains several features of the HEI-2005, in that it (1) contains 12 components, many unchanged, including 9 adequacy components (dietary components to increase) and 3 moderation components (dietary components to decrease); (2) uses a density approach to set standards; and (3) utilizes least-restrictive standards (easiest to achieve). Updates to the index include the following: (1) "greens and beans" replaces "dark green and orange vegetables and legumes"; (2) "seafood and plant proteins" was added to reflect the new recommendation for seafood; (3) "fatty acids" (a ratio of polyunsaturated and monounsaturated to saturated fatty acids) replaces "oils and saturated fat" based on the recommendation to replace saturated fat with monounsaturated and polyunsaturated fatty acids; and (4) a moderation component ("refined grains") replaces the adequacy component ("total grains") to assess overconsumption (Guenther et al. 2013). Table 9.11 compares the HEI-2005 and HEI-2010 components and scoring allotments.

The HEI-2010 reflects the key recommendations of the 2010 *Dietary Guidelines* and will continue to be used to assess the diet quality of Americans, in evaluating interventions, in dietary pattern research, and to evaluate the food environment (Guenther et al. 2013). As one example, the HEI-2010 was used to assess the quality of American children's diets between 2003 and 2008 (US Department of Agriculture 2013). As shown in Table 9.12, the quality of children's diets remains poor, with total scores ranging from 47 to 50 (a score of 100 indicates that the recommendations, on average, were met or exceeded). Although the average scores for all components of the HEI-2010 were below the standards across all years, there were small but significant increases in consumption of total fruit (which includes 100% fruit juice) and whole fruit, and small but significant decreases in consumption of empty calories (US Department of Agriculture 2013).

MYPLATE FOOD GUIDANCE SYSTEM

Following the release of the 2010 *Dietary Guidelines for Americans* in 2011, MyPlate replaced MyPyramid. The two-page graphic (Figure 9.3) was developed by the USDA's CNPP.

MyPlate is both an icon and an interactive food guidance system designed to remind and support Americans in making better food choices and building a healthy plate at mealtimes. MyPlate emphasizes the fruit, vegetable, grains, protein, and dairy food groups, and encourages individuals to seek more information at the accompanying website, http://choosemyplate.gov. With MyPlate, the USDA hopes to provide an easy-to-understand icon that translates the key consumer actions identified in the 2010 *Dietary Guidelines*. These messages include the following:

- Balance calories.
  - Enjoy your food, but eat less.
  - Avoid oversized portions.

TABLE 9.11

Comparison of the Healthy Eating Index 2005 and Healthy Eating Index 2010 Components and Scoring Allotments

HEI-2005		HEI-2010	
Component	Maximum Points	Component	Maximum Points
Adequacy (Higher Score Indicates Higher Consumption)			
Total fruit[a]	5	Total fruit[a]	5
Whole fruit[b]	5	Whole fruit[b]	5
Total vegetables[c]	5	Total vegetables[c]	5
Dark green and orange vegetables and legumes[c]	5	Greens and beans[c]	5
Total grains	5	Whole grains	10
Whole grains	5		
Milk[d]	10	Dairy[d]	10
Meat and beans[e]	10	Total protein foods[e]	5
		Seafood and plant proteins[e,f]	5
Oils[g]	10	Fatty acids[h]	10
Moderation (Higher Score Indicates Lower Consumption)			
Saturated fat	10	Refined Grains	10
Sodium	10	Sodium	10
Calories from SoFAAS[i]	20	Empty calories[i,j]	20

Source: Guenther, P.M. et al., *J. Acad. Nutr. Diet*, 113, 2013.

a Includes fruit juice.
b Includes all forms except juice.
c Includes any beans and peas (called "legumes" in HEI-2005) not counted as total protein foods (called "meat and beans" in HEI-2005).
d Includes all milk products, such as fluid milk, yogurt, and cheese, and fortified soy beverages.
e Beans and peas are included here (and not with vegetables) when the Total Protein Foods (called Meat and Beans in HEI-2005) standard is otherwise not met.
f Includes seafood, nuts, seeds, soy products (other than beverages), as well as beans and peas counted as Total Protein Foods.
g Includes nonhydrogenated vegetable oils and oils in fish, nuts, and seeds.
h Ratio of polyunsaturated and monounsaturated fatty acids to saturated fatty acids.
i Calories from solid fats, alcoholic beverages, and added sugars.
j Threshold for counting alcohol is >13 g/1000 kcal.

- Foods to increase.
  - Make half your plate fruits and vegetables.
  - Switch to fat-free or low-fat (1%) milk.
  - Make at least half your grains whole grains.
- Foods to reduce.
  - Compare sodium (salt) in foods like soup, bread, and frozen meals, and choose foods with lower numbers.
  - Drink water instead of sugary drinks (US Department of Agriculture 2011a).

Development of MyPlate

MyPlate was the result of a formative research project conducted by the USDA in 2010 to develop a next-generation food icon and nutrition messaging based on the 2010 *Dietary Guidelines for*

TABLE 9.12

Diet Quality of American Children, Ages 2–17, as Measured by the Healthy Eating Index 2010

Dietary Component (Maximum Score)	2003–2004 Score	2005–2006 Score	2007–2008 Score
Adequacy (Higher Score Indicates Higher Consumption)			
Total fruit (5)	3.3	3.4	4.0*
Whole fruit (5)	2.9	3.4	4.6*
Total vegetables (5)	2.3	2.3	2.3
Greens and beans (5)	0.7	0.8	0.9
Whole grains (10)	1.6	1.7	1.8
Dairy (10)	8.6	8.4	8.3
Total protein foods (5)	4.0	4.1	4.2
Seafood and plant proteins (5)	2.4	2.4	2.1
Fatty acids (10)	3.1	2.9	3.0
Moderation (Higher Score Indicates Lower Consumption)			
Refined grains (10)	4.5	4.3	4.6
Sodium (10)	5.5	5.1	5.0
Empty calories (20)	8.0	8.3	9.0**
Total (100)	46.9	47.1	49.8

Source: US Department of Agriculture, Center for Nutrition Policy and Promotion, *Nutrition Insight*, 52, 2013. Available at http://www.cnpp.usda.gov/sites/default/files/nutrition_insights_uploads/Insight52.pdf, accessed February 2, 2015.

*Significantly different from 2003–2004 and 2005–2006 ($P < .05$).

**Significantly different from 2003–2004 ($P < .05$).

Americans. Although MyPyramid was only 5 years old at the time, it was already critiqued for being both too complicated and too simplistic. In addition, confusion arose with some still using the "old pyramid" (Food Guide Pyramid) and others using the "new pyramid" (MyPyramid). Concerns also arose that consumers, being so familiar with the pyramid shape, were not paying attention to the icon or implementing its messages. In May 2010, the White House Childhood Obesity Task Force recommended a "next generation Food Pyramid," though some felt that a completely new image was needed to refocus attention on healthy eating (US Department of Agriculture 2011b).

The USDA undertook a comprehensive research approach to develop consumer nutrition messages and test potential food icons. This research included interviews with federal nutrition education staff, such as those in the USDA, HHS, and Department of Education; analysis of media coverage surrounding the 2005 *Dietary Guidelines*; an environmental scan of six existing communication programs intended to change consumers' knowledge, attitudes, and behaviors around diet and exercise; a literature review of reports, articles, and commercial research on consumer food preferences, attitudes, and habits; consumer focus groups; and a quantitative survey to test language and graphic images. During the focus groups, consumers were shown images of MyPyramid, an abstract pyramid with a triumphant figure on top, a plate depicting food groups, and a thought bubble depicting food groups. Although no single graphic appealed to everyone, most groups preferred the plate and the thought bubble. Ultimately, the plate was chosen because it is a familiar eating symbol, despite concerns expressed by focus group members outlined in Table 9.13 (US Department of Agriculture 2011b).

The USDA acknowledges that the MyPlate icon will not teach all nutrition concepts or change consumer behavior on its own. Rather, its focused purpose is to grab consumers' attention to eat

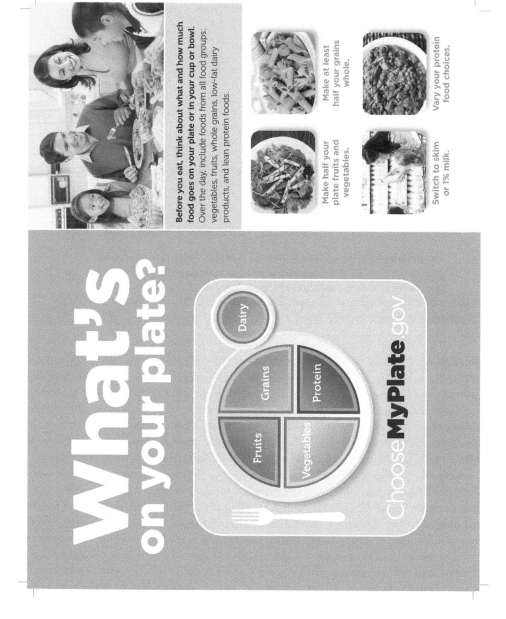

FIGURE 9.3 MyPlate. (From US Department of Agriculture, Center for Nutrition Policy and Promotion, MyPlate Mini Poster. Available at http://www.choosemyplate .gov/downloads/mini_poster_English_final.pdf, accessed February 2, 2015.)

(*Continued*)

Cut back on sodium and empty calories from solid fats and added sugars

Look out for salt (sodium) in foods you buy. Compare sodium in foods and choose those with a lower number.

Drink water instead of sugary drinks. Eat sugary desserts less often.

Make foods that are high in solid fats—such as cakes, cookies, ice cream, pizza, cheese, sausages, and hot dogs—occasional choices, not every day foods.

Limit empty calories to less than 260 per day, based on a 2,000 calorie diet.

Be physically active your way

Pick activities you like and do each for at least 10 minutes at a time. Every bit adds up, and health benefits increase as you spend more time being active.

Children and adolescents: get 60 minutes or more a day.

Adults: get 2 hours and 30 minutes or more a week of activity that requires moderate effort, such as brisk walking.

Vegetables	Fruits	Grains	Dairy	Protein Foods
Eat more red, orange, and dark-green veggies like tomatoes, sweet potatoes, and broccoli in main dishes.	Use fruits as snacks, salads, and desserts. At breakfast, top your cereal with bananas or strawberries; add blueberries to pancakes.	Substitute whole-grain choices for refined-grain breads, bagels, rolls, breakfast cereals, crackers, rice, and pasta.	Choose skim (fat-free) or 1% (low-fat) milk. They have the same amount of calcium and other essential nutrients as whole milk but less fat and calories.	Eat a variety of foods from the protein food group each week, such as seafood, beans and peas, and nuts as well as lean meats, poultry, and eggs.
Add beans or peas to salads (kidney or chickpeas), soups (split peas or lentils), and side dishes (pinto or baked beans), or serve as a main dish.	Buy fruits that are dried, frozen, and canned (in water or 100% juice), as well as fresh fruits.	Check the ingredients list on product labels for the words "whole" or "whole grain" before the grain ingredient name.	Top fruit salads and baked potatoes with low-fat yogurt.	Twice a week, make seafood the protein on your plate.
Fresh, frozen, and canned vegetables all count. Choose "reduced sodium" or "no-salt-added" canned veggies.	Select 100% fruit juice when choosing juices.	Choose products that name a whole grain first on the ingredients list.	If you are lactose intolerant, try lactose-free milk or fortified soymilk (soy beverage).	Choose lean meats and ground beef that are at least 90% lean. Trim or drain fat from meat and remove skin from poultry to cut fat and calories.

For a 2,000-calorie daily food plan, you need the amounts below from each food group.
To find amounts personalized for you, go to ChooseMyPlate.gov.

Eat 2½ cups every day	Eat 2 cups every day	Eat 6 ounces every day	Get 3 cups every day	Eat 5½ ounces every day
What counts as a cup? 1 cup of raw or cooked vegetables or vegetable juice; 2 cups of leafy salad greens	**What counts as a cup?** 1 cup of raw or cooked fruit or 100% fruit juice; ½ cup dried fruit	**What counts as an ounce?** 1 slice of bread; ½ cup of cooked rice, cereal, or pasta; 1 ounce of ready-to-eat cereal	**What counts as a cup?** 1 cup of milk, yogurt, or fortified soymilk; 1½ ounces natural or 2 ounces processed cheese	**What counts as an ounce?** 1 ounce of lean meat, poultry, or fish; 1 egg; 1 Tbsp peanut butter; ½ ounce nuts or seeds; ¼ cup beans or peas

USDA
US Department of Agriculture • Center for Nutrition Policy and Promotion
August 2011
CNPP-25
USDA is an equal opportunity provider and employer

FIGURE 9.3 (CONTINUED) MyPlate. (From US Department of Agriculture, Center for Nutrition Policy and Promotion, MyPlate Mini Poster. Available at http://www.choosemyplate.gov/downloads/mini_poster_English_final.pdf, accessed February 2, 2015.)

TABLE 9.13

Focus Group Feedback Regarding Two Possible Food Guidance Icons

	Pros	Cons
Plate icon depicting food groups	• Conveys a nutrition message about family mealtime and making half the plate fruits and vegetables. • A good reminder to model this plate at dinnertime and to eat healthy.	• Plate applies more to dinner than breakfast, lunch, or snacks. • Does not convey what choices are best within food groups. • Conveys proportionality between groups, but not the amounts that should be eaten. • Difficult to apply to combination foods prevalent in various cultures (e.g., fajitas, lasagna, stir-fry). • Does not represent a total day or diet.
Thought bubble depicting food groups	• Effective reminder to think about healthy eating over the day.	• Provides less information on how to eat using the food groups.

Source: US Department of Agriculture, Center for Nutrition Policy and Promotion, Development of 2010 *Dietary Guidelines for Americans* Consumer Messages and New Food Icon: Executive Summary of Formative Research, June 2011. Available at http://www.choosemyplate.gov/food-groups/downloads/MyPlate/ExecutiveSummaryOfFormative Research.pdf, accessed February 2, 2015.

healthfully at mealtime and prompt further knowledge seeking. Additional resources, along with strategic and consistent messaging and communications, are necessary to provide all the information consumers need to eat a healthy diet (US Department of Agriculture 2011b). ChooseMyPlate. gov contains these resources and messages for a variety of audiences, including children, college students, dieters, pregnant and breastfeeding women, educators and teachers, healthcare professionals, and partners. Printable materials, videos, sample menus and recipes, daily food plans, diet analysis tools, and games are among the many resources available on the website, with more being added over time (US Department of Agriculture, http://www.choosemyplate.gov/).

Criticism

In an effort to address weaknesses they perceive in MyPlate, faculty members at the Harvard School of Public Health have developed their own graphic, Harvard's Healthy Eating Plate (Figure 9.4).

In contrast to MyPlate, Harvard's version provides detailed guidance on the healthiest choices in the major food groups, providing basic nutrition advice to help consumers choose a healthy diet. To illustrate, Harvard's Healthy Eating Plate goes beyond the simple MyPlate visual by specifying that people should choose whole grains and limit refined grains, as well as choose fish, poultry, beans, and nuts while limiting red meat, cheese, bacon, cold cuts, and other processed meats. Harvard's plate also distinguishes between potatoes and other vegetables, stating that "potatoes and French fries don't count" (Harvard School of Public Health, http://www.hsph.harvard.edu/nutritionsource /healthy-eating-plate/).

Other major differences between MyPlate and Harvard's Healthy Eating Plate lie in the food groups represented. For example, Harvard's version incorporates a bottle of healthy oil and encourages consumers to use olive, canola, and other plant oils while limiting butter and avoiding trans fat. Information on fat of any kind is not included in MyPlate. Conversely, Harvard's plate does not include the dairy group depicted in MyPlate. Rather, Harvard's plate replaces dairy with water, explaining that consumers should limit their intake of milk to 1–2 servings a day given the little evidence supporting high dairy intake as protective against osteoporosis and the considerable

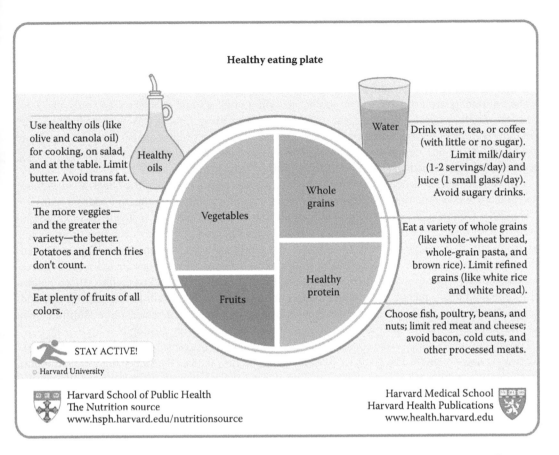

Healthy eating plate

Use healthy oils (like olive and canola oil) for cooking, on salad, and at the table. Limit butter. Avoid trans fat.

Healthy oils

Water

Drink water, tea, or coffee (with little or no sugar). Limit milk/dairy (1-2 servings/day) and juice (1 small glass/day). Avoid sugary drinks.

Whole grains

Vegetables

Healthy protein

Fruits

The more veggies— and the greater the variety—the better. Potatoes and french fries don't count.

Eat plenty of fruits of all colors.

Eat a variety of whole grains (like whole-wheat bread, whole-grain pasta, and brown rice). Limit refined grains (like white rice and white bread).

Choose fish, poultry, beans, and nuts; limit red meat and cheese; avoid bacon, cold cuts, and other processed meats.

STAY ACTIVE!

© Harvard University

Harvard School of Public Health
The Nutrition source
www.hsph.harvard.edu/nutritionsource

Harvard Medical School
Harvard Health Publications
www.health.harvard.edu

FIGURE 9.4 Harvard's Healthy Eating Plate. As printed in image and © Harvard University. For more information visit: http://www.health.harvard.edu. (Reprinted with permission from Harvard School of Public Health. Available at http://www.hsph.harvard.edu/nutritionsource/healthy-eating-plate.)

evidence indicating that high intakes may be harmful. Harvard's Healthy Eating Plate recommends drinking water and other calorie-free beverages while limiting juice and soda. Still another difference is the "stay active" message included in Harvard's plate but absent in MyPlate. This message serves as a reminder that eating a balanced meal and staying active is the best combination for good health (Harvard School of Public Health, http://www.hsph.harvard.edu/nutritionsource /healthy-eating-plate-vs-usda-myplate/).

DIETARY GUIDELINES FOR AMERICANS, 2015*

The final (seventh) meeting of the 2015 *Dietary Guidelines* Advisory Committee (DGAC) was held on December 15, 2014. Submission of public comments to the 2015 DGAC closed on December 30, 2014, but comments submitted to the committee remain viewable and searchable. In February 2015, the DGAC sent its report to the secretaries of HHS and USDA (Department of Health and Human Services 2015). The DGAC report contains the committee's dietary *and other* recommendations and systematic reviews of the peer-reviewed literature that supports their recommendations. Soon thereafter, a Federal Register notice was published announcing the DGAC report's available at

---

* Information for this section was obtained from reports at www.DietaryGuidelines.gov of the last meeting of the 2015 Dietary Guidelines Advisory Committee Meeting, held on December 15, 2014.

http://www.dietaryguidelines.gov. That site serves as the web platform for all materials related to the 2015 revision process, including announcements, archived webcasts of the public meetings, and the submitting/viewing of public comments. The public comments database is available at http://www.health.gov/dietaryguidelines/dga2015/comments/readComments.aspx. The public comments database reopened to accept public comments for 75 days, through early May 2015.

The comments are available to the public, including students and scholars who study the genesis of the *Dietary Guidelines* and contrast and compare the positions of various stakeholders (the food industry, nonprofit organizations, academics, and healthcare professionals). On the basis of the report and the public's comments, HHS and USDA jointly prepare the *Dietary Guidelines* policy document to be published and released as the eighth edition, ideally in late 2015.*

Although not yet published at the time of this writing, the eighth edition of the *Dietary Guidelines* is expected to make quantitative recommendations for saturated fats, sodium, and added sugar.

The 2010 *Dietary Guidelines* identified sodium, saturated fat, and added sugars as food factors of concern, and the 2015 DGAC determined that a reexamination of the evidence on these topics was necessary to evaluate whether revisions to the guidance were warranted. Sodium, saturated fats, and added sugars are of public health importance because they are associated with negative health outcomes when overconsumed. At the same time, the committee acknowledged that a potential unintended consequence of a recommendation on added sugars might be that consumers and manufacturers replace added sugars with low-calorie sweeteners. As a result, the committee also examined evidence on low-calorie sweeteners to inform statements on this topic.

The committee encourages the consumption of healthy dietary patterns that are low in saturated fat, added sugars, and sodium. The goals for the general population are less than 2300 mg dietary sodium per day (or age-appropriate DRI amount), less than 10% total calories from saturated fat per day, and a maximum of 10% of total calories from added sugars per day. Rather than focusing purely on reduction, emphasis should be placed on replacement and shifts in food intake and overall dietary patterns. Policies and programs at local, state, and national levels in both the private and public sector are necessary to support reduction efforts. The committee supports efforts in labeling and other campaigns to increase consumer awareness and understanding of sodium, saturated fats, and added sugars in foods and beverages. In particular, the DGAC recommends limiting marketing to children of "unhealthy" foods, such as those with added sugars and unhealthy fats. Also recommended is changing food labels to make them more useful to consumers, such as requiring larger, bolder letters and specifying the amount of sugar added to the food product. See Figure 5.4, which is the FDA's proposal for a new food label.

Although the overall themes of the 2010 DGA are not likely to change in the 2015 DGA (such as balancing calories to maintain a healthy weight and increasing consumption of fruits and vegetables) key differences are expected between previous editions of the DGA and the 2015 version.

It is expected that the 2015 *Dietary Guidelines* will make recommendations that set it apart from its forebears. The Report reverses nearly four decades of nutrition policy that placed priority on reducing total fat consumption throughout the population. A maximum fat intake of 35% of calories is recommended in the 2010 DGA. The 2015 Report recommends dropping the guideline regarding total dietary fat entirely, although not dismissing recommendations for individual lipids, such as unsaturated and saturated fat. The DGAC found that there is no need to continue restricting dietary cholesterol. Previously, the recommendation was to limit cholesterol to no more than 300 mg a day. For reference, one large egg has approximately 175–185 mg of cholesterol. The DGAC recommends that added sugars make up no more than 10% of total daily calories. Thus, a person whose diet provides 2000 calories in a day could get up to 200 calories of added sugars per day. As sugar delivers about four calories per gram and there are 15 g in a teaspoon, the total amount of added sugar would be 50 g, or just over 3 teaspoons. To put this in context, one 12-ounce can of a SSB has about 33 g of added sugar, more than 60% of the maximum amount of added sugar recommended for one day. For

---

* PowerPoint slides regarding the 2015 edition of the *Dietary Guidelines for Americans* are available for textbook adopters. Current information is also available at the *Dietary Guidelines* home page: http://health.gov/dietaryguidelines/.

the first time in the history of the *Dietary Guidelines*, sustainability is included as a focus area. The DGAC reviewed and analyzed the current scientific findings regarding food sustainability and food safety as they relate to current and long-term food security. Their rationale was that it is important to develop and maintain a food system that is safe and sustainable to ensure current and future food security. Food security exists when all people at all times have access to sufficient, safe, nutritious, and culturally appropriate food to maintain a healthy and active life (see Chapter 11 for more on food security). Understanding the link between how food is grown, caught, produced, processed, and transported and the health of humans and the environment will enable public health practitioners to inform policies related to dietary guidance, agriculture, and aquaculture, with the goal of developing "dietary guidance that supports human health and the *health of the planet* [emphasis added] over time." To that end, the *Advisory Report* calls for a reduction in meat consumption.

Factions with competing or conflicting interests lobby to have their interests supported (or at least not thwarted) by the government's 2015 edition of the *Dietary Guidelines for Americans*. To see this for yourself, read through some of the thousands of comments the DGAC received, which are available online at http://www.health.gov/dietaryguidelines/2015.asp.

DISEASE PREVENTION GUIDANCE FROM FEDERAL AND VOLUNTARY HEALTH ORGANIZATIONS

The seven leading causes of death in the US are, in order, heart disease, cancer, chronic lower respiratory diseases, stroke, accidents, Alzheimer's disease, and diabetes (Centers for Disease Control and Prevention 2012). Of these, heart disease, some forms of cancer, and type 2 diabetes correlate to poor nutrition. Escalating rates of obesity and the corresponding increases in morbidity, mortality, and healthcare costs necessitate a focus by public health practitioners on prevention of CVD, diabetes, and cancer through education and outreach.

CARDIOVASCULAR DISEASE

The AHA's 2006 Diet and Lifestyle Recommendations provide a foundation for a public health approach to CVD risk reduction. The plan includes recommendations for healthy eating and other health-promoting behaviors for healthy Americans 2 years of age or older. The recommendations are intentionally flexible to meet the unique needs for growth, development, and aging. In particular, the document presents guidelines for a healthy diet; healthy weight; cholesterol, blood pressure, and fasting blood sugar control; physical activity; and avoidance of tobacco, as detailed in Table 9.14 (Lichtenstein et al. 2006).

Compared to the AHA's previous guidelines released in 2000, the 2006 edition includes a significantly more restrictive fat intake recommendation. The recommendation for saturated fat was reduced from less than 10% of energy in 2000 to less than 7% of energy in 2006 (Krauss et al. 2000).

In addition to recommendations for individuals, the 2006 AHA statement contains strategies for practitioners, restaurants, the food industry, schools, and local governments to facilitate adoption of the AHA Diet and Lifestyle Recommendations (Box 9.15).

A more recent AHA statement from 2012 (Mozaffarian et al. 2012) provides evidenced-based, population-level strategies for improving diet, physical activity, and smoking habits. Strategies fall into six domains: media and educational campaigns; labeling and consumer information; taxation, subsidies, and other economic incentives; school and workplace approaches; local environmental changes; and direct restrictions and mandates. Table 9.15 lists examples from each of these domains for improving dietary habits.

Thus, AHA has been informed by the ecological model of health behavior change, which identifies multiple levels of influence on a person's behavior. These multiple levels include intrapersonal factors, interpersonal processes and primary groups, institutional factors, community factors, and public policy. The ecological model has been found to bring about population improvements in health, as we have learned from the campaigns for tobacco control (Sallis et al. 2008).

TABLE 9.14

AHA 2006 Recommendations and Strategies for CVD Risk Reduction

Strategy (Process Objective)	Recommendation (Outcome Objective)
Choose lean meats and vegetable alternatives; select fat-free (skim), 1% fat, and low-fat dairy products; and minimize intake of partially hydrogenated fats.	Reduce saturated fats to <7% of energy, *trans* fatty acids to <1% of energy, and cholesterol to <300 mg per day.
Choose and prepare foods with little or no salt.	Reduce sodium intake to no more than 2300 mg daily. Middle-aged and older adults, African Americans, and those with hypertension are advised to reduce sodium intake to 1500 mg of sodium daily.
Minimize the intake of food and beverages with added sugars.	Read labels to minimize consumption of foods with one or more of these ingredients: high-fructose corn syrup, corn syrup, raisin syrup, dextrose, honey, sucrose, fructose, maltose, concentrated fruit juice.
Strive to be physically active and control weight.	Adults should aim for >30 minutes of physical activity most days of the week. At least 60 minutes of physical activity most days of the week is recommended for adults who are attempting to lose weight or maintain weight loss and for children.
Aim for a diet rich in vegetables, fruits (not fruit juices), and whole-grain foods.	Follow the eating plan. Blood pressure may be further lowered by replacing some carbohydrates with either protein from plant sources or monounsaturated fat.
Achieve and maintain healthy cholesterol, blood pressure, and blood glucose levels.	Achieve and maintain a low-density lipoprotein (LDL) cholesterol level of <100 mg/dL; blood pressure of 120 mm Hg and a diastolic BP 80 mm Hg or less; and a fasting blood glucose level of <100 mg/dL.
	Avoid use of and exposure to tobacco products.
If alcohol is consumed, it should be at a moderate level.	Limit alcohol intake to not more than one drink per day for women and two drinks per day for men (1 drink = 12 oz. of beer, 4 oz. of wine, 1.5 oz. of 80-proof distilled spirits, or 1 oz. of 100-proof spirits).
Follow AHA Diet and Lifestyle Recommendations even when eating food that is prepared outside of the home.	

Source: Lichtenstein, A.H. et al., *Circulation*, 114, 2006.

Hypertension

Hypertension (blood pressure of 140/90 mm Hg or higher) affects approximately 31% of noninstitutionalized adults ages 20 and over in the US (National Center for Health Statistics 2013). As the population ages, the prevalence of hypertension will increase even more unless broad and effective preventive measures are implemented. The relationship between high blood pressure and risk of CVD events is independent of other risk factors: the higher the blood pressure, the greater the chance of heart attack, heart failure, stroke, and kidney disease.

Prehypertension

Prehypertension (blood pressure between 120/80 mm Hg and 139/89 mm Hg) signals the need for increased education of both healthcare professionals and the public to reduce blood pressure levels and prevent the development of hypertension in the general population. Hypertension prevention strategies are available to achieve this goal (National High Blood Pressure Education Program 2004).

**BOX 9.15   STRATEGIES FOR FACILITATING ADOPTION
OF THE AHA DIET AND LIFESTYLE RECOMMENDATIONS**

1. Practitioners should promote the AHA Diet and Lifestyle Recommendations to their patients, along with encouraging regular physical activity, discussing body mass index (BMI), and encouraging alcohol and tobacco control.
2. Restaurants should facilitate their customers' adherence to AHA recommendations by offering menu labeling; reducing portion sizes; reformulated recipes to reduce fat and sodium, providing more fruit and vegetable options prepared with minimally added salt, fat, and sugar; allowing patrons to substitute reduced-fat options for high-fat side dishes (such as French fries and potato salad); and providing whole-grain products.
3. The food industry should reduce the salt and sugar content of processed foods; replace saturated and *trans* fats in prepared foods and baked goods with low-saturated-fat liquid vegetable oils; increase the proportion of whole-grain foods available; package foods in smaller individual portion sizes; and develop packaging that allows for greater stability, preservation, and palatability of fresh fruits and vegetables without added sodium and that reduces refrigeration needs in grocery stores.
4. Schools should adopt HealthierUS School Challenge policies, such as limiting foods high in added sugar, saturated and *trans* fat, sodium, and calories while encouraging consumption of fruits, vegetables, whole-grain foods, and low-fat or fat-free dairy in all food sold outside of the reimbursable school lunch.
5. Local government should develop and implement a Safe Routes to School plan, implement land-use practices that promote nonmotorized transportation (walking and biking), and promote policies that increase availability of healthy foods, for example, use of public land for farmers' markets and full-service grocery stores in low-income areas.

Source: Lichtenstein, A.H. et al., *Circulation,* 114, 2006.

Public health approaches, such as reducing calories, saturated fat, and salt in processed foods; increasing community and school opportunities for physical activity; and other recommendations proposed by the AHA (see previous section on CVD) can achieve a downward shift in the distribution of the blood pressure in the US population, potentially reducing morbidity, mortality, and the lifetime risk of an individual becoming hypertensive. A population-based approach is an important component for any comprehensive plan to prevent hypertension. Even a small shift in the distribution of systolic blood pressure is likely to result in a substantial reduction in the burden of blood pressure-related illness (Stamler 1991).

Dietary Approaches to Stop Hypertension and Prevention

Adoption of healthy lifestyles by all persons is critical for the prevention of high blood pressure and is an indispensable part of the management of those with hypertension. Major lifestyle modifications shown to lower blood pressure include weight reduction in those individuals who are overweight or obese, dietary sodium reduction, physical activity, moderation of alcohol consumption, and adoption of the Dietary Approaches to Stop Hypertension (DASH) eating plan, which is rich in potassium and calcium. The DASH eating plan is outlined in Table 9.16.

Lifestyle modifications reduce blood pressure, enhance antihypertensive drug efficacy, and decrease cardiovascular risk. A 1600-mg-sodium DASH eating plan has effects similar to single-drug therapy and can decrease systolic blood pressure 8–14 mm Hg; combinations of two or more

TABLE 9.15

Selected Examples of Evidence-Based Population Approaches for Improving Diet

Domain	Examples
Media and education	• Sustained, focused media and educational campaigns for increasing consumption of specific healthful foods or reducing consumption of specific less healthful foods or beverages.
	• On-site supermarket and grocery store educational programs to support purchase of healthier foods.
Labeling and information	• Mandated Nutrition Facts panels or front-of-pack labels/icons to influence industry behavior and product formulations.
Economic incentives	• Subsidy strategies to lower prices of more healthful foods and beverages.
	• Tax strategies to increase prices of less healthful foods and beverages.
Schools and workplaces	• Multicomponent interventions focused on improving both diet and physical activity, including specialized educational curricula, trained teachers, supportive school policies, a formal physical education program, healthy food and beverage options, and a parental/family component.
	• Comprehensive work site wellness programs with nutrition, physical activity, and tobacco cessation/prevention components.
Local environment	• Increased availability of supermarkets near homes.
Restrictions and mandates	• Restriction on television advertisements for less healthful foods or beverages advertised to children.
	• Regulatory policies to reduce specific nutrients in foods (e.g., trans fats, salt, certain fats).

Source: Mozaffarian, D. et al., *Circulation*, 126, 2012.

lifestyle modifications can achieve even better results, as indicated in Table 9.17 (National High Blood Pressure Education Program 2004).

Diabetes

All recommendations to prevent the development of diabetes are based on the Diabetes Prevention Program (DPP), a major clinical trial that found that decreasing diabetes risk factors can prevent diabetes. The DPP, conducted at 27 centers nationwide, is the first major trial to show that lifestyle changes can effectively delay diabetes in a diverse population of overweight American adults with impaired glucose tolerance (IGT). Sponsored by the National Institute of Diabetes and Digestive and Kidney Diseases (NIDDK), an institute within the National Institutes of Health, the DPP compared three approaches to normalizing blood sugar—lifestyle modification, treatment with an oral hypoglycemic agent (metformin), and standard medical advice—in 3234 overweight people with IGT. The lifestyle modification manuals used in the study are available on the DPP website at http://www.bsc.gwu.edu/dpp/manuals.htmlvdoc (Box 9.16).

The DPP demonstrated that for every seven people with prediabetes who are treated for 3 years, one case of diabetes could be prevented. Thus, it should also be possible to delay or prevent the development of complications, substantially reducing the individual and public health burden of diabetes (Knowler et al. 2002).

Community screening programs, as well as primary care physicians, have an opportunity to identify individuals at high risk for developing diabetes and provide primary prevention strategies. The American Diabetes Association (ADA) recommends that individuals with normoglycemia have repeat screenings at 3-year intervals. However, for people with prediabetes, modest weight loss

TABLE 9.16
DASH Eating Plan

Food Groups	Servings per Day				Serving Sizes
	1600 Calories per Day	2000 Calories per Day	2600 Calories per Day	3100 Calories per Day	
Grains[a]	6	6–8	10–11	12–13	1 slice bread; 1 oz dry cereal;[b] 1/2 cup cooked rice, pasta, or cereal[b]
Vegetables	3–4	4–5	5–6	6	1 cup raw leafy vegetable; 1/2 cup cut-up raw or cooked vegetable; 1/2 cup vegetable juice
Fruits	4	4–5	5–6	6	1 medium fruit; 1/4 cup dried fruit; 1/2 cup fresh, frozen, or canned fruit; 1/2 cup fruit juice
Fat-free or low-fat milk and milk products	2–3	2–3	3	3–4	1 cup milk or yogurt; 1.5 oz. cheese
Lean meats, poultry, and fish	3–4 or less	6 or less	6 or less	6–9	1 oz. cooked meats, poultry, or fish; one egg[c]
Nuts, seeds, and legumes	3–4 per week	4–5 per week	1	1	1/3 cup or 1.5 oz. nuts; 2 tbsp. peanut butter; 2 tbsp. or 0.5 oz seeds; 1/2 cup cooked legumes (dry beans and peas)
Fats and oils	2	2–3	3	4	1 tsp. soft margarine; 1 tsp. vegetable oil; 1 tbsp. mayonnaise; 2 tbsp. salad dressing[d]
Sweets and added sugars	3 or less per week	5 or less per week	2 or less	2 or less	1 tbsp. sugar; 1 tbsp. jelly or jam; 1/2 cup sorbet or gelatin; 1 cup lemonade

Source: US Department of Health and Human Services, National Institutes of Health, National Heart, Lung, and Blood Institute, Following the DASH Eating Plan. Available at http://www.nhlbi.nih.gov/health/health-topics/topics/dash /followdash.html, accessed February 2, 2015.

[a] Whole grains are recommended for most grain servings as a good source of fiber and nutrients.

[b] Serving sizes vary between 1/2 cup and 1 1/4 cups, depending on cereal type. Check the product's Nutrition Facts label.

[c] Limit egg yolk intake to no more than four per week; two egg whites have the same protein content as 1 oz. of meat.

[d] Fat content determines the serving size for fats and oils, e.g., 1 tbsp. of regular salad dressing = 1 serving; 1 tbsp. of low-fat dressing = 0.5 serving; and 1 tbsp. of a fat-free dressing = 0 serving.

and a regular physical exam are advised in order to prevent or delay diabetes (American Diabetes Association 2013).

Prediabetes

Information learned thus far about the natural history and pathogenesis of diabetes indicates that this disease has a prolonged prediabetic phase. The ADA has identified an intermediate group of patients who have blood glucose values higher than the defined normal level but not high enough to meet the diagnostic criteria for diabetes. This group includes patients with impaired fasting glucose (IFG) or IGT.

- IFG is defined as fasting plasma glucose (FPG) values of 100–125 mg/dL (5.6–6.9 mmol/L); normal FPG values are below 100 mg/dL.
- IGT is defined as 2-hour, 75 g OGTT values of 140–199 mg/dL (7.8–11.0 mmol/L); normal values on this test are below 140 mg/dL.

TABLE 9.17

Lifestyle Modifications Recommended by the Joint National Committee to Manage Hypertension

Modification	Recommendation	Approximate Range of Systolic Blood Pressure Reduction
Weight reduction	Maintain normal body weight (BMI = 18.5–24.9 kg/m²)	5–20 mm Hg per 10 kg weight loss
DASH eating plan	Consume a diet rich in fruits, vegetables, and low-fat dairy products with a reduced content of saturated and total fat	8–14 mm Hg
Dietary sodium reduction	Reduce dietary sodium intake to no more than 2.4 g sodium or 6 g sodium chloride	2–8 mm Hg
Physical activity	Engage in regular aerobic physical activity, such as brisk walking, at least 30 minutes per day most days of the week	4–9 mm Hg
Moderation of alcohol consumption	Limit consumption to no more than two drinks per day in most men and to no more than one drink per day in women and lighter-weight persons (1 drink = 24 oz. beer, 10 oz. wine, or 3 oz. 80-proof whiskey)	2–4 mm Hg

Source: National High Blood Pressure Education Program, *The Seventh Report of the Joint National Committee on Prevention, Detection, Evaluation, and Treatment of High Blood Pressure,* US Department of Health and Human Services, National Institutes of Health, National Heart, Lung, and Blood Institute, NIH publication no. 04-5230, August 2004, http://www.nhlbi.nih.gov/guidelines/hypertension/jnc7full.pdf, accessed February 2, 2015.

- Individuals with a hemoglobin A1c value between 5.7% and 6.4% are also considered prediabetic; normal hemoglobin A1c values are below 5.7%.
- Diabetes is diagnosed when hemoglobin A1c levels are 6.5% or above; FPG levels are 126 mg/dL (7.0 mmol/L) or higher; 2-hour plasma glucose levels are 200 mg/dL (11.1 mmol/L) or higher during a 75 g OGTT; or classic symptoms of hyperglycemia are present. In the absence of unequivocal hyperglycemia, the results of any of these tests should be confirmed by repeat testing on different days (American Diabetes Association 2013).

People with IGT or IFG are at significant risk for diabetes. Other risk factors include history of diabetes in a first-degree relative, overweight, sedentary lifestyle, hypertension, dyslipidemia, history of gestational diabetes or delivery of a large-for-gestational-age infant, and polycystic ovary syndrome (PCOS). Blacks, Latin Americans, Native Americans, and Asian/Pacific Islanders also are at increased risk for diabetes (Box 9.17) (American Diabetes Association 2013).

Adults with a BMI of 25 kg/m² or higher and who have one or more additional risk factors, and those without risk factors who are 45 years of age or older, are candidates for screening to detect type 2 diabetes and prediabetes. Children who are overweight (BMI > 85th percentile for age and sex, weight for height > 85th percentile, or weight > 120% of ideal for height) and have two or more other risk factors should be considered for screening. To test for diabetes or prediabetes, the hemoglobin A1c, FPG, or 75 g 2-hour OGTT is appropriate. Screenings should be carried out in the healthcare setting due to the need for follow-up and discussion of abnormal results (American Diabetes Association 2013).

Prevention

People with IGT, IFG, or an elevated hemoglobin A1c should be given counseling on weight loss as well as instruction for increasing physical activity. Follow-up counseling appears important for success, and monitoring for the development of diabetes should be performed annually. Close attention

BOX 9.16   DIABETES PREVENTION PROGRAM

DPP participants ranged from age 25–85, with an average age of 51 years. Forty-five percent of DPP participants were from minority groups that suffer disproportionately from type 2 diabetes: African Americans, Hispanic Americans, Asian Americans and Pacific Islanders, and American Indians. The trial also recruited other groups at higher risk for type 2 diabetes, including individuals aged 60 or older, women with a history of gestational diabetes, and people with a first-degree relative with type 2 diabetes. Upon entering the study, all had IGT as measured by an oral glucose tolerance test (OGTT), and all were overweight, with an average body mass index (BMI) of 34, and were randomly assigned to one of the following groups:

- Treatment through lifestyle modification with the aim of reducing weight by 7% through a low-fat diet and exercising for 150 minutes a week. Participants in this arm received training in diet, exercise (most chose walking), and behavior modification skills.
- Treatment with the drug metformin (850 mg twice a day) plus information about diet and exercise, but no intensive motivational counseling.
- Treatment with a placebo instead of metformin, plus information about diet and exercise, but no intensive motivational counseling.

About 29% of the DPP group given information about diet and exercise and the placebo developed diabetes during the average follow-up period of 3 years, and 22% of the group given metformin and diet and exercise information developed diabetes. (Metformin lowers blood glucose mainly by decreasing the liver's production of glucose).

In contrast, only 14% of the lifestyle modification arm developed diabetes. Those in the lifestyle modification arm met the study goal—an average of 7%, or 15 lb., weight loss—in the first year and generally sustained a 5% total loss for the study's duration.

Lifestyle intervention worked equally well in men and women and in all ethnic groups. It was most effective in people ages 60 and older, whose risk of developing diabetes decreased by 71%. Metformin was also effective in both sexes and in all ethnic groups, but it was relatively ineffective in those who were less overweight or older. Both interventions lowered fasting blood glucose levels, but lifestyle changes more effectively lowered blood glucose levels 2 hours after a glucose drink. Also, about twice as many people in the lifestyle group compared to placebo regained normal glucose tolerance, showing that diet and exercise can reverse IGT.

Source: Knowler, W.C. et al., *N. Engl. J. Med.*, 346, 2002.

should be given to, and appropriate treatment given for, other CVD risk factors such as hypertension and dyslipidemia, as well as for tobacco use.

National Diabetes Education Program

The National Diabetes Education Program (NDEP) is jointly sponsored by HHS's NIDDK and the Centers for Disease Control and Prevention's (CDC's) Division of Diabetes Translation, with the participation of over 200 partner organizations at the federal, state, and local levels. NDEP's "Small Steps. Big Rewards. Prevent Type 2 Diabetes" initiative is the first national diabetes prevention campaign (Figure 9.5). Its goal is to promote subfederal primary prevention programs and to develop and disseminate tailored messages and materials that can be adopted for use in those diabetes prevention programs. NDEP has produced copyright-free campaign tools to help promote diabetes prevention and control. The "Small Steps. Big Rewards. Prevent Type 2 Diabetes" diet and lifestyle

**BOX 9.17   MODIFIABLE AND NONMODIFIABLE
CONDITIONS ASSOCIATED WITH DIABETES**

Nonmodifiable factors
- Age greater than 45 years.
- Diabetes in a first-degree relative.
- Race/ethnicity (African American, Asian American, Latino, Native American, or Pacific Islander).
- History of cardiovascular disease.

Modifiable lifestyle factors
- Overweight (body mass index [BMI] ≥ 25 kg/m^2).
- Physical inactivity.

Clinical conditions
- Hemoglobin A1c ≥ 5.7%, IGT, or IFG on previous testing.
- Hypertension (blood pressure at least 140/90 mm Hg or on therapy for hypertension).
- Dyslipidemia (high-density lipoprotein [HDL] cholesterol > 35 mg/dL and/or triglycerides > 250 mg/dL).
- History of gestational diabetes or women who delivered a baby weighing > 9 lb.
- PCOS.
- *Acanthosis nigricans* (a dermatalogic presentation characterized by hyperpigmented, velvety plaques of body folds; caused by hyperinsulinemia, a consequence of insulin resistance associated with obesity).

Source: American Diabetes Association, *Diabetes Care*, 36, 2013.

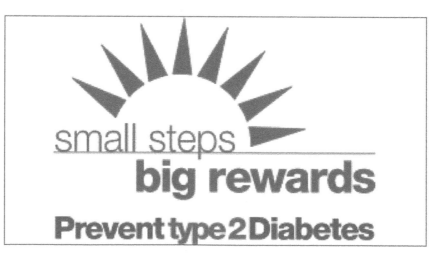

FIGURE 9.5   *Small Steps. Big Rewards. Prevent Type 2 Diabetes.* Campaign logo. (From US Department of Health and Human Services, National Institutes of Health, National Diabetes Education Program, *Small Steps. Big Rewards. Prevent Type 2 Diabetes*, Campaign logo. Available at http://www.ndep.nih.gov /partners-community-organization/campaigns/SmallStepsBigRewards.aspx, accessed September 17, 2013.)

recommendation is summarized in one sentence: By losing a modest amount of weight through 30 minutes of physical activity 5 days a week and eating healthier, people with prediabetes can delay or prevent the onset of type 2 diabetes (US Department of Health and Human Services, http://ndep.nih.gov/partners-community-organization/campaigns/smallstepsbigrewards.aspx).

CANCER

The possible relationship between the consumption of fruits and vegetables and reduced risk of cancer was a hot topic of research in the 1980s and 1990s, leading to an expert panel report convened by the World Cancer Research Fund (WCRF)/American Institute for Cancer Research (AICR) (World Cancer Research Fund 1997) concluding in 1997 that there was "convincing" evidence that high intakes of fruit and/or vegetables decrease the risk for mouth and pharynx, esophagus, stomach, colorectal, and lung cancers. However, the same organization published an updated report in 2007 downgrading "convincing" to either "probable" or "limited-suggestive" (World Cancer Research Fund 2007), as newer results from large prospective studies did not confirm the earlier, mostly case–control study, results (Key 2011). Nonetheless, the 2007 report affirmed "convincing" evidence as to red and processed meat and some cancers. Therefore, along with the dietary recommendation to reduce red and processed meat comes the corollary of increasing plant-food consumption, in part because weight gain and body fatness also show "convincing" evidence of increased cancer risk in the 2007 report. Thus, organizations such as the National Cancer Institute (NCI) and the AICR work to promote dietary change, based on the *Dietary Guidelines for Americans*. These organizations also support research into detection, prevention, and cures.

National Cancer Institute

Founded in 1991 as a partnership between the NCI and the Produce for Better Health Foundation (PBHF), the "5 a Day for Better Health" program was a national initiative to increase the consumption of fruits and vegetables by all Americans to at least five servings a day as a means of reducing the risk of many cancers, high blood pressure, heart disease, diabetes, stroke, and other chronic diseases. The program sought to do this by increasing public awareness of the importance of eating at least five servings of fruits and vegetables every day; by providing consumers with specific information about how to include more servings of fruits and vegetables in their daily routines; and by increasing the availability of fruits and vegetables at home, school, work, and other places where food is served (Centers for Disease Control and Prevention 2005).

Since its inception, the "5 a Day" program has gone through several changes. In 2005, the NCI transferred lead federal agency and health authority for the "5 a Day" program to the CDC. As the *Dietary Guidelines'* recommended intake of fruits and vegetables increased, the campaign followed suit by increasing its recommendations from a daily intake of at least five servings to the suggested intake of five to nine. Consequently, the PBHF (http://www.pbhfoundation.org/about/history/) relaunched its campaign in 2007 to reflect the escalating recommendation. The rebranded program, "Fruits & Veggies—More Matters (http://www.fruitsandveggiesmorematters.org/about-fruits-and-veggies-more-matters)," supports the recommendations made by the 2010 *Dietary Guidelines for Americans* and MyPlate of making half the plate fruits and vegetables, and now replaces "5 a Day" (Figure 9.6). Fruit and vegetable information, along with meal planning ideas, recipes, activities for children, and additional resources, can be found on the campaign's website, http://www.fruitsandveggiesmorematters.org/.

American Institute for Cancer Research

Founded in 1982, AICR offers cancer prevention education programs and supports research into the role of diet and nutrition in the prevention and treatment of cancer. In 1997, AICR partnered with the WCRF to publish their first expert report, *Food, Nutrition, and the Prevention of Cancer: A Global Perspective*. This report stimulated a surge of research and advancement in the field of diet and cancer prevention. Their second expert report, *Food, Nutrition, Physical Activity, and*

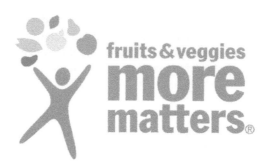

FIGURE 9.6 *Fruits & Veggies—More Matters.* Campaign logo. (Reprinted with permission from the Produce for Better Health Foundation.)

BOX 9.18   WCRF/AICR FOOD, NUTRITION, AND PHYSICAL ACTIVITY RECOMMENDATIONS FOR CANCER PREVENTION

1. Be as lean as possible without becoming underweight.
2. Be physically active for at least 30 minutes every day.
3. Limit consumption of energy-dense foods. Avoid sugary drinks.
4. Eat more of a variety of vegetables, fruits, whole grains, and beans.
5. Limit intake of red meat (beef, pork, lamb) and avoid processed meat.
6. If consumed at all, limit alcoholic drinks to two drinks a day for men and one drink a day for women.
7. Limit consumption of salty foods and foods processed with salt.
8. Aim to meet nutritional needs through diet alone. Dietary supplements are not recommended for cancer prevention.
   Special population recommendations:
9. Aim to breastfeed infants exclusively for 6 months and continue with complementary feeding thereafter.
10. After treatment, cancer survivors should follow the recommendations for cancer prevention.

Source: World Cancer Research Fund International, Our Cancer Prevention Recommendations. Available at http://www.wcrf.org/int/research-we-fund/our-cancer-prevention-recommendations, accessed February 2, 2015.

---

the *Prevention of Cancer: A Global Perspective,* was published in 2007 and sets out 10 public health goals and personal recommendations for cancer prevention (World Cancer Research Fund 2007). These recommendations to reduce the risk of developing cancer are similar to the 2010 *Dietary Guidelines for Americans.* These recommendations are now being updated through a continuous effort and published at http://www.wcrf.org/int/research-we-fund/our-cancer-prevention -recommendations (Box 9.18).

New American Plate

Three strategies are suggested for achieving the cancer prevention and weight management components of AICR's guidelines: eat a greater proportion of plant foods, keep physically active, and maintain a healthy weight. AICR developed the "New American Plate" as a way to help people achieve these goals. The New American Plate promotes a healthy proportion of plant foods to animal protein, attained by gradually making the transition to a plate that contains at least two-thirds vegetables, fruits, whole grains, and beans, and no more than one-third meat or dairy products.

The second step of the New American Plate suggests gradually reducing portion size as an additional way to reduce calories (American Institute for Cancer Research, http://www.aicr.org/new-american-plate/). For portion control, a medium-sized plate about the size of a Frisbee is suggested. As a weight-loss strategy, the "healthy plate" (half vegetables and fruit, a quarter healthy starches, and a quarter lean meats and alternates) has been adopted by *MOVE!*—a national weight management program designed by the Veterans Administration's National Center for Health Promotion and Disease Prevention (http://www.move.va.gov/). See also Chapter 4 for a discussion of collaborative prevention efforts by the ACS, ADA, and AHA.

CONCLUSION

The federal government has been providing food and nutrition guidance to the public and for use by public health professionals since the early twentieth century. Although guidance originally focused on food and prevention of deficiency, it gradually refocused on nutrients and prevention of chronic disease, with the nature of the guidance changing in response to the nutritional status of the population.

Primary tools for nutrition guidance include the *Dietary Guidelines for Americans* and MyPlate. The process of maintaining and updating this information is complex and ongoing, requiring input from both subject-matter experts and the general public. Because the *Dietary Guidelines* sets the standard for federal nutrition policy, nutrition assistance programs (such as WIC), and assessment (such as HEI), the federal government is able to speak with one consistent voice on nutrition issues. At present, a major focus of both private and public health organizations is on chronic diseases such as CVD, cancer, and diabetes, the risks for which are strongly correlated with poor diet and lifestyle choices. Accordingly, the 2015 *Dietary Guidelines* are expected to make quantitative recommendations concerning saturated fat, sodium, and added sugar. The influence of US dietary guidance extends beyond an individual's health, and an appreciation of our food production practices may be informative in developing guidance that promotes the health of all.

Michael Pollan, the coauthor of the quotation at the beginning of this chapter, offers his own irreverent dietary guidance (Pollan 2007).

Flagrantly Unscientific Rules of Thumb Regarding How to Eat

- Eat food. Don't eat anything your great-great-grandmother wouldn't recognize as food.
- Avoid food products with health claims. Not only are these foods likely to be heavily processed, the claims on them are often questionable.
- Avoid food products containing more than five ingredients that are unfamiliar and polysyllabic. Also avoid foods that contain high fructose corn syrup. All of these ingredients indicate the food is highly processed.
- Get out of the supermarket whenever possible so you can find fresh whole foods picked at the peak of nutritional quality.
- Pay more (better food costs more) and eat less (stop when you're 80% full).
- Eat mostly plants, especially leaves.
- Eat by following the dietary rules of a traditional culture; copy how the cultural group eats as well as what they eat.
- Cook and (if you can) plant a garden.
- Eat like an omnivore. Try to add new species, not just new foods, to your diet.

ACRONYMS

ACS	American Cancer Society
ADA	American Diabetes Association
AHA	American Heart Association
AI	Adequate Intake
AICR	American Institute for Cancer Research

AMDR	Acceptable Micronutrient Distribution Range
BMI	Body mass index
CDC	Centers for Disease Control and Prevention
CNPP	Center for Nutrition Policy and Promotion (within USDA)
CVD	Cardiovascular disease
DASH	Dietary Approaches to Stop Hypertension
DGAC	Dietary Guidelines Advisory Committee
DPP	Diabetes Prevention Program
DRI	Dietary Reference Intake
EAR	Estimated Average Requirement (for groups)
EER	Estimated Energy Requirement
FDA	Food and Drug Administration (within HHS)
FPG	Fasting plasma glucose
HDL	High-density lipoprotein
HEI	Healthy Eating Index
HHS	Department of Health and Human Services
IFG	Impaired fasting glucose
IGT	Impaired glucose tolerance
IOM	Institute of Medicine
NAS	National Academy of Sciences
NCI	National Cancer Institute
NDEP	National Diabetes Education Project
NDL	Nutrient Data Laboratory
NHANES III	Third National Health and Nutrition Examination Survey
NIDDK	National Institute of Diabetes and Digestive and Kidney Diseases
NRC	National Research Council
NSLP	National School Lunch Program
OGTT	Oral glucose tolerance test
PBHF	Produce for Better Health Foundation
PCOS	Polycystic ovary syndrome
RDA	Recommended Dietary Allowance
RNI	Recommended Nutrient Intake (Canada)
SBP	School Breakfast Program
SNAP	Supplemental Nutrition Assistance Program
SoFAAS	Solid fats, alcohol, and added sugars
UL	Tolerable Upper Intake Level
USDA	United States Department of Agriculture
WCRF	World Cancer Research Fund
WHO	World Health Organization (of the United Nations)
WIC	Special Supplemental Nutrition Program for Women, Infants, and Children

STUDENT ASSIGNMENTS AND ACTIVITIES DESIGNED TO ENHANCE LEARNING AND STIMULATE CRITICAL THINKING

1. Consider W.O. Atwater's quote in the first section of the chapter. Written more than a 100 years ago, describe the significance of this quote in the twenty-first century.
2. In reviewing Table 9.1, why have the food group categories changed over time? For someone who is not knowledgeable about nutrition, which of the eight food guides listed in this table would be the easiest to understand and/or prove most useful? Which would be the most challenging/least useful? Explain your answer.

3. Compare and contrast the 1992 USDA *Food Guide Pyramid* graphic (http://www.nal.usda .gov/fnic/Fpyr/pyramid.gif), the *MyPyramid* graphic (http://www.choosemyplate.gov/food -groups/downloads/MiniPoster.pdf), and the *MyPlate* graphic (http://www.choosemyplate.gov /downloads/mini_poster_English_final.pdf). Of these three graphics, which best exemplifies the principles of designing a food guide, described in the section "Food Guide Pyramid, 1992–2005." Explain your answer.

4. Using MyPlate, develop a lesson plan to teach a group of third-grade students about healthy eating. Describe what you would do differently to teach a group of college students.

5. Several years after the release of MyPlate, the USDA has asked you to help redesign the next food guide graphic. Outline the steps you would take in creating this graphic, including any information you might gather and the source(s) of that information. Propose a new graphic (be sure to include a mock-up), and describe the reasons behind your design.

6. Review Figure 9.2, and complete the table for the 2005, 2010, and 2015 *Dietary Guidelines*. Discuss how the *Dietary Guidelines* have changed over time. How has the wording changed? What effect might this have on the meaning and messages of the guidelines?

7. View the public comments submitted to the *Dietary Guidelines* Advisory Committee in the development of the 2010 *Dietary Guidelines for Americans,* available at http://162.79.16.124. Find one comment from a trade group, one from a nutrition professional, and one from a consumer. Compare and contrast the comments from each of these three stakeholders. Include in your discussion which, if any, of the recommendations from these three stakeholders was included in the final version of the *Dietary Guidelines*. Based on the comments and your own ideas, what changes, if any, would you recommend for the 2015 *Dietary Guidelines for Americans*? Explain your answer.

8. Is the Healthy Eating Index (HEI) a useful tool? Why or why not?

9. What observations and interpretations can you make from the HEI and HEI-2010 data presented in Tables 9.5 and Table 9.11 respectively?

10. List the uses and limitations of the Dietary Reference Intakes (DRIs).

11. Estimating the calorie and fat content of meals is no easy task. Even dietitians have difficulty (see the *NY Times* article, "Losing Count of Calories as Plates Fill Up" at http://www.nytimes.com/1997/04/02/garden/losing-count-of-calories-as-plates-fill-up .html?pagewanted=all&src=pm). Record your food and beverage intake at lunch for one day. Be sure to include condiments, seasonings, preparation methods, and estimated portion sizes. How many calories do you think this meal contained? How many grams of fat and fiber? How many milligrams of sodium?

Using the Nutrient Data Laboratory (NDL, http://ndb.nal.usda.gov/), determine the calorie, fat, fiber, and sodium content of your lunch meal. Was your estimation close to what the NDL estimated? Describe your experience using the NDL and any surprises you found with your results.

12. What are the benefits and possible consequences of having *disease-related* dietary guidance along with *federal* dietary guidance? Is having multiple guidance systems optimal, or should we have just one? Explain your answer.

REFERENCES

American Diabetes Association. Position statement: Standards of medical care in diabetes—2013. *Diabetes Care.* 2013;36(Suppl 1):S11–S66.

American Institute for Cancer Research. The New American Plate. Available at http://www.aicr.org/new -american-plate/, accessed February 2, 2015.

Aubrey A. Why we got fatter during the fat-free boom. *NPR,* March 28, 2014. Available at http://www.npr.org /blogs/thesalt/2014/03/28/295332576/why-we-got-fatter-during-the-fat-free-food-boom, accessed January 12, 2015.

Basiotis PP, Carlson A, Gerrior SA, Juan WY, Lino M. *The Healthy Eating Index: 1999–2000*. US Department of Agriculture, Center for Nutrition Policy and Promotion. CNPP-12, December 2002. Available at http://www.cnpp.usda.gov/sites/default/files/healthy_eating_index/HEI99-00report.pdf, accessed February 2, 2015.

Centers for Disease Control and Prevention. *5 A Day Works!* Atlanta: US Department of Health and Human Services, 2005. Available at http://www.cdc.gov/nccdphp/dnpa/nutrition/health_professionals/programs /5aday_works.pdf, accessed February 2, 2015.

Centers for Disease Control and Prevention. Leading Causes of Death, 2012. Available at http://www.cdc.gov /injury/wisqars/pdf/leading_causes_of_death_by_age_group_2012-a.pdf, accessed February 2, 2015.

Davis C, Saltos E. Dietary recommendations and how they have changed over time. In Frazao E, ed. *America's Eating Habits: Changes and Consequences*. Washington, DC: Economic Research Service. US Department of Agriculture. Agriculture Information Bulletin No. 750, 1999, pp. 33–50. Available at http:// www.ers.usda.gov/publications/aib-agricultural-information-bulletin/aib750.aspx#.UgENZ1OISUc, accessed February 2, 2015.

Department of Health and Human Services. Office of Disease Prevention and Health Promotion. Dietary Guidelines for Americans, 2015. Available at http://www.health.gov/dietaryguidelines/2015.asp#meetings, accessed February 2, 2015.

Dietary Guidelines Advisory Committee. Report of the Dietary Guidelines Advisory Committee on the Dietary Guidelines for Americans, 2010, Appendix E-4, History of the Dietary Guidelines for Americans, 2010. Available at http://www.cnpp.usda.gov/sites/default/files/dietary_guidelines_for_americans/2010DGAC Report-camera-ready-Jan11-11.pdf, accessed February 12, 2015.

Dietary Guidelines Advisory Committee. Report of the Dietary Guidelines Advisory Committee on the Dietary Guidelines for Americans, 2005, August 19, 2004. Available at http://www.health.gov/dietaryguidelines /dga2005/report/, accessed February 2, 2015.

Dwyer JT. Nutrition guidelines and education of the public. *J Nutr.* 2001;131(11 Suppl):3074S–3077S.

Fruits & Veggies More Matters. About Us. Available at http://www.fruitsandveggiesmorematters.org/about -fruits-and-veggies-more-matters, accessed February 2, 2015.

Guenther PM, Casavale KO, Reedy J et al. Update of the Healthy Eating Index: HEI-2010. *J Acad Nutr Diet.* 2013;113(4):569–580.

Harvard School of Public Health. Healthy Eating Plate & Health Eating Pyramid. Available at http://www.hsph .harvard.edu/nutritionsource/healthy-eating-plate/, accessed February 2, 2015.

Harvard School of Public Health. Healthy Eating Plate vs. USDA's MyPlate. Available at http://www.hsph .harvard.edu/nutritionsource/healthy-eating-plate-vs-usda-myplate/, accessed January 2, 2015.

HealthierUS.gov (web archive). Available at http://webarchive.library.unt.edu/eot2008/20080916003723/http: /healthierus.gov/, accessed February 2, 2015.

Kant AK. Consumption of energy-dense, nutrient-poor foods by adult Americans: Nutritional and healthy implications. The Third National Health and Nutrition Examination Survey, 1988–1994. *Am J Clin Nutr.* 2000;72(4):929–936.

Kant AK. Reported consumption of low-nutrient-density foods by American children and adolescents. Nutritional and health correlates, NHANES III, 1988 to 1994. *Arch Pediatr Adolesc Med.* 2003;157(8):789–796.

Kennedy ET, Ohls J, Carlson S, Flemming K. The healthy eating index: Design and applications. *J Am Diet Assoc.* 1995;95(10):1103–1108.

Key TJ. Fruit and vegetables and cancer risk. *Br J Cancer.* 2011;104:6–11.

Knowler WC, Barrett-Connor E, Fowler SE et al. Reduction in the incidence of type 2 diabetes with lifestyle intervention or metformin. *N Engl J Med.* 2002;346(6):393–403.

Krauss RM, Eckel RH, Howard B et al. AHA Dietary Guidelines: Revision 2000: A statement for health-care professionals from the Nutrition Committee of the American Heart Association. *Circulation.* 2000;102(18):2284–2299.

Kuehn BM. Experts charge new US dietary guidelines pose daunting challenge for the public. *JAMA.* 2005;293(8):918–920.

Lanou AJ, Berkow SE, Barnard ND. Calcium, dairy products, and bone health in children and young adults: A reevaluation of the evidence. *Pediatrics.* 2005;115(3):736–743.

Lichtenstein AH, Appel LJ, Brands M et al. Diet and lifestyle recommendations revision 2006: A scientific statement from the American Heart Association Nutrition Committee. *Circulation.* 2006;114(1):82–96.

Light L. A fatally flawed food guide. *Whole Life Times*, November 2004. Available at http://u2.lege.net/whale .to/a/light.html, accessed February 2, 2015.

Mozaffarian D, Afshin A, Benowitz NL et al. Population approaches to improve diet, physical activity, and smoking habits: A scientific statement from the American Heart Association. *Circulation.* 2012;126(12):1514–1563.

National Center for Health Statistics. Health, United States, 2012: With Special Feature on Emergency Care. Table 64: Hypertension among Adults Aged 20 and Over, by Selected Characteristics: United States, Selected Years 1988–1994 through 2007–2010. Hyattsville, MD, 2013, pp. 207–208.

National High Blood Pressure Education Program. *The Seventh Report of the Joint National Committee on Prevention, Detection, Evaluation, and Treatment of High Blood Pressure.* US Department of Health and Human Services, National Institutes of Health, National Heart, Lung, and Blood Institute. NIH Publication No. 04-5230, August 2004. Available at http://www.nhlbi.nih.gov/guidelines/hypertension /jnc7full.pdf, accessed February 2, 2015.

National Nutrition Monitoring and Related Research Act of 1990 (7 USC. 5341), Public Law, 101–445. Available at http://www.gpo.gov/fdsys/pkg/USCODE-2009-title7/html/USCODE-2009-title7-chap84.htm, accessed February 2, 2015.

National Research Council. *Dietary Reference Intakes: Applications in Dietary Assessment.* Washington, DC: The National Academies Press, 2000.

National Research Council. *Dietary Reference Intakes: Applications in Dietary Planning.* Washington, DC: The National Academies Press, 2003a.

National Research Council. *Dietary Reference Intakes: Guiding Principles for Nutrition Labeling and Fortification.* Washington, DC: The National Academies Press, 2003b.

National Research Council. *Dietary Reference Intakes: The Essential Guide to Nutrient Requirements.* Washington, DC: The National Academies Press, 2006.

National Research Council, Commission on Life Science, Food and Nutrition Board, Committee on Diet and Health. *Diet and Health: Implications for Reducing Chronic Disease Risk.* Washington, DC: National Academy Press, 1989.

Nestle M. *Food Politics: How the Food Industry Influences Nutrition and Health.* Berkeley, CA: University of California Press, 2002.

Pollan M. Unhappy meals. *The New York Times Magazine,* January 28, 2007, p. 38.

Produce for Better Health Foundation. About PBH: History. Available at http://www.pbhfoundation.org/about /history/, accessed February 2, 2015.

Report of a Joint WHO/FAO Expert Consultation. *Diet, Nutrition and the Prevention of Chronic Diseases.* WHO Technical Report Series 916. Geneva, Switzerland: World Health Organization, 2003. Available at http://www.who.int/dietphysicalactivity/publications/trs916/en/, accessed February 2, 2015.

Sallis JF, Owen N, Fisher EB. Ecological models of health behavior. In Glanz K, Rimer BK, Viswanath K, eds. *Health Behavior and Health Education: Theory, Research, and Practice,* 4th ed. San Francisco: Jossey-Bass, 2008, pp. 465–486.

Schneeman BO, Mendelson R. Dietary guidelines: Past experience and new approaches. *J Am Diet Assoc.* 2002;103(10):1498–1500.

Stamler R. Implications of the INTERSALT study. *Hypertension.* 1991;17(Suppl 1):I16–I20.

US Congress, Senate Select Committee on Nutrition and Human Needs. *Dietary Goals for the United States,* 1st ed. Washington, DC: US Government Printing Office, 1977a.

US Congress, Senate Select Committee on Nutrition and Human Needs. *Dietary Goals for the United States, Supplemental Views.* Washington, DC: US Government Printing Office, 1977b.

US Congress, Senate Select Committee on Nutrition and Human Needs. *Dietary Goals for the United States,* 2nd ed. Washington, DC: US Government Printing Office, 1977c.

US Department of Health and Human Services, Public Health Service. *The Surgeon General's Report on Nutrition and Health.* DHHS (PHS) Publication No. 88-50210, 1988. Available at http://profiles.nlm.nih .gov/NN/B/C/Q/G/, accessed February 2, 2015.

US Department of Health and Human Services. National Diabetes Education Program. Small Steps. Big Rewards. Prevent type 2 Diabtes Campaign. Available at http://ndep.nih.gov/partners-community -organization/campaigns/smallstepsbigrewards.aspx, accessed February 17, 2015.

US Department of Agriculture, US Department of Health and Human Services. *Nutrition and Your Health: Dietary Guidelines for Americans.* Home and Garden Bulletin No. 232, February 1980. Available at http://www.health.gov/dietaryguidelines/1980thin.pdf, accessed February 2, 2015.

US Department of Agriculture, US Department of Health and Human Services. *Nutrition and Your Health: Dietary Guidelines for Americans,* 2nd ed. Washington, DC: Home and Garden Bulletin No. 232, 1985. Available at http://www.health.gov/dietaryguidelines/1985thin.pdf, accessed February 2, 2015.

US Department of Agriculture, US Department of Health and Human Services. *Nutrition and Your Health: Dietary Guidelines for Americans,* 3rd ed. Washington, DC: Home and Garden Bulletin No. 232, November 1990. Available at http://www.health.gov/dietaryguidelines/1990thin.pdf, accessed February 2, 2015.

US Department of Agriculture, Center for Nutrition Policy and Promotion. *The Food Guide Pyramid*. Home and Garden Bulletin No. 252, August 1992, revised October 1996. Available at http://www.cnpp.usda.gov/sites/default/files/archived_projects/FGPPamphlet.pdf, accessed February 2, 2015.

US Department of Agriculture, US Department of Health and Human Services. *Nutrition and Your Health: Dietary Guidelines for Americans*, 4th ed. Washington, DC: Home and Garden Bulletin No. 232, December 1995. Available at http://www.health.gov/dietaryguidelines/dga95/default.htm, accessed February 2, 2015.

US Department of Agriculture, US Department of Health and Human Services. *Nutrition and Your Health: Dietary Guidelines for Americans*, 5th ed. Washington, DC: Home and Garden Bulletin No. 232, 2000. Available at http://www.health.gov/dietaryguidelines/dga2000/document/frontcover.htm, accessed February 2, 2015.

US Department of Agriculture, US Department of Health and Human Services. *Dietary Guidelines for Americans, 2005*, 6th ed. Washington, DC: HHS Publication number: HHS-ODPHP-2005-01-DGA-A. USDA Publication number: Home and Garden Bulletin No. 232, January 2005a. Available at http://www.health.gov/dietaryguidelines/dga2005/document/default.htm, accessed February 2, 2015.

US Department of Agriculture, Center for Nutrition Policy and Promotion. *MyPyramid*, CNPP-15, April 2005b. Available at http://www.choosemyplate.gov/food-groups/downloads/MiniPoster.pdf, accessed February 2, 2015.

US Department of Agriculture, US Department of Health and Human Services. *Dietary Guidelines for Americans, 2010*, 7th ed. Washington, DC: US Government Printing Office, December 2010. Available at http://www.health.gov/dietaryguidelines/dga2010/dietaryguidelines2010.pdf, accessed February 2, 2015.

US Department of Agriculture. Press Release: First Lady, Agriculture Secretary Launch *MyPlate* Icon as a New Reminder to Help Consumers to Make Healthier Food Choices. Washington, DC, June 2, 2011a. Available at http://www.usda.gov/wps/portal/usda/usdamediafb?contentid=2011/06/0225.xml&printable=true&contentidonly=true, accessed February 2, 2015.

US Department of Agriculture, Center for Nutrition Policy and Promotion. Development of *2010 Dietary Guidelines for Americans* Consumer Messages and New Food Icon: Executive Summary of Formative Research, June 2011b. Available at http://www.choosemyplate.gov/food-groups/downloads/MyPlate/ExecutiveSummaryOfFormativeResearch.pdf, accessed February 2, 2015.

US Department of Agriculture, Center for Nutrition Policy and Promotion. Diet quality of children age 2–17 years as measured by the healthy eating index-2010. *Nutr Insight*. 2013;52:1–2. Available at http://www.cnpp.usda.gov/sites/default/files/nutrition_insights_uploads/Insight52.pdf, accessed August 22, 2013.

US Department of Health and Human Services. News Release: HHS and USDA announce the appointment of the 2015 *Dietary Guidelines* Advisory Committee, May 31, 2013. Available at http://www.health.gov/dietaryguidelines/2015DGAC-Announcement-Release.pdf, accessed February 2, 2015.

Welsh SO, Davis C, Shaw A. *USDA's Food Guide: Background and Development*. US Department of Agriculture, Human Nutrition Information Service, Nutrition Education Division. Hyattsville, MD. Miscellaneous Publication No. 1514, September 1993. Available at http://www.cnpp.usda.gov/sites/default/files/archived_projects/FGPBackgroundAndDevelopment.pdf, accessed February 2, 2015.

White B. Dietary fatty acids. *Am. Fam. Physician*. 2009;80(4):345–350.

Willett WC. *Eat, Drink, and Be Healthy*. New York: Simon and Schuster Source, 2001, p. 139.

World Cancer Research Fund, American Institute for Cancer Research. *Food, Nutrition and the Prevention of Cancer: A Global Perspective*. Washington, DC: American Institute for Cancer Research, 1997.

World Cancer Research Fund, American Institute for Cancer Research. *Food, Nutrition, Physical Activity, and the Prevention of Cancer: A Global Perspective*. Washington DC: AICR, 2007.

Zelman K, Kennedy E. Naturally nutrient rich…putting more power on Americans' plates. *Nutr Today*. 2005;40(2):60–68.

10 Food and Nutrition Assessment of the Community

Despite how central food is to our lives, most of us know very little about where the food we eat comes from, how it is grown, and how it reaches our plates. This lack of knowledge is true not only for individuals but also for communities as a whole.

Hassanein and Jacobson (2004)

INTRODUCTION

Assessment, policy development, and assurance are the three core functions of public health, whether at the federal, state, or local level. Assessment, the focus of this chapter, refers to the systematic collection, assembly, analysis, and dissemination of information about the health of a community. Policy development involves the creation of comprehensive public health policies based on scientific knowledge. Assurance is the pledge to constituents that services necessary to achieve agreed-upon goals are provided by encouraging the action of others (private or public), by stipulating action through regulation, or by providing the service directly (The Committee for the Study of the Future of Public Health 1988).

Every public health agency must ensure that assessment occurs either directly or through intergovernmental or interagency cooperation. Accurate information on the health status of a community and a clear understanding of the available resources is requisite to making informed decisions about which areas should have priority, which policies might be effective, or which interventions might be possible to implement. In addition, monitoring must be either ongoing or undertaken at regular intervals to provide a baseline understanding of the community's health in order to evaluate how well any new policies or interventions improve health, how cost-effective one option is over another, or how long a program might continue (Institute of Medicine et al. 1996).

Community health assessment includes the following:

- Determining the health needs of the community by establishing a systematic process that periodically provides pertinent health information.
- Investigating adverse health events and health hazards by conducting timely investigations that identify the magnitude of health problems, including their duration, trends, location, and at-risk populations.
- Analyzing the determinants of identified health problems to discover the reasons why certain populations are at risk for adverse health outcomes.

A component of the community health assessment is assessment of food and nutrition status. In performing their role of assessment, public health agencies monitor food- and nutrition-related health in order to identify and solve health problems associated with diet. In addition to diagnosing the community's health status, state and local public health agencies must

- Identify food- and nutrition-related threats to health.
- Periodically collect, analyze, and publicize information on access, utilization, costs, and outcomes of nutrition services.
- Focus on the vital statistics and nutrition-related health status of specific groups at higher risk than the population as a whole.

The primary goal of this chapter is to introduce the information needed to conduct food and nutrition assessments within a community. A secondary goal is to help readers appreciate the value of ongoing collaboration between local health assessment coordinators and nutritionists, and state and local food and nutrition assessment efforts.

COMMUNITY ASSESSMENT

There are three types of food- and nutrition-related assessments discussed in this chapter. They are the *community nutrition assessment*, the *community food assessment* (sometimes referred to as a *food system assessment*), and the *community food security assessment*. In clinical practice, the counterpart to the food assessment would be the diet history.

The purpose of any kind of assessment is to collect and analyze information in order to identify problems and suggest solutions to ameliorate them. In the clinic, assessment forms the basis for developing and implementing an individual's care plan or course of medical nutrition therapy. In the community, assessment forms the basis for subsequent program planning and evaluation.

Regardless of the specific focus of the assessment—or who initiates the process or assumes major responsibility for carrying it out—the goals of food and nutrition assessments in the community are to

- Improve the health of the people in a defined area by building the capacity of local health jurisdictions to reduce nutritional risk and promote optimal nutritional health of community members.
- Raise official awareness of food and nutrition issues to promote the inclusion of nutrition questions in local health assessments and otherwise get food and nutrition issues on the local agenda.
- Determine how to allocate limited resources.
- Evaluate the efficacy of food and nutrition programs and services in the community.
- Identify current and potential food and nutrition problems in the community.

Three basic kinds of information are gathered during any community assessment. These include a statistical community profile, qualitative data on the experiences of the population, and an assessment of local resources and assets (The Washington State Community Nutrition Assessment Education Project, http://depts.washington.edu/commnutr/home/index.htm). Termed an *assets-based approach* (Kretzmann and McKnight 1993), this type of assessment recognizes and employs individual and community talents, skills, and assets, rather than focusing on problems and needs. Such an approach imparts a sense of ownership to community members participating in the process (Box 10.1).

In every community there are groups who care about nutrition: churches, healthcare institutions, government agencies, breastfeeding support groups, Head Start, schools, parents, and healthcare providers. A thoughtful compilation of assets prevents an assessment from becoming a compendium of morbidity and mortality statistics.

The successful community assessment includes understanding current issues confronting families and individuals, evaluating local capacities for supporting health and nutrition needs, and building community support for implementing changes. To conduct a community assessment, it is necessary to (The Washington State Community Nutrition Assessment Education Project, http://depts.washington.edu /commnutr/home/index.htm)

1. Organize a planning group.
2. Define community boundaries.
3. Gather quantitative data that include a statistical profile of the community and a compendium of community resources.

BOX 10.1   THE COMMUNITY TOOL BOX

The Community Tool Box is a project that promotes community health and development by connecting people, ideas, and resources. The Community Tool Box provides practical skill-building information on over 300 different topics, including step-by-step instruction, examples, checklists, and related resources. Maintained by the Work Group for Community Health and Development at the University of Kansas, the development of the Community Tool Box has been ongoing since 1994, and its utilization rates have grown over time, from about 17,000 user sessions in 1997 to over 1 million user sessions in 2006. Current uses of the Community Tool Box include providing guidance for community work, training, technical assistance, university instruction, certification, and building capacity for funded initiatives. Additional information can be found at http://ctb.ku.edu.

4. Collect qualitative data that reflect the food and nutrition concerns of representatives of key community groups.
5. Analyze and prioritize common issues, high-risk individuals and populations, and unmet needs.

THE COMMUNITY NUTRITION ASSESSMENT

A nutrition assessment of a community is initiated and implemented by professionals to examine a broad range of nutrition-related issues and assets in order to improve the community's nutrition services system. The nutrition assessment is part of the larger community health assessment. During the assessment process, relationships are forged between individuals and organizations that may result in enhanced opportunities for collaboration and funding. An overarching goal of the community nutrition assessment is a movement away from a categorical and programmatic view of nutrition services and programs to a focus on the role of nutrition in the community as a whole.

The New York State Department of Health (NYSDOH, http://www.health.ny.gov/statistics/chac/) Community Health Assessment Clearinghouse, the Washington State Community Nutrition Assessment Project (http://depts.washington.edu/commnutr/home/index.htm), the Public Health/ Community Nutrition dietetic practice group of the Academy of Nutrition and Dietetics (AND), and others have compiled knowledge, skills, tools, and resources for nutrition professionals and local health assessment coordinators to use when conducting a community nutrition assessment (Boxes 10.2 and 10.3).

BOX 10.2   COMMUNITY HEALTH ASSESSMENT CLEARINGHOUSE

The NYSDOH has compiled resources to use when performing a community health assessment. The NYSDOH Community Health Assessment Clearinghouse is a *one-stop* resource for community health planners, practitioners, and policy developers. Community Health Indicator Reports are available at the state, regional, and county levels, and provide easy access to 250 health indicators for 15 health topic areas. Guidance documents; examples of community health assessments; and links to national, state, and county public health data resources are also provided. The Community Health Assessment Clearinghouse is available at http://www.health.ny.gov/statistics/chac/.

BOX 10.3   ONLINE SOURCES FOR COMMUNITY NUTRITION ASSESSMENT

When planning a community nutrition assessment, be sure to investigate the growing number of online sources. For example, the Washington State Community Nutrition Assessment Project website, developed in 1999 by the Washington State Department of Health and University of Washington, contains a wealth of information, including case studies, sources of data, questions for surveys, documents, and other resources (http://depts.washington.edu/commnutr/home/). Still another resource is the online book, *Moving to the Future*, a product of the Association of State and Territorial Public Health Nutrition Directors. The tools available at this website are geared toward planning nutrition and physical activity programs, and include information, surveys, and worksheets for conducting a community assessment (http://www.movingtothefuture.org).

A nutrition assessment examines, in particular, the health and nutrition status of community members, including

- Pregnancy-related status, including pre-pregnancy weight, weight gain during pregnancy, and anemia.
- Prevalence of diseases affected by nutrition.
- Physical activity and food-related behaviors.
- Food intake, such as amount of fruits and vegetables consumed.
- Dental health.
- Food security.

Local Nutrition Surveillance

For effective nutrition programming, planning, and policymaking, state and community leaders require timely objective information on the current and changing nutrition condition of the populations they serve. Providing such information is the goal of nutrition surveillance, which collects nutrition indicators from a representative sample of a particular locality. Examples of measurements used in nutrition surveillance include self-reported height and weight and brief food frequency questionnaires (FFQs). The inclusion in surveillance studies of questions regarding knowledge, attitudes, and behavior can help in developing target strategies for dietary messages. Indicators of dietary practices in the community, such as comparing the amount of supermarket shelf space for whole vs. low-fat and fat-free milk, may also be used. The problems identified through surveillance can help generate timely interventions (Byers 1998).

Nutrition surveillance comprises four types of activities: timely warning and intervention, problem identification, policy and program planning, and management and evaluation. As an example, in 1984, New York State began a Nutrition Surveillance Program (NSP), the first phase of which was connected to the Supplemental Nutrition Assistance Program (SNAP), Special Supplemental Food Program for Women, Infants, and Children (WIC), and a new program that supported over 1000 emergency food programs in the state, and also expanded home-delivered meals to the frail elderly. The NSP gathered information about the characteristics and unmet nutritional needs of these populations, which was then used for funding requests and program development. The second phase of the NSP began in 1988, identifying and characterizing populations at nutritional risk and evaluating the status of current nutrition programs. Results of this assessment included the addition of a nutrition component to the Dental Survey of School Children and the development of an inventory of information sources in all state agencies. The third phase, a policy and planning phase, monitored the Healthy People 2000 objectives and the 5-year plan of the state's Food and Nutrition Policy Council (Dodds and Melnik 1993). Additional information about the New York State NSP can be found at http://www.ncbi.nlm.nih.gov/pmc/articles/PMC1403366.

THE COMMUNITY FOOD ASSESSMENT

A community food assessment is a participatory and collaborative process spearheaded by members of the community rather than health professionals. Community members along with officials representing public and private agencies examine a broad range of food-related issues and community assets in order to improve the community's food system. Through such an assessment, diverse stakeholders work together to research their local food system, publicize their findings, and take action. A number of communities, such as those described in the next three sections, have successfully planned and implemented community food assessments, gathered a wide range of data, and used the results to generate tangible outcomes. Their endeavors demonstrate that assessments in diverse settings can generate a variety of results, including new policies and programs, as well as produce benefits such as new partnerships and capacity development (Pothukuchi et al. 2002).

A community food assessment relies on the participation of diverse stakeholders, including community residents, to plan and implement the assessment and emphasizes shared leadership and collaborative decision making. In addition, it fosters education and empowerment strategies, such as training young people in survey methods. Significantly, this type of assessment focuses on meeting the needs of low-income and other marginalized populations, examines a variety of issues and the connections between them, and generates specific recommendations and actions aimed at improving the local food system (Community Food Security Coalition n.d.).

A community food assessment includes four components (Pothukuchi et al. 2002):

- *Organization* to identify key stakeholders, arrange initial meetings, determine the group's interest in conducting an assessment, identify and recruit other participants representing diverse interests and skills, and continue to coordinate and engage constituents throughout the project.
- *Planning* to review other assessments that have been conducted; determine assessment purpose and goals; develop an overall plan and decision-making process and clarify roles; define geographic population boundaries; and identify and secure grants, in-kind resources, and/or project sponsors.
- *Research* to develop questions and indicators, identify existing data and information needed, develop research tools, collect and analyze data, and compile and summarize findings.
- *Advocacy* to discuss findings with community and develop recommendations; create action plans to implement priority recommendations; determine whether additional partners should be recruited; develop media strategy; disseminate findings to the public, policymakers, and journalists; urge policymakers and others to take action based on recommendations; and evaluate the assessment project.

Community Food Assessment Projects

Whereas community food assessments are undertaken for a variety of reasons and in diverse communities, a review of nine community food assessment projects—from Austin, TX to Somerville, MA, outlined in Table 10.1—conducted between 1993 and 2003 (Pothukuchi 2004) revealed these common characteristics:

- *Focused on the needs of low-income residents* and shared a concern for the problems they face with respect to food security. Recommendations from the studies included such strategies as instituting a new bus route connecting low-income neighborhoods to large supermarkets, the development of year-round farmers' markets, and improved coordination of food assistance efforts throughout the county.
- *Shared concerns about the sustainability of the food system* relevant to their own communities. In these studies, sustainability included creating closer links between two or more food system activities (for example, production, processing, distribution, consumption, and

TABLE 10.1
Nine Community Food Assessments

Site	Assessment Goals	Issues Examined	Outcomes
Austin, TX	Raise awareness of community needs, problems Inform systematic action on community food problems	Food access problems in central Austin, coping strategies Quality of food available in a poor neighborhood	New grocery bus route Legislation allowing public lands for community gardens, farmers' markets Grocery store renovation Awareness of food access Food policy council established
Berkeley, CA	Enhance community knowledge, awareness of local food systems Study feasibility of new ways to link farmers' markets and communities	Local food production: farms and urban gardens Food retail Role of educational institutions Public policies related to above issues	Formalized collaboration between Berkeley Food Policy Council and area producers, retailers, and community-based nonprofit (including youth) organizations Links between local producers and Berkeley school cafeterias Dissemination of study tools nationally
Detroit, MI	Support community food security planning, actions Create university–community partnerships on community food issues	Food in local economy (including contribution to local economy; grocery store locations; food access, availability in poor neighborhoods) Nutrition, food insecurity Neighborhood improvement, including community gardens Regional agriculture	Collaboration by nonprofit organizations in nutrition, social services, greening, community development, etc., to develop community food projects Greater public, private, nonprofit, university collaboration on community food issues National dissemination of study tools, findings Production, dissemination of *Detroit Food Handbook* for local planning
Los Angeles, CA	Assess food insecurity in inner city, following 1993 unrest, adequacy of federal food programs, and role of food industry in inner city community-based strategies for change Propose framework for community food security planning	Community food access, availability, prices Hunger and food insecurity Food retail structure Sustainable production, distribution models Current food policies; alternative approaches	Formation of Los Angeles Community Food Security Network, Los Angeles food policy council Growth of community gardens, farmers' markets, food stamp outreach Food assessments in other communities Catalyst for community food security movement in the United States

(Continued)

TABLE 10.1 (CONTINUED)
Nine Community Food Assessments

Site	Assessment Goals	Issues Examined	Outcomes
Madison, WI	Increase knowledge, understanding of local food system Inform strategies for improving food security Establish university, community partnerships	Conventional food system (production, processing, wholesale, retail) and its impacts on environment, food access, availability Antihunger resources Coping strategies of low-income residents Alternatives to conventional system Policies helping, hurting community food security	Development of Dane County REAP (Research, Education, Action, and Policy) Food Group Greater visibility of food issues in Madison Increased networking, collaboration among individuals and organizations around food issues Madison Food System Working Paper series National dissemination of assessment tools
Milwaukee, WI	Examine root causes of hunger Develop partnerships to promote food security and systemic change in Milwaukee County	Population characteristics Food access and transportation Food retail: locations, availability, prices Antihunger and alternative food sources Perceptions and experiences of poor individuals and families	Formation of Milwaukee Farmers' Market Association Development of Fondy Food Center Project (market, kitchen incubator, information center) Overhaul of emergency pantry network, community meal program coalition, and inclusion of new types of technical assistance and guidelines Expansion of WIC Farmers' Market Nutrition Program (FMNP) to all farmers' markets Increased university–community partnerships National dissemination of study tools, findings
North Country Region, NY	Mobilize and engage a broad network of country residents Improve access to healthful, locally produced foods while strengthening economic viability of regional agricultures	Demographics, health, economy, agriculture, food availability Sources of food, eating patterns Ways to build a stronger community through alternative management of local food resources Visions for how local food system should look and work in 5 years Visions for 20 years	Development of an extension staff position to continue work Increased networks among community, agency members Creation of a fellowship kitchen to serve all community members, including needy and vulnerable households in Essex County Program to provide donations of venison and beef to local food pantries in Lews and St. Lawrence counties Establishment of weekly farmers' market in Jefferson County Improved food distribution networks between the community action programs of Jefferson and Franklin Counties Increased storage and trucking facilities through joint efforts of a food security committee

(Continued)

TABLE 10.1 (CONTINUED)
Nine Community Food Assessments

Site	Assessment Goals	Issues Examined	Outcomes
San Francisco, CA	Identify and promote strategies to improve food access to nutritious foods in Bayview Hunters Point neighborhood Provide job training for neighborhood youth	Food sources for residents, barriers to access, consumption Preferred alternatives for food procurement	Creation of a new Bayview Community Farmers' Market Commitments on the part of corner store owners to stock fresh produce Transit authority agreement to provide transit shuttles to food sources Skills development, empowerment of neighborhood youth
Somerville, MA	Strengthen planning and policy for community-based food and nutrition resources for low-income residents	Food and nutrition needs, resources	Publication of an extensive community food and nutrition guide Cooking classes for low-income residents Implementation of a Community Kitchen Task Force to examine the feasibility of commercial kitchen facilities Formation of a Public Health Nutrition Task Force to conduct community food and nutrition strategic planning

Source: Adapted from Pothukuchi K., *J Plan Educ Res.* 2004;23(4):356–77.

waste disposal); making specific food system practices more environmentally friendly; including previously excluded categories, such as low-income consumers and small farmers; and educating community residents about their participation in food systems and ways to enhance sustainability.

- *Viewed the community as a source of strength* that held solutions to problems of food access.
- *Focused on assets in the community*, such as existing resources, infrastructure, and motivated and talented individuals and their networks.
- *Relied on extant data from multiple sources*, including social, economic, demographic, and health data from censuses; community directories; and primary information derived from surveys, focus groups, and interviews.

Beneficial and tangible outcomes from these community food assessments are reviewed in *What's Cooking in Your Food System?* (Pothukuchi et al. 2002). In addition, this guide discusses problems with our present food system and their relevance to food security, details the process of planning and conducting a community assessment, and reviews how to implement changes based on assessment results. Process-oriented benefits resulting from the featured programs include development of networks and coalitions, community participation and collaboration, and capacity development.

Food and Farming in Missoula County

In 2003, two professors from the University of Montana formed a steering committee of stakeholders from the community that included farmers, county planning officials, and food bank representatives to identify the most vital research questions related to food and farming in Missoula County. Next, the faculty members designed a multidisciplinary university course, engaging 21 students in gathering information regarding food production, distribution, and consumption in the county (*Missoula County Community Food Assessment* 2004). The results of this research are compiled in two reports: *Our Foodshed in Focus* (Community Food and Agriculture Coalition of Missoula County, http://www.missoulacfac.org/ourfoodshedinfocus.html) uses existing statistical data, primarily from US census reports and other government sources, to describe patterns in the local food system, and how these have changed over time. Seven chapters, all authored by students, detail relevant trends in the following areas: demographics, agricultural production, environment, food distribution, employment in farming and food-related businesses, consumption, and food security and access. Each chapter also discusses why these trends might be occurring and explains why these measures are important. Appendices include both the raw data and the data sources used for each chapter. Additional reference material is provided at the end of each chapter. *Grow, Eat, Know* (Community Food and Agriculture Coalition of Missoula County, http://www.missoulacfac.org/resourceguide.html) is a resource guide of food and farming in the county.

The next phase of the project sought input from county agricultural producers and county residents. Representatives of the agricultural community were asked to comment on the future of farming in the county, whereas residents of various income levels were asked to identify their concerns regarding food quality, cost, and access. The research was designed to answer questions that the steering committee asked about Missoula County's food system. It includes the following:

- What is needed for viable and sustainable commercial food production in the county?
- What are the existing assets and barriers to creating a more viable and sustainable production system?
- What concerns do county residents at various income levels have about food, including quality, access, transportation to food outlets, cost, eating behaviors, and choices?
- What do residents perceive as their county's food-related assets?

Original data were collected during the spring of 2004. The results of these interviews and recommendations for action are compiled in a report entitled *Food Matters* (Community Food and

Agriculture Coalition of Missoula County, http://www.missoulacfac.org/foodmatters.html). The report also offers recommendations designed to generate a community dialogue about the future of the food and farming system in the county.

Food System Sustainability in Concord

In 2011, a group of nearly 30 Concord, MA citizens, town officials, and local experts formed a steering and advisory committee to discuss ways to promote a sustainable local food system. Committee members represented farmers, educators, business owners, local policymakers, chefs, and representatives of local organizations. In order to answer one member's question (what is our food story and where do we go from here?), the committee partnered with the Conway School—a graduate program in sustainable landscape planning and design—to prepare a community food report for the town. The goal of the assessment was to assist community members in their effort to understand the complexities of localizing their food system. Primary objectives were to explore interactions between a local food system and social, ecological, and economic health in Concord; encourage a community-wide conversation about Concord's participation in its regional food system; and recommend next steps and future projects.

The final report, *Building Local Food Connections* (2012), provides an assets- and needs-based assessment of Concord's food system resources, including land use, food production, distribution, processing, storage, preparation, consumption, and food waste recovery. The report includes a history of agriculture in Concord, *local leader* profiles, informative data, pictures, maps, graphs, charts, and six critical recommendations for Concord's local food system:

• Establish a local food policy council.
• Implement farm-to-institution programs.
• Promote a town-wide gardening movement.
• Revitalize animal husbandry in Concord.
• Match farmers and growers with suitable land in Concord.
• Permanently protect farmland for agriculture use.

The Community Food Security Assessment

The food security assessment collects information to determine the extent to which existing community resources provide adequate, culturally acceptable foods to households in the area. Although many elements overlap, a community *food security* assessment more specifically focuses on communities at risk for low food security than does a community *food* assessment (Box 10.4).

The US Department of Agriculture (USDA) has developed a toolkit of instructions and materials for conducting a community food security assessment (Cohen et al. 2002). The kit contains standardized measurement tools for assessing various aspects of community food security. These tools focus on examining basic assessment components: profiling general community characteristics and community food resources, assessment of household food security, food resource accessibility, food

---

BOX 10.4   WHAT IS A COMMUNITY FOOD SECURITY ASSESSMENT?

"A community food security assessment is a unique type of community assessment. It includes the collection of various types of data to provide answers to questions about the ability of existing community resources to provide sufficient and nutritionally sound amounts of culturally acceptable foods to households in the community."

Source: Cohen B et al., *Community Food Security Assessment Toolkit.* Economic Research Service. E-FAN-02-013, July 2002. Available at http://www.ers.usda.gov/media/327699/efan02013_1_.pdf, accessed January 16, 2015.

availability and affordability, and food production resources. Appendices to the toolkit provide tips for developing data tables, materials and guides for conducting focus groups, and materials for conducting food store surveys.

Community Food Security Assessment Projects

Obtaining Affordable, Nutritious Food in East Austin, Texas

Access Denied (Sustainable Food Center 1995) describes the food system of East Austin, Texas, and how it failed to meet community needs. The analysis revealed that access to nutritious affordable food was difficult for much of the community. At the time of the study, these shopping realities limited consumer selection and increased the cost of food for people who could least afford it. The area studied had just two supermarkets—both smaller and one more expensive than similar stores in other parts of the town. Securing transportation to these food outlets was often difficult; for many, hiring a taxi was the only way to buy food at the supermarket. As a result of being unable to access supermarkets, many low-income shoppers relied on expensive corner convenience stores. Wholesale grocery companies rarely served these smaller stores, which forced owners to charge higher prices and offer limited selections. There were 38 convenience stores in the community, but only 5 stocked the ingredients for a balanced meal. All of the convenience stores stocked alcoholic beverages, but only 18 carried milk. There were 20 agencies that distributed emergency food in the area studied.

This assessment of food resource accessibility and availability demonstrated that the resources did exist to improve the food system and to overcome obstacles to getting good food. The report suggests community resources and solutions in access, store quality, alternative retail formats, local food production, and food education. The authors of the report list such options as forming grocer cooperatives that could take advantage of group purchasing and shared warehousing for small store owners; forming neighborhood food-buying clubs; initiating shopper shuttles, reduced fares, and other transportation solutions to help people get to stores; supporting farmers' markets and produce stands; and producing local food through community gardening programs and urban farms.

Community Food Security Assessments in Sacramento County, California

In 1999–2000, the Sacramento Hunger Commission conducted a pilot project to study food access needs in Del Paso Heights and North Sacramento, two low-income neighborhoods in Sacramento County, California. The goal of the assessment was to systematically examine access to nutritious, affordable food in communities impacted by hunger; increase the awareness of barriers to food security; and facilitate improved access to nutritious food. Their subsequent report, *Breaking Barriers: A Road to Improved Food Access* (2000), outlined recommendations made by low-income residents about how to improve food access in their community. The assessment identified a need for improved public transportation to markets supplying fresh, nutritious, affordable food. In response, the commission received funding to implement some of the recommendations in the report. The group's research and advocacy helped implement a neighborhood shuttle and generated a new bus route connecting underserved neighborhoods to a grocery store on the opposite side of a freeway.

In the fall of 2003, the Sacramento Hunger Commission proposed a community food security assessment of Avondale/Glen Elder, a low-income neighborhood in the southern part of the city. Avondale/Glen Elder was chosen because of its manageable size and relatively effective organization. Nonetheless, it proved a difficult area to assess because of its diversity of cultures and languages. A VISTA (Volunteer in Service to America) volunteer and a Hunger Commission intern developed a comprehensive plan and then gathered a plethora of information on the area's food security and food access status. A steering committee of active community residents oversaw and contributed to the assessment. They surveyed *food closet* clients, senior home-delivered meal recipients, and other community residents and evaluated each food resource in the neighborhood to determine its effectiveness in providing affordable, nutritious, culturally appropriate food. The data were then evaluated and presented in a comprehensive report (Box 10.5) (Salcone 2004).

BOX 10.5   RECOMMENDATIONS FROM THE AVONDALE/GLEN ELDER ASSESSMENT

- Establish a closer full-service grocery store.
- Improve shuttle bus route to connect individuals with services and food resources.
- Increase public transit information outreach to immigrant populations.
- Create a grocery store carpool network.
- Arrange a farmers' market carpool system and bus field trip.
- Allow use of Electronic Benefit Transfer (EBT) card at farmers' markets.
- Coordinate food closet services for alternate days and times
- Arrange cooking classes and include nutrition and health information in activities.
- Preserve and protect open spaces that can be used as community gardens.
- Develop a community-organized, food-buying cooperative.
- Improve outreach for public assistance programs.
- Increase the number of WIC farmers' market vouchers available, as well as the number of WIC staff.
- Expand farm-to-school and school garden programs.
- Stagger lunch periods in middle and high schools to reduce line lengths.
- Set length for elementary school lunch periods.
- Provide nonmilk beverage options for lactose-intolerant youth.
- Encourage teachers to set a positive example.

Source: Salcone, J. *The Avondale/Glen Elder Community Food Assessment: Food Security in a South Sacramento Neighborhood.* The Sacramento Hunger Commission, 2004.

Food Availability, Accessibility, Affordability, and Quality in Fresno County

In 2002, Fresno Metro Ministry, a faith-based nonprofit organization, began the planning process for a community food assessment of Fresno County, a culturally diverse California county with over 800,000 residents. Although it is the most productive agricultural county in the US, Fresno has some of the highest unemployment and poverty rates in California (Jessup 2004). The Fresno Metro Ministry trained more than 80 local neighborhood leaders, conducted over 850 survey assessments of consumers, and surveyed 131 retail stores with the goal of identifying key factors in food availability, accessibility, affordability, and quality in the county. The objectives of the community food assessment were to assess a number of districts, involve local residents and community volunteers in the survey process, empower community members to make food policy recommendations to local officials (via a food policy council), and create an action plan based on the collected data. Various data collection methods were used, including surveys, assessment software, geographic information system (GIS) mapping tools (described later in the chapter), and local task forces (Ver Ploeg et al. 2009).

Conducted between 2003 and 2005, the Fresno Fresh Access Community Food Assessment was funded at $200,000 for 2 years by the USDA. Results included the following findings:

- Low-income residents purchase fresh produce at flea markets, but some lack enough money to buy fresh food.
- Healthy, culturally appropriate foods are not available in some neighborhoods.
- About one-third of weekly meals consist of fast food.
- Many low-income residents are not accessing federal nutrition programs even though they may be eligible and require healthier foods for their families.
- Food acquisition habits vary by ethnicity.

Based on the results and recommendations of the Fresno Fresh Access Community Food Assessment, several outcomes ensued (WhyHunger, http://www.whyhunger.org/getinfo/showArticle/articleId/629#3), including

- Establishment of a Food and Built Environment Policy Group. As a direct result of the assessment, Fresno Metro Ministry went on to coordinate this group, with the county health department and California State University as partners and funding from the California Endowment.
- Improvements in the food and physical activity environments. Fresno Metro Ministry received a grant to plan an intervention to improve the environment for access to food and physical activity in a specific neighborhood of southeast Fresno.
- Adoption of a comprehensive Wellness Policy by Fresno Unified School District, the fourth largest school district in California.

CONDUCTING AN ASSESSMENT

Despite varying goals and a somewhat different focus, any community assessment entails many of the same components, some of which may occur simultaneously or be repeated in a feedback loop (Box 10.6).

The Centers for Disease Control and Prevention (CDC, http://www.cdc.gov/stltpublichealth/cha/assessment.html) at the Community Health Assessment Gateway identifies the following common elements to assessment and planning frameworks:

1. Organize and plan.
2. Engage the community.
3. Develop a goal or vision.
4. Conduct community health assessment(s).
5. Prioritize health issues.
6. Develop a community health improvement plan.
7. Implement and monitor the community health improvement plan.
8. Evaluate processes and outcomes.

The Community Health Assessment Gateway also provides numerous planning models, frameworks, and tools. One that may be of particular interest is Community Health Assessment and Group Evaluation (CHANGE). Authored by the CDC, it is described as a tool for all communities interested in creating social and built environments that support healthy living. The focus is on gathering and organizing data on community assets to prioritize needs for policy changes. Users complete an action plan (Centers for Disease Control and Prevention, http://www.cdc.gov/stltpublichealth/cha/assessment.html).

BOX 10.6 ASSESSMENT, PLANNING, IMPLEMENTATION, AND EVALUATION

Problem solving can be distilled into four basic tasks: assessment, planning, implementation, and evaluation. It is a lucky break for nutritionists that these sequential tasks can be remembered using the acronym APIE. When faced with a problem, the first action one must take is to analyze the situation. Based on that assessment, the second step consists of planning a course of action. Next, the plan is implemented. Finally, the intervention's effectiveness is evaluated. The process can repeat itself as many times as necessary, with the results of the evaluation determining the plan for the next cycle.

Source: Spark, A. Neologisms and mnemonics: linguistic tools in nutrition education and communication. Presented at the annual meeting of the American Dietetic Association, October 22, 1996.

This section, unless otherwise noted, is based on *What's Cooking in Your Food System?* (Pothukuchi et al. 2002) and the *Community Food Security Assessment Toolkit* (Cohen et al. 2002).

Organize a Team

A community assessment is envisioned, planned, conducted, and used by people living and working in the community. Representation from different segments of a community increases access to data, improves the likelihood of participation by their constituencies, ensures a focus on community concerns and goals, and can lead to positive and lasting change. In addition to community representation, assessment participants should provide diversity, expertise, experience, availability, and a capacity for decision making.

A team should have 8–12 members to be comprehensive without becoming unwieldy. Team members can be recruited from local government agencies, educational institutions, community- and faith-based organizations, health providers, food retailers, residents, and farmers. It is imperative to convince potential members of the importance of the assessment's goals, the need for that individual's particular skills or knowledge, the clarity of the assessment plan, and the intention to implement change based on results.

A review of the literature indicates that health outcomes are improved through community empowerment, with *empowerment domains* defined to include participation, community-based organizations, local leadership, resource mobilization, assessment of problems, links with other people and organizations, and program management. Those with power or with access to it (for example, a health practitioner) and those who desire it (for example, a client) must work together to create the necessary conditions to achieve empowerment, as in a community assessment (Laverack 2006).

Once constituted, the team works together to

- Clarify goals and interests.
- Agree on a planning and decision-making process.
- Define the community to be assessed.
- Identify funds and other resources.
- Plan and conduct the research.
- Prepare and disseminate findings.
- Evaluate the findings.
- Implement follow-up actions in response to the findings.

Define the Community and the Scope of the Assessment

Defining the geographical boundaries of the community to be assessed is fundamental to a community food assessment. Will you be assessing an entire county as in the Missoula County Foodshed study, or smaller urban neighborhoods as done by the Hunger Commission in Sacramento?

If conducting a community food assessment or food security assessment, consider the parts of the food system to be examined. Is the study wide ranging: linking aspects of the food system to health or sustainability? Or is it more narrowly focused on food access in a particular low-income neighborhood? Knowing what and whom you are going to assess helps to refine planning and the development of tools, such as surveys and questionnaires.

Preliminary Research

Community characteristics provide a socioeconomic and demographic profile of the people in the community. Such a profile usually includes total population, age, race, ethnicity, household structure, educational attainment, employment status, occupation, income, and poverty status. Demographic and socioeconomic data such as these are some of the easiest to collect because they are assembled by federal, state, or county agencies. Because these data have been systematically collected, they are almost always reliable and valid. Most are available on the Internet, in the local public library, or from the state or county agency. Relying on existing information for the community profile is the least expensive way to gather statistics and provides consistent data that can be used easily for comparative purposes. Any additional types of data that may be available may also be illustrative. For example, the ability to discern if households with occupants over 65 years of age tend to be clustered in one area may provide insight into needed public transportation routes (Box 10.7).

BOX 10.7   COMPONENTS OF A DEMOGRAPHIC PROFILE OF A COMMUNITY

Total Population ___
Gender
Number of people   Male ___ Female ___ Other/No Response ___
Household Structure
Total number of households ___   Persons per household ___
Family Households (*number of households*) ___
Number of married-couple families ___
Number of single-parent families with a male head of household ___
Number of single-parent families with a female head of household ___
Nonfamily Households (*total number*) ___
Number of people who live alone ___
Number of people in households who are ≥65 years ___
(Depending on numbers, consider subset by gender/location)
Race/ethnicity
Number of people

| White ___ | Asian/Pacific Islander ___ | Hispanic origin (of any race) ___ |
| American Indian ___ | African American ___ | Other ___ |

Age (in years)
Number of people

<5	18–21	36–49	65–74
5–12	22–25	50–54	75–84
13–17	26–35	55–64	≥85

Median Household Income ___
Poverty Status
Number of people of all ages below poverty level ___
Number of related children <18 years of age in poverty ___
Number of related children ages 5 to 17 years in families in poverty ___
(If enough data, consider subset by location)
Employment Status
Number of people ≥16 years of age

| In labor force ___ | Civilian ___ | Not employed ___ |
| In armed forces ___ | Employed ___ | Not in labor force ___ |

(If enough data, consider additional age brackets)

The Washington State Community Nutrition Education Project website provides health statistics, nutrition program data, and community resources (see http://depts.washington.edu/commnutr/assess/dsource-tables.htm).

Collect Data

Data collection is vital to the assessment process. Evaluation of results must be based on accurate and reliable information. When selecting data sources or developing questions for surveys, bear in mind the goals of the assessment. Not all data that can be gathered will be pertinent to a particular assessment; conversely, it is important not to overlook useful data sources or replicate research.

These data collection methods are commonly used in community assessments:

- Surveys, questionnaires.
- Focus groups.
- Interviews (e.g., informal, semistructured, standardized open-ended, key informant, etc.).
- Community meetings, public hearings.
- Direct or participant observation.
- Document analysis.
- Photo documentation, photo novella, photovoice.
- Community asset/problem mapping.

Some of these methods are discussed in the following sections. Each has its strengths and weaknesses. Ultimately, the method used will depend on the assessment's particular goals and the resources available.

Focus Groups

Focus groups are an effective means of gaining additional insight into a community and for developing appropriate survey questions to be administered to a larger audience. One study conducted a series of focus groups involving specifically targeted segments within a multicultural community. Despite differences in ethnicity, age, and length of residence, community members voiced similar concerns about the advantages and difficulties of living in a multiethnic, multilingual neighborhood; about housing and other environmental issues; and about problems accessing healthcare. In addition, participation in the focus group increased participation in other community endeavors (Clark et al. 2003).

Members of each focus group should be fairly homogeneous and be familiar with the topic under discussion. A number of focus groups may need to be convened so that all subgroups within the defined community are represented. Focus groups are conducted by a trained facilitator.

Surveys, Questionnaires, and Observation

Surveys aid data gathering from larger numbers of people than possible through focus groups and thus help ensure representativeness. Survey responses are collected by interview, written response, or observation. Questions can be close-ended as in multiple choice, or scaled answers or open-ended, allowing the respondent or observer to answer freely.

The Food Store Survey provided in the USDA Community Food Security Assessment Toolkit (http://www.ers.usda.gov/media/327699/efan02013_1_.pdf) is an example of an observational survey. The observer can complete this survey at a store without direct contact with other people.

With training in data collection, many surveys can be administered by nonprofessional volunteers. Questionnaires used in nutritional assessment of individuals are generally, though not always, administered one-on-one by trained personnel and are thus more costly and more time-consuming. Nutritional assessment questionnaires include food diaries, 24-hour dietary recalls, FFQs, and diet histories (Box 10.8).

BOX 10.8   DIETARY COLLECTION AND ANALYSIS

There are a variety of techniques to assess dietary intake, each with their own strengths and weaknesses. All dietary assessment methods are limited and absolute validity is difficult to determine. It sometimes makes sense to collect dietary intake data, even if the information is flawed. Keep in mind that collection and assessment of dietary intake is burdensome to subjects and staff, and is very costly. Carefully consider how you will use the data and if they are really essential for your study.

- *Multiple-Day Food Diary.* Study participants are asked to measure or weigh everything they eat for a specified number of days. Subject burden is high, but food diaries are useful for motivating people in intervention studies and are considered the gold standard in dietary assessment. A quantitative assessment is possible with food diaries.
- *24-Hour Dietary Recall.* A retrospective detailed interview conducted by a registered dietitian to determine a subject's dietary intake from the preceding 24-hour period. The burden to the volunteer is low, but you must collect serial recalls to adequately characterize usual intake. A quantitative assessment is possible with 24-hour recalls.
- *Food Frequency Questionnaire.* Standardized forms inquiring about the frequency of intake of different foods or food groups. FFQs are not as accurate as other measures but are useful in large population studies or when studying the association of a specific food and a disease. Several validated questionnaires exist, and the most appropriate one will depend on your study. Some questionnaires can be scanned and quantitatively assessed.
- *Diet History.* An in-depth interview conducted by a registered dietitian to determine the volunteer's usual meal patterns and other details of dietary intake. Diet histories typically provide qualitative rather than quantitative information. The type of information collected can be tailored to meet the needs of your study.

Source: Adapted from the University of Vermont Clinical Research Center, Bionutrition Services. Nutrition Assessment. Available at http://www.uvm.edu/medicine/clinicalresearch/?Page=nutriassessment.html&SM=submenu1 .html, accessed February 11, 2015.

To the extent possible, communities need to be helped in identifying assessment methods that are comparable with other surveys (Byers et al. 1997). For example, when FFQs and food security questionnaires are used, asking the same questions as are used in national surveys can help make local survey results comparable with national data.

Profile Food Resource Availability, Accessibility, and Affordability

Sustained economic and social adversity in low-income neighborhoods may make it difficult for residents to obtain nutritious, affordable food. A community food resource assessment determines how well-equipped the community is to meet the food-related needs of its residents. A profile of all existing resources must be created to determine the adequacy of the extant community food resources, pinpoint possible barriers to food security, and increase access to nutritious food in the community.

Community food resources include retail food stores, farmers' markets, food cooperatives, and food assistance programs. Access to these resources depends on both their presence at reasonable distances from home and the ability to physically get to these resources using a private vehicle or public transportation. Four key areas are investigated in an assessment of food resource accessibility and food availability:

- Identifying retail stores and other places to purchase food in order to determine availability of authorized federal SNAP retailers; number, type, and location of retail food stores; number and location of consumer food cooperatives; and number and location of farmers' markets and community supported agriculture (CSA) associations.
- Identifying the number and location of schools that participate in the National School Lunch Program (NSLP) and School Breakfast Program (SBP); Child and Adult Care Food Program (CACFP) providers; Summer Food Service Program (SFSP) sites; WIC Farmers' Market Nutrition Program (FMNP) sites; and WIC clinics.
- Identifying the community's emergency food assistance providers, including the number, location, and times of operation of food banks, food pantries, emergency kitchens, and distribution sites for The Emergency Food Assistance Program (TEFAP), Commodity Supplemental Food Program (CSFP), and Food Distribution Program on Indian Reservations (FDPIR).
- Describing the rate of participation in federal food assistance programs: WIC, SNAP, NSLP and SBP, CACFP, SFSP, WIC FMNP, TEFAP, CSFP, FDPIR, and Nutrition Services Incentives Program (NSIP) (see Chapter 11 for a description of these programs).

Defining the spatial relationship between housing and food outlets is an important part of a community food assessment. Groups undertaking an assessment frequently prepare maps of the community to visualize the physical connection or disconnection between residents and various types of food sources. To illustrate, a series of maps for Eugene, Oregon, is available at http://www-personal.umich.edu/~copyrght/image/solstice/sum04/schlossberg/.

Measure Household Food Security

Accurate measurement of household food security can help public officials, policymakers, service providers, and community groups assess the need for assistance, judge the effectiveness of existing programs designed to help such households, and identify population subgroups with unusually low levels of food security (Box 10.9). One main question drives this assessment: is low household food security a problem directly or personally experienced by a significant number of people in the community?

One way to collect household food security data is to conduct a representative household food security survey, as described in the USDA's *Guide to Measuring Household Food Security, Revised 2000* (Bickel et al. 2000). The assessment is predicated on the Core Module, a measurement tool developed to gather data on household food security.

Current Population Survey Food Security Supplement and the Core Module

The Core Module has been used both in national surveys, such as the Current Population Survey-Food Security Supplement (CPS-FSS), and in community food security assessments conducted on the local level (Carlson et al. 1999). The module can form the basis for a sophisticated measurement of four levels of food security as experienced and reported by household members.

Local studies using either the 18-question Core Module or the standard abbreviated 6-item subset can document the level of food security in the community. Appendix 10.1 provides the 18-question Core Module, followed by the abbreviated 6-item subset and information on scoring.

The CPS-FSS is the source of national- and state-level statistics on food security used in the USDA's annual reports on household food security. The CPS is a monthly labor force survey of about 50,000 households conducted by the Census Bureau for the Bureau of Labor Statistics. Once each year, after answering the labor force questions, the same households are asked a series of questions (the Food Security Supplement) about food security, food expenditures, and use of food and

---

**BOX 10.9   DEFINITIONS OF FOOD SECURITY
AND HUNGER IN THE UNITED STATES**

In 2006, the USDA introduced new language to describe ranges of severity of food insecurity. Despite the new labels, the methods used to assess households' food security remained unchanged, so statistics for 2005 and later years are directly comparable with those for earlier years for the corresponding categories.

- High food security (*old label* = *Food security*): no reported indications of food-access problems or limitations.
- Marginal food security (*old label* = *Food security*): one or two reported indications—typically of anxiety over food sufficiency or shortage of food in the house; little or no indication of changes in diets or food intake.
- Low food security (*old label* = *food insecurity without hunger*): reports of reduced quality, variety, or desirability of diet; little or no indication of reduced food intake.
- Very low food security (*old label* = *food insecurity with hunger*): reports of multiple indications of disrupted eating patterns and reduced food intake.

The USDA also differentiates between low/very low food security and hunger.

- *Low/very low food security*: a household-level economic and social condition of limited or uncertain access to adequate food.
- *Hunger*: an individual-level physiological condition that may result from low/very low food security.

Source: US Department of Agriculture, Economic Research Service. Definitions of Food Security. Available at http://www.ers.usda.gov/topics/food-nutrition-assistance/food-security-in-the-us/definitions-of-food-security.aspx, accessed January 13, 2015.

---

nutrition assistance programs. Food security data have been collected by the CPS-FSS annually since 1995 (US Department of Agriculture, http://www.ers.usda.gov/data-products/food-security -in-the-united-states/documentation.aspx). The survey consists of questions about several general types of household food conditions, events, and behaviors. They include

- Anxiety that the household food budget or food supply may be insufficient to meet basic needs.
- Perceptions that the food eaten by household members is inadequate in quality or quantity.
- Reported instances of reduced food intake or consequences of reduced food intake (such as the physical sensation of hunger or reported weight loss) for adults in the household.
- Reported instances of reduced food intake or its consequences for children in the household.

When used to collect data on a periodic basis, the questionnaire can provide systematic monitoring of the community's progress in addressing food security needs in the community.

Assessment of Food Production Resources

A community's agricultural system can boost the effectiveness of federal food assistance and education programs. Local agriculture can play a role in community food security when implemented together with a strong federal nutrition safety net and emergency food assistance programs. This can increase the availability of high-quality, affordable food within a community, offering small farmers an opportunity to maintain economic viability by supplying the local market with fresh foods, strengthening economic and social ties between farms and urban residents, and channeling a larger share of residents' food spending back into the local economy. Several key questions might be asked in an assessment of food production resources:

- Does the community have food production or food distribution resources? Who is served by these resources?
- Do low-income households have the opportunity to participate in community gardens or other food production activities?
- Are there any school-based gardening programs?
- Are locally produced foods sold through local food retailers and restaurants?
- Does the local school district purchase foods from local producers?
- Are locally produced foods used by other institutional food service outlets, such as colleges, prisons, and hospitals?

Securing Funding and Developing Budgets

Unfortunately, the scope and scale of an assessment is often determined by the available budget. Although volunteers and in-kind resources can reduce the actual cash outlay needed to conduct an assessment, some expenses must be met directly. Below are some assessment expenses to consider:

- Site and refreshments for meetings.
- Reimbursement for participation in community outreach.
- Support staff.
- Research personnel.
- Office space, phones, photocopying.
- Fund-raising.
- Printed materials such as flyers and survey forms.

Funding for community assessments may be difficult to obtain at the federal level, although the USDA Community Food Projects Competitive Grants Program (CFPCGP) has funded some projects. Community development block grants and SNAP education (SNAP-Ed) funds might prove a fruitful source. Locally, government agencies dedicated to nutrition, health, or community development, for example, may provide some assistance. Community and other private foundations, if you frame your assessment goals to match their interests, may also help with funding. Chapter 14 offers help in writing grants for funding.

Analyze and Present Data

Analysis of data is both quantitative (such as demographic data) and qualitative (from interviews and focus groups). In addition, the approach used depends on the assessment's goals, whether to compare your community to national data or to develop an action plan to improve food access. Presenting these data to stakeholders, policymakers, and the general public is integral to the assessment process.

The presentation should be easy to understand, with graphic displays such as maps and tables used whenever possible to clarify and amplify narrative presentations. Table 10.2 provides the demographic profile of Power County, ID and that of the state as a whole, courtesy of the US Census. Figure 10.1 plots the location of food markets on a map of Eugene, Oregon.

An assessment report that incorporates the data analysis can assume many identities other than that of a written report: a series of newsletter articles, a media or policy brief, a research or professional paper, resource guides or databases, a community presentation, or a study guide. Regardless

TABLE 10.2

Demographic Profile of Power County, Idaho, and Idaho State

People Quick Facts	Power County	Idaho
Population, 2013 estimate	7719	1,612,843
Population, percent change, April 1, 2010 to July 1, 2013	−1.3%	2.9%
Population, 2010	7817	1,567,582
Persons under 5 years old, percent, 2013	9.7%	7.0%
Persons under 18 years old, percent, 2013	30.5%	26.5%
Persons 65 years old and over, percent, 2013	13.4%	13.8%
Female persons, percent, 2013	49.0%	49.9%
White persons, percent, 2013[a]	93.4%	93.7%
Black persons, percent, 2013[a]	1.0%	0.8%
American Indian and Alaska Native persons, percent, 2013[a]	2.9%	1.7%
Asian persons, percent, 2013[a]	0.5%	1.4%
Native Hawaiian and other Pacific Islander, percent, 2013[a]	0.2%	0.2%
Persons reporting two or more races, percent, 2013	2.1%	2.2%
Persons of Hispanic or Latino origin, percent, 2013[b]	31.2%	11.8%
White persons, not Hispanic, percent, 2013	64.6%	83.1%
Living in same house 1 year and over, percent, 2009–2013	89.8%	82.8%
Foreign-born persons, percent, 2009–2013	13.4%	5.9%
Language other than English spoken at home, percentage 5+, 2009–2013	26.9%	10.4%
High school graduate, percent of persons age 25+, 2009–2013	80.3%	88.8%
Bachelor's degree, percent of persons age 25+, 2009–2013	15.9%	25.1%
Veterans, 2009–2013	478	122,955
Mean travel time to work (minutes), workers age 16+, 2009–2013	17.3	20.0
Housing units, 2013	2916	676,192
Homeownership rate, 2009–2013	70.8%	69.8%
Housing units in multi-unit structures, percent, 2009–2013	5.0%	14.9%
Median value of owner-occupied housing units, 2009–2013	$125,600	$162,100
Households, 2009–2013	2568	579,797
Persons per household, 2009–2013	2.99	2.68
Per capita money income in the past 12 months (2013 dollars), 2009–2013	$17,684	$22,568
Median household income, 2009–2013	$44,212	$46,767
Persons below poverty level, percent, 2009–2013	13.9%	15.5%

Source: US Census Bureau. State & County Quick Facts: Power County, Idaho. Last revised February 5, 2015. Available at http://quickfacts.census.gov/qfd/states/16/16077.html, accessed February 11, 2015.

[a] Includes persons reporting only one race.

[b] Hispanics may be of any race, so also are included in applicable race categories.

of the form the report takes, it should include an overview of the community and its food system (if applicable), a description of your assessment process, highlights and discussion of key findings, and recommendations for change.

Implement Findings

Of course, the ultimate purpose of an assessment is to make positive change. However, once an assessment is complete, the same general process, although focused on change, called for by the assessment, will need to be repeated. Types of action may include, for example, community mobilization through door-to-door canvassing, community education through media coverage or bilingual

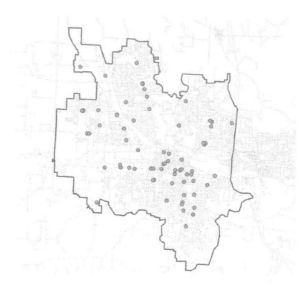

FIGURE 10.1   Access to food outlets in Eugene, Oregon. (Reproduced from Schlossberg M. Visualizing Accessibility II: Access to Food. Available at http://www-personal.umich.edu/~copyrght/image/solstice /sum04/schlossberg/, accessed April 22, 2013. With permission.)

brochures, program or activity development, and public policy advocacy. A recent, innovative instrument for advocacy is the food policy council (Box 10.10).

GEOGRAPHIC INFORMATION SYSTEMS

GIS is a computerized system for the storage, retrieval, manipulation, analysis, and display of geographically referenced data (Box 10.11). This technology provides a useful way to map and display spatial and temporal relationships. Geomapping is a valuable tool for conducting needs assessments, targeting specific populations for outreach, and examining program outcomes. GIS is used by many federal agencies, including the US Departments of Agriculture (USDA), Commerce, Education, Health and Human Services, Housing and Urban Development, Interior, Transportation, Veterans Affairs, and others (*Mapping the Nation* 2012). As one example, the USDA (http://www.ers.usda.gov /data-products.aspx#.UYur6oLLep4) provides access to several mapping programs, including

- Atlas of Rural and Small-Town America: maps county-level data on people, jobs, agriculture, and county classifications.
- Farm Program Atlas: provides access to county-level data on federal farm programs.
- Food Access Research Atlas: allows mapping of multiple indicators of food store access, such as supermarket accessibility and vehicle access, at the census tract level.
- Food Environment Atlas: maps county-level indicators that help determine and reflect a community's access to affordable, healthy food.
- SNAP Data System: provides data on state- and county-level estimates of SNAP participation and benefits, as well as sociodemographic characteristics of the population.

As GIS can include physical, biological, cultural, demographic, or economic information, it is a valuable tool in the natural, social, medical, and engineering sciences as well as in business and planning. Researchers, public health professionals, policymakers, and others use GIS to better understand geographic relationships that affect health outcomes, public health risks, disease transmission, access to healthcare, and other public health concerns. For example, the CDC uses GIS to

BOX 10.10   FOOD POLICY COUNCIL

A food policy council is a group of food system stakeholders who advise a city, county, or state government, as well as residents, on policies and programs related to agriculture, food distribution, hunger, food access, and nutrition. Most governments take actions that affect their local food system, such as zoning laws that affect grocery store placement and school nutrition policies. Yet these policies are often fragmented, and the negative health, social, environmental, and economic impacts of the food system are typically addressed in a piecemeal fashion. Food policy councils exist to examine these issues in a more holistic fashion, bringing together diverse stakeholders to collaboratively obtain previously unknown information about the food system and develop projects and policies to improve it. Current councils serve as advisory commissions to state and city governments, within departments of health, and as nonprofit organizations. Members may be formally appointed by the council or by government officials, or selected from an application process. Members may also be informally chosen through a self-selection process. Food policy councils are typically composed of community residents and representatives from the five food sectors: production, processing, distribution, consumption, and waste management. Increasingly, food policy councils have also reached out to community partners in the private and public sectors, such as urban and regional planners. These diverse coalitions often must educate themselves about their members' specialties and overcome their stereotypes in order to be effective.

Food policy councils address a variety of issues, and they are often created in response to a pressing need. Several main objectives of a food policy council are to

- Advocate for policy change to improve a community's food system.
- Develop programs that address gaps in a community's food system.
- Research and analyze the existing conditions of a community's food system.
- Communicate information about a community's food system.
- Foster partnerships among a community's five food sectors.

Food policy councils perform a variety of tasks, from researching food production, food access, and nutrition in their area to designing and implementing projects and policies to address those issues. One common issue many food policy councils face is how to increase residents' access to grocery stores. Food policy councils will examine the interrelated causes of the problem by considering such things as infrastructure (e.g., availability and adequacy of public transportation to existing grocery stores), economic development (e.g., existence of banks that will loan money to new grocery stores), built environment (e.g., identification of zoning codes or regulations that could be changed to allow grocery stores closer to residential areas), and alternatives or supplemental programs (e.g., ability of a farmers' market or home delivered meals program to fill service gaps). Additional examples include

- Conducting food system assessments and land-use inventories.
- Drafting backyard beekeeping or chicken ordinances.
- Researching local produce purchasing programs for detention centers.
- Identifying outdated land-use regulations or restrictive zoning codes.
- Finding applicable funding sources for food system programs, such as the Community Development Block Grant (CDBG) funds.
- Educating the public and policymakers about food, nutrition, hunger, and agricultural issues through discussion groups, position papers, and public meetings.

Source: DiLisio C and Hodgson K. *Food Policy Councils: Helping Local, Regional, and State Governments Address Food System Challenges.* Food system planning briefing paper. Chicago: American Planning Association; 2011. Available at http://ucanr.edu/sites/MarinFoodPolicyCouncil/files/178441.pdf, accessed January 20, 2015.

BOX 10.11   GEOGRAPHIC INFORMATION SYSTEMS (GIS) DEFINITIONS

Geocode—A code that represents the spatial characteristics of an *entity*, for example, a *coordinate point* or a *postcode*. A geocode may be a 5- or a 9-digit zip code, area code, county, state, or health-service area; census block or tract, global positioning system (GPS) reading; or a set of longitudinal–latitudinal coordinates.

Geocoding—The cross-referencing between specifically recorded x,y-coordinates of a location, relative to a standard reference grid such as the US National Grid, and nongeographic data such as addresses or postcodes. In this way, the accessing of the nongeographic data allows locations to be accurately mapped. Geocoding refers to collecting information to enable GIS presentation of data.

Georeference—To establish the relationship between page coordinates on a planar map and known real-world coordinates. Georeferenced data can be tied to a specific location or place, such as an area code, street address, or other census and political boundaries.

Source: Sommer S and Wade T, eds. *A to Z GIS: An Illustrated Dictionary of Geographic Information Systems.* Redlands, CA: ESRI Press, 2006.

provide maps and data on public health issues in the US, including heart disease, stroke, tobacco use in youth, and injury-related mortality. A list of CDC GIS web applications can be found at http://www.cdc.gov/gis/applications.htm (Box 10.12).

Although a young field that began in the 1960s, the antecedents of GIS go back hundreds of years in the fields of cartography and mapping. The history of GIS parallels that of computation in general, with mapping and geographic studies being early beneficiaries of the increasing power of computers (Ricketts 2003). In 2003, the US National Library of Medicine (NLM) added the term *geographic information systems* to its controlled vocabulary thesaurus known as MeSH (medical

BOX 10.12   SELECTED SOURCES OF INTERNATIONAL, NATIONAL, AND STATE GEOGRAPHIC INFORMATION SYSTEM (GIS) MAPS AND RESOURCES

- The University of Colorado, Boulder provides links to international, national, state, and regional (within Colorado) GIS maps and resources: http://ucblibraries.colorado.edu/map/links/gis.htm.
- Geo.Data.gov provides access to over 400,000 maps, datasets, and services from 172 agencies across the federal government: http://geo.data.gov.
- Esri, a GIS software and services company, provides access to US maps and commonly used nationwide map layers from various federal data sources: http://govmaps.org.
- The University of Maryland provides links to GIS maps and resources for several US government agencies and by state, as well as links to GIS organizations, portals, software, map servers, and other software and applications: http://lib.guides.umd.edu/content.php?pid=130101&sid=1115901.
- Links to GIS maps and resources by state are available through many institutions of higher education, including The University of Oregon (http://library.uoregon.edu/map/map_section/map_Statedatasets.html) and The University of Arkansas (http://libinfo.uark.edu/GIS/us.asp).

subject headings), reflecting the importance and growing use of GIS in health and healthcare research and practice (Boulos 2004).

Today, GIS is a multibillion dollar-per-year high technology industry. Worldwide spending on GIS software in 2004 was $1.8 billion, of which $544 million was spent by US federal, state, and local government agencies (Welsh 2005). By 2017, it is projected that the electric utility industry alone will spend $3.7 billion on GIS services, software, and tools (Box 10.12) (Pike Research 2012).

The geographic data in a GIS consist of a series of map layers that contain information about features located in specific locations. GIS links multiple sets of geospatial data and graphically displays that information as maps, with potentially many different layers of information. Assuming that all the information is at the same scale and has been formatted according to the same standards, users can overlay spatial information about any number of specific topics to examine how the layers interrelate. Each layer of a GIS map represents a particular *theme* or feature, and one layer could be derived from a data source completely different from the other layers.

As illustrated in Figure 10.2, one layer or *theme* could represent all the streets in a specified area. Another could correspond to all the buildings in the same area, and others could show vegetation or water resources. Additional themes could be census tract boundaries with sociodemographic variables collected by the US Census, WIC clinic locations and associated information, such as hours of operation or capacity, or ZIP code boundaries with data on low-birth-weight or Medicaid-eligible populations. As long as standard processes and formats have been arranged to facilitate integration, each of these themes could be based on data originally collected and maintained by a separate organization.

Analyzing this layered information as an integrated whole can significantly aid decision makers in considering complex choices, such as where to locate a WIC center to best serve the greatest number of eligible people (Koontz 2003). Table 10.3 describes the data themes for the lead agencies that engage in nutrition-related mapping activities.

Use of geocoding in health data systems provides the basis for cost-effective disease surveillance and intervention. A 2012 US Department of the Interior report estimated that the federal government spends billions of dollars annually to collect, maintain, and use geospatial information, yet

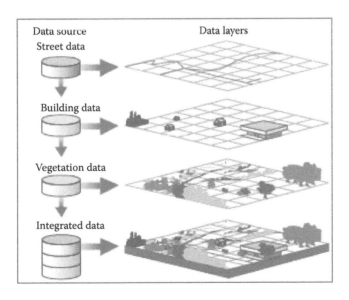

FIGURE 10.2 GIS layers or themes. (Reproduced from Figure 1 Visual Representation of Themes in a GIS, in *Geospatial Information: OMB and Agencies Need to Make Coordination a Priority to Reduce Duplication.* GAO-13-94. November 2012. Available at http://www.gao.gov/assets/660/650293.pdf, accessed February 1, 2015.)

TABLE 10.3

Data Themes, Descriptions, and Lead Federal Agencies for Food and Nutrition-Related Mapping Activities

Data Theme	Lead Agency	Description
Governmental units	Department of Commerce/ US Census Bureau	These data describe the official boundary of federal, state, local, and tribal governments as reported to the Census Bureau for purposes of reporting the nation's official statistics.
Geographic data	Department of Housing and Urban Development	Geographic data on homeownership rates, location of various forms of housing assistance, underserved areas, and race.
Public health	Department of Health and Human Services	Public health themes relate to the protection, improvement, and promotion of the health and safety of all people. For example, public health databases include spatial data on deaths and births, infectious and notifiable diseases, incident cancer cases, behavioral risk factor and tuberculosis surveillance, hazardous substance releases, and health effects, hospital statistics, and similar data.
Buildings and facilities	General Services Administration	Includes federal sites or entities with a geospatial location deliberately established for designated activities; a facility database might describe a factory, military base, college, hospital, power plant, fishery, national park, office building, space command center, or prison.
Transportation	Department of Transportation	Transportation data are used to model the geographic locations, interconnectedness, and characteristics of the transportation system within the United States. The transportation system includes both physical and nonphysical components representing all modes of travel that allow the movement of goods and people between locations.

Source: Adapted from Table 4 OMB Circular A-16 Data Themes, Descriptions, and Lead Agencies, in *Geospacial Information: Better Coordination Needed to Identify and Reduce Duplicative Investments.* GAO-04-703. June 2004. Available at http://www.gao.gov/new.items/d04703.pdf, accessed February 11, 2015.

duplication is common and millions of dollars are wasted as a result. Understanding the importance of geospatial information in the decision making and support of many governmental functions, the US Government Accountability Office (GAO) recommends improved coordination and reduced duplication through the development of a national strategy for coordinating geospatial investments (Geospatial Information 2012).

Examples of GIS in Food and Nutrition Programs

A community assessment project in Hinds County, Mississippi used GIS to select survey centers for a target population, evaluate sample representation, and perform a geography-based community health assessment. Survey centers focused on either a general population or a specific group within the population. Potential survey centers (such as local grocery stores or large discount stores) were overlaid on block groups to verify their location as a center. Only after the center for a target population had been identified were in-person surveys conducted. Geographic representation involved address geocoding of participants' residences and analysis of the geographic distribution samples in relation to the selected survey centers, demographics, and economic characteristics of the county. Finally, maps were created to depict the geographic distribution of variables such as health status, healthcare access, availability of transportation, and types of healthcare facilities available (Faruque et al. 2003).

The authors of the study concluded that traditional methods of surveying may disproportionately collect samples from a few, nonrepresentative areas, whereas using GIS to determine survey centers results in better representation of the study center, as long as the GIS infrastructure is available (Faruque et al. 2003).

CONCLUSION

Conducting a community assessment, whether it focuses on nutritional status, food access, or food security, involves a tremendous commitment of time, energy, and resources, yet there is significant payback in terms of heightened understanding of the assets and barriers that exist within a community. It is important to approach an assessment with clearly defined goals, to seek active participation from the diverse groups within the community, and to plan to create positive change.

Numerous tools are available to collect, analyze, and present data; however, the tools selected depend on the goals of the assessment as well as available funding. Most significantly, the information and knowledge attained through an assessment are only as useful as the change they impel.

ACRONYMS

AND　　　Academy of Nutrition and Dietetics
APIE　　　Assessment, Planning, Implementation, Evaluation
CACFP　　Child and Adult Care Food Program
CDBG　　Community Development Block Grant
CDC　　　Centers for Disease Control and Prevention
CFPCGP　Community Food Projects Competitive Grants Program
CHANGE　Community Health Assessment and Group Evaluation
CPS-FSS　Current Population Survey–Food Security Supplement
CSA　　　Community supported agriculture
CSFP　　Commodity Supplemental Food Program
EBT　　　Electronic Benefit Transfer
FDPIR　　Food Distribution Program on Indian Reservations
FFQ　　　Food frequency questionnaire
FMNP　　Farmers' Market Nutrition Program
GAO　　　United States Government Accountability Office
GIS　　　Geographic Information System
GPS　　　Global Positioning System
MeSH　　Medical Subject Headings
NLM　　　National Library of Medicine
NSIP　　Nutrition Services Incentive Program
NSLP　　National School Lunch Program
NSP　　　Nutrition Surveillance Program
NYSDOH　New York State Department of Health
SBP　　　School Breakfast Program
SFSP　　Summer Food Service Program
SNAP　　Supplemental Nutrition Assistance Program
SNAP-Ed　Supplemental Nutrition Assistance Program Education

TEFAP   The Emergency Food Assistance Program
USDA   United States Department of Agriculture
VISTA   Volunteers in Service to America
WIC   Special Supplemental Program for Women, Infants, and Children

STUDENT ASSIGNMENTS AND ACTIVITIES DESIGNED TO ENHANCE LEARNING AND STIMULATE CRITICAL THINKING

1. Describe how a community food assessment would be beneficial to have on hand in the event of an emergency.
2. You have been invited to talk to members of your local school's Parent Teacher Association (PTA). You would like to ask the PTA members what they think about school foods on campus, and if the students are allowed off campus, food in the immediate environment that might be patronized by the students. Which method would you choose: focus groups or questionnaires? Justify your answer, including the strengths and weaknesses of each method.
3. Search for a community nutrition assessment, community food assessment, or a community food security assessment of your hometown. If one is not available, look at neighboring towns, the county, or the state. Summarize the assessment in terms of the following:
   • Who initiated and performed the assessment, and why?
   • When was the assessment performed?
   • What type of assessment was performed (i.e., nutrition, food, or food security)?
   • What information was sought, and how was it obtained?
   • What were the findings?
   • What recommendations were made? Have any of these recommendations been implemented? If so, which one(s)?
4. Using the Appendix to the chapter, administer both the full (18-item) and abbreviated (6-item) US Household Food Security Survey to three individuals of different decades (e.g., one person each in their 20s, 40s, and 60s.) In order to maintain anonymity, label surveys with initials only—do not use full names. Score each survey. You should have a total of six scores, two per person—one for the full survey and one for the short form. Answer the following questions:
   • For each individual, do the two surveys indicate the same level of food security? If not, why might that be? What implications would this have for large surveys using only the short form?
   • Using the scoring method, describe the food security status for each individual you surveyed. Discuss differences by age, if any.
   • Describe your experience in administering and scoring these surveys, including answers to the following: Did the individual easily understand the questions, or did s/he ask for clarification? Did you find the instructions clear? Why or why not? Was the scoring easy or difficult? Why? How might the survey be modified to make it easier to understand, administer, and/or score?
5. You have been asked to initiate a community nutrition assessment in the county where you currently live. As you begin, the following questions need to be answered:
   • Who will you recruit for your assessment team?
   • How will you define your community?
   • Based on this definition, conduct a search for demographics on your community. See the text for sample demographic information to collect.
   • What other data/information will you need to include in the assessment? How will you obtain this information? Which methods will you use?
6. Using a county of your choice, first perform a web-based assessment of food resource availability, accessibility, and affordability by choosing one of the four key areas listed in the

section, Food Resource Availability, Accessibility, and Affordability. Then, use the USDA Food Environment Atlas (http://www.ers.usda.gov/data-products/food-environment-atlas/go-to-the-atlas.aspx#.UZDpF4LLep4) to create a set of maps showing relevant county-level data. Answer the following questions:

- How does the information you gathered from the web-based assessment compare to the maps you generated from the USDA Food Environment Atlas? Are the maps consistent with the data you gathered, or are there inconsistencies? Which method of data presentation do you prefer (lists vs. maps), and why?
- Looking at the maps, how does your county compare to surrounding counties on the various measures you chose?
- Based on this partial assessment, list three recommendations you might make to improve food resource availability, accessibility, and/or affordability in your county.

7. Answer the six questions listed in the section, Assessment of Food Production Resources, with regard to your current residential county.
- Does the community have food production or food distribution resources? Who is served by these resources?
- Do low-income households have the opportunity to participate in community gardens or other food production activities?
- Are there any school-based gardening programs?
- Are locally produced foods sold through local food retailers and restaurants?
- Does the local school district purchase foods from local producers?
- Are locally produced foods used by other institutional food service outlets, such as colleges, prisons, and hospitals?

8. Visit one of the following local programs and volunteer for two hours during mealtime:

Adult Day Care Program	Food Pantry	Jail/Prison
Church Kitchen	Head Start Program	School
Family Resource Center	Homeless Shelter	Soup Kitchen

Describe your experience. Include in your description the following information:
- Name and address of the program, type of program, and date and time of your visit.
- What is the purpose (mission, goals, objectives) of the program?
- Describe the population served by the program.
- How many people were served while you were on-site?
- How long did it take for everyone to be served?
- List the foods and beverages that were available. Were most or all food groups represented?
- Did participants have food options to choose from? If so, what were the options?
- Were options available for those with dietary or religious restrictions? Provide examples.
- If foods were prepared, how were they prepared (e.g., raw, baked, grilled, fried, etc.)?
- Was there enough food for everyone?
- How was the food served (e.g., self-service, table service, family style, buffet, etc.)?
- Were the participants charged for food? If so, how much?
- Was the staff friendly? Why or why not?
- Was the facility clean? If not, provide examples.
- Did food servers wear hairnets/caps and wash their hands before serving and/or wear gloves?
- How would you rate the overall quality of the program in terms of its efficiency, customer service, nutritional quality, food safety, and ability to meet its mission or purpose?

APPENDIX 10.1 US HOUSEHOLD FOOD SECURITY SURVEY MODULE, SHORT FORM SURVEY, AND CODING RESPONSE

HOUSEHOLD FOOD SECURITY SURVEY MODULE

Questionnaire Transition into Module (Administered to all households):
These next questions are about the food eaten in your household in the last 12 months, since (current month) of last year and whether you were able to afford the food you need.
Optional USDA Food Sufficiency Question/Screener: Question HHI (This question is optional. It is not used to calculate any of the food security scales. It may be used in conjunction with income as a preliminary screener to reduce respondent burden for high income households.)

HH1. Which of these statements best describes the food eaten in your household in the last 12 months:
- Enough of the kinds of food (I/we) want to eat;
- Enough, but not always the <u>kinds</u> of food (I/we) want;
- Sometimes <u>not enough</u> to eat; or,
- <u>Often</u> not enough to eat?
  [1] Enough of the kinds of food we want to eat
  [2] Enough but not always the kinds of food we want
  [3] Sometimes not enough to eat
  [4] Often not enough
  [ ] Don't Know or Refused

Household Stage 1: Questions HH2–HH4 (asked of all households; begin scale items)

HH2. Now I'm going to read you several statements that people have made about their food situation. For these statements, please tell me whether the statement was <u>often</u> true, <u>sometimes</u> true, or <u>never</u> true for (you/your household) in the last 12 months—that is, since last (name of current month).
The first statement is "(I/We) worried whether (my/our) food would run out before (I/we) got money to buy more." Was that <u>often</u> true, <u>sometimes</u> true, or <u>never</u> true for (you/your household) in the last 12 months?
[ ] Often true [ ] Sometimes true [ ] Never true [ ] Don't know or Refused
HH3. "The food that (I/we) bought just didn't last, and (I/we) didn't have money to get more." Was that <u>often</u>, <u>sometimes</u>, or <u>never</u> true for (you/your household) in the last 12 months?
[ ] Often true [ ] Sometimes true [ ] Never true [ ] Don't Know or Refused
HH4. "(I/we) couldn't afford to eat balanced meals." Was that <u>often</u>, <u>sometimes</u>, or <u>never</u> true for (you/your household) in the last 12 months?
[ ] Often true [ ] Sometimes true [ ] Never true [ ] Don't Know or Refused

Screener for Stage 2 Adult-Referenced Questions: If affirmative response (i.e., "often true" or "sometimes true") to one or more of Questions HH2–HH4, OR, response [3] or [4] to question HH1 (if administered), then continue to *Adult Stage 2*; otherwise, if children under age 18 are present in the household, skip to *Child Stage 1*, otherwise skip to *End of Food Security Module.*
Adult Stage 2: Questions AD1–AD4 (asked of households passing the screener for Stage 2 adult-referenced questions).

AD1. In the last 12 months, since last (name of current month), did (you/you or other adults in your household) ever cut the size of your meals or skip meals because there wasn't enough money for food?
[ ] Yes [ ] No (Skip AD1a) [ ] Don't Know (Skip AD1a)

AD1a. [IF YES ABOVE, ASK] How often did this happen—almost every month, some months but not every month, or in only 1 or 2 months?
[ ] Almost every month [ ] Some months but not every month [ ] Only 1 or 2 months
[ ] Don't Know
AD2. In the last 12 months, did you ever eat less than you felt you should because there wasn't enough money for food?
[ ] Yes [ ] No [ ] Don't Know
AD3. In the last 12 months, were you ever hungry but didn't eat because there wasn't enough money for food?
[ ] Yes [ ] No [ ] Don't Know
AD4. In the last 12 months, did you lose weight because there wasn't enough money for food?
[ ] Yes [ ] No [ ] Don't Know

Screener for Stage 3 Adult-Referenced Questions: If affirmative response to one or more of questions AD1 through AD4, then continue to *Adult Stage 3*; otherwise, if children under age 18 are present in the household, skip to *Child Stage 1*; otherwise skip to *End of Food Security Module.*
Adult Stage 3: Questions AD5–AD5a (asked of households passing screener for Stage 3 adult-referenced questions).

AD5. In the last 12 months, did (you/you or other adults in your household) ever not eat for a whole day because there wasn't enough money for food?
[ ] Yes [ ] No (Skip AD5a) [ ] Don't Know (Skip AD5a)
AD5a. [IF YES ABOVE, ASK] How often did this happen—almost every month, some months but not every month, or in only 1 or 2 months?
[ ] Almost every month [ ] Some months but not every month [ ] Only 1 or 2 months
[ ] Don't Know

Child Stage 1: Questions CH1–CH3 (Transitions and questions CH1 and CH2 are administered to all households with children under age 18) Households with no child under age 18, skip to *End of Food Security Module.*
Transition into Child-Referenced Questions:
Now I'm going to read you several statements that people have made about the food situation of their children. For these statements, please tell me whether the statement was OFTEN true, SOMETIMES true, or NEVER true in the last 12 months for (your child/children living in the household who are under 18 years old).

CH1. "(I/we) relied on only a few kinds of low-cost food to feed (my/our) child/the children) because (I was/we were) running out of money to buy food." Was that often, sometimes, or never true for (you/your household) in the last 12 months?
[ ] Often true [ ] Sometimes true [ ] Never true [ ] Don't Know or Refused
CH2. "(I/We) couldn't feed (my/our) child/the children) a balanced meal, because (I/we) couldn't afford that." Was that often, sometimes, or never true for (you/your household) in the last 12 months?
[ ] Often true [ ] Sometimes true [ ] Never true [ ] Don't Know or Refused
CH3. "(My/Our child was/The children were) not eating enough because (I/we) just couldn't afford enough food." Was that often, sometimes, or never true for (you/your household) in the last 12 months?
[ ] Often true [ ] Sometimes true [ ] Never true [ ] Don't Know or Refused

Screener for Stage 2 Child Referenced Questions: If affirmative response (i.e., "often true" or "sometimes true") to one or more of questions CH1–CH3, then continue to *Child Stage 2*; otherwise skip to *End of Food Security Module.*

Child Stage 2: Questions CH4–CH7 (asked of households passing the screener for stage 2 child-referenced questions).

> CH4. In the last 12 months, since (current month) of last year, did you ever cut the size of (your child's/any of the children's) meals because there wasn't enough money for food?
> [ ] Yes [ ] No [ ] Don't Know
>
> CH5. In the last 12 months, did (CHILD'S NAME/any of the children) ever skip meals because there wasn't enough money for food?
> [ ] Yes [ ] No (Skip CH5a) [ ] Don't Know (Skip CH5a)
>
> CH5a. [IF YES ABOVE ASK] How often did this happen—almost every month, some months but not every month, or in only 1 or 2 months?
> [ ] Almost every month [ ] Some months but not every month [ ] Only 1 or 2 months
> [ ] Don't Know
>
> CH6. In the last 12 months, (was your child/were the children) ever hungry but you just couldn't afford more food?
> [ ] Yes [ ] No [ ] Don't Know
>
> CH7. In the last 12 months, did (your child/any of the children) ever not eat for a whole day because there wasn't enough money for food?
> [ ] Yes [ ] No [ ] Don't Know

End of Food Security Module

Source: US Department of Agriculture, Economic Research Service. *U.S. Household Food Security Survey Module: Three-Stage Design, With Screeners.* September 2012. Available at http://www.ers.usda.gov/data-products/food-security-in-the-united-states/data-files/food-security-survey-modules/household.aspx, accessed January 15, 2015.

Short Form of the Food Security Survey Module

For surveys that cannot implement the 18-question module above, this "Short Form" 6-item scale provides a reasonably reliable substitute. It uses a subset of the standard 18 items.

Transition into Module:

These next questions are about the food eaten in your household in the last 12 months, since (current month) of last year and whether you were able to afford the food you need.

> HH3. I'm going to read you several statements that people have made about their food situation. For these statements, please tell me whether the statement was <u>often</u> true, <u>sometimes</u> true, or <u>never</u> true for (you/your household) in the last 12 months—that is, since last (name of current month).
> The first statement is, "The food that (I/we) bought just didn't last, and (I/we) didn't have money to get more." Was that <u>often</u>, <u>sometimes</u>, or <u>never</u> true for (you/your household) in the last 12 months?
> [ ] Often true [ ] Sometimes true [ ] Never true [ ] Don't Know or Refused
>
> HH4. "(I/we) couldn't afford to eat balanced meals." Was that <u>often</u>, <u>sometimes</u>, or <u>never</u> true for (you/your household) in the last 12 months?
> [ ] Often true [ ] Sometimes true [ ] Never true [ ] Don't Know or Refused
>
> AD1. In the last 12 months, since last (name of current month), did (you/you or other adults in your household) ever cut the size of your meals or skip meals because there wasn't enough money for food?
> [ ] Yes [ ] No (Skip AD1a) [ ] Don't Know (Skip AD1a)

AD1a. [IF YES ABOVE, ASK] How often did this happen—almost every month, some months but not every month, or in only 1 or 2 months?
[ ] Almost every month [ ] Some months but not every month [ ] Only 1 or 2 months
[ ] Don't Know

AD2. In the last 12 months, did you ever eat less than you felt you should because there wasn't enough money for food?
[ ] Yes [ ] No [ ] Don't Know

AD3. In the last 12 months, were you ever hungry but didn't eat because there wasn't enough money for food?
[ ] Yes [ ] No [ ] Don't Know

Source: US Department of Agriculture, Economic Research Service. *U.S. Household Food Security Survey Module: Six-Item Short Form.* September 2012. Available at http://www.ers.usda.gov/data -products/food-security-in-the-united-states/data-files/food-security-survey-modules/short.aspx, accessed January 12, 2015.

Coding Responses and Assessing Household Food Security Status from the US Household Food Security Survey Module and Short Form

Responses of "yes," "often," "sometimes," "almost every month," and "some months but not every month" are coded as affirmative. The sum of affirmative responses to a specified set of items is referred to as the household's raw score on the scale comprising those items. Households with high or marginal food security are classified as food secure. Those with low or very low food security are classified as food insecure.

For the full US Household Food Security Survey Module[1]:

- Questions HH2 through CH7 comprise the US Household Food Security Scale (questions HH2 through AD5a for households with no child present). Specification of food security status depends on raw score and whether there are children in the household (i.e., whether responses to child-referenced questions are included in the raw score).
  - For households with one or more children:
    – Raw score zero—High food security
    – Raw score 1–2—Marginal food security
    – Raw score 3–7—Low food security
    – Raw score 8–18—Very low food security
  - For households with no child present:
    – Raw score zero—High food security
    – Raw score 1–2—Marginal food security
    – Raw score 3–5—Low food security
    – Raw score 6–10—Very low food security

For the Six-Item Short Form,[2] food security status is assigned as follows:

- Raw score 0–1—High or marginal food security (raw score 1 may be considered marginal food security, but a large proportion of households that would be measured as having marginal food security using the household or adult scale will have raw score zero on the six-item scale)
- Raw score 2–4—Low food security
- Raw score 5–6—Very low food security

Source:

[1]Data from US Department of Agriculture, Economic Research Service. *U.S. Household Food Security Survey Module: Three-Stage Design, With Screeners.* September 2012. Available at http://www.ers.usda.gov/data-products/food-security-in-the-united-states/data-files/food-security-survey-modules/household.aspx, accessed January 22, 2015.

[2]Data from US Department of Agriculture, Economic Research Service. *U.S. Household Food Security Survey Module: Six-Item Short Form.* September 2012. Available at http://www.ers.usda.gov/data-products/food-security-in-the-united-states/data-files/food-security-survey-modules/short.aspx, accessed January 22, 2015.

REFERENCES

Bickel G, Nord M, Price C, Hamilton W, Cook J. *Measuring Food Security in the United States: Guide to Measuring Household Food Security, Revised 2000.* Alexandria, VA: Food and Nutrition Service, U.S. Department of Agriculture, March 2000. Available at http://www.fns.usda.gov/guide-measuring-household-food-security-revised-2000, accessed January 16, 2015.

Boulos MN. Towards evidence-based, GIS-driven national spatial health information infrastructure and surveillance services in the United Kingdom. *Int J Health Geogr.* 2004;3:1.

Breaking Barriers: A Road to Improved Food Access. Sacramento, CA: The Sacramento Hunger Commission, 2000.

Byers T. Nutrition monitoring and surveillance. In Willett W, ed. *Nutritional Epidemiology*, 2nd ed. New York: Oxford University Press, 1998, chap. 14.

Byers T, Serdula M, Kuester S, Mendlein J, Ballew C, McPherson RS. Dietary surveillance for states and communities. *Am J Clin Nutr.* 1997;65(4 Suppl):1210S–1214S.

Carlson SJ, Andrews MS, Bickel GW. Measuring food insecurity and hunger in the United States: Development of a national benchmark measure and prevalence estimates. *J Nutr.* 1999;129(2 Suppl):510S–516S.

Centers for Disease Control and Prevention. State, Tribal, Local, and Territorial Public Health Professionals Gateway. Community Health Assessment. Assessment & Planning Models, Frameworks & Tools. Available at http://www.cdc.gov/stltpublichealth/cha/assessment.html, accessed February 12, 2015.

Clark MJ, Cary S, Diemert G et al. Involving communities in community assessment. *Pub Health Nurs.* 2003;20(6):456–463.

Cohen B, Andrews M, Kantor LS. *Community Food Security Assessment Toolkit.* Economic Research Service, U.S. Department of Agriculture. E-FAN-02-013, July 2002. Available at http://www.ers.usda.gov/media/327699/efan02013_1_.pdf, accessed January 16, 2015.

The Committee for the Study of the Future of Public Health. *The Future of Public Health.* Division of HealthCare Services. Institute of Medicine. Washington, DC: National Academy Press, 1988.

Community Food Security Coalition. *Community Food Security Programs: What Do They Look Like?* Venice, CA: Community Food Security Coalition, n.d. Available at http://www.mainecf.org/portals/0/pdfs/shared/CFS_projects.pdf, accessed January 16, 2015.

Dodds JM, Melnik TA. Development of the New York State Nutrition Surveillance Program. *Public Health Rep.* 1993;106(2):230–240.

Esri. *Mapping the Nation: Government and Technology Making a Difference.* Redlands, CA: ESRI Press, 2012.

Faruque FS, Lofton SP, Doddato TM, Mangum C. Utilizing geographic information systems in community assessment and nursing research. *J Comm Health Nurs.* 2003;20(3):179–191.

Food Matters: Farm Viability and Food Consumption in Missoula County. Available at http://www.missoulacfac.org/foodmatters.html, accessed January 16, 2015.

Grow, Eat, Know: A Resource Guide to Food and Farming in Missoula County. Available at http://www.missoulacfac.org/resourceguide.html, accessed January 16, 2015.

Hassanein N, Jacobson M, Atthowe H et al. *Missoula County Community Food Assessment,* 2004. Available at http://www.missoulacfac.org/missoulacountycommunityfoodassessment.html, accessed January 16, 2015.

Hassanein N, Jacobson M, Diaz L et al. *Our Foodshed in Focus: Missoula County Food and Agriculture by the Numbers.* Missoula County, MO, 2004. Available at http://www.missoulacfac.org/ourfoodshedinfocus.html, accessed June 30, 2015.

Institute of Medicine, Stoto MA, Abel C, Dievler A, eds. *Healthy Communities: New Partnerships for the Future of Public Health.* Washington, DC: National Academy Press, 1996. Available at http://www.nap.edu/openbook.php?isbn=030905625X, accessed January 16, 2015.

Jessup E. Fresno fresh access engages diverse communities and local policymakers. *Community Food Security News*. Spring 2004, p. 3. Available at http://www.whyhunger.org/getinfo/showArticle/articleId/3634, accessed January 16, 2015.

Koontz LD. Geographic Information Systems: Challenges to Effective Data Sharing. GAO-03-874T, June 10, 2003. Available at http://www.gao.gov/new.items/d03874t.pdf, accessed January 16, 2015.

Kretzmann JP, McKnight JL. *Building Communities from the Inside Out: A Path toward Finding and Mobilizing a Community's Assets*. Chicago: ACTA Publications, 1993.

Laverack G. Improving health outcomes through community empowerment: A review of the literature. *J Health Popul Nutr*. 2006;24(1):113–120.

New York State Department of Health. Community Health Assessment Clearinghouse. Available at http://www.health.ny.gov/statistics/chac/, accessed January 16, 2015.

Our Foodshed in Focus: Missoula County Food and Agriculture by the Numbers. Available at http://www.missoulacfac.org/ourfoodshedinfocus.html, accessed January 16, 2015.

Pike Research. Annual Utility Spending on GIS Tools and Services Will Reach $3.7 Billion by 2017, 2012. Available at http://www.navigantresearch.com/newsroom/annual-utility-spending-on-gis-tools-and-services-will-reach-3-7-billion-by-2017, accessed January 13, 2015.

Pothukuchi K. Community food assessment: A first step in planning for community food security. *J Plan Educ Res*. 2004;23(4):356–377.

Pothukuchi K, Joseph H, Burton H, Fisher A. *What's Cooking in Your Food System? A Guide to Community Food Assessment*. Venice, CA: Community Food Security Coalition, 2002.

Powner DA. Geospatial Information: OMB and Agencies Need to Make Coordination a Priority to Reduce Duplication. GAO-13-94, November 2012. Available at http://www.gao.gov/assets/660/650293.pdf, accessed January 15, 2015.

Ricketts TC. Geographic information systems and public health. *Annu Rev Public Health*. 2003;24:1–6.

Salcone J. *The Avondale/Glen Elder Community Food Assessment: Food Security in a South Sacramento Neighborhood*. Sacramento, CA: The Sacramento Hunger Commission, 2004.

Sustainable Food Center. *Access Denied: An Analysis of Problems Facing East Austin Residents in Their Attempts to Obtain Affordable, Nutritious Food*. Austin, TX: Sustainable Food Center, 1995. Available at http://sustainablefoodcenter.org/about/reports, accessed January 16, 2015.

US Department of Agriculture, Economic Research Service. Food Security in the United States: CPS Food Security Supplement. Available at http://www.ers.usda.gov/data-products/food-security-in-the-united-states/documentation.aspx, accessed January 16, 2015.

US Department of Agriculture, Economic Research Service. Data Products. Available at http://www.ers.usda.gov/data-products.aspx#.UYur6oLLep4, accessed January 6, 2015.

Ver Ploeg M, Breneman V, Farrigan T et al. *Access to Affordable and Nutritious Food—Measuring and Understanding Food Deserts and Their Consequences: Report to Congress*. Economic Research Service, U.S. Department of Agriculture. AP-036, June 2009, p. 141. Available at http://www.ers.usda.gov/publications/ap-administrative-publication/ap-036.aspx#.UXmfRoIn9bw, accessed January 15, 2015.

The Washington State Community Nutrition Assessment Education Project. Available at http://depts.washington.edu/commnutr/home/index.htm, accessed January 16, 2015. [The 12-step approach was developed by Carolyn Gleason, MS, RD, Regional Nutrition Consultant, DHHS/HRSA Seattle Field Office. 206-615-2486, Fax 206-615,2500, cleason@hrsa.dhhs.gov.]

Welsh W. Location, location, location. *Washington Technology*, April 14, 2005. Available at http://washingtontechnology.com/articles/2005/04/14/location-location-location.aspx?sc_lang=en, accessed January 13, 2015.

WhyHunger. Community Food Assessment: Program Profiles. Available at http://www.whyhunger.org/getinfo/showArticle/articleId/629#3, accessed January 25, 2015.

11 Promoting Food Security

The trouble with being poor is that it takes up all your time.

William de Kooning (1904–1997)

INTRODUCTION

At the household level, food security means that all family members have access at all times to enough food for an active, healthy life. Certain groups of Americans are more at risk of material hardship than others. These groups, which include the unemployed and underemployed, disabled, racial and ethnic minorities, single-parent households, women, children, and the elderly, often are the focus of the nation's domestic food and nutrition assistance programs that promote food for an active, healthy life. People living in poverty are at risk of having inadequate resources for food and other necessities. Children account for about a third of poor people. Although less than 9% of the elderly are poor, poverty rates for older women are higher than the average for older people. In addition to tax-supported efforts to help feed low-income people, the private sector also plays a large role in addressing hunger and community-level solutions in the United States; but this chapter focuses on the role of the federal government's nutrition safety net to protect individuals and families from malnutrition, hunger, and food insecurity. After defining food security, we review the extent of poverty and food insecurity in the United States, and examine the varied and numerous federal nutrition assistance programs.

PARSING FOOD SECURITY

Over the years, *food security* has referred variously to (1) price supports that ensure the continued ability of farmers to produce a food supply adequate to feed the nation, (2) protection of our food supply from both unintentional and intentional contamination (see Chapter 13), and (3) access at all times to enough food for an active, healthy life.

Using the phrase *food security* to describe farm supports has gone out of favor. The 1985 Farm Bill (P.L. 99-198), also known as the *Food Security Act of 1985*, was the last bill introduced in Congress with *food security* in the title.

Today, public health practitioners speak of food security at the household, community, and world levels:

- *Household food security* is defined as access, at all times, to enough food for an active, healthy life for all household members. The US Department of Agriculture (USDA) monitors food security through an annual survey of about 53,000 US households, conducted as a supplement to the US Census Bureau's nationally representative Current Population Survey (CPS). As the survey is sent to homes, the USDA is monitoring food security at the household (not individual) level. According to the USDA's Economic Research Service (ERS), 14.3% of American households were food-insecure at least some time during 2013, and 5.6% suffered very low food security (Coleman-Jensen et al. 2014).
- *Community food security* is a relatively newer concept with roots in community nutrition, nutrition education, public health, sustainable agriculture, and anti-hunger and community development (see also Chapter 12). There is no universally accepted definition of

community food security, though it is an extension of household food security (Cohen et al. 2002). In the broadest terms, it describes a prevention-oriented approach that supports the development and enhancement of sustainable, community-based strategies to improve access of low-income households to healthful nutritious food supplies, to increase the self-reliance of communities in providing for their own food needs, and to promote comprehensive responses to local food, farm, and nutrition issues (Kantor 2001). Community food security is also described as a community in which all residents obtain a safe, culturally acceptable, nutritionally adequate diet through a sustainable food system that maximizes self-reliance and social justice (Hamm and Bellows 2003), and a sustainable community food system that improves the health of the community, environment, and individuals over time, involving a collaborative effort to build locally based, self-reliant food systems (McCullum et al. 2005).

- *World food security* describes the universal right of everyone to have access to safe and nutritious food, consistent with the right to adequate food and the fundamental right of everyone to be free from hunger. In 1996, 180 nations met for the World Food Summit and signed the Rome Declaration on World Food Security, pledging their common commitment to achieving food security for all and to an ongoing effort to eradicate hunger in all countries, with a pledge of reducing the number of undernourished people by half (to about 400 million) no later than 2015 (Rome Declaration on World Food Security 1996). The latest United Nation's Food and Agricultural Organization (FAO) reports indicate that although this target is not being met, global hunger continues to be reduced. About 805 million people are estimated to be chronically undernourished in 2012–2014 (FAO et al. 2014).

POVERTY IN THE UNITED STATES

The source of official poverty estimates is the CPS' Annual Social and Economic Supplement, a sample survey of approximately 100,000 households nationwide. Historically, poverty rates have differed, depending on race and Hispanic origin, age, type of household, and residence. For example, blacks and Hispanics have poverty rates that greatly exceed the national average. The poverty rate for all blacks and Hispanics remained near 30% during the 1980s and mid-1990s, and thereafter began to fall. In 2000, the rate for blacks dropped to 22.5%, and in 2006, the rate for Hispanics fell to 20.6%—the lowest rate for both groups since the United States began measuring poverty in 1959. Unfortunately, the rate for blacks has increased since 2000, reaching 27.2% in 2013. The poverty rate for Hispanics crept up again to 26.5% in 2010 and has receded slightly to 23.5% as of 2013. In contrast, the poverty rate for non-Hispanic whites has always been below the overall poverty rate; and in comparison, in 2000, the rate for non-Hispanic whites was 7.4%, in 2006 the rate was 8.2%, and in 2013 it was 9.6% (DeNavas-Walt and Proctor 2013). Poverty rates among black and Hispanic children are much higher than among white children and have been so since at least 1977 when the Census Bureau began making separate estimates. In 1979, the average central city poverty rate was 15.7%; at its highest point, in 1993, it was 21.5% (US Bureau of the Census, http://www.census.gov /hhes/www/poverty/data/historical/hstpov8.xls).

As indicated in Table 11.1, the official poverty rate in 2013 was 14.5%, with 45.3 million people living in poverty (the highest since 1959 was 46.3 million people in 2010). Those who defined themselves as black only or as black and some other race had the highest rates (27.2%), followed by those of Hispanic origin of any race (23.5%), Asians (10.5%), and non-Hispanic whites (9.6%). Among children under 18 years of age, 19.9% lived in poverty, contrasted with 9.5% of those over 65 years. Of all family groups, poverty is highest among those headed by single women. Poverty rates also depend on where people live. The average poverty rates are greatest inside principal cities and lowest outside the principal cities. The poverty rate is greatest in the south and lowest in the northeast (DeNavas-Walt and Proctor 2014).

TABLE 11.1

**Selected Characteristics of Individuals in Poverty
in the United States, 2013**

Description	Percent	Number (in Thousands)
All	14.5	45,318
Sex		
Female	15.8	159,605
Male	13.1	153,361
Age (in years)		
Under 18	19.9	14,659
18–64	13.6	26,429
65 and over	9.5	4231
Race/Ethnicity		
Black	27.2	11,041
Hispanic (any race)	23.5	12,744
White	12.3	29,936
White, non-Hispanic	9.6	18,796
Asian	12.3	1785
Region		
South	16.1	18,870
West	14.7	10,812
Midwest	12.9	8590
Northeast	12.7	7046

Source: DeNavas-Walt C and Proctor BD. Income and Poverty in the United States: 2013. Current Population Reports. US Census Bureau. Table 3 People in Poverty by Selected Characteristics: 2012 and 2013. Available at https://www.census.gov/content/dam/Census/library/publications/2014/demo/p60-249.pdf, accessed February 15, 2015.

Table 11.2 displays 5-year averages of the poverty rate and the number in poverty for seven mutually exclusive racial categories (six race-alone categories and the two or more races category), the Hispanic origin group of any race, and the non-Hispanic white group in the United States from 2007 to 2011. The Census Bureau uses 5-year averages to allow for the analysis of poverty rates by race and Hispanic origin for many levels of geography, as well as detailed race and origin groups in the cities and towns with the largest populations of these groups. For example, in 2007–2011, among the Asian population, poverty rates were highest for Vietnamese (14.7%) and Koreans (15.0%), and lowest for Filipinos (5.8%). For Hispanics, national poverty rates ranged from a low of 16.2% for Cubans to a high of 26.3% for Dominicans (Macartney et al. 2013).

NUTRITION AND HEALTH CHARACTERISTICS OF LOW-INCOME POPULATIONS

In 2004, the USDA published the four-volume *Nutrition and Health Outcomes Study.* The study contains analyses of data from the Third National Health and Nutritional Examination Survey (NHANES-III) conducted in 1988–1994, comparing the nutrition and health characteristics of Food Stamp Program (FSP, now called the Supplemental Nutrition Assistance Program, SNAP) and Special Supplemental Nutrition Program for Women, Infants, and Children (WIC) participants with their higher-income counterparts and with people who were eligible but did not participate in the FSP and WIC. The study also examined low-income school-age children and older Americans, comparing them with their higher-income counterparts. In essence, the study

TABLE 11.2

Poverty Rates and Number in Poverty by Race and Hispanic Origin Using 5-Year Averages, 2007–2011

Race and Hispanic Origin[a]	5-Year Average, 2007–2011			
Description	Percentage (Estimate)	90% Confidence Interval (±)[b]	Number (Estimate)	90% Confidence Interval (±)[b]
All races	14.3	0.1	42,739,924	277,336
White alone	11.6	0.1	25,659,922	193,148
White alone, non-Hispanic	9.9	0.1	18,959,814	152,602
Black or African American alone	25.8	0.1	9,472,583	50,241
American Indian and Alaska Native alone	27.0	0.4	651,226	9734
Asian alone	11.7	0.1	1,663,303	19,470
Asian Indian	8.2	0.3	224,343	7718
Chinese	13.4	0.2	424,332	7305
Filipino	5.8	0.2	146,113	4685
Japanese	8.2	0.3	64,553	2727
Korean	15.0	0.3	206,241	5340
Vietnamese	14.7	0.4	228,381	6674
Native Hawaiian and other Pacific Islander alone	17.6	0.7	85,346	3634
Native Hawaiian	14.4	1.0	21,937	1485
Samoan	17.6	1.6	17,606	1616
Tongan	18.1	3.0	7221	1421
Guamanian or Chamorro	11.6	1.4	8197	1007
Fijians	6.4	1.8	1738	488
Other Pacific Islander	29.7	2.3	28,647	2643
Some other race alone	24.6	0.2	3,792,156	47,496
Two or more races	18.7	0.2	1,415,388	13,717
Hispanic origin (any race)	23.2	0.2	11,197,648	77,014
Mexican	24.9	0.2	7,744,050	65,971
Guatemalan	24.9	0.6	262,575	7506
Salvadoran	18.9	0.5	323,317	8870
Cuban	16.2	0.4	279,011	5969
Dominican	26.3	0.5	364,523	6591
Puerto Rican	25.6	0.3	1,142,216	13,907

Source: Macartney S et al., US Census Bureau. *Poverty Rates for Selected Detailed Race and Hispanic Groups by State and Place: 2007–2011*. American Community Survey Briefs, ACSBR/11-17. Washington, DC: US Census Bureau; 2013: Table 1. Available at http://www.census.gov/prod/2013pubs/acsbr11-17.pdf, accessed February 15, 2015.

[a] Federal surveys give respondents the option of reporting more than one race. Therefore, two basic ways of defining a race group are possible. A group such as Asian may be defined as those who reported Asian and no other race (the race-alone or single-race concept) or as those who reported Asian regardless of whether they also reported another race (the race-alone-or-in-combination concept). Whereas this table shows data using the race-alone approach, note that about 2.5% of people reported more than one race. Information on those who reported more than one race during 2007–2011, such as American Indian and Alaska Native alone or in combination, or Asian alone or in combination, is available from the February 2013 American Community Survey Brief (http://www.census.gov/prod/2013pubs/acsbr11-17.pdf). Because Hispanics may be of any race, data in this table for Hispanics overlap with data for race groups.

[b] A 90% confidence interval is a measure of an estimate's variability. The larger the confidence interval in relation to the size of the estimate, the less reliable the estimate.

highlights the health characteristics of low-income people (less than 130% of the poverty level) by comparing them with their counterparts who have more money (more than 130% of the poverty level).

Specifically, data from NHANES-III were used to compare the nutrition and health characteristics of FSP participants along with a group of nonparticipants with higher incomes (income above 130% of poverty) (Fox et al. 2004a). This research was designed to establish a baseline from which to monitor over time the nutritional and health characteristics of FSP participants and nonparticipants. FSP participants and their higher-income nonparticipant counterparts are compared on the basis of diet quality (based on Healthy Eating Index [HEI] scores), body mass index (BMI), nutritional biochemistries, bone density, infant feeding practices, physical activity, and chronic health conditions. Significant disparities were noted between the two groups for all nutrition and health characteristics cited and are highlighted below.

- *Healthy Eating Index Scores.* FSP participants were more likely than higher-income nonparticipants to consume poor diets (24% vs. 15%) and less likely to consume *good* diets (6% vs. 12%).
- *Dietary nutrient intake.* FSP participants consumed more food energy than income-eligible nonparticipants (95% of the 1989 recommended energy allowance vs. 91%). FSP participants were less likely than higher-income nonparticipants to consume adequate amounts of iron (91% vs. 95%), zinc (80% vs. 88%), and calcium (73% vs. 83%).
- *Body weight.* Adult and teenage female FSP participants had significantly greater BMIs than high-income nonparticipants (28.3% vs. 26.4% and 19.8% vs. 19.2%, respectively). Female FSP participants were less likely to be at a healthy weight (28% vs. 49%) and more likely to be obese (42% vs. 22%) than higher-income nonparticipants.
- *Bone density.* FSP participants over 80 years were almost twice more likely to have severely reduced bone density than higher-income nonparticipants (42% vs. 24%).
- *Nutritional status (biochemistries).* Female FSP participants were more likely than higher-income nonparticipants to be iron deficient (14% vs. 6% for 20 to 29 year olds and 20% vs. 9% for 30 to 39 year olds). FSP participants were less likely than higher-income nonparticipants to have low red blood cell folate levels (11% vs. 6%). Overall, the prevalence of anemia among FSP participants was double that of higher-income nonparticipants (4% vs. 2%).
- *Infant feeding practices.* FSP participants were less likely than higher-income nonparticipants to have breastfed their infants (45% vs. 63%). Among those who breastfed, fewer FSP participants (36% vs. 44%) breastfed for at least 6 months. More FSP participants than higher-income nonparticipants started their infants on solid food earlier than 4 months (20% vs. 24%).
- *Physical activity.* In comparison with higher-income nonparticipating children, FSP children were less likely to engage in vigorous physical activity (mean times per week: 4.4 vs. 4.8), engage in physical activity at least three times per week (74% vs. 81%), and be involved in team sports or other organized exercise programs (50% vs. 68%). Fewer FSP children than higher-income nonparticipating children 5–16 years of age limited television watching to no more than 2 hours per day (55% vs. 68%). Fewer FSP adults than higher-income nonparticipating adults were physically active three or more times per week (37% vs. 60%) or five or more times per week (28% vs. 46%).
- *Chronic health conditions.* FSP participants were more likely than higher-income nonparticipants to report having diabetes (10% vs. 5%), to having had a heart attack (5% vs. 3%) or a stroke (4% vs. 2%), and to actually have high blood pressure, based on physician assessment (23% vs. 18%) (Fox et al. 2004a).

FOOD INSECURITY IN THE UNITED STATES

Since 1995, the USDA has monitored food security in the nation's households through an annual, nationally representative survey conducted by the Census Bureau. Information about households' food expenditures and sources of food assistance is also collected.

The physiological phenomenon of hunger is defined as an uneasy or painful sensation caused by not having access to enough food (Bickel et al. 2000). In 2013, one or more family members in an estimated 5.6% of American households did not have enough food to eat at least some time during the year (Coleman-Jensen et al. 2014). Unlike the situation in some developing nations where famine is widespread among young children, and hunger manifests itself as *kwashior-kor* and *marasmus*, hunger generally manifests itself in a less severe form in the United States. This is in part because the USDA food assistance programs help to provide a food safety net for many low-income individuals and families. Whereas starvation seldom occurs in the United States, children and adults do go hungry and chronic mild undernutrition occurs when financial resources are low.

Food insecurity describes widespread but less severe hunger problems. Food insecurity means that a household had (1) limited or uncertain availability of food or (2) limited or uncertain ability to acquire foods in socially acceptable ways (in other words, without resorting to emergency food supplies, scavenging, stealing, or other unusual coping strategies). Since 2006, the USDA has recognized two levels of food insecurity:

- *Low food security*: reports of multiple indications of food access problems, but few, if any, indications of reduced food intake.
- *Very low food security*: reports of multiple indications of reduced food intake and disrupted eating patterns due to inadequate resources for food. In most, but not all households with very low food security, respondents report feeling hungry at some time during the year but did not eat because there was not enough money for food (Box 11.1).

PREVALENCE OF FOOD INSECURITY IN THE UNITED STATES

National prevalence rates from 1999 to 2013 (odd years) for food security and food insecurity appear in Table 11.3. In 2013, 85.7% of American households were food secure, 8.7% exhibited low food security, and 5.6% had very low food security. Food insecurity has increased over time, from 10.1% in 1999 to a peak of 14.9% in 2011 (Coleman-Jensen et al. 2014). In comparing changes in averages from 2001–2003 to 2011–2013, food insecurity increased the most—by 6.2–7.0% points—in Nevada (7.0%), Missouri (6.5%), Tennessee (6.5%), Mississippi (6.2%), and Delaware (6.2%). Missouri has the dubious distinction of also being the state with the highest increase—4.5%—in very low food security (Coleman-Jensen et al. 2014).

Historically, the prevalence of food insecurity follows a discernible geographic pattern; states with the highest rates border the Atlantic Ocean, Mexico, and the Gulf of Mexico. In 2011–2013, the rates of food insecurity (low or very low food security) were the highest—17.3–21.2% of the population—in Arkansas (21.2%), Missouri (21.1%), Texas (18%), Tennessee (17.4%), and North Carolina (17.3%) (Coleman-Jensen et al. 2014).

During 2011–2013, 7.0–8.4% of the population in seven states experienced very low food security. The rates were highest in Arkansas (8.4%) and Missouri (8.1%), with the next two closest states being Ohio and Mississippi (Coleman-Jensen et al. 2014). Children in US households do not usually experience reduced food intake unless reduced food intake among adults reaches severe levels. Nevertheless, in about 1.0% of households, one or more children were subject to reduced food intake and disrupted eating patterns (very low food security) at some time during 2013. In some households with very low food security among children, only older children

BOX 11.1 USDA: FOOD SECURITY AND HUNGER

Prior to 2006, reports on food security used the following general classifications: *food secure, food insecure without hunger,* and *food insecure with hunger.* Households with low food security were described as "food insecure without hunger," and households with very low food security were described as "food insecure with hunger." However, in 2006, the National Research Council's Committee on National Statistics (CNSTAT) recommended that the USDA make a clear and explicit distinction between *food insecurity* and *hunger.* CNSTAT stated in its final report that food insecurity is a household-level economic and social condition of limited or uncertain access to adequate food. Hunger, on the other hand, is an individual level physiological condition that may result from food insecurity. The word *hunger* refers to a potential consequence of food insecurity that, because of prolonged, involuntary lack of food, results in discomfort, illness, weakness, or pain that goes beyond the usual uneasy sensation. CNSTAT advised that the food security survey does not measure hunger, which would require collecting detailed and extensive information on physiological experiences of individual household members. In response to CNSTAT's recommendations, the USDA introduced new language to describe ranges of severity of food insecurity, as depicted in the chart below. The labels "food insecurity without hunger" and "food insecurity with hunger" were replaced by *low food security* and *very low food security,* respectively. The defining characteristic of very low food security is that, at times during the year, the food intake of household members was reduced and their normal eating patterns were disrupted because the household lacked money and other resources for food. Because the criteria used to classify households did not change, statistics reported since 2006 are directly comparable with those for earlier years for the corresponding categories.

General Categories (unchanged)	Detailed Categories		
	Old Label (prior to 2006)	New Label (since 2006)	Description of Household Conditions
Food security	Food security	High food security	No reported indications of food access problems or limitations
		Marginal food security	1 or 2 reported indications— typically of anxiety over food sufficiency or shortage of food in the house. Little or no indication of changes in diets or food intake.
Food insecurity	Food insecurity *without hunger*	Low food security	Reports of reduced quality, variety, or desirability of diet. Little or no indication of reduced food intake
	Food insecurity *with hunger*	Very low food security	Reports of multiple indications of disrupted eating patterns and reduced food intake.

Source: National Research Council. Food Insecurity and Hunger in the United States: An Assessment of the Measure. Panel to Review US Department of Agriculture's Measurement of Food Insecurity and Hunger. Wunderlich GS, Norwood JL, Eds. Committee on National Statistics, Division of Behavioral and Social Sciences and Education. Washington, DC: The National Academies Press, 2006. Washington, DC. Available at http://www.nap.edu/catalog .php?record_id=11578, accessed January 10, 2015. Coleman-Jensen A, Nord M, Andrews M, Carlson S. *Household Food Security in the United States in 2011.* ERR-141, US Department of Agriculture, Economic Research Service, 2012. Available at: http://www.ers.usda.gov/media/884525/err141.pdf, accessed June 29, 2015.

TABLE 11.3
Number and Prevalence Rates of Food Security and Food Insecurity by Category, 1999–2013 (Odd Years)

				Prevalence of Food Security and Food Insecurity, by Category and Year						
					Food Insecure					
Year	**Total[a]**	**Food Secure**		**All**		**Low Food Security**		**Very Low Food Security**	
	1000	1000	%	1000	%	1000	%	1000	%
				Households					
2013	122,579	105,070	85.7	17,509	14.2	10,664	8.7	6845	5.6
2011	119,484	101,631	85.1	17,853	14.9	11,014	9.2	6839	5.7
2009	118,174	100,820	85.3	17,354	14.7	10,601	9.0	6753	5.7
2007	117,100	104,089	88.9	13,011	11.1	8262	7.0	4749	4.1
2005	114,437	101,851	89.0	12,586	11.0	8158	7.1	4428	3.9
2003	112,214	99,631	88.8	12,583	11.2	8663	7.7	3920	3.5
2001	107,824	96,303	89.3	11,521	10.7	8010	7.4	3511	3.3
1999	104,684	94,154	89.9	10,529	10.1	7420	7.1	3109	3.0
				Individuals (by Food Security Status of Household)[b]					
2013	310,853	261,775	84.2	49,078	15.8	31,974	10.3	17,104	5.5
2011	305,893	255,773	83.6	50,120	16.4	33,232	10.9	16,888	5.5
2009	301,750	251,588	83.4	50,162	16.6	32,499	10.8	17,663	5.9
2007	297,042	260,813	87.8	36,229	12.2	24,287	8.2	11,942	4.0
2005	291,501	256,373	87.9	35,128	12.1	24,349	8.4	10,779	3.7
2003	286,410	250,155	87.3	36,255	12.7	26,622	9.3	9633	3.4
2001	276,661	243,019	87.8	33,642	12.2	24,628	8.9	9014	3.3
1999	270,318	239,304	88.5	31,015	11.5	23,237	8.6	7779	2.9
				Adults (by Food Security Status of Household)[b]					
2013	237,219	203,913	86.0	33,306	14.0	21,115	8.9	12,191	5.1
2011	231,385	197,923	85.5	33,462	14.5	21,371	9.2	12,091	5.2
2009	227,543	194,579	85.5	32,964	14.5	20,741	9.1	12,223	5.4
2007	223,467	199,672	89.4	23,795	10.6	15,602	7.0	8193	3.7
2005	217,897	195,172	89.6	22,725	10.4	15,146	7.0	7579	3.5
2003	213,441	190,451	89.2	22,990	10.8	16,358	7.7	6632	3.1
2001	204,340	183,398	89.8	20,942	10.2	14,879	7.3	6063	3.0
1999	198,900	179,960	90.5	18,941	9.5	13,869	7.0	5072	2.5

Year	**Total[c]**	**Food-Secure Households**		**Food-Insecure Households[d]**		**Households with Food-Insecure Children[e]**		**Households with Very Low Food Security Among Children**	
	1000	1000	%	1000	%	1000	%	1000	%
				Households with Children					
2013	38,486	30,978	80.5	7508	19.5	3814	9.9	360	0.9
2011	38,803	30,814	79.4	7989	20.6	3862	10.0	374	1.0
2009	39,525	31,114	78.7	8411	21.3	4208	10.6	469	1.2
2007	39,390	33,160	84.2	6230	15.8	3273	8.3	323	0.8
2005	39,601	33,404	84.4	6197	15.6	3244	8.2	270	0.7

(Continued)

TABLE 11.3 (CONTINUED)

Number and Prevalence Rates of Food Security and Food Insecurity by Category, 1999–2013 (Odd Years)

Prevalence of Food Security and Food Insecurity, by Category and Year

Households with Children

2003	40,286	33,575	83.3	6711	16.7	3606	9.0	207	0.5
2001	38,330	32,141	83.9	6189	16.1	3225	8.4	211	0.6
1999	37,884	32,290	85.2	5594	14.8	3089	8.2	219	0.6

Children (by Household Food Security Status)[b]

2013	73,634	57,862	78.6	15,772	21.4	8585	11.7	765	1.0
2011	74,508	57,850	77.6	16,658	22.4	8565	11.5	845	1.1
2009	74,207	57,010	76.8	17,197	23.2	8957	12.1	988	1.3
2007	73,575	61,140	83.1	12,435	16.9	6766	9.2	691	0.9
2005	73,604	61,201	83.1	12,403	16.9	6718	9.1	606	0.8
2003	72,969	59,704	81.8	13,265	18.2	7388	10.1	420	0.6
2001	72,321	59,620	82.4	12,701	17.6	6866	9.5	467	0.6
1999	71,418	59,344	83.1	12,074	16.9	6996	9.8	511	0.7

Source: Calculated by USDA, Economic Research Service using Current Population Survey Food Security Supplement data; Coleman-Jensen A et al., *Household Food Security in the United States in 2013*. ERR-173, US Department of Agriculture, Economic Research Service, September 2014. Available at http://www.ers.usda.gov/media/1565415 /err173.pdf, accessed February 15, 2015.

[a] Totals exclude households whose food security status is unknown because they did not give a valid response to any of the questions in the food security scale. In 2013, these represented 433,000 households with children (0.4% of all households).

[b] The food security survey measures food security status at the household level. Not all individuals residing in food-insecure households were directly affected by the households' food insecurity. Similarly, not all individuals in households classified as having very low food security were subject to the reductions in food intake and disruptions in eating patterns that characterize this condition. Young children, in particular, are often protected from effects of the households' food insecurity.

[c] Totals exclude households whose food security status is unknown because they did not give a valid response to any of the questions in the food security scale. In 2013, these represented 150,000 households (0.4% of all households with children).

[d] Food-insecure households are those with low or very low food security among adults or children or both.

[e] Households with food-insecure children are those with low or very low food security among children.

may have experienced the more severe effects of food insecurity, while younger children were protected from those effects (Coleman-Jensen et al. 2014). The mental and physical changes that accompany inadequate food intake can have harmful, lasting effects on a child's learning, physical and psychological health, and overall quality of life (Alaimo et al. 2001; Casey et al. 2005; Kleinman et al. 2002).

An indicator of how adequately households meet their food needs is the amount of money spent on food. In 2011, the median US household spent $47.50 per person for food each week, about 15% higher than the cost of the USDA's Thrifty Food Plan, a low-cost food *market basket* that meets dietary standards, taking into account household size and the age and sex of household members. The name *Thrifty Food Plan* refers to the diet required to feed a family of 4 persons (a man and a woman aged 19–50, a child aged 6–8, and a child aged 9–11). The typical food-insecure household spent 6% less than suggested by the Thrifty Food Plan, whereas the typical food-secure household spent 17% more than the cost of the plan (or almost one-quarter more than the typical food-insecure household) (Coleman-Jensen et al. 2014).

FEDERAL NUTRITION ASSISTANCE PROGRAMS

Federal nutrition assistance programs increase food security by providing children and low-income people access to food, a healthful diet, and nutrition education. The Food and Nutrition Service (FNS) within the USDA administers 15 food assistance programs, including SNAP (formerly FSP), WIC, and the child nutrition programs.

The proposed budget for fiscal year (FY) 2015, which began in October 1, 2014, includes just over $112 billion for programs aimed at promoting food security and preventing hunger, allocated as follows:

- $84.246 billion for SNAP.
- $20.537 billion for child nutrition programs, including the National School Lunch Program (NSLP), School Breakfast Program (SBP), Summer Food Service, Special Milk, and Child and Adult Care Food Programs (CACFP).
- $6.82 billion for WIC (US Department of Agriculture 2015).

The USDA has the vast majority of responsibility for providing food assistance programs in the United States. In partnership with the USDA, at least three other cabinet-level departments are charged with the responsibility for administering food assistance programs in the United States.

- The Department of Health and Human Services (HHS) administers Head Start, a school readiness program that provides meals and snacks to infants and preschool-age children. HHS is also home to the Administration on Aging (AoA), which administers the Nutrition Services Incentive Program (NSIP), a food assistance program for the elderly, although it receives commodity foods and financial support from the USDA's FNS.
- The Department of Defense (DoD) and USDA maintain a partnership that takes advantage of the DoD's large-scale buying power to provide fresh fruit and vegetables to the NSLP.
- The Department of Homeland Security and USDA work together as part of the efforts to protect America's food supply.

All federal departments are required to prepare 5-year strategic plans that identify their key goals and objectives, their strategies for attaining them, and measures of progress. One of the USDA's four strategic goals for FY 2014–2018 is to ensure that all US children have access to safe, nutritious, and balanced meals, which is one of the same strategic goals as stated for FY 2010–2015 (US Department of Agriculture, http://www.usda.gov/documents/usda-strategic-plan-fy-2014-2018.pdf). As part of this strategic goal for FY 2010–2015, the USDA (http://www.ocfo.usda.gov/usdasp/sp2010 /sp2010.pdf) aimed to reduce to zero the number of households with very low food security among children, increase to 75% the eligible people who participate in SNAP, and increase to 60% and 25% the proportion of eligible children who participate in the NSLP and SBP, respectively, by 2015.

For FY 2014–2018, the USDA aims to reduce to zero the number of households with very low food security among children, increase to 79% the eligible people who participate in SNAP, increase to 59.7% the eligible people participating in the NSLP, and increase to 17.5% the annual percentage of children who participate in the free/reduced-price NSLP and also participate in summer feeding programs, by 2018.

The USDA, illustrated by the organizational chart in Figure 11.1, maintains seven offices, each administered by its own Under Secretary. The office of Food, Nutrition, and Consumer Services

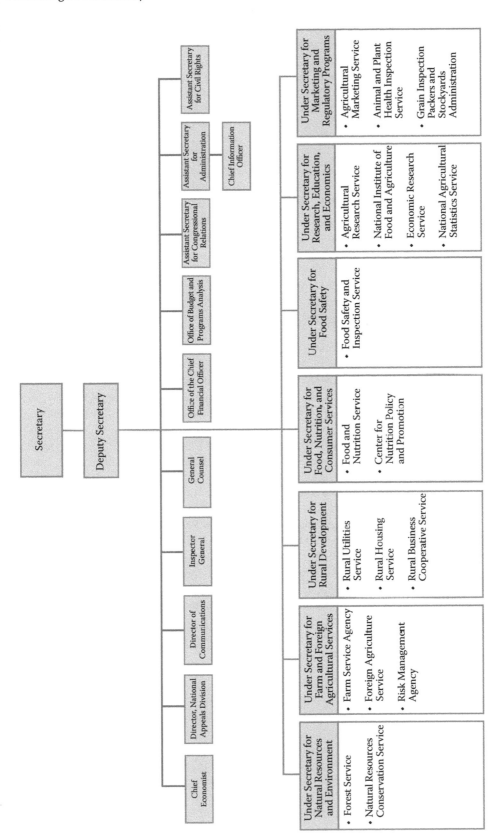

FIGURE 11.1 USDA organization chart. (From United States Department of Agriculture. USDA Organization Chart. Available at http://www.usda.gov/wps/portal /usda/usdahome?navid=USDA_ORG_CHART. Accessed May 30, 2013.)

(FNCS) works to "harness the Nation's agricultural abundance to end hunger and improve health in the United States" (US Department of Agriculture, http://www.usda.gov/wps/portal/usda/usdahome ?contentidonly=true&contentid=missionarea_FNC.xml). Within FNCS, the FNS administers federal domestic nutrition assistance programs aimed at increasing food security and reducing hunger. The other agency, Center for Nutrition Policy and Promotion (CNPP), created in 1994, works to improve the health and well-being of Americans by developing and promoting dietary guidance that links scientific research to the nutrition needs of individuals (US Department of Agriculture 2014).

Food and Nutrition Service

The mission of the FNS is "to increase food security and reduce hunger in partnership with cooperating organizations by providing children and low-income people access to food, a healthful diet, and nutrition education in a manner that supports American agriculture and inspires public confidence." For FY 2014, FNS identified the following Strategic Priorities (US Department of Agriculture 2014):

- Help Americans eat smart and maintain a healthy weight.
- Preserve public trust in our programs.
- FNCS is "the employer of choice."
- Reduce food insecurity by helping feed those in need.
- Implement the Farm Bill.
- Communicate our mission and work to the public.

To that end, FNS administers 15 domestic food and nutrition assistance programs that, in partnership with state and tribal governments, serve one in four Americans each year. Table 11.4 summarizes the major programs, and some programs are highlighted in more detail in the following pages.

Expenditures for the 15 food assistance programs totaled $108.9 billion in FY 2013 (October 1, 2012 to September 30, 2013), an increase of 2% from FY 2012 and the 13th consecutive year in which food and nutrition assistance expenditures exceeded the previous historical record. These programs account for 72% of the USDA's annual budget. Five of the programs alone accounted for 96% of the USDA's total expenditures for food and nutrition assistance: SNAP, NSLP, WIC, SBP, and CACFP (*The Food Assistance Landscape: FY 2013 Annual Report* 2014).

For ease of reference, FNS programs with unifying characteristics may be grouped together, as organized on the FNS website under programs (US Department of Agriculture, http://www .fns.usda.gov): SNAP, WIC, Child Nutrition Programs, and Food Distribution Programs. Child Nutrition Programs include the Fresh Fruit and Vegetable Program (FFVP), Special Milk Program (SMP), and Summer Food Service Program (SFSP), in addition to CACFP, NSLP, and SBP. Food Distribution Programs include Commodity Supplemental Food Program (CSFP), Food Distribution Program on Indian Reservations (FDPIR), NSIP, and The Emergency Food Assistance Program (TEFAP). Disaster Relief falls into its own category (Box 11.2).

Supplemental Nutrition Assistance Program

As the cornerstone of the USDA's nutrition assistance programs, SNAP plays a vital role in helping to improve nutrition among low-income individuals. The program provides nutrition assistance benefits and nutrition education services to needy households and to those making the transition from welfare to work. It serves as the first line of defense against hunger and enables low-income families to buy nutritious food with Electronic Benefits Transfer (EBT) cards. The program operates in 50 states, the District of Columbia, Guam, and the US Virgin Islands. The federal government oversees the state operation of SNAP through state and local SNAP offices. In FY 2014, over 46 million individuals in over 22 million households participated in the program.

TABLE 11.4

Annual Summary of Food and Nutrition Service Programs, FY 2008–2012

	FY 2010	FY 2011	FY 2012	FY 2013	FY 2014
Supplemental Nutrition Assistance Program[a]					
People participating (thousands)	40,302	44,709	46,609	47,636	46,536
Households participating (thousands)	18,618	21,072	22,330	23,052	22,700
Value of benefits ($ millions)	64,702	71,811	74,619	76,066	70,000
Average monthly benefit per person ($)	133.79	133.85	133.41	133.07	125.35
Average monthly benefit per household ($)	289.60	283.99	278.48	274.98	256.98
Total cost ($ millions)	68,284	75,687	78,411	79,929	74,126
Puerto Rico Grant ($ millions)[b]	2001	2001	2001	2001	2061
National School Lunch Program[c]					
Children participating (thousands)	31,753	31,840	31,621	30,674	30,339
Total lunches served (millions)	5278	5275	5213	5098	5008
Percent free (%)	55.9	58.1	59.6	62.1	63.5
Percent reduced-price (%)	9.4	8.4	8.6	8.3	8.0
Total after-school snacks served (millions)	219	226	230	220	220
Cash payments ($ millions)	9752	10,105	10,414	11,057	11,319
Commodity costs ($ millions)	1128	1195	1164	1163	1302
Total cost ($ millions)	10,880	11,300	11,578	12,220	12,621
School Breakfast Program[c]					
Children participating (thousands)	11,669	12,175	12,868	13,200	13,555
Total breakfasts served (millions)	1968	2048	2145	2223	2266
Percent free or reduced price (%)	83.5	83.7	84.2	84.8	84.9
Total cost ($ millions)	2859	3034	3277	3514	3673
Special Milk Program[d]					
Total half-pints served (millions)	72	67	61	55	50
Total cost ($ millions)	12	12	12	11	10
Child/Adult Care Feeding Program[e]					
Average daily attendance (thousands)	3411	3426	3547	3680	3889
Total meals served (millions)	1910	1929	1945	1957	1979
Child care centers (millions)	1248	1276	1306	1337	1370
Day care homes (millions)	595	583	569	551	538
Adult care centers (millions)	67	70	70	70	71
Percent free or reduced price (%)	82.1	81.7	81.6	81.7	81.9
Cash payments ($ millions)	2398	2472	2590	2721	2850
Commodity costs ($ millions)	94	103	114	124	133
Total costs ($ millions)	2638	2724	2855	2994	3126
Summer Food Service Program[f]					
Average daily attendance (thousands)	2304	2278	2348	2427	2646
Total meals served (millions)	134	137	144	151	160
Total cost (millions)	359	373	398	428	464
Child Nutrition State Administration ($ millions)[g]	183	193	210	225	212
WIC (Special Supplemental Food)[h]					
Women, infants, and children participating (thousands)	9175	8961	8908	8663	8259
Food cost ($ millions)	4562	5,020	4,810	4,497	4326
Average monthly food cost per person ($)	41.44	46.69	45.00	43.26	43.65
Total cost ($ millions)	6691	7179	6800	6478	6296

(*Continued*)

TABLE 11.4 (CONTINUED)
Annual Summary of Food and Nutrition Service Programs, FY 2008–2012

	FY 2010	FY 2011	FY 2012	FY 2013	FY 2014
Commodity Supplemental Food Program[i]					
Total participation (thousands)	519	588	594	580	574
Total cost ($ millions)	165	198	209	203	198
Food Distribution on Indian Reservations[i]					
Total participation (thousands)	85	78	77	76	85
Total cost ($ millions)	95	94	97	100	111
NSIP (Elderly Feeding)[j]					
Total meals served (millions)	NA	NA	NA	NA	NA
Total cost ($ millions)	2.5	1.7	2.8	2.7	2.7
The Emergency Food Assistance Program[k]					
Total pounds distributed (millions)	746	778	542	840	758
Total food cost ($ millions)	566	462	378	629	560
Total cost ($ millions)	631	532	444	693	629

Source: US Department of Agriculture. Overview. Food and Nutrition Service. Summary of Annual Data, FY 2010–2014. Available at http://www.fns.usda.gov/pd/overview, accessed February 15, 2015.

Note: FY 2014 data are preliminary and all data are subject to revisions.

[a] Participation data are 12-month averages. Total cost includes benefits, the federal share of state administrative expenses, and other federal costs (e.g., printing and processing stamps). SNAP was known as the Food Stamp Program prior to FY 2009.

[b] Puerto Rico's Nutrition Assistance Grant provides benefits analogous to SNAP. Smaller outlying areas with similar grants include American Samoa ($6.5 million in FY 2008) and the Northern Marianas ($16.2 million).

[c] NSLP and SBP participation data are 9-month averages (summer months are excluded). They represent average daily meals served adjusted by an attendance factor. School lunch costs include cash payments, entitlement commodities, bonus commodities (surplus foods donated by USDA), and cash-in-lieu of commodities. School breakfast costs are cash payments. Cash payments are federal reimbursements to state agencies based on meals served multiplied by reimbursement rates, which are adjusted annually to reflect changes in food costs. Free and reduced-price meals served to needy children are reimbursed at much higher rates than full-price meals.

[d] Special milk costs are cash payments based on an annually determined reimbursement rate and the actual cost of free milk (a small portion of the total—less than 7% for all years).

[e] Total costs include cash payments, entitlement and bonus commodities, cash-in-lieu of commodities, sponsor administrative costs, start-up costs, and audits.

[f] Average daily attendance is reported only for July, the peak month of activity. Costs include cash payments, entitlement and bonus commodities, and the federal share of state and sponsor administrative costs. The decline in meals served since FY 2001 is largely attributable to alternative summer meal service in the NSLP and SBP under Seamless Waiver provisions, which eased reporting requirements for sponsors.

[g] The federal share of state administrative costs for the NSLP, SBP, and CAFCP.

[h] Total costs include food benefits, nutrition services and administrative funds, the FMNP, infrastructure, breastfeeding promotion and peer counseling, program evaluation, and technical assistance.

[i] Includes commodity distribution costs (entitlement and bonus), the federal share of state administrative expenses, and other costs (such as storage and transportation, food losses and demo projects—national level only, unavailable prior to FY 1996).

[j] The NSIP was formerly called Nutrition Program for the Elderly. As of FY 2002, meals served are reported to the AoA (HHS) rather than FNS. In FY 2003, administration of cash grants was transferred to the AoA, and FNS costs were limited to the value of commodities distributed.

[k] Total cost includes commodities distributed (entitlement and bonus) and the federal share of state administrative expenses. Emergency food assistance is food made available to hunger relief organizations such as food banks and soup kitchens. It is not disaster relief.

BOX 11.2   FOOD ASSISTANCE FOR DISASTER RELIEF

FNS is responsible for providing nutrition assistance for disaster-affected areas requiring a federal response. In the aftermath of a major disaster or emergency, FNS coordinates with state, local, and voluntary organizations (as well as with other federal agencies) to determine potential nutrition assistance needs of disaster victims.

Agencies of the USDA help in many ways in a disaster, but perhaps the most immediate is to ensure that people who find themselves suddenly in need have enough to eat. The Food Distribution Division of the FNS has the primary responsibility of supplying food for disaster relief by providing commodity foods for shelters and other mass-feeding sites, distributing commodity food packages directly to households in need, and issuing emergency SNAP benefits.

In an emergency, disaster relief agencies such as the Red Cross and the Salvation Army request food and nutrition assistance through state agencies that run the USDA's nutrition assistance programs. The state agencies, in turn, notify the USDA of the types and quantities of food needed by the relief organizations for emergency feeding operations. Every state and US territory has on-hand stocks of commodity foods that are used for USDA-sponsored food programs, such as the NSLP, TEFAP, and FDPIR. In an emergency, the USDA can authorize states to release their food stocks to disaster relief organizations to feed people at shelters and mass-feeding sites. If the president declares a disaster, states can distribute commodity foods directly to households that are in need as a result of an emergency, and the USDA can authorize the issuance of emergency SNAP benefits when regular commercial food supply channels have been restored. The disaster SNAP (D-SNAP) system operates under a different set of eligibility and benefit delivery requirements than the regular SNAP; people who might not ordinarily qualify for SNAP benefits may be eligible under the D-SNAP. In 2012, over $43.7 million in D-SNAP benefits and more than 1.1 million pounds of USDA foods for congregate and household feeding in New York and New Jersey were provided in response to Hurricane Sandy.[1]

Guidance (updated in 2014) can be found here: http://www.fns.usda.gov/sites/default/files /D-SNAP_handbook_0.pdf

It is important to note that due to the unforeseen nature of disasters, spending for food assistance for disaster relief varies by year, potentially with some extremes. For example, in FY 2008, D-SNAP was operated almost every month, with 378 counties and parishes issuing over $447 million in benefits to nearly 1.2 million households. There were 72 major presidential disaster declarations in 2008, and it was the only year to have a major hurricane in nearly every month of the hurricane season. Disasters in 2008 ranged from wildfires in California; floods in Arkansas, Illinois, Indiana, Iowa, Nebraska, Oregon, Washington, and Wisconsin; tornadoes in Arkansas, Colorado, and Oklahoma; and Hurricanes Gustav and Ike that affected Louisiana and Texas.

Conversely, in FY 2009, D-SNAP was operated in response to tornadoes in Arkansas and Oklahoma and floods in Illinois and Minnesota. In total, 14 counties issued $12.7 million in D-SNAP benefits to 27,482 households, less than 3% of the number of households and benefits issued in 2008.[2]

Source:
[1]Data from US Department of Agriculture. Food and Nutrition Service. Food Assistance in Disaster Situations. Available at http://www.fns.usda.gov/disaster/food-assistance-disaster-situations, accessed February 17, 2015.
[2]Data from US Department of Agriculture. Food and Nutrition Service. FNS 2008 and 2009 Disaster Lessons Learned and Best Practices Report. December 2009. Available at http://www.fns.usda.gov/sites/default/files/2008 -2009_lessons.pdf, accessed February 17, 2015.

TABLE 11.5

Supplemental Nutrition Assistance Program Annual Summary, 2010–2014

Fiscal Year	Participation		Benefits Costs (Billions)	Average Monthly Benefit	
	Persons (Millions)	Households (Millions)		Per Person	Per Household
2014	46.5	22.7	$69.998	$125.35	$256.98
2013	47.6	23.1	$76.066	$133.07	$274.98
2012	46.6	22.3	$74.619	$133.41	$278.48
2011	44.7	21.1	$71.811	$133.85	$283.99
2010	40.3	18.6	$64.702	$133.79	$289.60
2009	33.5	15.2	$50.360	$125.31	$275.51
2008	28.2	12.7	$34.608	$102.19	$226.60

Source: US Department of Agriculture. Food and Nutrition Service. Program Data: Supplemental Nutrition Assistance Program. Annual State Level Data: FY 2009–2014. Available at http://www.fns.usda.gov/pd/supplemental-nutrition-assistance-program-snap, accessed February 15, 2015.

SNAP is an entitlement program; all those who qualify for benefits should receive them. The program provides a monthly benefit amount to eligible low-income families that can be used to purchase food. Eligibility for SNAP is based on household income and assets. Many able-bodied, childless, unemployed adults have time limits on their receipt of SNAP benefits.

Participation in SNAP generally peaks in periods of high unemployment, inflation, and recession. In 1994, participation reached an all-time high of 27.5 million before declining to about 17.2 million in 2000. By 2008, participation exceeded the 1994 rate at approximately 28.2 million and continued to increase annually through 2013, peaking at 47,636. As of 2014, participation had declined to 46,536, slightly less than participation in 2012. Table 11.5 illustrates SNAP participation from 2010 to 2014. In FY 2012, over half of SNAP participants were children or elderly. Forty-five percent of SNAP beneficiaries were children (under 18 years), 46% were non-elderly adults, and 9% were elderly adults (60 years and older) (Box 11.3) (Strayer et al. 2014).

Although SNAP is the federal name, state programs maintain flexibility to name the program on their own, though they are encouraged not to use FSP (US Department of Agriculture, http://www.fns.usda.gov/ORA/menu/Published/SNAP/SNAP.htm#Building). In fact, by March 2011, only seven states were using the name FSP: Alaska, Idaho, Indiana, Missouri, New Hampshire, New York, and Utah (US Department of Agriculture, http://www.fns.usda.gov/sites/default/files/state-chart.pdf). As of July 2013, Alaska, Idaho, Missouri, New Hampshire, and Utah still had not changed their programs' names.

Eligibility and Benefits

To be eligible to receive SNAP benefits, a household must meet certain standards regarding income and resources, work, and citizenship status. The amount of benefits an eligible household receives, called an *allotment*, depends on the age and number of people in the household and on the net monthly household income. Unless someone in the household is over 60 or receiving disability checks, a household may receive SNAP benefits if the gross income (before deductions) is 130% or less of the federal poverty level and net monthly income is 100% or less of federal poverty (US Department of Agriculture, http://www.fns.usda.gov/snap/eligibility).

Calculating the Maximum Monthly SNAP Benefit Allotment

The amount of benefits the household receives is known as an allotment. There are two steps for calculating the benefits for a household. First, the net monthly income of the household is multiplied

BOX 11.3 A BRIEF HISTORY OF SNAP

The SNAP program traces its origins to the Food Stamp Plan, which began in 1939 to help needy families during the Great Depression. A historical summary is available at http://www .fns.usda.gov/snap/rules/Legislation/about.htm. The modern program started as a pilot project in 1961 and was authorized as a permanent program in 1964. Expansion of the program occurred most dramatically after 1974, when Congress required all states to offer food stamps to low-income households. The legislation authorizing the current SNAP was enacted in 1977 (as the Food Stamp Act) and made significant changes in program regulations, such as tightening eligibility requirements and administration, and removing the requirement that food stamps be purchased by participants. Under the Food, Conservation, and Energy Act of 2008,[1] the food stamp program was officially renamed SNAP, and the Food Stamp Act of 1977 was renamed the Food and Nutrition Act of 2008. The name change was an effort to fight stigma, and reflected more recent updates made to the program, such as a focus on nutrition and an increase in benefit amounts. The Food, Conservation, and Energy Act of 2008 further increased program benefits and eligibility, as well as strengthened program integrity, simplified administration, maintained state flexibility, improved health through nutrition education, and improved access.

A history of US farm bills, including legislation, side-by-side comparisons, research articles, legislative histories, and other resources, can be found on the National Agricultural Law Center's website at http://www.nationalaglawcenter.org/farmbills/.

Source: [1]Food, Conservation, and Energy Act of 2008, Public Law 110-234, 122 Stat. (2008): 923–1551. Available at http://www.gpo.gov/fdsys/pkg/PLAW-110publ234/pdf/PLAW-110publ234.pdf, accessed January 18, 2015.

by 0.3 (because SNAP households are expected to spend about 30% of their resources on food). Next, the result is subtracted from the maximum allotment for the household size. See Table 11.6 for the allotment amounts per household size.

As an example, a household of three people with no income can receive up to $511 per month. For the most current maximum monthly allotments, go to the SNAP website on resources, income,

TABLE 11.6

SNAP Monthly Allotment by Household Size, October 1, 2014–September 30, 2015

People in Household	Maximum Monthly Allotment
1	$194
2	$357
3	$511
4	$649
5	$771
6	$925
7	$1022
8	$1169
Each additional person	$146

Source: US Department of Agriculture. Food and Nutrition Service. Supplemental Nutrition Assistance Program: Benefits. Available at http://www.fns.usda.gov/snap /eligibility, accessed February 15, 2015.

and benefits at http://www.fns.usda.gov/snap/eligibility. The income limits, maximum benefits, and calculation of benefits as well as current standards for eligibility to participate in the program are explained in detail on the SNAP website at http://www.fns.usda.gov/snap/.

In FY 2014, the average monthly per person benefits ranged from a low of $104.64 in Minnesota to a high of $225.38 in Hawaii (US Department of Agriculture, http://www.fns.usda.gov/sites /default/files/pd/18SNAPavg$PP.pdf). The states and territories with the highest average monthly household benefits were Guam ($583.75), Hawaii ($443.02), Alaska ($392.47), the Virgin Islands ($367.98), and California ($305.86) (US Department of Agriculture, http://www.fns.usda.gov/sites /default/files/pd/19SNAPavg$HH.pdf).

Using SNAP Benefits

The switch from paper coupons to EBT was completed nationwide in 2004, which helped increase program integrity, reduce fraud, and eliminate stigma. Each recipient household receives a plastic EBT card, similar to a bank debit card, which allows withdrawals for food purchases at any authorized SNAP retailer. Every month, the household's allotment is added to their EBT card; when benefits are posted, they are immediately available. SNAP benefits are accessed by swiping the EBT card at a point-of-sale terminal and entering a personal identification number (PIN). Funds are then transferred from the SNAP benefits account to the retailer's account.

SNAP recipients may only spend the amount in the account. Households can use their SNAP benefits to buy most foods, as well as seeds and plants that produce food for the household members to eat. Excluded items include alcoholic beverages, tobacco, pet foods, nonfood items (e.g., soap, paper products, household supplies), vitamin-mineral supplements, medicines, and hot foods and foods that will be eaten in the store. While the majority of SNAP benefits are redeemed in supermarkets and super stores, in some areas, restaurants can be authorized to accept SNAP benefits from qualified homeless, elderly, or disabled people in exchange for low-cost meals. In addition, the USDA authorizes farmers' markets, as well as direct marketing farmers and nonprofit food buying cooperatives that elect to do business via a community-supported agriculture (CSA) model, to accept EBT payments. Though they redeem less than 1% of all SNAP benefits nationwide, farmers' market redemptions increased 624% between FY 2007 and FY 2011, and the number of farmers' markets and direct marketing farmers increased 360% during that time (US Department of Agriculture 2011).

SNAP Quality Control

The EBT has been one of the most promising developments in the fight against SNAP benefit fraud because EBT creates an electronic record of each transaction, making fraud easier to detect. The USDA provides bonus awards to states whose compliance rate exceeds the national average; conversely, states with error rates greatly exceeding the national average pay cash sanctions. Effective management of SNAP helps ensure that those families and individuals most in need of nutrition assistance receive it, and the funds intended for this purpose are not diminished by waste or program abuse. To this end, the USDA monitors and works with all states to improve performance and assure that the SNAP quality control systems remain strong (*Supplemental Nutrition Assistance Program Quality Control Review Handbook* 2012).

To help support these efforts, FNS has undertaken several initiatives designed to increase payment accuracy, including

- Continued funding for state exchange activity.
- FNS national and regional payment accuracy conferences.
- Technical assistance to states.
- National and regional publications publicizing successful payment accuracy strategies implemented across the country.
- Continued examination of state agency application processes (*Supplemental Nutrition Assistance Program Quality Control Annual Report: Fiscal Year 2012* 2013).

In FY 2013, the payment error rate in SNAP was 3.20%, the lowest national payment error rate in the history of the program, the seventh year in a row that the error rate has been lower than the previous year (US Department of Agriculture and Food and Nutrition Service 2015), and well below the 4.18% target set by the US Office of Management and Budget (OMB) for 2013 (US Department of Agriculture, http://www.ocfo.usda.gov/usdasp/sp2010/StrategicPlanUpdate.pdf). The payment error rate is the sum of the overpayment and underpayment error rates.

The cost of overpayments, though small as a percentage of all payments (2.77 % in FY 2012, as an average across states, down from 2.99% in 2011), amounted to $2.1 billion in FY 2012. Similarly, the cost of underpayments—the value of benefits that should have been paid to eligible participants but were not—is small as a percentage of total payments (0.65%), although still substantial ($485 million). In 2012, the net cost to the government of erroneous payments—the cost of overpayments less the cost of underpayments—was over $1.5 billion (*Supplemental Nutrition Assistance Program Quality Control Annual Report: Fiscal Year 2012* 2013).

Virtually all (98%) households receiving SNAP are eligible for some benefit. The problem of erroneous payments is thus not as much an issue of determining eligibility as it is of correctly targeting benefits to the changing circumstances of low-income households. Neither overpayment nor underpayment errors have much effect on overall household purchasing power. In fact, most overpayments to eligible households are small relative to household income and official poverty standards. On average, 51 million individuals were eligible for SNAP benefits each month in FY 2012, and 42 million (83%) chose to participate. Thus, 17% of low-income people who would have qualified for SNAP did not participate in FY 2012, meaning that about 9 million people lost out on SNAP benefits (Eslami 2014).

The participation rate by individuals in SNAP is significant for communities as well, since every $1 in new SNAP benefits generates up to $1.80 in economic activity (US Department of Agriculture et al. 2012). Analysis by the FNS found that, if SNAP served an additional 5% of those eligible in FY 2009, 2.2 million more low-income people would have an additional $859 million in benefits per year, generating $1.5 billion in new economic activity nationwide (US Department of Agriculture, http://www.fns.usda.gov/snap/outreach/business-case.htm).

SNAP Participation

An important measure of a program's performance is its ability to reach its target population. Each year, FNS estimates the rate of participation in SNAP among those eligible for benefits. The participation rate is a ratio of the number of program participants to the number of eligible people. Counts of the number of participants are obtained from administrative records, and counts of the number of people eligible for benefits are estimated based on national survey data and a variety of other sources.

In 2011, participation rates were the highest for Maine, Oregon, and Washington with 100% of eligible individuals participating in SNAP; the District of Columbia and Michigan at 99% and Vermont at 97%. The lowest rates (61% or less) were found in Hawaii, California, and Wyoming (Cunnyngham 2014).

Outreach initiatives are being implemented to increase program participation by making more eligible people aware of SNAP. Although SNAP reaches 83% of eligible people, 96% of available benefits were provided, because individuals eligible for larger benefits tend to participate in SNAP at higher rates than those eligible for smaller benefits. As a result, SNAP appears to be reaching the neediest eligible individuals (Eslami 2014).

The Food and Nutrition Act of 2008 provides that state SNAP agencies have the opportunity to inform low-income households about the availability, eligibility requirements, application procedures, and benefits of SNAP and are reimbursed 50% for allowable administrative program costs of such informational activities (US Department of Agriculture and Food and Nutrition Services 2009). FNS also makes SNAP outreach materials available for free, including tool kits for community partners, SNAP agencies, and retailers; posters and flyers in English and Spanish; brochures and handouts in 37 different languages; suggestions for outreach activities; pre-screening tools; promising practices; photo gallery; and radio and television public service announcements. These resources are available at http://www.fns.usda.gov/snap/outreach/.

Two populations are of particular interest for increasing participation in SNAP, namely legal immigrants and the elderly.

- *Legal immigrants.* The eligibility rules for SNAP, including eligibility for legal nonciti-zens, changes from time to time. Since the inception of the current SNAP in 1977, undoc-umented immigrants and noncitizens in the United States temporarily, such as students, have not been eligible for benefits, although legal immigrants were eligible. The mid-1990s was a period of welfare reform, and major changes to the FSP were enacted through The Personal Responsibility and Work Opportunity Reconciliation Act of 1996 (PRWORA), including eliminating eligibility of most legal immigrants to food stamps (US Department of Agriculture, http://www.fns.usda.gov/snap/short-history-snap). However, by 2000, a quarter of low-income children in the United States had immigrant parents. In the major-ity of low-income immigrant families, the children were eligible for SNAP because they were citizens, whereas their parents were often barred from eligibility because they were undocumented or ineligible legal noncitizens. Thus, as part of the 2002 Farm Bill, SNAP was expanded to include noncitizen children, elders, and disabled individuals who entered the United States before enactment of the PRWORA in 1996 (Capps et al. 2004). FNS embarked on a major outreach initiative to publicize this change. Nevertheless, in FY 2012, the participation rate for eligible noncitizens was 56% compared to national rates of 83% among all eligible individuals (Eslami 2014). Information about SNAP policy for noncitizens who qualify outright or qualify after a certain waiting period is available on the SNAP website at http://www.fns.usda.gov/snap/snap-policy-non-citizen-eligibility.
- Although SNAP has special provisions to facilitate participation by low-income elderly people (US Department of Agriculture, http://www.fns.usda.gov/snap/applicant_recipients /eligibility.htm), the participation rate in FY 2012 was only 42% for eligible elderly (Eslami 2014). As indicated in Table 11.7, as the age of the individual increases, the rate of partici-pation in SNAP decreases. In 2012, only 42% of eligible older adults participated in the program, compared to 85% of eligible adults less than 60 years of age and 100% of eligible children under the age of 18 years (Eslami 2014). Low participation rates by seniors appear motivated by a low expected benefit level, lack of awareness regarding eligibility, and the use of other food assistance programs, such as group and home-delivered meals. Despite the low SNAP participation rate, elderly eligible nonparticipants are, on average, more food secure, spend more money on food, and eat more nutritiously than other participants (Yanyuan Wu 2009).

SNAP Nutrition Education

All 50 states, the District of Columbia, and the Virgin Islands provide nutrition education for SNAP recipients and other low-income individuals. The goal of SNAP Education (SNAP-Ed) is to increase the likelihood that people eligible to receive SNAP benefits will make healthy food choices within a limited budget and choose physically active lifestyles consistent with the current edition of the *Dietary Guidelines for Americans* and USDA food guidance (e.g., MyPlate). Under the Healthy, Hunger-Free Kids Act of 2010 (P.L. 111-296), Section 241, the federal government established SNAP-Ed as the Nutrition Education and Obesity Prevention Grant Program, which calls for SNAP-Ed to include an emphasis on obesity prevention. SNAP-Ed funds may be used for evidence-based activities delivered through individual and group-based strategies, comprehen-sive multilevel interventions, and/or community and public health approaches. USDA encourages

TABLE 11.7

Supplemental Nutrition Assistance Program Participation Rates for Individuals by Demographic Characteristics, 2012

	Participating (QC)	Eligible (CPS)	Participation Rate (QC/CPS)
Individuals in all households	42,129,048	50,708,090	83.08
Age of individual children under age 18	18,903,254	18,737,826	100.80
Preschool-age	6,270,986	5,929,889	105.75
School-age	12,632,268	12,807,937	98.63
Adults age 18–59	19,505,506	23,025,637	84.71
Elderly age 60 and over	3,720,288	8,944,627	41.59
Living alone	2,802,738	5,082,993	55.14
Living with others	917,551	3,861,634	23.76
Nondisabled childless adults subject to work registration	3,142,504	3,359,103	93.55
Noncitizens	1,556,861	2,795,163	55.70
Citizen children living with noncitizen adults	3,519,770	4,705,523	74.80
Employment status of nonelderly adults			
Employed	5,403,236	7,183,987	75.21
Not employed	14,102,269	15,841,650	89.02
Individuals by household composition			
Households with children	29,715,405	31,651,590	93.88
One adult	15,741,622	12,204,869	128.98
Married household head	7,293,357	11,430,877	63.80
Other households with children	6,680,427	8,015,844	83.34
Households without children	12,413,643	19,056,500	65.14
Gender of individual			
Male	18,328,080	22,387,840	81.87
Female	23,800,968	28,320,250	84.04
Metropolitan status			
Urban	33,858,282	41,243,154	82.09
Rural	8,270,766	9,464,936	87.38

Source: Eslami E. *Trends in Supplemental Nutrition Assistance Program Participation Rates: Fiscal Year 2010 to Fiscal Year 2012.* Washington, DC: Mathematica Policy Research, Inc.; 2014. Table A.3. Available at http://www.fns.usda .gov/sites/default/files/ops/Trends2010-2012.pdf, accessed February 15, 2015.

Note: Participating and eligible totals represent monthly averages. Participation rates over 100% are the result of discrepancies between the estimates of eligible and participating individuals and households, including the data from which they are estimated. The totals in this table do not include participants who received disaster assistance or were ineligible for SNAP. Also excluded are some categorically eligible participants who did not meet the federal SNAP income or asset rules. CPS: Current Population Survey; QC: quality control.

states to focus their efforts on three behavioral outcomes consistent with the *Dietary Guidelines for Americans*:

- Make half your plate fruits and vegetables, and at least half your grains whole grains, and switch to fat-free and low-fat milk and milk products.
- Increase physical activity and reduce time spent in sedentary behaviors as part of a healthy lifestyle.
- Maintain appropriate calorie balance during each stage of life—childhood, adolescence, adulthood, pregnancy and breastfeeding, and older age.

States may address other behavioral outcomes consistent with the goal and focus of SNAP-Ed and other *Dietary Guidelines for Americans* principles such as consuming smaller portions, drinking fewer sugary beverages, and reducing sodium, but the primary emphasis should remain on establishing healthy eating habits and physically active lifestyles to promote health and prevent disease, including obesity (US Department of Agriculture 2015). In order to receive a grant for SNAP-Ed activities, a state agency must submit a SNAP-Ed plan that includes

- The methods the state will use to notify eligible individuals about the availability of SNAP-Ed activities.
- A description of the SNAP-Ed services to be provided and how the state will deliver those services.
- The methods the state will use to identify its target audience.
- A description of how the state will coordinate activities with national, state, and local nutrition education and health promotion initiatives and interventions.
- An operating budget for the federal FY.

Guidelines for developing the SNAP-Ed plan are detailed in the SNAP-Ed guidance report. A SNAP-Ed toolkit is also available to assist states in selecting appropriate, evidence-based obesity prevention interventions (US Department of Agriculture 2014). In 2010, $379.1 million in federal funds was approved for SNAP-Ed activities; the smallest grant was awarded to Vermont ($69,250) and the largest—nearly a third of all SNAP-Ed funds—to California ($118.9 million) (Box 11.4) (US Department of Agriculture, http://snap.nal.usda.gov/snap/ApprovedFederalFundsSNAP-Ed01202010.pdf).

SNAP-Ed providers are supported by the online resource system known as the SNAP-Ed Connection, funded by the FNS of the USDA and maintained by the National Agricultural Library's Food and Nutrition Information Center (FNIC) in collaboration with the University of Maryland. The SNAP-Ed Connection provides information on training and continuing education resources; curricula, lesson plans, and other education materials developed for low-income families; recipes appropriate for low-income audiences; photographs for nutrition education and outreach materials; and a semi-annual e-Bulletin detailing programmatic updates and success stories from state and implementing agencies (US Department of Agriculture, http://snap.nal.usda.gov/about-snap-ed-connection-0).

School Food Programs

School food programs include the NSLP, the SBP, afterschool snacks, and summer feeding programs. Feeding the nation's children is a daunting task, primarily administered by the USDA, with some assistance from the DoD. Many meals are subsidized based on children's income eligibility, and there is a movement to introduce universal free breakfast in all schools. All meals served through these programs must meet minimum nutrition standards. Team Nutrition within the USDA provides assistance in improving nutrition and nutrition education. Alternative sources of food, such as locally grown produce, are being investigated to aid in the effort to improve food quality (Box 11.5).

National School Lunch Program

Although school food service began in the United States as long ago as the mid-1850s (Gunderson 1971), it was not until 1946 that the National School Lunch Act (NSLA) (US Social Security Administration 1946) authorized the NSLP. The NSLA asserts that national security depends on encouraging the domestic consumption of nutritious agricultural commodities and safeguarding the health and well-being of the nation's children (Box 11.6). Indeed, it has been stated repeatedly that the NSLP legislation came about in response to the claims that many American men had been rejected for World War II military service because of diet-related health problems (Fox et al. 2004b).

**BOX 11.4   DETERMINATION OF STATE ALLOCATIONS
FOR SNAP-ED GRANTS, FY 2013 AND BEYOND**

FNS will allocate SNAP-Ed grants by

- Determining annually each state's share of the $375 million allocated for SNAP-Ed for FY 2011.
- Adjusting grant allocations for inflation from FY 2012 and annually thereafter.
- Allocating the available funding each FY using a formula that factors in state shares of the base 2009 federal SNAP-Ed expenditures, building annually to a 50/50 weighting of expenditures to national SNAP participation from FY 2014 to FY 2018 and beyond.

State allocations for SNAP-Ed grants were determined for FY 2013 and beyond follows:

- For FY 2013, the state's percentage of national SNAP-Ed expenditures for FY 2009, as reported in February 2010.
- For FY 2014, 90% based on the state's percentage of national SNAP-Ed expenditures for FY 2009, as reported in February 2010, plus 10% based on the state's percentage of national SNAP participation for the 12-month period February 1, 2012 to January 31, 2013.
- For FY 2015, 80% based on the state's percentage of national SNAP-Ed expenditures for FY 2009, as reported in February 2010, plus 20% based on the state's percentage of national SNAP participation for the 12-month period February 1, 2013 to January 31, 2014.
- For FY 2016, 70% based on the state's percentage of national SNAP-Ed expenditures for FY 2009, as reported in February 2010, plus 30% based on the state's percentage of national SNAP participation for the 12-month period February 1, 2014 to January 31, 2015.
- For FY 2017, 60% based on the state's percentage of national SNAP-Ed expenditures for FY 2009, as reported in February 2010, plus 40% based on the state's percentage of national SNAP participation for the 12-month period February 1, 2015 to January 31, 2016.
- For FY 2018 and thereafter, 50% based on the state's percentage of national SNAP-Ed expenditures, plus 50% based on the state's percentage of national SNAP participation for the previous 12-month period ending January 31.

Source: Federal Register. 78 (66) April 5, 2013. Available at http://www.gpo.gov/fdsys/pkg/FR-2013-04-05/xml /FR-2013-04-05.xml. Accessed February 15, 2015.

School lunch, the oldest and second largest of the USDA's food assistance programs, is the cornerstone of the largely school-based child nutrition programs. The NSLA has been amended numerous times. In 2000, the National School Lunch Act of 1946 was renamed the Richard B. Russell National School Lunch Act in recognition of the senator from Georgia who proposed the legislation and played a key role leading to its passage by Congress and ultimate approval by President Truman. In 2010, the Healthy, Hunger-Free Kids Act (US Government Publishing Office 2010) amended the Richard B. Russell National School Lunch Act and the Child Nutrition Act of 1966. The NSLP is celebrated each year during the National School Lunch Week during the week beginning on the second Sunday of October.

BOX 11.5   TEAM NUTRITION

Team Nutrition is an initiative of the FNS to promote the nutritional health of the nation's school children. Team Nutrition supports the child nutrition programs through three strategies: (1) training and technical assistance for foodservice professionals to enable them to prepare and serve nutritious and appealing meals; (2) nutrition education in schools to reinforce positive nutrition messages and encourage students to make healthy food and physical activity choices; and (3) building school and community support for creating healthy school environments. The nutrition education messages and materials developed by Team Nutrition can be used consistently throughout the country and focus on five behavior outcomes: (1) eat a variety of foods; (2) eat more fruits, vegetables, and grains; (3) eat lower fat foods more often; (4) get your calcium-rich foods; and (5) be physically active. Nutrition education messages are delivered through six reinforcing communication channels to reach children where they live, learn, and play, as well as the adults who care for them: food service initiatives, classroom activities, school-wide events, home activities, community programs and events, and media events and coverage. Resources such as graphics, brochures, newsletters, posters, nutrition education materials, and training and technical assistance manuals are available for download and/or upon request from the Team Nutrition website at http://teamnutrition.usda.gov/.

Source: US Department of Agriculture. Food and Nutrition Service. Team Nutrition. Available at http://www.fns .usda.gov/tn/join-team, accessed January 8, 2015.

BOX 11.6   COMMODITY PROGRAMS

The commodity program began in the early 1930s as an outgrowth of federal agricultural policies designed to increase the revenue that farmers received from their produce. By buying large quantities of food and, thus, removing large quantities of food from the open market, government was able to keep prices up while making food available to feed people whose jobs were lost during the Depression. Through its commodity programs, the USDA still helps farmers while providing food to people in need. Currently, the USDA supports farmers by purchasing foods that are surplus or in need of price support, and then makes these commodities available to schools and other outlets to feed children, the elderly, and the needy.

Source: US Department of Agriculture. Food and Nutrition Service. Food Distribution Programs History and Background. Available at http://www.fns.usda.gov/fdd/aboutfd/history.htm, accessed January 24, 2015.

Public and nonprofit private schools and residential child care institutions may participate in the NSLP. The program operates in public and nonprofit private schools and residential child care institutions. Nutritionally balanced meals are provided to children each school day. The meals must be available at no cost or for a reduced price for children who meet certain income levels. After-school snacks are also offered in sites that meet eligibility requirements. Schools that offer school lunch receive cash reimbursements and donated foods from the USDA for each meal served meeting federal nutrition requirements. In 2008, virtually all public schools and 94% of public and private schools combined participated in the program nationwide (Ralston et al. 2008).

Participation in the program varies with income and age; students certified to receive free or reduced-price meals are more likely to participate than those who are not certified to receive meal benefits, and elementary school children participate at a greater rate than secondary school students (Fox and Condon 2012). Students eligible for free lunches and snacks are those from families with incomes at or below 130% of the federal poverty guidelines, as outlined in Table 11.8. Of

TABLE 11.8

USDA Food and Nutrition Service FY 2015 Income Eligibility Guidelines Effective from July 1, 2014 to June 30, 2015

Household Size	130% Federal Poverty Guideline					Household Size	185% Federal Poverty Guideline				
	Annual	Monthly	Twice per Month	Every Two Weeks	Weekly		Annual	Monthly	Twice per Month	Every Two Weeks	Weekly
1	15,171	1265	633	584	292	1	21,590	1800	900	831	416
2	20,449	1705	853	787	394	2	29,101	2426	1213	1120	560
3	25,727	2144	1072	990	495	3	36,612	3051	1526	1409	705
4	31,005	2584	1292	1193	597	4	44,123	3677	1839	1698	849
5	36,283	3024	1512	1396	698	5	51,634	4303	2152	1986	993
6	41,561	3464	1732	1599	800	6	59,145	4929	2465	2275	1138
7	46,839	3904	1952	1802	901	7	66,656	5555	2778	2564	1282
8	52,117	4344	2172	2005	1003	8	74,167	6181	3091	2853	1427
Each additional family member	5278	440	220	203	102	Each additional family member	7511	626	313	289	145

Source: Adapted from Federal Register 79(43) March 2014. Available at http://www.fns.usda.gov/sites/default/files/2014-04788.pdf, accessed February 15, 2015.

the 5 billion lunches served in school year (SY) 2014, 63.5% were served free and 8.0% to children who paid a reduced price (Box 11.7) (US Department of Agriculture, http://www.fns.usda.gov /pd/36slmonthly.htm).

Those eligible for reduced-price lunches and snacks are from families with incomes between 130% and 185% of poverty. (For SY 2014–2015, 130% of the poverty level was $31,005 for a family of 4; 185% was $44,123.) Children eligible for reduced-price meals cannot be charged more than $0.40 per lunch. All other children pay full price, which is less than the retail value of the meal, because all meal service programs that participate in the NSLP must operate on a nonprofit basis. Afterschool snacks are provided to children on the same income eligibility basis as school meals. However, in schools where at least 50% of students are eligible for free or reduced-price meals, snacks may be served for free (US Department of Agriculture, http://www.fns.usda.gov/sites /default/files/NSLPFactSheet.pdf).

Federal Assistance

The program is administered by the FNS on the national level, by state agencies (usually state departments of education) at the state level, and by school districts at the local level. States receive federal reimbursement and other assistance in establishing, maintaining, and operating the program. State agencies provide local districts with reimbursements and monitor their programs. Federal assistance is provided in the form of cash reimbursement and commodity food donation.

- *Cash reimbursements.* The cash reimbursements schools receive are based on the number of lunches and snacks, established reimbursement rates, and poverty level of participating students. A cash subsidy is provided for every program lunch and snack served. Additional cash subsidies are provided for children who qualify for free or reduced-price meal benefits. During SY 2014–2015, reimbursement rates were $2.93 for free lunches, $2.53 for reduced-price lunches, and $0.28 for children who paid full price for their meals. Snacks were reimbursed at rates of $0.80, $0.40, and $0.07, respectively. Schools that are certified to be in compliance with the updated meals requirements will receive an additional 6 cents for each meal served. This bonus will be adjusted for inflation in subsequent years. Higher reimbursement rates are also provided to Alaska and Hawaii, and for schools with high percentages of low-income students (60% or more of the students receive free or reduced price meals) (US Department of Agriculture, http://www.fns.usda.gov/sites/default/files /NSLPFactSheet.pdf).

BOX 11.7   MEASURING POVERTY

There are two slightly different versions of the federal poverty measure.

- *Poverty thresholds* are the original version of the federal poverty measure. The thresholds are updated each year by the Census Bureau and are used mainly for statistical purposes—for instance, preparing estimates of the number of Americans in poverty each year.
- *Poverty guidelines* are the other version of the federal poverty measure. They are issued each year in the Federal Register by the HHS. The guidelines are a simplification of the poverty thresholds for use for administrative purposes—for instance, determining financial eligibility for certain federal programs.

Source: US Department of Health and Human Services. Office of the Assistant Secretary for Planning and Evaluation. 2015 Poverty Guidelines. Available at http://aspe.hhs.gov/poverty/15poverty.cfm, accessed February 15, 2015.

- *Commodities.* Schools are entitled to receive commodity foods, called *entitlement foods*, at a value of 23.25 cents for each meal served in FY 2012–2013. Schools can also get *bonus* commodities—considered those over and above entitlement foods—as they become available through agricultural surpluses. They are then offered to states on a fair-share basis and do not count against a state's regular entitlement dollars. The type and quantity of bonus commodities distributed by the USDA in a given year are dictated by agricultural surpluses and market conditions. Commodity foods include more than 180 different kinds of products. Entitlement foods available in SY 2013–2014 for the Schools/Child Nutrition Commodity Programs included fruits and vegetables, meats, eggs, fish, dry and canned beans, cheese, vegetable oils, rice, pasta products, flour, and other grain products (US Department of Agriculture, http://www.fns.usda.gov/fdd/mobile/foods-available/foods-available-list.html).

Over the years, the USDA has worked to improve the quality and nutritional content of the products it purchases. In 1980, it required that all fruits be packed in light syrup or natural juices, and also eliminated the use of tropical oils for all its products. In 1985, consistent with the School Meals Initiative for Healthy Children, which stipulates that the NSLP meals must not only provide one-third of recommended nutrients but also be consistent with the *Dietary Guidelines for Americans*, the department promoted the development of new products that were lower in fat, such as beef patties with a 10–11% fat content and bulk ground beef and bulk ground pork with the fat content lowered from 22–24% to 17–19%; increased its offerings of poultry products; and added new lower fat items such as ground turkey and turkey sausage, reduced-fat cheddar cheese, *lite* mozzarella cheese, canned salsa, and fully cooked beef patties. In 1993–1994, the USDA more than doubled the quantity of a variety of fresh fruits and vegetables distributed to schools (US Department of Agriculture and Farm Service Agency 1995).

Nutrition Standards

Meals served under the NSLP have historically been required to meet specific federal nutrition standards in order to qualify for federal and state cash reimbursements and federal commodities. Under the Healthy, Hunger-Free Kids Act of 2010 (HHFKA), the USDA was directed to update the NSLP's meal pattern and nutrition standards (the first major changes in school meals in 15 years) based on the latest *Dietary Guidelines for Americans*. The new meal pattern increases the availability of fruits, vegetables, and whole grains on the school menu; sets calorie limits to ensure age-appropriate meals; and gradually reduces the sodium content of meals. Table 11.9 lists the nutrition standards by school grade, which went into effect at the beginning of SY 2012–2013. Although school lunches must meet these federal standards, local schools or districts make the decisions about what foods to serve and how to prepare them.

Obesity Prevention

The increase in childhood obesity and reduction in physical activity is leading to a number of health problems for many children. Once they occur, some of these health problems will follow children into adulthood. Many of these problems can be prevented or alleviated by improved nutrition. The HHFKA (US Government Publishing Office 2010) calls for a number of initiatives to address childhood obesity prevention. Designed to improve nutrition in school meals programs, the act

- Requires USDA to establish updated meal pattern regulations and nutrition standards for the school lunch program.
- Provides an additional 6 cents per lunch for schools that are certified to be in compliance with the new meal pattern regulation.
- Removes the previous requirement that schools serve milk in a variety of fat contents and instead requires that schools offer a variety of fluid milk consistent with the *Dietary Guidelines for Americans*.

TABLE 11.9

Nutrition Standards in the National School Lunch and School Breakfast Programs

	Breakfast Meal Pattern			Lunch Meal Pattern		
Meal Pattern	Grades K–5	Grades 6–8	Grades 9–12	Grades K–5	Grades 6–8	Grades 9–12
Amount of Food[a] Per Week (Minimum per Day)						
Fruits (cups)[b,c]	5 (1)[d]	5 (1)[d]	5 (1)[d]	2 1/2 (1/2)	2 1/2 (1/2)	5 (1)
Vegetables (cups)[b,c]	0	0	0	3 3/4 (3/4)	3 3/4 (3/4)	5 (1)
Dark green[e]	0	0	0	1/2	1/2	1/2
Red/orange[e]	0	0	0	3/4	3/4	1 1/4
Beans/peas (legumes)[e]	0	0	0	1/2	1/2	1/2
Starchy[e]	0	0	0	1/2	1/2	1/2
Other[e,f]	0	0	0	1/2	1/2	3/4
Additional veg to reach total[g]	0	0	0	1	1	1 1/2
Grains (oz. eq.)[h]	7–10 (1)	8–10 (1)	9–10 (1)	8–9 (1)	8–10 (1)	10–12 (2)
Meats/meat alternates (oz. eq.)	0[i]	0[i]	0[i]	8–10 (1)	9–10 (1)	10–12 (2)
Fluid milk (cups)[j]	5 (1)	5 (1)	5 (1)	5 (1)	5 (1)	5 (1)
Other Specifications: Daily Amount Based on the Average for a 5-Day Week						
Min-max calories (kcal)[k,l]	350–500	400–550	450–600	550–650	600–700	750–850
Saturated fat (% total calories)[l]	<10	<10	<10	<10	<10	<10
Sodium (mg)[l,m]	≤430	≤470	≤500	≤640	≤710	≤740
Trans fat[l]	Nutrition label or manufacturer specifications must indicate zero grams of trans fat per serving					

Source: US Department of Agriculture. Food and Nutrition Service. Final Rule Nutrition Standards in the National School Lunch and School Breakfast Programs, January 2012. Available at http://www.fns.usda.gov/cnd/Governance /Legislation/dietaryspecs.pdf, accessed February 15, 2015.

[a] Food items included in each food group and subgroup and amount equivalents. Minimum creditable serving is 1/8 cup.

[b] One-quarter cup of dried fruit counts as 1/2 cup of fruit; 1 cup of leafy greens counts as 1/2 cup of vegetables. No more than half of the fruit or vegetable offerings may be in the form of juice. All juice must be 100% full strength.

[c] For breakfast, vegetables may be substituted for fruits, but the first two cups per week of any such substitution must be from the dark green, red/orange, beans, and peas (legumes) or "Other vegetables" subgroups as defined in §210.10(c)(2)(iii).

[d] The fruit quantity requirement for the SBP (5 cups/week and a minimum of 1 cup/day) is effective July 1, 2014 (SY 2014–2015).

[e] Larger amounts of these vegetables may be served.

[f] This category consists of "Other vegetables" as defined in §210.10(c)(2)(iii)(E). For the purposes of the NSLP, "Other vegetables" requirement may be met with any additional amounts from the dark green, red/orange, and beans/peas (legumes) vegetable subgroups as defined in §210.10(c)(2)(iii).

[g] Any vegetable subgroup may be offered to meet the total weekly vegetable requirement.

[h] All grains must be whole grain-rich in both the NSLP and the SBP beginning July 1, 2014 (SY 2014–2015).

[i] There is no separate meat/meat alternate component in the SBP. Schools may substitute 1 oz. eq. of meat/meat alternate for 1 oz. eq. of grains after the minimum daily grains requirement is met.

[j] Fluid milk must be low fat (1% milk fat or less, unflavored) or fat-free (unflavored or flavored).

[k] The average daily amount of calories for a 5-day school week must be within the range (at least the minimum and no more than the maximum values).

[l] Discretionary sources of calories (solid fats and added sugars) may be added to the meal pattern if within the specifications for calories, saturated fat, trans fat, and sodium. Foods of minimal nutritional value and fluid milk with fat content greater than 1% milk fat are not allowed.

[m] Final sodium specifications are to be reached by SY 2022–2023 or July 1, 2022. Intermediate sodium specifications are established for SY 2014–2015 and 2017–2018. See required intermediate specifications in §210.10(f)(3) for lunches and §220.8(f)(3) for breakfast.

- Requires schools to make free potable water available where meals are served.
- Requires USDA to establish regulations for local school wellness policies and to provide technical assistance to states and schools in consultation with the US Department of Education and the Centers for Disease Control and Prevention. Local school wellness policies must include, at a minimum
  - Goals for nutrition promotion and education, physical activity, and other school-based activities that promote student wellness.
  - Nutrition guidelines for all foods available on each school campus during the school day that are consistent with federal regulations and that promote student health and reduce childhood obesity.
  - A requirement allowing parents, students, school food representatives, physical education teachers, school health professionals, the school board, school administrators, and the general public to participate in the development, implementation, and review and update of the local school wellness policy.
  - A requirement that the public be informed about the content, implementation, and periodic assessment of the local school wellness policy.
- Requires USDA to establish science-based nutrition standards for all foods sold in schools at any time during the school day outside the school meals programs (allows exemptions for school-sponsored fundraisers if the fundraisers are approved by the school and are infrequent).
- Requires local educational agencies to report in a clear and accessible manner information about the school nutrition environment to USDA and to the public, including information on food safety inspections, local wellness policies, school meal program participation, nutritional quality of program meals, etc.
- Establishes an organic food pilot program that provides competitive grants to schools for programs to increase the quantity of organic foods provided to schoolchildren.
- Requires USDA to identify, develop, and disseminate model product specifications and practices for food offered in school programs. USDA must analyze the quantity and quality of nutrition information available to schools about food products and commodities and submit a report to Congress on the results of the study and recommend legislative changes necessary to improve access to information.
- Requires USDA to provide technical assistance and competitive grants that do not exceed $100,000 to schools, state and local agencies, Indian tribal organizations (ITOs), agricultural producers, and nonprofit entities for farm-to-school activities. The federal share of project costs cannot exceed 75% of the total cost of the project.
- Requires USDA to establish a program of required education, training, and certification for school food service directors; criteria and standards for selection of School Nutrition State Agency Directors; and required training and certification for local school food service personnel (US Government Publishing Office 2010).

Alternative Sources of School Food

In the mid-1990s, farm-to-cafeteria programs began to arise in response to dissatisfaction with the quality of the food provided by the NSLP (Okie 2005), the proliferation of *competitive foods* in schools, and a concern about the impact of conventional agricultural practices on the environment. Complementary movements and initiatives include school gardens, farm-to-preschool, and farm-to-college programs.

Farm-to-cafeteria is defined as a program (and movement) to serve locally produced foods from area farmers in institutional cafeterias. Farm-to-cafeteria programs are seen as a huge win: farmers benefit from increased business; the community is able to keep money within the region; and consumers enjoy the taste, freshness, and nutrients of local produce (WhyHunger, http://www.whyhunger.org/getinfo/showArticle/articleId/92). In 2013, 2470 school districts in all 50 states were operating an estimated 2571 farm-to-school programs, up from 400 programs in 2004, 6 in 2001, and 2 in the 1996–1997 SY (Martinez et al. 2010).

Interest in local foods has also grown from the environmental movement, which considers long-distance transportation of foods as a contributor to greenhouse gas emissions, as well as consumers' interests in better understanding the origin of their foods (Martinez et al. 2010). Thus, the movement is not simply about food and nutrition but also about education and care of the environment. Taste, nutrition, and protection of the environment are considerations in food service. How foods are grown and how livestock is treated matter. For example, grass-fed lambs have a distinctly different flavor from that of corn-fed lambs raised in feedlots. When buying from local farmers, food service directors and chefs can talk directly to farmers about their farming practices. In addition, transportation from local venues uses less fossil fuel, and the food remains fresh and flavorful. Quality produce may cost more up front, but if it results in less plate waste, it can end up being less expensive (Biemiller 2005). One Washington state school district found increased consumption of fresh fruits and vegetables by both elementary school students and staff after introducing a salad bar offering locally grown, organic food (Flock et al. 2003).

Whereas a limited number of studies have found organic and sustainably grown food to be higher in antioxidants (Benbrook 2005), iron, magnesium, and phosphorous than conventionally grown foods, and lower in levels of nitrates and heavy metals (Worthington 2001), Gussow (1996) and Nestle (2006) contend that organically grown produce are better, not necessarily for nutritional reasons, but rather owing to the fact that organic farming conserves natural resources and reduces pollution of air, water, and soil (Box 11.8).

Issues that arise in farm-to-cafeteria programs in K-12 schools include obtaining funds to support farm-to-school initiatives and infrastructure (food service staff trainings, student educational activities, equipment, etc.); understanding USDA's school food procurement requirements; building farm-to-school stakeholder networks to facilitate community, share experience, and build relationships; increasing awareness of existing USDA efforts to support local and regional food systems; and developing evaluation systems to measure the impact of farm-to-school programs on farmers, school food service, and students' health and behaviors (US Department of Agriculture et al. 2011). The sample programs described next have each addressed some of these issues in various ways.

- *New North Florida Cooperative Association, Inc.*—begun in 1995 and the granddaddy of the farm-to-school movement, this collective of farmers in Florida, Georgia, Alabama, Mississippi, and Arkansas sells washed, cut, and packaged vegetables to local school districts. Since it began the farm-to-school program, the cooperative has served over 1 million students in 72 school districts. At any given time, 60–100 farmers are involved in the cooperative, and in each case, the farmer is connected with the local school district or the one that is closest to the farmer's operation. Start-up resources included several loans and grants, and since 2002, the cooperative has funded itself through direct sales and consulting work. A key to the cooperative's success is in the offering of minimally processed, value-added products that do not require additional washing or cutting by the food service

---

BOX 11.8   BUY LOCAL CONCEPTS

- *Sustainability*—the ability to provide for the needs of the current population without damaging the ability of future generations to provide for themselves. A sustainable process can be carried out again and again without negative environmental effects or exorbitant cost to anyone involved.
- *Buy local*—a green politics goal of buying locally produced goods and services, paralleling the phrase *think globally, act locally*.
- *Food miles*—the distance food travels from where it is grown or raised to where consumers purchase it, an indicator for the environmental impact of the food and its components.

staff. These products—such as raw sweet potato sticks, bagged and washed collard greens, peas, ground goat meat, strawberries, blackberries, watermelon, okra, turnip greens, and green beans—are primarily used as side dishes to the main entrée. The cooperative is also involved in educational work with the farmers and at the schools.

- *Farm-to-School Salad Bar Program, Riverside, California*—launched in 2005, the Farm-to-School Salad Bar Program began at Jefferson Elementary School with support from the California Endowment and in partnership with the Center for Food & Justice. The salad bar was started with grant funds, though it was later fully integrated into the school meal program and food service budget. Since its inception, the program has expanded to 29 of the district's 31 elementary schools. A daily salad bar is offered as an alternative to the hot lunch meal, and includes local fruits and vegetables such as lettuce, strawberries, broccoli, kiwi, spinach, apples, oranges, celery, cucumbers, and jicama. Commodity protein, dairy, and grain items are also available. Evaluation results show that the program has had a positive impact on schools, students, and farmers: school meal participation by both students and faculty has increased, leading to increased school revenues; about a quarter of students choose the salad bar lunch over hot lunch each day, and those that do take an average of almost one extra serving of fruits and vegetables per meal; and farmers are benefiting from increased revenues and school relationships.

- *Get Smart, Eat Local, NH Farm-to-School Program*—focusing on the procurement of just one local product, the NH farm-to-school program connects schools with state apple farmers. Because apples and apple cider do not require significant washing or prepping, no major changes to kitchen infrastructure or staffing were required at the school level. In addition, the cost of buying New Hampshire apples was negotiated so that it was not higher than other available sources. Since the program's inception in 2003, students have started identifying apples as a NH product, and the number of schools ordering apples and cider has increased to over 300. Some schools are also purchasing other local products, such as greens, root vegetables, berries, and honey. Starting in 2006, the NH farm-to-school program launched a pilot to work with eight seacoast NH school districts to make more direct links with local growers and increase the amount of locally grown foods served at the schools (Joshi et al. 2006).

School Gardens. Arguably the jewel in the crown of the farm-to-cafeteria movement, school gardens provide experiential learning, increased physical activity, and a source of fresh food (Gottlieb and Azuma, http://www.niehs.nih.gov/about/visiting/events/pastmtg/assets/docs_n_z /supplementary_informationoverviewgottlieb.pdf). A study of elementary school gardeners in Wisconsin found an increased willingness among children to try new fruits and vegetables compared to nongardeners (Meinen et al. 2012). A separate study of second graders found that students receiving both nutrition education and hands-on gardening were more likely to choose and consume vegetables in the school lunch than those receiving nutrition education only (Parmer et al. 2009).

- *Edible Schoolyard*—Established in Berkeley, California, in 1995 with the help and vision of Alice Waters, this one-acre, asphalt-coated abandoned lot next to a middle school was transformed into an oasis of seasonal produce, herbs, vines, berries, and flowers, surrounded by fruit trees. The garden is wholly integrated into the school's curriculum and lunch program. This approach fosters awareness and appreciation for nourishment, the community, and stewardship of the land. Since the founding of the Edible Schoolyard Berkeley, six additional Edible Schoolyard programs have been established in cities such as Greensboro, North Carolina; Lake Placid, New York; Los Angeles; New Orleans; New York City; and San Francisco (The Edible Schoolyard Project, http://edibleschoolyard.org/).

Farm to Pre-School. An expansion of the farm-to-school model, farm-to-preschool programs serve a variety of early child care settings: preschools, Head Start, daycare centers, programs in

K–12 school districts, nurseries, and family home care facilities. Program goals include influencing the eating habits of young children when their food preferences are forming; creating healthy lifestyles through good nutrition and experiential opportunities (e.g., gardening); improving healthy food access at home and within the community; and influencing policies to address childhood obesity. Farm-to-preschool programs may include sourcing local foods for school meals and snacks; promoting and increasing access to local foods for child care providers and families; offering nutrition and/or garden-based curricula; school gardening; food preparation demonstrations and taste testing; field trips to farms, farmers' markets, and community gardens; parent workshops; and influencing policies at the local, state, or national level (Farm to Preschool, http://www.farmtopreschool .org/whatisfarmtopreschool.html). A description of successful farm-to-preschool programs is provided by the Farm to Preschool subcommittee of the National Farm to School Network at http:// www.farmtopreschool.org/programmodels.html.

Farm-to-college programs. Like farm-to-school programs, farm-to-college programs connect institutions of higher education with area producers to provide local farm products for campus meals and events. Over 175 schools have farm-to-college programs. Nearly 4000 students at more than 350 universities and schools have joined the Real Food Challenge since 2008, a campaign to increase the procurement of *real food* on college and university campuses. In the fall of 2011, the Real Food Campus Commitment campaign started with the aim of getting campuses to formally commit to a 20% real food goal by 2020 (California Student Sustainability Coalition, http://www .sustainabilitycoalition.org/projects/west-coast-real-food-challenge). Unlike K–12 schools, colleges are more active throughout the year, allowing them to take advantage of the summer growing months. In addition, they are perhaps, among all academic institutions, most receptive to the potential public relations advantages of using locally and sustainably grown food; most able to meet potentially higher costs; and most likely to have receptive constituents (Box 11.9) (Murray 2005).

Barriers to change and some solutions. A number of barriers exist to farm-to-cafeteria programs. These include seasonality, a disjuncture between production capacity and supply requirements of institutions, and a workable payment mechanism. Purchasing locally grown food in the face of prime vendor agreements requires not only dedication to the concept but a solid understanding of the purchasing process. Liability insurance required by vendors can be prohibitive. Further, one-to-one purchasing and ordering take longer, and smaller nearby farms may not be able to offer competitive prices or the quantities needed by large institutions (Biemiller 2005).

Solutions to these barriers include menus that take seasonality into account, using produce such as onions and potatoes that have a stable shelf-life and are minimally processed, farm producer cooperatives to enhance efficiency and consistency, farm grower cooperatives to meet volume

---

BOX 11.9   THE YALE SUSTAINABLE FOOD PROJECT

The arrival at Yale University of Alice Waters' daughter Fanny (born 1983) meshed perfectly with the student organization Food from the Earth, whose members promoted organic food in the dining halls, a farm, and institutional composting. Out of this relationship emerged, in 2002, the Yale Sustainable Food Project, a joint endeavor of the university's dining services, students, faculty, and administrators. Designed to nourish the interconnected pleasures of growing, cooking, and sharing food, it is the Ivy League, college-level version of the Edible Schoolyard. The dining service actively develops working relationships with local farmers who promote the vitality of soil, seed, and ecosystem; ranchers who care for their livestock using humane and ecological methods; and food distributors who can trace their products to responsible sources.

Source: Yale University. Yale Sustainable Food Project. History. Available at http://www.yale.edu/sustainablefood /about_history.html, accessed January 20, 2015.

needs, and educating farmers about purchasing and billing procedures (Sullivan 2003). Overcoming *consumer reluctance* may be a matter of education. A study of 560 K–4 grade students found that after being taught about the history and lore of nutritious, plant-based foods, children in an intervention group ate between 3 and 20 times more new food than children in the control group. The students also proved to be agents of change in their families (Demas 1998).

Legislation. Several recent pieces of legislation contain provisions of importance for the farm-to-cafeteria movement. Section 4302 of the 2008 Farm Bill (Food, Conservation, and Energy Act of 2008, P.L. 110-234) (US Government Publishing Office 2008) requires that the Secretary of Agriculture encourage schools participating in the NSLP and SBP to purchase unprocessed, locally grown, and locally raised food to the maximum extent practicable and appropriate. This section also allows schools to use a geographic preference for the procurement of unprocessed agricultural products. Section 4303 of the same act establishes a pilot program for high-poverty schools that provide hands-on vegetable gardening and nutrition education as part of a school-based or summer program (US Government Publishing Office 2008).

Section 243 of the Healthy, Hunger-Free Kids Act of 2010 (P.L. 111-296) (US Government Publishing Office 2010) requires the Secretary of Agriculture to carry out a program to assist eligible schools, state and local agencies, ITOs, agricultural producers or groups of agricultural producers, and nonprofit entities through competitive grants and technical assistance to implement farm-to-school programs that improve access to local foods in eligible schools. These grants may be used for training, supporting operations, planning, purchasing equipment, developing school gardens, developing partnerships, and implementing farm-to-school programs.

School Breakfast Program

The Child Nutrition Act of 1966 established the SBP, a federally assisted meal program that provides nutritionally balanced, low- or no-cost breakfasts to children in public and nonprofit private schools and residential child care institutions. SBP began as a pilot project in 1966 and was made permanent in 1975. The program is administered at the federal level by the FNS. At the state level, the program is usually administered by state education agencies, which operate the program through agreements with local school food authorities in more than 89,000 schools and institutions. SBP operates in a similar manner as the NSLP. Generally, public or nonprofit private schools of high-school grade or under and public or nonprofit private residential child care institutions may participate. School districts and independent schools that choose to take part receive cash subsidies (but not commodity foods) from USDA for each meal they serve. In return, they must serve breakfasts that meet the federal requirements summarized in Table 11.9, and they must offer free or reduced price breakfasts to eligible children. Children from families with incomes at or below 130% of the federal poverty level are eligible for free meals. Those with incomes between 130% and 185% of the poverty level are eligible for reduced-price meals. Children from families with incomes over 185% of poverty pay full price, though their meals are still subsidized to some extent. The poverty guidelines are presented in Table 11.8 as previously noted.

Most of the support the USDA provides to schools in the SBP comes in the form of a cash reimbursement for each breakfast served. For SY 2012–2013, the basic cash reimbursement rates were $1.55, $1.25, and $0.27 for free, reduced-price, and paid breakfasts, respectively. Schools that are certified to be in compliance with the meal pattern requirements will receive an additional 6 cents for each meal served. This bonus will be adjusted for inflation in subsequent years. Higher reimbursement rates are also provided to Alaska and Hawaii, and for schools who qualify for higher *severe need* reimbursements—40% or more of their lunches are served free or at a reduced price. Severe need payments are up to 30 cents higher than the normal reimbursements for free and reduced-price breakfasts. About 77% of the breakfasts served in the SBP receive severe need payments. Schools may charge no more than 30 cents for a reduced-price breakfast. Schools set their own prices for breakfasts served to students who pay the full meal price (paid), though they must operate their meal services as nonprofit programs. Participation has slowly but steadily grown over the years from half a million in 1970 to 7.5 million in 2000. In FY 2011, over 12.1 million children participated every day. Of those, over 10.1 million received their meals free or at a reduced price. For FY 2011, the program cost $3.0 billion, up from $1.9 billion in FY 2005 (US Department of Agriculture, http://www.fns.usda.gov/sites/default/files/SBPfactsheet.pdf).

Section 105 of the Healthy, Hunger-Free Kids Act of 2010 (P.L. 111-296) (US Government Publishing Office 2010) authorizes appropriations for competitive grants to state educational agencies for subgrants to local education agencies to establish, maintain, or expand the SBP at qualifying schools. Priority will be given to local educational agencies with qualifying schools in which at least 75% of the students are eligible for free or reduced price lunches. Grants may be used to establish, promote, or expand an SBP of the qualifying school, including a nutritional education component; extend the period during which school breakfast is available at the qualifying school; provide school breakfast to students of the qualifying school during the school day; or for other appropriate purposes as determined by the Secretary of Agriculture.

Universal Free Breakfast

Fewer low-income children participate in the SBP than in the NSLP. There is concern that low-income children might be coming to school without eating breakfast and still not be participating in the SBP for a variety of reasons, including perceived stigma associating school breakfast participation with poverty. One approach to increasing participation in the SBP is to offer universal free breakfast to all students, regardless of their household income. This option, known as Provision 2, is usually offered at schools that have a high percentage (greater than 75%) of students who qualify for free or reduced price meals. Many schools find that using Provision 2 at breakfast increases participation, reduces stigma, improves attendance, and increases test scores (US Department of Agriculture, http://www.fns.usda.gov/sites/default/files/breakfast_talkingpoints.pdf).

In 2003, the New York City Department of Education, which serves almost a million meals a day, became one of the first large urban school districts to make school breakfast free to all students regardless of their ability to pay. Analysis of New York City's universal school breakfast policy indicates a considerable improvement in student participation across income levels: 5%, 20%, and 35% increase in breakfast participation among students eligible for free, reduced price, and paid meals, respectively. Growth in breakfast participation may be due to reduced stigma or an improvement in food quality or efficiency. In addition, there were small but significant gains in attendance for black students eligible for free school lunch and for Asian students not eligible for free lunch (Leos-Urbel et al. 2013).

Breakfast in Classroom

As another tactic to increase participation in the SBP, there is a growing trend toward breakfast in the classroom programs. This initiative provides universal free breakfast to all students, usually during homeroom. Students eat together in the classroom after the first bell, making it easier and more likely that students will participate. Little teaching time is lost, since breakfast takes only 10–15 minutes to eat and that time can be simultaneously used to take attendance, collect homework, make announcements, or read to the class. Many teachers feel this is a valuable use of time and that their classes are more productive when students have a healthy breakfast. The USDA provides additional strategies for increasing SBP participation at http://www.fns.usda.gov/cnd/breakfast/expansion/default.htm.

Summer Feeding Programs

Summer feeding programs were created to continue providing nutritious meals free of charge to children from low-income areas during periods when schools are closed for vacation. In both the SFSP and the Seamless Summer Feeding Option (SSO), the meals served must conform to federal nutrition and meal pattern requirement standards as illustrated in Table 11.10. The programs, which operate in low-income areas, may feed children through 18 years of age. The meals served are

TABLE 11.10
SFSP Meal Patterns

Breakfast

Select all three components for a reimbursable breakfast

One serving milk	
Fluid milk	1 cup
One serving fruit/vegetable	
Juice,[a] fruit, and/or vegetable	1/2 cup
One serving grains/bread[b]	
Bread or	1 slice
Cornbread or biscuit or roll or muffin or	1 serving
Cold dry cereal or	3/4 cup
Hot cooked cereal or	1/2 cup
Pasta or noodles or grains	1/2 cup

Snack

Select two of the four components for a reimbursable snack

One serving milk	
Fluid milk	1 cup
One serving fruit/vegetable	
Juice,[a,c] fruit, and/or vegetable	3/4 cup
One serving grains/bread[b]	
Bread or	1 slice
Cornbread or biscuit or roll or muffin or	1 serving
Cold dry cereal or	3/4 cup
Hot cooked cereal or	1/2 cup
Pasta or noodles or grains or	1/2 cup
One serving meat/meat alternate	
Lean meat or poultry or fish[d] or	1 oz.
Alternate protein product or	1 oz.
Cheese or	1 oz.
Egg or	1/2 large egg
Cooked dry beans or peas or	1/4 cup
Peanut or other nut or seed butters or	2 tbsp.
Nuts and/or seeds or	1 oz.
Yogurt[e]	4 oz.

Lunch or Supper

Select all four components for a reimbursable meal

One serving milk	
Fluid milk	1 cup
Two servings fruits/vegetables	
Juice,[a] fruit, and/or vegetable	3/4 cup
One serving grains/bread[b]	
Bread or	1 slice
Cornbread or biscuit or roll or muffin or	1 serving
Hot cooked cereal or	1/2 cup
Pasta or noodles or grains	1/2 cup
One serving meat/meat alternate	
Lean meat or poultry or fish[d] or	2 oz.

(Continued)

TABLE 11.10 (CONTINUED)
SFSP Meal Patterns

Alternate protein product or	2 oz.
Cheese or	2 oz.
Egg or	1 large egg
Cooked dry beans or peas or	1/2 cup
Peanut or other nut or seed butters or	4 tbsp.
Nuts and/or seeds[f] or	1 oz.
Yogurt[e]	8 oz.

Source: US Department of Agriculture. Food and Nutrition Service. Summer Food Service Program Meals and Snack Patterns. Available at http://www.fns.usda.gov/cnd/summer/Administration/meal_patterns.html, accessed February 15, 2015.

[a] Fruit or vegetable juice must be full strength.

[b] Breads and grains must be made from whole grain or enriched meal or flour. Cereal must be whole grain or enriched or fortified.

[c] Juice cannot be served when milk is the only other snack component.

[d] A serving consists of the edible portion of cooked lean meat or poultry or fish.

[e] Yogurt may be plain or flavored, unsweetened or sweetened.

[f] Nuts and seeds may meet only one-half of the total meat/meat alternate serving and must be combined with another meat/meat alternate to fulfill the lunch or supper requirement.

reimbursed based on the number of reimbursable meals served multiplied by the combined operating and administrative rate for that meal. For summer 2013, the maximum reimbursement rate per meal in the 48 contiguous states was $1.98 per breakfast, $3.47 per lunch or supper, and $0.82 per snack in self preparation-rural sites; and $1.94 per breakfast, $3.41 per lunch or supper, and $0.80 per snack in other types of sites (vended-urban) (US Department of Agriculture, http://www.fns.usda.gov/cnd/summer/FAQs.htm).

At most sites, children receive either one or two meals per day, with a snack counting as a meal option. Allowable meals may include breakfast, morning snack, lunch, afternoon snack, and supper. Up to two types of meals per day can be reimbursed (three for migrant sites and camps).

Summer Food Service Program

The SFSP is authorized under Section 13 of the NSLA (42 U.S.C. 1761). Although millions of children depend on nutritious free and reduced-price meals and snacks at school for 9 months out of the year, just a fraction of that receive the free meals provided by the SFSP. Federal resources are available for local sponsors who want to combine a feeding program with a summer activity program. All sponsors receive training before starting the program to learn how to plan, operate, and monitor a successful food service program. The payments that sponsors receive are based on the number of meals served and the documented costs of running the program. SFSP sponsors receive payments for serving healthy meals and snacks to children and teenagers, 18 years and younger, at approved sites in low-income areas. Schools, public agencies, and private nonprofit organizations may apply to sponsor the program. They include

- Public or private nonprofit schools.
- Units of local, municipal, county, tribal, or state government.
- Private nonprofit organizations.
- Public or private nonprofit camps.
- Public or private nonprofit universities or colleges.

Since 1969, the program has grown from 1200 sites serving 2.2 million meals at a cost of a third of a million dollars to 39,800 sites in 2012 serving 143.7 million meals at a cost of almost $400 million, which includes cash payments for meals served, sponsor administrative costs, state administrative expenses, and health inspection costs. In 2012, over 2.3 million children per day were served during the peak month of July (US Department of Agriculture, http://www.fns .usda.gov/sites/default/files/pd/sfsummar.pdf). More than one-third of the program's daily attendance was accounted for by four states: New York (458,966), Texas (177,981), Florida (155,570), and California (115,841), and New York alone accounts for about one-fifth of attendance (US Department of Agriculture, http://www.fns.usda.gov/pd/04sffypart.htm). Nevertheless, only one in seven of the low-income children who participated in school lunch during the school year participated in the summer feeding programs (both SFSP and SSO) in July 2012, due in large part to budget cuts at the state and local levels. As a result, the USDA made summer feeding a top priority, with the goal of serving 5 million more meals in summer 2013. USDA has taken a number of steps to achieve this goal, including

- Intensively targeting five states (Arkansas, California, Colorado, Rhode Island, and Virginia) and targeting support to another 10 states with significant room for growth (Alabama, Iowa, Kansas, Kentucky, Louisiana, Mississippi, Nevada, North Dakota, Oklahoma, and Texas).
- Bringing together national and state stakeholders to collaborate and strategize on ways to grow the summer feeding programs.
- Reaching out to potential new sponsors and sites through webinars, conference calls, and new outreach and informational materials.
- Holding its third annual SFSP Awareness Week (week of June 10th) to promote and raise awareness of the program.
- Utilizing social media to host twitter town halls with hunger organizations and others (Burke et al. 2013).

Seamless Summer Feeding Option

The SSO is a permanent option for school districts participating in the NSLP or SBP. In essence, schools operate SFSP as an extension of the NSLP. Authorized by the Child Nutrition and WIC Reauthorization Act of 2004, the option combines features of the NSLP, SBP, and SFSP, streamlining the administrative and monitoring requirements for operating in the school districts. The SSO is designed to reduce paperwork and administrative burden, making it easier for schools to feed children from low-income areas during the traditional summer vacation periods and for year-round schools, long school vacation periods (generally exceeding 2–3 weeks). School districts and nonschool settings must apply to operate an SSO Program. The various types of sites allowed to participate in this option include

- *Open sites*—all children eat free in communities where at least 50% of the children are eligible for free or reduced-price school meals.
- *Restricted open sites*—meet the open site criteria, but are later restricted for safety, control, or security reasons.
- *Closed enrolled sites*—may be in any community for an enrolled group of low-income children and meet the 50% criteria for open sites. This excludes academic summer schools.
- *Migrant sites*—serving children of migrant families.
- *Camps*—residential or nonresidential camps (US Department of Agriculture, http://www .fns.usda.gov/cnd/seamless_summer.htm).

All eligible meals provided under the SSO are paid at the NSLP/SBP applicable free rates and must follow the same meal patterns as those required by the NSLP/SBP. A comparison chart of how the SSO differs from the SFSP and NSLP/SBP can be found at http://www.fns.usda.gov/sites/default/files/SFSP_SeamlessComparisonChart.pdf.

The SSO Program began as a pilot program in California and Florida. It expanded to all states in 2002 and was originally set to end in 2004. However, in 2004, this program became a permanent option for school districts to operate a feeding program during the summer months.

Supplemental Nutrition Program for Women, Infants, and Children (WIC)

WIC serves to safeguard the health of low-income women, infants, and children up to age 5 years who are at nutritional risk by providing (1) nutritious foods to supplement diets (see Tables 11.11 and 11.12 describing the monthly packages of food); (2) nutrition education and counseling; and (3) screening and referrals to other health, welfare, and social services.

WIC was launched in 1972 to meet the special nutritional needs of low-income pregnant, breast-feeding, and postpartum non-breastfeeding women; infants; and children up to 5 years of age who are at nutritional risk. What started as a pilot project has expanded to serve all 50 states, the District of Columbia, Puerto Rico, Guam, American Samoa, the American Virgin Islands, Northern Mariana, and 34 ITOs. The 90 WIC state agencies administer the program through approximately 1836 local agencies and 9000 clinic sites.

WIC serves over half of all infants born in the United States, and more than 8.5 million people get WIC benefits each month. In 1974, the first year WIC was permanently authorized, 88,000 people participated. Average participation for FY 2014 was approximately 8.26 million (US Department of Agriculture, http://www.fns.usda.gov/pd/wisummary.htm). Children have always been the largest category of WIC participants. Of the 8.26 million people who received WIC benefits in FY 2014, more than half (4.32 million) were children and about a quarter each were infants (1.96 million) and women (1.97 million) (US Department of Agriculture, http://www.fns.usda.gov/pd/37WIC_Monthly.htm).

WIC's goal is to improve birth outcomes and support the growth and development of infants. WIC provides supplemental foods and nutrition education—including breastfeeding promotion and support—through payment of cash grants to state agencies that administer the program through local agencies at no cost to eligible persons. The program serves as an adjunct to good healthcare

---

TABLE 11.11
WIC Food Package—Maximum Monthly Allowances for Infants

Foods	Fully Formula-Fed Infants			Partially Breastfed Infants				Fully Breastfed Infants	
	0–3 Months	4–5 Months	6–11 Months	0–1 Month	1–3 Months	4–5 Months	6–11 Months	0–5 Months	6–11 Months
WIC Formula[a]	806 fl. oz.	884 fl. oz.	624 fl. oz.	1 can powder	364 fl. oz.	442 fl. oz.	312 fl. oz.		
Infant cereal			24 oz.				24 oz.		24 oz.
Baby food fruits and vegetables			128 oz.				128 oz.		256 oz.
Baby food meat									77.5 oz.

Source: Adapted from US Department of Agriculture. Food and Nutrition Service. WIC Program. Benefits and Services. SNAPSHOT of the WIC Food Packages—Maximum Monthly Allowances of Supplemental Foods for Infants. Available at http://www.fns.usda.gov/sites/default/files/Snapshot-WIC-InfantFoodPkgs.pdf, accessed February 15, 2015.

[a] Fluid ounces are based on reconstituted liquid concentrate.

TABLE 11.12
WIC Food Package—Maximum Monthly Allowances for Children and Women

	Children	Women		
Foods	Children 1–4 Years	Pregnant and Partially Breastfeeding (Up to 1 Year Postpartum)	Postpartum (Up to 6 Months Postpartum)	Fully Breastfeeding (Up to 1 Year Postpartum)
Juice, single strength	128 fl. oz.	144 fl. oz.	96 fl. oz.	144 fl. oz.
Milk[a]	16 qt.	22 qt.	16 qt.	24 qt.
Breakfast cereal[b]	36 oz.	36 oz.	36 oz.	36 oz.
Cheese				1 lb.
Eggs	1 dozen	1 dozen	1 dozen	2 dozen
Fruits and vegetables	$6.00 in cash value vouchers	$10.00 in cash value vouchers	$10.00 in cash value vouchers	$10.00 in cash value vouchers
Whole wheat bread[c]	2 lb.	1 lb.		1 lb.
Fish (canned)[d]				30 oz.
Legumes (dry or canned) and/or peanut butter	1 lb. (64 oz. canned) or 18 oz.	1 lb. (64 oz. canned) and 18 oz.	1 lb. (64 oz. canned) or 18 oz.	1 lb. (64 oz. canned) and 18 oz.

Source: Adapted from US Department of Agriculture. Food and Nutrition Service. WIC Program. Benefits and Services. SNAPSHOT of the WIC Food Packages—Maximum Monthly Allowances of Supplemental Foods for Children and Women. Available at http://www.fns.usda.gov/sites/default/files/Snapshot-WIC-Children-WomenFoodPkgs.pdf, accessed February 15, 2015.

[a] Allowable options for milk alternatives are cheese, soy beverage, and tofu.

[b] At least one half of the total number of breakfast cereals on state agency food lists must be whole grain.

[c] Allowable options for whole wheat bread are whole-grain bread, brown rice, bulgur, oatmeal, whole-grain barley, soft corn, or whole wheat tortillas.

[d] Allowable options for canned fish are light tuna, salmon, sardines, and mackerel.

during critical times of growth and development in order to prevent the occurrence of health problems and to improve the health status of the women, infants, and children identified at nutritional risk. WIC is supplementary to SNAP and any other program that distributes foods to needy families, such as soup kitchens, shelters, or other forms of emergency food assistance (Montana Department of Public Health and Human Services 2011).

Supplemental foods are made available monthly in the form of seven different WIC food packages. Most WIC participants access the food packages by redeeming vouchers or checks to obtain specific foods at participating retail outlets. The use of electronic cards is growing, and as a result of the Healthy, Hunger-Free Kids Act of 2010 (US Government Publishing Office 2010), all WIC state agencies are required to implement WIC EBT statewide by October 1, 2020. A few state agencies distribute WIC foods through warehouses or deliver foods to participants' homes (US Department of Agriculture, http://www.fns.usda.gov/sites/default/files/wic/wic-fact-sheet.pdf). WIC also provides nutrition counseling and referrals to health and other social services to participants at no charge.

WIC is not an entitlement program; that is, Congress does not set aside funds to allow every eligible individual to participate in the program. Instead, WIC is a federal grant program for which Congress authorizes a specific amount of funding each year for program operations. FNS, which administers the program at the federal level, provides these funds to WIC state agencies (state health departments or comparable agencies) to pay for WIC foods, nutrition counseling and education, and administrative costs. Eligible women and their infants and children must meet income guidelines, a state residency requirement, and must be individually determined to be at *nutrition risk* by a health professional. To be eligible on the basis of income, applicants' income must fall at or below 185% of the federal poverty level (see Table 11.8). A person who participates, or has family members who participate, in certain other benefit programs, such as SNAP, Medicaid, or Temporary Assistance for Needy Families (TANF), automatically meets the income eligibility requirement. Two major types of nutrition risk are recognized for WIC eligibility:

- *Medically based risks* such as anemia, underweight, overweight, maternal age, history of pregnancy complications, or poor pregnancy outcomes.
- *Dietary risks* such as failure to meet the *Dietary Guidelines for Americans* or inappropriate nutrition practices.

Nutrition risk is determined by a health professional such as a physician, nutritionist, or nurse and is based on federal guidelines. This health screening is free to program applicants.

WIC Food Benefits

In most WIC state agencies, WIC participants receive checks or vouchers to purchase specific foods each month that are designed to supplement their diets. The foods provided are high in one or more of the following nutrients: protein, calcium, iron, and vitamins A and C. These are the nutrients frequently lacking in the diets of the program's target population. As illustrated in Tables 11.11 and 11.12, different food packages are provided for different categories of participants. WIC foods include iron-fortified infant formula and infant cereal, iron-fortified adult cereal, vitamin-C rich fruit or vegetable juice, eggs, milk, cheese, peanut butter, dried and canned beans/peas, and canned fish. Soy-based beverages, tofu, fruits and vegetables, baby foods, whole wheat bread, and other whole-grain options were added in 2009 to better meet the nutritional needs of WIC participants (Box 11.10). Special therapeutic infant formulas and medical foods are provided when prescribed by a physician for a specified medical condition (Box 11.10) (US Department of Agriculture 2014).

WIC Appropriations and Priorities

Congress appropriated $6.522 billion for WIC in FY 2013 (US Department of Agriculture 2014). The average food benefit per month in FY 2013 was $43.26 (US Department of Agriculture, http://www.fns.usda.gov/pd/wic-program). Almost $4.5 billion was spent toward food costs and $1.8 billion on nutrition services and administration (NSA). Approximately two-thirds of NSA costs are used to provide nutrition education, breastfeeding promotion and support, and linkages to health and other client services (for example, immunization; drug, alcohol, and tobacco education; referrals to family and child health social programs). The remaining third is used for traditional management functions (US Department of Agriculture, http://www.fns.usda.gov/pd/37WIC_Monthly.htm).

EBT development has been a key long-term goal of FNS and of the WIC program. The challenge has been in finding technological solutions that are both affordable and can meet the functional needs of a relatively complex nutrition program. Nevertheless, the Healthy, Hunger-Free Kids Act of 2010 (US Government Publishing Office 2010) provides technical changes to WIC EBT requirements, including requiring the Secretary of Agriculture to establish national technical standards, minimum standards for installing WIC EBT equipment, and limitations on the imposition of costs on vendors. In addition, the Act mandates that all WIC state agencies implement EBT systems by October 1, 2020, and requires states to report their EBT implementation status annually to USDA. The proposed rule (Special Supplemental Nutrition Program for Women, Infants and Children 2013) addressing these and other EBT-related provisions was published in the Federal Register on February 28, 2013, and public comments were accepted until June 29, 2013.

WIC cannot serve all eligible people, so a system of priorities has been established for filling program openings. Once a local WIC agency has reached its maximum caseload, vacancies are filled in the order of the following priority levels:

BOX 11.10   UPDATING THE WIC FOOD PACKAGES

In 2003, FNS contracted with the Institute of Medicine (IOM) to independently review the WIC food packages. FNS charged IOM with recommending specific changes based on current information about the nutrition needs of WIC participants without affecting the cost of the WIC food packages. The IOM issued two reports: the initial report (2004)[1] describes nutrient needs for the WIC target population and establishes criteria for new food packages; the final report (2005)[2] offers specific recommendations for food package changes.

It was the recommendation of the IOM in 2004 that the new food package should reduce the prevalence of inadequate and excessive nutrient intakes in participants, contribute to an overall dietary pattern that is consistent with the *Dietary Guidelines for Americans* or to a diet that is consistent with dietary recommendations for infants and children younger than 2 years of age, and encourage and support breastfeeding. Foods in the package should be available in forms suitable for low-income persons who may have limited transportation, storage, and cooking facilities; be acceptable, readily available, and commonly consumed; take into account cultural food preferences; and provide incentives for families to participate in the WIC program. Care should be taken to consider the effects on vendors and WIC of changes in the package.[1]

In October 2009, the USDA instituted its first major revisions to the WIC food packages in the 35 years since the program's inception. The changes reflect the IOM's recommendations almost in their entirety. The revised food packages include the addition of fresh fruits, vegetables, and whole grains, and also include the final report's recommendation to substitute foods in an effort to meet the needs of the diverse WIC population. All changes are cost-neutral, since the additions made to the packages are balanced by reduced amounts of juice and dairy products.[3] Going forward, the Healthy, Hunger-Free Kids Act of 2010[4] requires that WIC food packages be reviewed every 10 years.

The current WIC food packages and the regulatory requirements for WIC-eligible foods are described in the *Code of Federal Regulations* (7 CFR Part 246.10) and on the WIC website at http://www.fns.usda.gov/wic/benefitsandservices/foodpkg.HTM.

Source:
[1]Data from Institute of Medicine. *Proposed Criteria for Selecting the WIC Food Packages.* Washington, DC: National Academies Press; 2004. Available at http://www.iom.edu/Reports/2004/Proposed-Criteria-for-Selecting-the-WIC-Food-Packages.aspx, accessed January 9, 2015.
[2]Data from Institute of Medicine. *WIC Food Packages: Time for a Change.* Washington, DC: National Academies Press; 2005. Available at http://www.iom.edu/Reports/2005/WIC-Food-Packages-Time-for-a-Change.aspx, accessed January 9, 2015.
[3]Data from Institute of Medicine. Actions Taken: USDA Revises WIC Food Packages for First Time. Available at http://www.iom.edu/Reports/2005/WIC-Food-Packages-Time-for-a-Change/Actions-Taken.aspx, accessed January 9, 2015.
[4]Data from Healthy, Hunger-Free Kids Act of 2010, Public Law 111-296, 124 Stat. (2010): 3183–3266. Available at http://www.gpo.gov/fdsys/pkg/PLAW-111publ296/pdf/PLAW-111publ296.pdf, accessed January 9, 2015.

- Priority I. Pregnant women, breastfeeding women, and infants determined to be at nutrition risk because of a nutrition-related medical condition such as anemia, underweight, overweight, or pre-term birth.
- Priority II. Infants up to 6 months of age whose mothers participated in WIC or could have participated and had nutrition-related medical conditions.
- Priority III. Children at nutrition risk because of a nutrition-related medical problem.
- Priority IV. Pregnant or breastfeeding women and infants at nutrition risk because of an inadequate dietary pattern.
- Priority V. Children at nutrition risk because of an inadequate dietary pattern.

- Priority VI. Non-breastfeeding, postpartum women with any nutrition risk (medical or diet-related).
- Priority VII. Current WIC participants who, without WIC foods, could continue to have medical and/or dietary problems.

Note that state agencies can decide to place homeless and migrant participants in Priorities IV–VII and place postpartum women in Priorities III–V. Any priority can be subdivided by the states into subcategories of risk using factors such as income or age (US Department of Agriculture, http://www.fns.usda.gov/wic/howtoapply/eligibilityprioritysystem.htm).

Breastfeeding

Mothers participating in WIC are encouraged to breastfeed their infants if possible, and those that do receive breastfeeding educational materials and counseling, follow-up support through peer counselors, and an enhanced food package (for those who exclusively breastfeed) and are eligible to participate in WIC longer than non-breastfeeding mothers. In addition, breastfeeding mothers can receive breast pumps, breast shells, or nursing supplementers to help support the initiation and continuation of breastfeeding. The Healthy, Hunger-Free Kids Act of 2010 requires data collection on the number of fully and partially breastfed infants at the state and local level, a program to recognize exemplary breastfeeding practices at local agencies, and provides performance bonuses for states with highest and most improved breastfeeding rates (US Government Publishing Office 2010). Data from the first 2 years since the Act was signed indicate a 1.5% increase in the number of WIC infants reported as breastfed between FY 2010 and FY 2011 (28.2%), and a 0.9 percentage increase to 29.0% in FY 2012 (12.1% were fully breastfed and 16.9% were partially breastfed) (US Department of Agriculture 2012).

The WIC Infant Formula Rebate System

For mothers who cannot or choose not to breastfeed their infants, WIC state agencies provide infant formula. In fact, between 57% and 68% of all infant formula sold in the United States in 2004–2006 was purchased through WIC (Oliveira et al. 2010). WIC state agencies are required by law to have competitively bid infant formula rebate contracts with infant formula manufacturers, and contracts are awarded to the bidder offering the lowest total monthly net wholesale price. In these contracts, WIC state agencies agree to provide one brand of infant formula, and in return, the manufacturer gives the state agency a rebate for each can of infant formula purchased by WIC participants. The brand of infant formula provided by WIC varies from one state agency to another, depending on which company has the rebate contract in a particular state. Rebates are generally large, averaging about 85% of the wholesale price. Thus, by negotiating rebates with formula manufacturers, states are able to serve more people. For example, without the rebates, infant formula would be the single most expensive food item provided by WIC, accounting for 44% of all food costs in FY 2005 versus only 17% after taking into account the savings from rebates (Oliveira et al. 2010). For FY 2010, rebate savings were $1.7 billion, supporting an average of 1.9 million participants each month or 20.5% of the estimated average monthly caseload (US Department of Agriculture, http://www.fns.usda.gov/wic/frequently-asked-questions-about-wic#7). While rebates substantially reduce the price of infant formula paid by WIC, they are only one part of the cost equation. Other factors, such as the net wholesale price of the primary contract formula, can lead to increased costs (Box 11.11).

WIC Farmers' Market Nutrition Program

The WIC Farmers' Market Nutrition Program (FMNP) provides fresh, unprepared, locally grown fruits and vegetables from local farmers' markets and roadside stands to WIC recipients (over 4 months of age). The federal food benefit level for FMNP recipients is $10–30 per year per recipient, but state agencies may supplement the benefit level. The farmers, farmers' markets, or roadside stands then submit the coupons to the bank or state agency for reimbursement.

BOX 11.11   CONSEQUENCES OF POLICY ON WIC INFANT FORMULA COSTS

Before 2004, infant formula manufacturers could submit a bid for the WIC rebate contract based on any formula in their product line as long as it was suitable for routine use by the majority of healthy, full-term infants. WIC state agencies were responsible for identifying the specific infant formulas in the winning manufacturer's product line to be used in the state's WIC program. As a result, the contract formulas provided to WIC participants in a particular state would not necessarily include the primary contract-brand product specified in the manufacturer's bid. For example, some of the winning bids in 2003 identified the primary contract brand as the newly developed and more expensive formulas supplemented with the fatty acids docosahexaenoic acid (DHA) and arachidonic acid (ARA), which some studies have linked to improved vision and cognitive development in infants. Nevertheless, some states chose not to offer the DHA/ARA-supplemented formulas to their participants, instead choosing an unsupplemented formula.

As a result of the Child Nutrition and WIC Reauthorization Act of 2004 (P.L. 108-265), for all contracts based on bid solicitations issued after September 2004, state agencies must use the primary contract infant formula for which the manufacturer submitted its bid (and for which the contract was awarded) as the first choice of issuance, with all other infant formulas issued as an alternative. Therefore, if the winning bid is based on a DHA/ARA-supplemented formula, the WIC state agency must offer that formula to the WIC participants in the state. After the legislation was enacted, nearly all bids submitted by formula manufacturers identified DHA/ARA-supplemented formulas as the primary contract infant formula. Consequently, all WIC state agencies now offer DHA/ARA-supplemented formulas to their WIC recipients.

Because WIC accounts for most of the infant formula sales in the United States, the 2004 legislation has ensured large sales volumes for these supplemented products while increasing their visibility to non-WIC consumers. In fact, DHA/ARA-supplemented formulas accounted for 98% of all formula sales in 2008, up from 69% in 2004 (the first DHA/ARA-supplemented formula was introduced in 2002). By requiring that states issue the primary contract infant formula (determined by the manufacturer) as the first choice of issuance, P.L. 108-265 has contributed to the rapid growth of DHA/ARA-supplemented formulas and the near disappearance of unsupplemented formulas from the marketplace. In addition, the net wholesale price of infant formula increased by an average of 73% between states' contracts in effect in December 2008 and the states' previous contracts. Most (72%) of this increase was due to the higher wholesale prices of DHA/ARA-supplemented formulas compared to unsupplemented formulas. (The remaining 28% of the increase was due to a decrease in rebates.) As a result, WIC state agencies spent about $127 million more on infant formula over the course of a year. This is equivalent to the cost of supporting 134,200 persons in WIC for a year, or about 2% of all women, infants, and children participating in WIC in FY 2008.

Source: Oliveira V, Frazao E, Smallwood D. *Rising Infant Formula Costs to the WIC Program: Recent Trends in Rebates and Wholesale Prices.* ERS-93, US Department of Agriculture, Economic Research Service, 2010. Available at http://www.ers.usda.gov/media/136568/err93_1_.pdf, accessed February 15, 2015.

A variety of fresh, nutritious, unprepared, locally grown fruits, vegetables, and herbs may be purchased with FMNP coupons. State agencies may limit sales to specific foods grown within the state borders to encourage FMNP recipients to support state farmers. Nutrition education is provided to FMNP recipients by the state agency, often through an arrangement with the local WIC agency. Other educators and program partners may provide nutrition education and/or educational information to FMNP recipients, such as cooperative extension programs, local chefs, farmers or farmers' markets associations, and various other nonprofit or for-profit organizations. These educational arrangements help to encourage FMNP recipients to improve and expand their diets by adding fresh fruits and vegetables, as well as educate them on how to select, store, and prepare the fresh produce they buy with their FMNP coupons.

During FY 2011, 18,487 farmers, 4079 farmers' markets, and 3184 roadside stands were authorized to accept FMNP coupons, which resulted in over $16.4 million in revenue to farmers. In FY 2011, 1.9 million WIC participants received benefits. For FY 2012, $16.5 million was appropriated for the program (US Department of Agriculture, http://www.fns.usda.gov/sites/default/files/WIC -FMNP-Fact-Sheet.pdf).

Child and Adult Care Food Program

After an extension of the 1968 Special Food Service Program for Children's 3-year demonstration project, the Child Care Food Program was authorized in 1975, becoming a permanent program in 1978. The name was officially changed to CACFP in 1989 to reflect the adult component of this program. CACFP plays a vital role in improving the quality of day care for children and elderly adults by making care more affordable for many low-income families. CACFP supports nutritious meals and snacks in child care centers, Head Start, family or group day care homes, *at-risk* afterschool care programs, emergency shelters, and adult day care centers (Box 11.12).

Through CACFP, more than 3.3 million infants and children (birth through age 18 years) and 120,000 chronically impaired adults or people over age 60 at adult day care centers receive nutritious meals and snacks each day as part of their day care. CACFP reaches even further to provide meals to children residing in emergency shelters, and snacks and suppers to youths participating in eligible after-school care programs. Free meals are provided to adults who receive SNAP, FDPIR, Social Security Income, or Medicaid; children whose families receive benefits from SNAP, FDPIR, or state programs funded through TANF, or who are income-eligible participants of Head Start or Early Head Start; or children who live in emergency shelters.

The USDA's FNS administers CACFP through grants to states. The program is administered within most states by the state educational agency. The child care component and the adult day care component of CACFP may be administered by different agencies within a state, at the discretion of the governor. Independent centers and sponsoring organizations enter into agreements with their administering state agencies to assume administrative and financial responsibility for CACFP operations. Participating programs are required to provide meals and snacks according to the nutrition standards set by USDA. Table 11.13 lists the CACFP meal and snack patterns for children older than 1 year. Meals served to infants (ages birth through 11 months) must meet the requirements that are outlined in Table 11.14.

CACFP provides cash reimbursement for meals served to children and adults in day care centers based upon the participant's eligibility for free, reduced-price, or paid meals. The reimbursement rates vary, based on the type of meal (lunches have a higher reimbursement rate than snacks) and the type of institution. FNS also provides funds to state agencies for administrative expenses incurred in supervising and giving technical assistance to institutions participating in CACFP. In addition, USDA (http://www.fns.usda.gov/cnd/care/cacfp/aboutcacfp.htm) makes donated agricultural foods or cash-in-lieu of donated foods available to institutions participating in CACFP. CACFP is an entitlement program. In FY 2014, preliminary data show that participation in the program averaged 3.88 million with a total of 1.98 billion subsidized meals and snacks at a federal cost of $2.99 billion (US Department of Agriculture, http://www.fns.usda.gov/pd/ccsummar.htm).

Community-based programs that offer enrichment activities for at-risk children and youth after school, such as Feeding America's Kids Cafes (Feeding America, http://feedingamerica.org/how-we -fight-hunger/programs-and-services/child-hunger/kids-cafe.aspx), can provide free meals and snacks through CACFP. Programs receiving benefits must be offered in areas where at least 50% of the children are eligible for free and reduced-price meals, based upon school data. To help meet the need for ongoing training of CACFP staff in the nutritional needs of infants, USDA publishes an infant feeding guide. The book contains information about infant development, nutrition for infants,

BOX 11.12 HEAD START CHILD NUTRITION PERFORMANCE STANDARDS

Head Start is a federal school-readiness program for low-income preschool-aged children up to age 5 years. Many Head Start programs also provide Early Head Start, which serves infants, toddlers, pregnant women, and their families who have incomes below the federal poverty level. Head Start programs provide comprehensive services to enrolled children and their families, which include health, nutrition, and social services. Programs may be based in centers or schools that children attend for part-day or full-day services, family child care homes, or children's own homes where a staff person visits once a week to provide services. The Office of Head Start (OHS), within the Administration of Children and Families of the HHS, awards competitive grants to public and private agencies to provide these services to specific communities. Head Start programs must meet a number of performance standards, which can be found on the OHS website at http://eclkc.ohs.acf.hhs.gov/hslc/standards/Head Start Requirements.

The performance standards specific to child nutrition (45 CFR §1304.23) are listed below:

Identification of nutritional needs. Staff and families must work together to identify each child's nutritional needs, taking into account staff and family discussions concerning

- Any relevant nutrition-related assessment data, such as height, weight, hemoglobin, or hematocrit.
- Information about family eating patterns, including cultural preferences, special dietary requirements for each child with nutrition-related health problems, and the feeding requirements of infants and toddlers and each child with disabilities.
- For infants and toddlers, current feeding schedules and amounts and types of food provided, including whether breast milk or formula and baby food is used, meal patterns, new foods introduced, food intolerances and preferences, voiding patterns, and observations related to developmental changes in feeding and nutrition must be shared with parents and updated regularly.
- Information about major community nutritional issues, as identified through the Community Assessment or by the Health Services Advisory Committee or the local health department.

Nutritional services. Grantee and delegate agencies must design and implement a nutrition program that meets the nutritional needs and feeding requirements of each child, including those with special dietary needs and children with disabilities. Also, the nutrition program must serve a variety of foods, which consider cultural and ethnic preferences and also broaden the child's food experience.

- All Early Head Start and Head Start programs must use funds from the USDA Food and Consumer Services Child Nutrition Programs as the primary source of payment for meal services. Early Head Start and Head Start funds may be used to cover those allowable costs not covered by the USDA.
- Each child in a part-day center-based program must receive meals and snacks that provide at least a third of the child's daily nutritional needs. Each child in a full-day center-based program must receive meals and snacks that provide half to two-thirds of the child's daily nutritional needs, depending on the length of the program day.
- All children in morning center-based programs, who have not received breakfast at the time they arrive at the program, must be served a nourishing breakfast.
- Each infant and toddler in center-based programs must receive food appropriate to their nutritional needs, developmental readiness, and feeding skills, as

recommended in the USDA meal pattern or nutrient standard menu planning requirements outlined in 7 CFR parts 210, 220, and 226 (available at http://www .fns.usda.gov/cnd/Governance/regulations.htm and http://www.fns.usda.gov/cnd /Care/Regs-Policy/Regulations.htm).

- For 3 to 5 year olds, foods served must be high in nutrients and low in fat, sugar, and salt. The quantities and kinds of food served must conform to recommended serving sizes and minimum standards for meal patterns recommended in the USDA meal pattern or nutrient standard menu planning requirements outlined in 7 CFR parts 210, 220, and 226 (available at http://www.fns.usda.gov /cnd/Governance/regulations.htm and http://www.fns.usda.gov/cnd/Care/Regs -Policy/Regulations.htm).

- Meal and snack periods in center-based programs must be appropriately scheduled and adjusted, where necessary, to ensure that individual needs are met. Infants and young toddlers who need it must be fed *on demand* to the extent possible or at appropriate intervals.

- Home-based programs must provide appropriate snacks and meals to each child during group socialization activities.

- Staff must promote effective dental hygiene among children in conjunction with meals.

- Parents and appropriate community agencies must be involved in planning, implementing, and evaluating the program's nutritional services.

Meal service. Grantee and delegate agencies must ensure that nutritional services in center-based settings contribute to the development and socialization of enrolled children by providing that

- A variety of food is served, which broadens each child's food experiences.

- Food is not used as punishment or reward, and that all children are encouraged, but not forced, to eat or taste their food.

- Sufficient time is allowed for each child to eat.

- All toddlers and preschool children and assigned classroom staff, including volunteers, eat together family-style and share the same menu to the extent possible.

- Infants are held while being fed and are not laid down to sleep with a bottle.

- Medically based diets or other dietary requirements are accommodated.

- As developmentally appropriate, opportunity is provided for the involvement of children in food-related activities.

Family assistance with nutrition. Parent education activities must include opportunities to assist individual families with food preparation and nutritional skills.

Food safety and sanitation. Head Start programs must post evidence of compliance with all applicable federal, state, tribal, and local food safety and sanitation laws, including those related to the storage, preparation, and service of food and the health of food handlers. In addition, agencies must contract only with food service vendors that are licensed in accordance with state, tribal, or local laws.

- For programs serving infants and toddlers, facilities must be available for the proper storage and handling of breast milk and formula.

Source: US Department of Health and Human Services. Administration for Children and Families. Office of Head Start. Early Childhood Learning and Knowledge Center. "Head Start Program Performance Standards and Other Regulations: Child Nutrition." Title 45 *Code of Federal Regulations*, §1304.23. Revised January 8, 2008. Available at http://eclkc.ohs.acf.hhs.gov/hslc/standards/Head Start Requirements/1304/1304.23 Child nutrition.htm, accessed January 20, 2015.

TABLE 11.13

CACFP Children's Meal Patterns for Breakfast, Snack, and Lunch/Supper

	Breakfast		
Select all three components for a reimbursable breakfast	**Ages 1–2**	**Ages 3–5**	**Ages 6–12[a]**
One serving milk[b]			
Fluid milk	1/2 cup	3/4 cup	1 cup
One serving fruit/vegetable			
Juice,[c] fruit, and/or vegetable	1/2 cup	1/2 cup	1/2 cup
One serving grains/bread[d]			
Bread or	1/2 slice	1/2 slice	1 slice
Cornbread or biscuit or roll or muffin or	1/2 serving	1/2 serving	1 serving
Cold dry cereal or	1/4 cup	1/3 cup	3/4 cup
Hot cooked cereal or	1/4 cup	1/4 cup	1/2 cup
Pasta or noodles or grains	1/4 cup	1/4 cup	1/2 cup

	Snack		
Select two of the four components for a reimbursable snack	**Ages 1–2**	**Ages 3–5**	**Ages 6–12[a]**
One serving milk[b]			
Fluid milk	1/2 cup	1/2 cup	1 cup
One serving fruit/vegetable			
Juice,[c,e] fruit, and/or vegetable	1/2 cup	1/2 cup	3/4 cup
One serving grains/bread[d]			
Bread or	1/2 slice	1/2 slice	1 slice
Cornbread or biscuit or roll or muffin or	1/2 serving	1/2 serving	1 serving
Cold dry cereal or	1/4 cup	1/3 cup	3/4 cup
Hot cooked cereal or	1/4 cup	1/4 cup	1/2 cup
Pasta or noodles or grains or	1/4 cup	1/4 cup	1/2 cup
One serving meat/meat alternate			
Meat or poultry or fish[f] or	1/2 oz.	1/2 oz.	1 oz.
Alternate protein product or	1/2 oz.	1/2 oz.	1 oz.
Cheese or	1/2 oz.	1/2 oz.	1 oz.
Egg[g] or	1/2 egg	1/2 egg	1/2 egg
Cooked dry beans or peas or	1/8 cup	1/8 cup	1/4 cup
Peanut or other nut or seed butters or	1 tbsp.	1 tbsp.	2 tbsp.
Nuts and/or seeds or	1/2 oz.	1/2 oz.	1 oz.
Yogurt[h]	2 oz.	2 oz.	4 oz.

	Lunch or Supper		
Select all four components for a reimbursable meal	**Ages 1–2**	**Ages 3–5**	**Ages 6–12[a]**
One serving milk[b]			
Fluid milk	1/2 cup	3/4 cup	1 cup
Two servings fruits/vegetables			
Juice,[c] fruit, and/or vegetable	1/4 cup	1/2 cup	3/4 cup
One serving grains/bread[d]			
Bread or	1/2 slice	1/2 slice	1 slice
Cornbread or biscuit or roll or muffin or	1/2 serving	1/2 serving	1 serving
Cold dry cereal or	1/4 cup	1/3 cup	3/4 cup
Hot cooked cereal or	1/4 cup	1/4 cup	1/2 cup
Pasta or noodles or grains	1/4 cup	1/4 cup	1/2 cup

(Continued)

TABLE 11.13 (CONTINUED)
CACFP Children's Meal Patterns for Breakfast, Snack, and Lunch/Supper

One serving meat/meat alternate

Meat or poultry or fish[f] or	1 oz.	11/2 oz.	2 oz.
Alternate protein product or	1 oz.	11/2 oz.	2 oz.
Cheese or	1 oz.	11/2 oz.	2 oz.
Egg or	1/2 egg	3/4 egg	1 egg
Cooked dry beans or peas or	1/4 cup	3/8 cup	1/2 cup
Peanut or other nut or seed butters or	2 tbsp.	3 tbsp.	4 tbsp.
Nuts and/or seeds[i] or	1/2 oz.	3/4 oz.	1 oz.
Yogurt[h]	4 oz.	6 oz.	8 oz.

Source: US Department of Agriculture. Food and Nutrition Service. Child and Adult Care Food Program. Meal Patterns. Available at http://www.fns.usda.gov/cnd/care/programbasics/meals/meal_patterns.htm, accessed February 15, 2015.

[a] Children age 12 and older may be served larger portions based on their greater food needs. They may not be served less than the minimum quantities listed in this column.

[b] Milk served must be low fat (1%) or nonfat (skim).

[c] Fruit or vegetable juice must be full strength.

[d] Breads and grains must be made from whole grain or enriched meal or flour. Cereal must be whole grain or enriched or fortified.

[e] Juice cannot be served when milk is the only other snack component.

[f] A serving consists of the edible portion of cooked lean meat or poultry or fish.

[g] A half egg meets the required minimum amount (1 oz. or less) of meat alternate.

[h] Yogurt may be plain or flavored, unsweetened or sweetened.

[i] Nuts and seeds may meet only one-half of the total meat/meat alternative serving and must be combined with another meat/meat alternate to fulfill the lunch or supper requirement.

breastfeeding and formula feeding, preventing tooth decay, feeding solid foods, drinking from a cup, choking prevention, sanitary food preparation and safe food handling, commercially prepared and home-prepared baby food, the storage and handling of breast milk, and infant meal patterns (*Feeding Infants: A Guide for Use in the Child Nutrition Programs* 2001).

Senior Farmers' Market Nutrition Program

The Senior Farmers' Market Nutrition Program (SFMNP) was established in FY 2001 to provide low-income seniors with coupons that can be exchanged for eligible foods at farmers' markets, roadside stands, and CSA programs. SFMNP awards grants to states, US territories, and federally recognized Indian tribal governments to provide low-income seniors with coupons that can be exchanged for fresh, nutritious, and unprocessed fruits, vegetables, honey, and fresh-cut herbs. The majority of grant funds may be used to support the costs of the foods provided under the SFMNP; state agencies may use up to 10% of their grants for program administrative costs.

Low-income seniors are generally defined as individuals who are at least 60 years old and who have household incomes of not more than 185% of the federal poverty income guidelines.

SFMNP benefits are provided to eligible recipients for use during the harvest season, which is generally May through October. (In some states, the SFMNP season is relatively short, because the growing season in that area is not very long. In other states with longer growing seasons, recipients have a longer period of time in which to use their SFMNP benefits.) The 2008 Farm Bill provided $20.6 million annually to operate the SFMNP through 2012. In FY 2011, over 863,000 low-income seniors received vouchers worth $20–50 per year (US Department of Agriculture, http://www.fns.usda.gov/sfmnp/overview).

TABLE 11.14
CACFP Meal Patterns for Infants through 11 Months of Age

Birth–3 Months	4–7 Months	8–11 Months
	Breakfast	
4–6 fl. oz. formula[a] or breast milk[b,c]	4–8 fl. oz. formula[a] or breast milk[b,c] and	6–8 fl. oz. formula[a] or breast milk[b,c] and
	0–3 tbsp. infant cereal[a,d]	2–4 tbsp. infant cereal[a] and
		1–4 tbsp. fruit or vegetable or both
	Snack	
4–6 fl. oz. formula[a] or breast milk[b,c]	4–6 fl. oz. formula[a] or breast milk[b,c]	2–4 fl. oz. formula[a] or breast milk,[b,c] or fruit juice[e] and
		0–1/2 bread[d,f] or 0–2 crackers[d,f]
	Lunch or Supper	
4–6 fl. oz. formula[a] or breast milk[b,c]	4–8 fl. oz. formula[a] or breast milk[b,c] and	6–8 fl. oz. formula[a] or breast milk[b,c] and
	0–3 tbsp. infant cereal[a,d] and	2–4 tbsp. infant cereal[a] and/or
	0–3 tbsp. fruit or vegetable or both[d]	1–4 tbsp. meat, fish, poultry, egg yolk, cooked dry beans or peas; or 1/2–2 oz. cheese; or 1–4 oz. (volume) cottage cheese; or 1–4 oz. (weight) cheese food or cheese spread, and
		1–4 tbsp. fruit or vegetable or both

Source: US Department of Agriculture. Food and Nutrition Service. Child and Adult Care Food Program. Meal Patterns. Available at http://www.fns.usda.gov/cnd/care/programbasics/meals/meal_patterns.htm, accessed February 15, 2015.

[a] Infant formula and dry infant cereal must be iron-fortified.

[b] Breast milk or formula, or portions of both, may be served; however, it is recommended that breast milk be served in place of formula from birth through 11 months.

[c] For some breastfed infants who regularly consume less than the minimum amount of breast milk per feeding, a serving of less than the minimum amount of breast milk may be offered, with additional breast milk offered if the infant is still hungry.

[d] A serving of this component is required when the infant is developmentally ready to accept it.

[e] Fruit juice must be full strength.

[f] A serving of this component must be made from whole grain or enriched meal or flour.

For FY 2013, grants were awarded to 52 state agencies and federally recognized ITOs. It should be noted that not all state agencies operate the SFMNP on a statewide basis. State agencies may limit SFMNP sales to specific foods that are locally grown in order to encourage SFMNP recipients to support the farmers in their own state. There are certain foods not eligible for purchase with SFMNP benefits, including dried fruits or vegetables, such as prunes (dried plums), raisins (dried grapes), sun-dried tomatoes, or dried chili peppers. Potted fruit or vegetable plants, potted or dried herbs, wild rice, nuts of any kind, maple syrup, cider, and molasses are also not allowed.

Nutrition education is provided to SFMNP recipients by the state agency, often through an arrangement with the local WIC agency. Nutrition education and/or education information may also be provided by program partners, such as cooperative extension programs, local Area Agencies on Aging, local chefs, farmers or farmers' market associations, and other nonprofit or for-profit organizations. These educational arrangements help encourage SFMNP recipients to improve and expand their diets by adding fresh fruits and vegetables, as well as educate them on how to select, store, and prepare the fresh produce they buy with their SFMNP coupons (US Department of Agriculture, http://www.fns.usda.gov/sfmnp/overview).

Special Milk Program

The Child Nutrition Act of 1966 authorized the SMP, which provides milk free of charge or at a low cost to children in schools and child care institutions that do not participate in other federal child nutrition meal service programs. This federally assisted program reimburses schools for the milk they serve. The federal reimbursement for each half-pint of milk sold to children in SY 2014–2015 was 23 cents (US Department of Agriculture, http://www.fns.usda.gov/school-meals/rates-reimbursement).

For children who receive their milk free, the USDA reimburses schools the net purchase price of the milk. Schools in the NSLP or SBP may also participate in the SMP to provide milk to children in half-day prekindergarten and kindergarten programs where children do not have access to the school meal programs (US Department of Agriculture, http://www.fns.usda.gov/cnd/milk/AboutMilk/SMPFactSheet.pdf).

Expansion of the NSLP and SBP, which include milk, has led to a substantial reduction in the SMP since its peak in the late 1960s. The program served nearly 3 billion half-pints of milk in 1969, 1.8 billion in 1980, and 181 million in 1990. In FY 2011, the program served over 66 million half-pints of milk at a cost of $12.3 million. Schools or institutions must offer only pasteurized fluid types of fat-free or low-fat (1%) milk that meet state and local standards. All milk should contain vitamins A and D at levels specified by the Food and Drug Administration (FDA) (US Department of Agriculture, http://www.fns.usda.gov/cnd/milk/AboutMilk/SMPFactSheet.pdf).

Nutrition Services Incentive Program

The NSIP provides funding to states, territories, and eligible ITOs that efficiently deliver nutritious meals to older adults. Funds are provided to purchase food or to cover the costs of food commodities provided by USDA for congregate and home-delivered nutrition programs. Funds are allotted to states and other entities based on each state's share of total meals served during the prior year. Although states may choose to receive the grant as cash, commodity foods, or a combination of cash and commodities, most states choose to receive their share of funds in cash rather than commodities. NSIP funds must be used exclusively to purchase food; funds may not be used for meal preparation or other nutrition-related services, such as nutrition education or administrative costs. Meals served under the NSIP must meet the most recent *Dietary Guidelines for Americans,* and each meal must provide at least one-third of the dietary reference intakes (DRIs). In FY 2014, $160 million was appropriated for the NSIP (Aussenberg and Colello 2014).

Age is the only factor used in determining eligibility for the NSIP. People at least 60 years of age, and their spouses (of any age), are eligible for NSIP benefits. ITOs may select an age below 60 for defining an *older* person for their tribes. Eligibility is also extended to disabled people under age 60 who live in elderly housing facilities where congregate meals are served, disabled people who reside at home and accompany elderly participants to meals, and volunteers who assist in the meal service (US Department of Agriculture, http://www.fns.usda.gov/fdd/programs/nsip/nsip_eligibility.htm).

Formerly the Nutrition Program for the Elderly (NPE), NSIP was established by Section 311 of the Older Americans Act (OAA) of 2000, as amended, and has been authorized in one form or another under the OAA since 1974. Originally, the program was administered by the USDA, which provided cash and/or commodities to supplement meals provided under the authority of the OAA. The Consolidated Appropriations Resolution, 2003, P.L. 108-7, amended the OAA to transfer the NSIP appropriation from the USDA to the AoA within HHS, which did not result in significant changes to the procedures for administering the program at the state, tribal, and local levels. The AoA administers the NSIP and provides state agencies funds to purchase food. All, or part, of these funds may be used to purchase food through the FNS within USDA. USDA (http://www.fns.usda.gov/fdd/programs/nsip/about_nsip.htm) also donates bonus foods to NSIP when feasible (Aussenberg and Colello 2014). Table 11.15 lists the USDA commodity foods available to state agencies that administered the NSIP in 2013.

Food Distribution Programs

The USDA administers several food distribution programs, including the school and child nutrition programs, which are designed to benefit both agriculture and low-income individuals. These programs serve the agricultural community by using surplus commodities purchased by the USDA from farmers and other producers. The programs help reduce federal food inventories and storage costs while also assisting the needy. Four of these programs are described next.

The Emergency Food Assistance Program

TEFAP helps supplement the diets of low-income Americans, including elderly people, by providing them with emergency food and nutrition assistance at no cost. Through TEFAP, the USDA purchases commodity foods, including processing and packaging, and makes them available to state agencies. The proportion of food each state receives from the total amount of food provided is based on the number of unemployed people and the number of people with incomes below the poverty level in the state. States then provide the food to local agencies, usually food banks, which in turn distribute the food to local organizations that directly serve the public, such as soup kitchens and food pantries. Two types of public or private nonprofit groups are eligible to receive assistance from TEFAP:

- Organizations that provide food and nutrition assistance to the needy through the distribution of food for home use or the preparation of meals to be served in a congregate setting. Organizations that distribute food for home use must determine the household's eligibility by applying the income standards that are set by the state.
- Organizations that provide prepared meals are eligible to receive commodities if they can demonstrate that they serve predominately low-income persons (US Department of Agriculture and Food and Nutrition Service 2014a).

Recipients of TEFAP include some of the most vulnerable populations, including the elderly, children, working families, and people who are homeless. Households that meet state eligibility criteria may also receive food for home use through TEFAP. Each state sets income standards for determining what households are eligible to receive food for home consumption. Income standards may, at the state's discretion, be met through participation in other existing federal, state, local food, health, or welfare programs for which eligibility is based on income, such as SNAP, NSP, or WIC. States can adjust the income criteria in order to ensure that assistance is provided only to those households most in need. However, recipients of prepared meals for home use are considered to be needy and are not subject to a means test (US Department of Agriculture and Food and Nutrition Service 2014a).

TEFAP was first authorized as the Temporary TEFAP in 1981 to distribute surplus commodities to households. The name was changed to The Emergency Food Assistance Program under the 1990 Farm Bill. Congress appropriated $318.25 million for TEFAP in FY 2014—$268.75 million to purchase food and another $49.401 million for administrative support for state and local agencies. In addition to commodity foods purchased with appropriated funds, TEFAP receives surplus foods from the USDA. In FY 2013, $228.5 million in surplus foods were made available to TEFAP (US Department of Agriculture and Food and Nutrition Service 2014a).

Food Distribution Program on Indian Reservations

The USDA provides financial assistance to Native Americans via an assortment of programs and services, one of which is the FDPIR, an alternative to SNAP. In 1973, Congress established FDPIR to provide supplemental food to low-income households living on or near rural American Indian reservations as an acceptable alternative to SNAP benefits. Because of the remote and geographically dispersed locations of many reservations and other Indian lands, many otherwise eligible American Indian families have been unable to participate in SNAP, as access to SNAP offices and

TABLE 11.15

Commodity Supplemental Food Program Commodities, 2013

Food Category	Examples
Canned vegetables	Green beans, vegetarian beans, carrots, whole kernel corn, peas, sliced potatoes, spaghetti sauce, spinach, sweet potatoes, tomatoes, mixed vegetables
Canned fruits	Applesauce, apricots, mixed fruit, peaches, pears, plums
Canned meats	Beef, chicken, salmon
Canned juices	Apple, cranapple, grape, orange, tomato
Dairy	Cheese blend, instant nonfat dry milk packages, 1% milk boxes, powdered infant formula cans
Boxed grains	Grits, farina, spaghetti, macaroni, oats, rice, whole grain rotini, infant rice cereal, ready-to-eat cereals (corn, oat, rice, wheat bran)
Packaged dry beans	Baby lima, light red kidney, great northern, pinto
Oils	Peanut butter in jars

Source: US Department of Agriculture. Food and Nutrition Service. *USDA Foods Available for 2013 Commodity Supplemental Food Program* (no longer available on the Internet).

authorized grocery stores has been difficult. Households may not participate in FDPIR and SNAP in the same month (US Department of Agriculture and Food and Nutrition Service 2014b).

Through FDPIR, commodity foods are provided to low-income households, including the elderly, living on Indian reservations, and to Native American families residing in designated areas near reservations or in Oklahoma (Box 11.13).

FDPIR is administered at the federal level by the FNS and locally by either an ITO or an agency of a state government. There are approximately 276 tribes receiving benefits under the FDPIR through 100 ITOs and 5 state agencies. The USDA purchases and ships commodities to the ITOs and state agencies based on their orders from a list of available foods. These administering agencies store and distribute the food, determine applicant eligibility, and provide nutrition education to recipients. Each month, participating households receive a food package to help them maintain a nutritionally balanced diet. Participants may select from over 70 products. The USDA provides the administering agencies with funds for program administrative costs (US Department of Agriculture and Food and Nutrition Service 2014b).

Average monthly participation for FY 2013 was 75,590 individuals. In FY 2014, $104 million was appropriated for FDPIR, approximately $40.2 million for the federal share of local level administrative costs, and the remainder for food purchases. The USDA purchases most foods distributed in the program with FDPIR appropriations; however, some commodities offered through FDPIR may be purchased under agricultural support programs (US Department of Agriculture and Food and Nutrition Service 2014b).

Unmet Needs

A study conducted by the US Commission on Civil Rights in 2003 examined federal funding of programs intended to assist Native Americans. The commission's report reveals that funding directed to Native Americans through FDPIR, as well as other programs, has not been sufficient to address the basic and urgent needs of indigenous peoples. For example, between 1995 and 1997, 22.2% of Native American households were hungry or on the edge of hunger (food insecure), more than twice the rate of the population as a whole. Recall that the USDA defines *food insecurity* as the limited or uncertain availability of food, or limited or uncertain ability to acquire foods in socially acceptable ways. Overall, 8.6% of the Native American households reported that they were suffering from hunger, also more than double the nationwide rate. The commission found that significant disparities in federal funding exist between Native Americans and other groups in the United States, as well as the general population. The commission recommended that the USDA and other

BOX 11.13   NATIVE AMERICANS' DIETS

Compared to other US population groups, Native Americans are more likely to be poor, unemployed, and experience high levels of food insecurity. As a result, many low-income Native American families rely on federal food programs, and commodity foods provided through some programs are higher in fat and calories and lower in fiber. Researchers from the USDA ERS and the University of Nevada Las Vegas American Indian Research and Education Center surveyed adults from tribes across the country to understand commodity food use patterns and food choice. Survey respondents reported multigenerational use of commodity foods, with 90% of respondents indicating they had grandparents and/or parents who used commodity foods while growing up. The consumption rate of commodity or purchased foods in comparison to foods obtained via traditional methods (hunting, fishing, gathering, or growing) indicates that most meals consist of commodity or purchased foods. Those who used commodity foods over the previous 5 years were significantly more likely to prefer and purchase canned fruit, canned meat, and boxed meals. The authors conclude that commodity foods are a mainstay, rather than a short-term supplement, of Native Americans' diets, and that regular and continued use of commodity foods over the life course may influence food preferences and practices. With growing rates of obesity and diet-related diseases among this population, the authors suggest that funds—rather than commodities—be donated so that more traditional foods, such as bison and other wild game instead of beef, and fresh fruits and vegetables instead of canned produce, can be ordered by reservation stores and food banks. Nutrition education programs should also focus on harvesting and preparing traditional, locally available foods. Future research can help explain how commodity foods affect the diets and health of Native Americans.

Source: Chino M et al., *Pimatisiwin: A Journal of Aboriginal and Indigenous Community Health*. 2009;7(2):279–289. Available at http://www.pimatisiwin.com/online/wp-content/uploads/2010/jan/07HaffChino.pdf, accessed January 15, 2015.

federal agencies administering Native American programs identify and regularly assess the unmet needs of American Indians. Through laws, treaties, and policies established over hundreds of years, the federal government is obligated to ensure that funding is adequate to meet these needs (US Commission on Civil Rights 2003).

Commodity Supplemental Food Program

The CSFP works to improve the health of low-income elderly persons at least 60 years of age by supplementing their diets with USDA foods. USDA purchases food and makes it available to CSFP state agencies along with funds for administrative costs. State agencies that administer CSFP are typically departments of health, social services, education, or agriculture. State agencies store the food and distribute it to public and nonprofit private local agencies; the local agencies determine the eligibility of applicants, distribute the foods, and provide nutrition education (US Department of Agriculture, http://www.fns.usda.gov/csfp/about-csfp).

This program originally targeted low-income pregnant women, children, and the elderly, all populations that are covered under other programs. One difference is that the CSFP provided food directly to the population (USDA commodity surplus foods), instead of vouchers or money. The overlap of populations served has been addressed, and as of February 6, 2014, new enrollment of women and children has ceased. Going forward, CSFP will only serve low-income elderly (US Department of Agriculture 2014).

CSFP food packages do not provide a complete diet, but rather include items that are good sources of the nutrients typically lacking in the diets of the target population (US Department of

Agriculture, http://www.fns.usda.gov/csfp/about-csfp). For the elderly, states establish an income limit that is at or below 130% of the federal poverty level. States may establish local residency requirements based on designated service areas or may require that participants be at nutritional risk as determined by a physician or local agency staff. For FY 2014, $202.682 million was appropriated for CSFP. In FY 2013, an average of more than 579,000 people each month participated in the program (US Department of Agriculture and Food and Nutrition Service 2014c).

ENDING HUNGER

In addition to the numerous federal food assistance programs providing a safety net, hundreds of nongovernmental, nonprofit organizations exist, which work to end hunger in the United States. We cannot possibly examine them all; thus, this section just briefly notes the history of Feeding America, a network of more than 200 member food banks and food-rescue organizations serving all 50 states, the District of Columbia, and Puerto Rico. This network supports approximately 50,000 local charitable agencies operating more than 94,000 programs, including food pantries, soup kitchens, emergency shelters, and after-school programs (Box 11.14).

BOX 11.14   THE FIRST FOOD BANK

John van Hengel was a soup-kitchen volunteer in 1967 when he founded the first food bank with a truckload of produce gleaned from Arizona farm fields and citrus groves. Soup kitchens and community food pantries have existed for more than a century, but the idea of a food bank took van Hengel's modest local efforts and made them bigger and more reliable. The key was creating a distribution network, convincing corporations that their donated food would be safely handled and would not be resold. In addition, businesses were able to cut the costs of disposing or storing unusable food, take a tax break, and satisfy multiple charities through a single point of contact. Van Hengel's idea grew into a nationwide network of food banks that converts food industry leftovers into meals for the poor. That network, Feeding America (formerly America's Second Harvest), distributes over 3 billion meals annually. Currently, the program supports over 60,000 charitable agencies, including food pantries, soup kitchens, emergency shelters, and after-school programs.

Working at a soup kitchen in Phoenix, van Hengel often searched in supermarket refuse bins for his own food. Van Hengel credited his seminal idea to a woman with 10 children and a husband on death row whom he met while *dumpster diving* for food in refuse bins behind grocery stores. She suggested that what was really needed was a place to both deposit food and check it out—*like a bank*. Finding edible, if not salable, food, he persuaded a grocery store manager, and then the manager's boss, to donate surplus food. Soon he and his helpers had more food than they could use, so they started delivering the excess to missions, alcoholism treatment centers, and abused women's shelters. He tried unsuccessfully to persuade several religious and nonprofit organizations in Phoenix to start a warehouse food bank. Finally, a downtown Phoenix church gave him an abandoned bakery, and church members contributed $3000 for utility bills. St. Mary's Food Bank, which still operates, distributed more than 250,000 lb. of food to 36 charities in its first year of operation. In 1975, van Hengel accepted a grant to set up 18 food banks; America's Second Harvest incorporated the next year. The timing was auspicious, as the new Tax Reform Act gave corporations tax benefits if they donated inventory to charity.

Sources: Feeding America. Our Food Bank Network. Available at http://feedingamerica.org/how-we-fight-hunger /our-food-bank-network.aspx, accessed January 15, 2015; St. Mary's Food Bank Alliance. Our History. Available at http://www.firstfoodbank.org/learn-more/our-history, accessed January 15, 2015; Sullivan P. Obituary. John van Hengel Dies at 83; Founded 1st Food Bank in 1967. *Washington Post.* October 8, 2005, p. B06.

CONCLUSION

Ensuring food security for at-risk populations, such as the elderly and low-income women and children, has become an enormous undertaking, operating largely under the aegis of the USDA and augmented by nongovernmental organizations such as Feeding America. Safety net programs range in type and population served; from WIC to SNAP to Head Start to adult day care for the elderly. The NSLP alone serves billions of meals each year. Due to the associations of negative health outcomes with food insecurity, it is not sufficient to provide just any food. Programs such as Team Nutrition have been instituted to improve nutrition education in schools receiving assistance from the USDA. In addition, efforts are being made to enhance the quality of the food itself by improving nutritional standards and supporting local farms and delivering fresh fruits and vegetables directly to schools.

ACRONYMS

AoA	Administration on Aging
ARA	Arachidonic acid
BMI	Body mass index
CACFP	Child and Adult Care Food Program
CNPP	Center for Nutrition Policy and Promotion
CNSTAT	Committee on National Statistics
CPS	Current Population Survey
CSA	Community supported agriculture
CSFP	Commodity Supplemental Food Program
DHA	Docosahexaenoic acid
DoD	Department of Defense
DRI	Dietary reference intake
D-SNAP	Disaster SNAP
EBT	Electronic benefits transfer
ERS	Economic Research Service
FAO	Food and Agricultural Organization
FDA	Food and Drug Administration
FDPIR	Food Distribution Program on Indian Reservations
FFVP	Fresh Fruit and Vegetable Program
FMNP	Farmers' Market Nutrition Program
FNCS	Food, Nutrition, and Consumer Services
FNIC	Food and Nutrition Information Center
FNS	Food and Nutrition Service
FSP	Food Stamp Program
FY	Fiscal year
HEI	Healthy Eating Index
HHFKA	Healthy, Hunger-Free Kids Act of 2010
HHS	Department of Health and Human Services
IOM	Institute of Medicine
ITO	Indian Tribal Organization
NHANES	National Health and Nutrition Examination Survey
NPE	Nutrition Program for the Elderly
NSA	Nutrition Services and Administration
NSIP	Nutrition Services Incentive Program
NSLA	National School Lunch Act
NSLP	National School Lunch Program

OAA	Older Americans Act
OHS	Office of Head Start
OMB	Office of Management and Budget
PIN	Personal identification number
PRWORA	Personal Responsibility and Work Opportunity Reconciliation Act
SBP	School Breakfast Program
SFMNP	Senior Farmers' Market Nutrition Program
SFSP	School Food Service Program
SMP	Special Milk Program
SNAP	Supplemental Nutrition Assistance Program
SNAP-Ed	Supplemental Nutrition Assistance Program Education
SSO	Seamless Summer Feeding Option
SY	School year
TANF	Temporary Assistance for Needy Families
TEFAP	The Emergency Food Assistance Program
USDA	United States Department of Agriculture
WIC	Special Supplemental Nutrition Program for Women, Infants, and Children

STUDENT ASSIGNMENTS AND ACTIVITIES DESIGNED TO ENHANCE LEARNING AND STIMULATE CRITICAL THINKING

1. Read the poverty measure summary by Gordon M. Fisher, The Development and History of the Poverty Thresholds, Social Security Bulletin, vol. 55, no. 4, Winter 1992, pp. 3–14, available at: http://www.ssa.gov/history/fisheronpoverty.html. Summarize the role that food cost has played in the development of the poverty thresholds.
2. Review the most recent *Household Food Security in the United States* report at http://www.ers.usda.gov/publications. How do the food security rates in your state differ from other states and the nation as a whole? How have rates changed over time? What might be some reasons for these trends?
3. Use the Internet to determine the minimum wage in your state. Based on the most current annual poverty threshold for an individual under 65 years old (without children, see http://www.census.gov/hhes/www/poverty/data/threshld/index.html), how many hours per week must one work at minimum wage to make 100% of the federal poverty level? 130%? 185%? 200%?
4. What is the current maximum daily SNAP allotment a person can receive if they live in a household of four people (assuming 30 days per month)? What is the allotment per meal (assuming 3 meals per day)? What do these figures tell you about SNAP?
5. SNAP benefits cannot be used to purchase alcoholic beverages, tobacco, hot foods and foods that will be eaten in the store, pet foods, and most nonfood items (seeds and plants that produce food are allowed). Are there any exceptions to these regulations? Given the high rates of obesity in the United States, should *junk foods* be added to this list? Present arguments on both sides of the issue, being sure to include your definition of *junk foods*.
6. In addition to education, list and discuss other strategies that can be used to increase SNAP participation.
7. Take a 3-day *SNAP challenge* to better understand what life can be like for millions of low-income Americans. Based on the current maximum SNAP benefit allotment, determine what your daily allotment would be as a single-person household. For example, in 2015, the maximum monthly allotment for one person was $194 (see Table 11.6). This averages out to $6.47 per day, assuming 30 days per month. All food and beverages purchased and

eaten during the challenge, including fast food and eating out, must be included in the total spending. In addition, during the challenge, only eat food that you purchased for the project; do not eat food that you already own (exceptions include spices and condiments). Avoid accepting free food from friends, family, or at work, including at receptions, briefings, or other events where food is served. Keep track of receipts on food spending and take note of your experiences throughout the 3 days. Once the challenge is over, summarize your experiences, being sure to answer the following questions:

    a. What types of foods and beverages did you eat most often during the week? What made you choose these items over others?

    b. What foods or beverages would you have liked to consume, but did not? Why?

    c. Describe any methods you used to decrease your food costs.

    d. Did you ever feel hungry during the week? If so, what did you do? How might food insecurity or lack of funds for adequate food affect daily activities?

    e. Describe the overall healthfulness of your weekly diet.

    f. Based on your experience, what suggestions do you have for policies or programs that could address any issues or barriers encountered during completion of the 3-day SNAP challenge?

8. Review the Team Nutrition resource library (http://teamnutrition.usda.gov/library.html). Identify a gap or need in what is already available, such as a specific topic or a specific audience, and develop a new resource. Describe the gap this resource is meant to fill, and how it fills the need.

9. Find another example (not already listed in the text) of a farm-to-school program, school gardens program, farm-to-preschool program, or farm-to-college program in the United States. Write a case study about this program, including details about the impetus for change, implementation process, solutions to challenges or barriers, and successes.

10. Find and compare the most recent participation rates for the NSLP and SBP. Describe at least three reasons why rates between the two programs differ.

11. In addition to breakfast in the classroom programs, describe three other ways schools and districts can increase participation in the SBP.

12. Given that breast milk is the optimal food for most infants, should women receiving WIC benefits be allowed to choose to formula feed? Present arguments on both sides of the issue.

13. What is the maximum number of federal food and nutrition programs each of the following individuals can participate in? Provide the names of the programs he/she is eligible for, as well as the reason(s) for eligibility.

    • 3-year-old female with anemia whose household income equals 125% of the poverty guideline.

    • 10-year-old male whose household income equals 175% of the poverty guideline.

    • 16-year-old pregnant female whose household income equals 100% of the poverty guideline.

    • 24-year-old male whose household income equals 150% of the poverty guideline.

    • 50-year-old female whose household income equals 130% of the poverty guideline.

    • 85-year-old male whose household income equals 120% of the poverty guideline.

14. Summarize changes to the various federal nutrition programs as a result of the most recent farm bill.

15. Visit a SNAP office, WIC center, NSLP/SBP-participating school, Head Start program, Adult Day Care Center, food pantry, or other local agency that implements one of the federal nutrition programs described in the chapter. Observe and/or volunteer at the location for at least 2 hours. Describe your experience, including your impressions of how well the location meets the mission or purpose of the nutrition program it implements.

REFERENCES

Alaimo K, Olson CM, Frongillo EA, Jr. Food insufficiency and American school-aged children's cognitive, academic, and psychosocial development. *Pediatrics.* 2001;108(1):44–53. Erratum in *Pediatrics.* 2001;108(3):824.

Aussenberg RA, Colello KJ. Domestic Food Assistance: Summary of Programs. Congressional Research Service, February 24, 2014. Available at http://www.ncsl.org/documents/statefed/Domestic_Food _Assistance.pdf, accessed February 15, 2015.

Benbrook C. Elevating Antioxidant Levels in Food through Organic Farming and Food Processing: An Organic Center State of Science Review. The Organic Center for Education and Promotion, 2005. Available at http://organic.insightd.net/reportfiles/Antioxidant_SSR.pdf, accessed January 24, 2015.

Bickel G, Nord M, Price C, Hamilton W, Cook J. *Measuring Food Security in the United States: Guide to Measuring Household Food Security, Revised 2000.* U.S. Department of Agriculture, Food and Nutrition Service, 2000. Available at http://www.fns.usda.gov/sites/default/files/FSGuide_0.pdf, accessed January 10, 2015.

Biemiller L. Fresh from the farm. *Chron Higher Ed.* 2005;52(14):A36–A38.

Blum-Kemelor DM, Molofsky AJ. *Feeding Infants: A Guide for Use in the Child Nutrition Programs.* FNS-258, U.S. Department of Agriculture, Food and Nutrition Service, 2001. Available at http://www.fns .usda.gov/tn/resources/feeding_infants.pdf, accessed January 20, 2015.

Burke M, Sims K, Anderson S, FitzSimons C, Hewins J. *Hunger Doesn't Take a Vacation: Summer Nutrition Status Report 2013.* Food Research and Action Center. Available at http://frac.org/pdf/2013_summer _nutrition_report.pdf, accessed February 15, 2015.

Capps R, Koralek R, Lotspeich K, Fix M, Holcomb P, Anderson JR. Assessing Implementation of the 2002 Farm Bill's Legal Immigrant Food Stamp Restorations: Final Report to the United States Department of Agriculture Food and Nutrition Service. The Urban Institute, 2004. Available at http://urban.org /UploadedPDF/411138_LegalImmigrantRestorations.pdf, accessed February 15, 2015.

Casey PH, Szeto KL, Robbins JM, Stuff JE, Connell C, Gossett JM, Simpson PM. Child health-related quality of life and household food security. *Arch Pediatr Adolesc Med.* 2005;159(1):51–56.

Cohen B, Andrews M, Kantor LS. *Community Food Security Toolkit.* EFAN-02-013, U.S. Department of Agriculture, Economic Research Service, 2002. Available at http://www.ers.usda.gov/media/327699 /efan02013_1_.pdf, accessed January 20, 2015.

Coleman-Jensen A, Gregory C, Singh A. *Household Food Security in the United States in 2013.* ERR-173, U.S. Department of Agriculture, Economic Research Service, September 2014. Available at http://www.ers .usda.gov/media/1565415/err173.pdf, accessed February 15, 2015.

Cunnyngham KE. *Reaching Those in Need: State Supplemental Nutrition Assistance Program Participation Rates in 2011.* Washington, DC: Mathematica Policy Research, 2014. Available at http://www.fns.usda .gov/sites/default/files/Reaching2011.pdf, accessed February 15, 2015.

Demas A. Low-fat school lunch programs: Achieving acceptance. *Am J Cardiol.* 1998;82(10):80T–82T.

DeNavas-Walt C, Proctor BD. Income and Poverty in the United States: 2013. Current Population Reports. US Census Bureau. Table B-1 Poverty Status of People, by Family Relationship, Race, and Hispanic Origin: 1959 to 2013. Available at https://www.census.gov/content/dam/Census/library/publications/2014/demo /p60-249.pdf, accessed February 15, 2015.

DeNavas-Walt C, Proctor BD. Income and Poverty in the United States: 2013. Current Population Reports. US Census Bureau. Table 3 People in Poverty by Selected Characteristics: 2012 and 2013. Available at https://www.census.gov/content/dam/Census/library/publications/2014/demo/p60-249.pdf, accessed February 15, 2015.

Eslami E. *Trends in Supplemental Nutrition Assistance Program Participation Rates: Fiscal Year 2010 to Fiscal Year 2012.* Washington, DC: Mathematica Policy Research, Inc., 2014. Available at http://www.fns.usda .gov/sites/default/files/ops/Trends2010-2012.pdf, accessed February 15, 2015.

FAO, IFAD, WFP. *The State of Food Insecurity in the World 2014. Strengthening the Enabling Environment for Food Security and Nutrition.* Rome: FAO, 2014. Available at http://www.fao.org/3/a-i4037e.pdf, accessed February 15, 2015.

Farm to Preschool. What Is Farm to Preschool. Available at http://www.farmtopreschool.org/whatisfarmtopreschool .html, accessed January 20, 2015.

Feeding America. Kids Café. Available at http://feedingamerica.org/how-we-fight-hunger/programs-and -services/child-hunger/kids-cafe.aspx, accessed February 15, 2015.

Flock P, Petra C, Ruddy V, Peterangelo J. A Salad Bar Featuring Organic Choices: Revitalizing the School Lunch Program, 2003. Available at http://www.farmtoschool.org/resources-main/a-salad-bar-featuring -organic-choices-revitalizing-the-school-lunch-program, accessed February 15, 2015.

Fox MK, Condon E. *School Nutrition Dietary Assessment Study-IV: Summary of Findings.* Washington, DC: Mathematica Policy Research, 2012. Available at http://www.fns.usda.gov/sites/default/files/SNDA-IV _Findings_0.pdf, accessed January 24, 2015.

Fox MK, Cole N, Lin B-H. *Nutrition and Health Characteristics of Low-Income Populations. Volume 1, Food Stamp Program Participants and Nonparticipants.* EFAN-04014-1, U.S. Department of Agriculture, Economic Research Service, 2004a. Available at http://webarchives.cdlib.org/sw12j6951w/http://www .ers.usda.gov/publications/efan04014-1/, accessed January 10, 2015.

Fox MK, Hamilton W, Lin B-H. *Effects of Food Assistance and Nutrition Programs on Nutrition and Health: Volume 3, Literature Review.* FANRR19-3, U.S. Department of Agriculture, Economic Research Service, 2004b. Available at http://www.ers.usda.gov/media/873018/fanrr19-3_002.pdf, accessed January 24, 2015.

Gottlieb R, Azuma A. Healthy Schools/Healthy Communities: Opportunities and Challenges for Improving School and Community Environments. Urban & Environmental Policy Institute, Occidental College. Available at http://www.niehs.nih.gov/about/visiting/events/pastmtg/assets/docs_n_z/supplementary_informationover viewgottlieb.pdf, accessed January 20, 2015.

Gunderson GW. *The National School Lunch Program: Background and Development.* 0-429-783. Washington, DC, 1971. Available at http://www.fns.usda.gov/nslp/history, accessed January 15, 2015.

Gussow J. Is organic food more nutritious? And, is that the right question? *Organic Farming Research Foundation Information Bulletin.* Fall 1996;3:1,10. Available at http://archive.sare.org/sanet-mg/archives /html-home/38-html/0190.html, accessed February 1, 2015.

Hamm MW, Bellows AC. Community food security and nutrition educators. *J Nutr Educ Behav.* 2003; 35(1):37–43.

Healthy, Hunger-Free Kids Act of 2010, Public Law 111-296, 124 Stat. (2010): 3183–3266. Available at http:// www.gpo.gov/fdsys/pkg/PLAW-111publ296/pdf/PLAW-111publ296.pdf, accessed January 24, 2015.

Joshi A, Kalb M, Beery M. *Going Local: Paths to Success for Farm to School Programs.* Developed by the National Farm to School Program, Center for Food & Justice, Occidental College, and Community Food Security Coalition, 2006. Available at http://www.farmtoschool.org/resources-main/going-local-paths -to-success-for-farm-to-school-programs, accessed February 15, 2015.

Kantor LS. Community food security programs improve food access. *Food Rev.* 2001;24(1):20–26.

Kleinman RE, Hall S, Green H, Korzec-Ramirez D, Patton K, Pagano ME, Murphy JM. Diet, breakfast, and academic performance in children. *Ann Nutr Metab.* 2002;46(Suppl 1):24–30.

Leos-Urbel J, Schwartz AE, Weinstein M, Corcoran S. Not just for poor kids: The impact of universal free school breakfast on meal participation and student outcomes. *Economics of Education Review.* 2013;36:88–107.

Macartney S, Bishaw A, Fontenot K. *Poverty Rates for Selected Detailed Race and Hispanic Groups by State and Place: 2007–2011.* American Community Survey Briefs, ACSBR/11-17. Washington, DC: U.S. Census Bureau, 2013: Table 1, February 2013. Available at http://www.census.gov/prod/2013pubs /acsbr11-17.pdf, accessed February 15, 2015.

Martinez S, Hand M, Da Pra M et al. *Local Food Systems: Concepts, Impacts, and Issues.* ERR-97, U.S. Department of Agriculture, Economic Research Service, 2010. Available at http://www.ers.usda .gov/media/122868/err97_1_.pdf, accessed February 15, 2015.

McCullum C, Desjardins E, Kraak VI, Ladipo P, Costello H. Evidence-based strategies to build community food security. *J Am Diet Assoc.* 2005;105(2):278–283.

Meinen A, Friese B, Wright W, Carrel A. Youth gardens increase healthy behaviors in young children. *J Hunger Environ Nutr.* 2012;7(2–3):192–204.

Murray SC. A Survey of Farm-to-College Programs: History, Characteristics and Student Involvement. University of Washington, 2005. Available at http://www.farmtocollege.org/Resources/Murraythesis _final_June2005.pdf, accessed January 24, 2015.

Nestle M. *What to Eat.* New York: North Point Press, 2006, p. 55.

Okie S. Eating lessons at school. In Okie S, ed. *Fed Up! Winning the War against Childhood Obesity.* Washington, DC: The National Academies Press, 2005, pp. 183–210.

Oliveira V. *The Food Assistance Landscape: FY 2013 Annual Report.* EIB-120, U.S. Department of Agriculture, Economic Research Service, February 2014. Available at http://www.ers.usda.gov/media/1282272/eib120 .pdf, accessed February 15, 2015.

Oliveira V, Frazao E, Smallwood D. *Rising Infant Formula Costs to the WIC Program: Recent Trends in Rebates and Wholesale Prices.* ERS-93, U.S. Department of Agriculture, Economic Research Service, 2010. Available at http://www.ers.usda.gov/media/136568/err93_1_.pdf, accessed February 15, 2015.

Parmer SM, Salisbury-Glennon J, Shannon D, Struempler B. School gardens: An experiential learning approach for a nutrition education program to increase fruit and vegetable knowledge, preference, and consumption among second-grade students. *J Nutr Ed Behav.* 2009;41(3):212–217.

Ralston K, Newman C, Clauson A, Guthrie J, Buzby J. *The National School Lunch Program: Background, Trends, and Issues*. ERR-61, U.S. Department of Agriculture, Economic Research Service, 2008. Available at http://www.ers.usda.gov/media/205594/err61_1_.pdf, accessed January 25, 2015.

Richard B. Russell National School Lunch Act, Public Law 79-396, 60 Stat. (1946): 239. Available at http://www.ssa.gov/OP_Home/comp2/F079-396.html, accessed January 24, 2015.

Rome Declaration on World Food Security and World Food Summit Plan of Action. FAO Corporate Document Repository, November 1996. Available at http://www.fao.org/docrep/003/W3613E/W3613E00.htm, accessed January 20, 2015.

"Special Supplemental Nutrition Program for Women, Infants and Children." Title 7 *Code of Federal Regulations*, §246.1. Revised September 28, 2011.

Strayer M, Eslami E, Leftin J. *Characteristics of Supplemental Nutrition Assistance Program Households: Fiscal Year 2012*. SNAP-12-CHAR, U.S. Department of Agriculture, Food and Nutrition Service, Office of Research and Analysis, 2014. Available at http://www.fns.usda.gov/sites/default/files/2012Characteristics Summary.pdf, accessed February 15, 2015.

Sullivan D. Expanding Farm-to-School Programs Create Opportunities for Farmers...and Children, 2003. Available at http://www.newfarm.org/depts/talking_shop/1203/farm-to-school.shtml, accessed January 24, 2015.

Supplemental Nutrition Assistance Program Quality Control Annual Report: Fiscal Year 2012. U.S. Department of Agriculture, Food and Nutrition Service, Program Accountability and Administration Division, Quality Control Branch, 2013. Available at http://www.fns.usda.gov/sites/default/files/snap/SNAP_QC_2012.pdf, accessed February 15, 2015.

Supplemental Nutrition Assistance Program Quality Control Review Handbook. FNS Handbook 310, U.S. Department of Agriculture, Food and Nutrition Service, October 2012. Available at http://www.fns.usda .gov/sites/default/files/FNS_310_Handbook.pdf, accessed January 20, 2015.

The Edible Schoolyard Project. Available at http://edibleschoolyard.org/, accessed February 15, 2015.

The Real Food Campus Commitment. Available at http://www.sustainabilitycoalition.org/projects/west-coast -real-food-challenge, accessed February 15, 2015.

US Bureau of the Census, Current Population Survey, Annual Social and Economic Supplements. Table 8. Poverty of People, by Residence: 1959 to 2013. Available at http://www.census.gov/hhes/www/poverty /data/historical/hstpov8.xls, accessed February 15, 2015.

US Commission on Civil Rights. A Quiet Crisis: Federal Funding and Unmet Needs in Indian Country, July 2003. Available at http://www.usccr.gov/pubs/na0703/na0204.pdf., accessed January 20, 2015.

US Department of Agriculture. About SNAP-Ed Connection. Available at http://snap.nal.usda.gov/about-snap -ed-connection-0, accessed January 29, 2015.

US Department of Agriculture, Farm Service Agency. Agricultural Marketing Service. Food and Consumer Service. Improving USDA Commodities. Tri-Agency Commodity Specification Review Report, 1995.

US Department of Agriculture. FNS. Available at http://www.fns.usda.gov, accessed February 15, 2015.

US Department of Agriculture. Food, Nutrition, and Consumer Services. Available at http://www.usda.gov /wps/portal/usda/usdahome?contentidonly=true&contentid=missionarea_FNC.xml, accessed February 15, 2015.

US Department of Agriculture, Food and Nutrition Service, Agricultural Marketing Service. USDA Farm to School Team 2010 Summary Report, 2011. Available at http://www.fns.usda.gov/sites/default/files/2010 _summary-report.pdf, accessed February 15, 2015.

US Department of Agriculture. Food and Nutrition Service. Approved Federal Funds for SNAP Education by Fiscal Year. Available at http://snap.nal.usda.gov/snap/ApprovedFederalFundsSNAP-Ed01202010.pdf, accessed January 24, 2015.

US Department of Agriculture. Food and Nutrition Service. Available at http://www.fns.usda.gov/fdd/mobile /foods-available/foods-available-list.html, accessed February 15, 2015.

US Department of Agriculture. Food and Nutrition Service. Child and Adult Care Food Program. About CACFP. Available at http://www.fns.usda.gov/cnd/care/cacfp/aboutcacfp.htm, accessed January 20, 2015.

US Department of Agriculture. Food and Nutrition Service. Child and Adult Care Food Program Annual Summary. Available at http://www.fns.usda.gov/pd/ccsummar.htm, accessed February 15, 2015.

US Department of Agriculture. Food and Nutrition Service. Commodity Supplemental Food Program. About CSFP. Available at http://www.fns.usda.gov/csfp/about-csfp, accessed February 15, 2015.

US Department of Agriculture, Food and Nutrition Service. Commodity Supplement Food Program Fact Sheet, June 2014c. Available at http://www.fns.usda.gov/sites/default/files/pfs-csfp.pdf, accessed February 15, 2015.

US Department of Agriculture. Food and Nutrition Service. Commodity Supplemental Food Program. Last updated September 4, 2014. Available at http://www.fns.usda.gov/csfp/commodity-supplemental-food-program-csfp, accessed September 9, 2014.

US Department of Agriculture. Food and Nutrition Service. Expanding School Breakfast. Talking Points. Available at http://www.fns.usda.gov/sites/default/files/breakfast_talkingpoints.pdf, accessed February 15, 2015.

US Department of Agriculture, Food and Nutrition Service. Food Distribution Program on Indian Reservations Fact Sheet, July 2014b. Available at http://www.fns.usda.gov/sites/default/files/pfs-fdpir, accessed February 15, 2015.

US Department of Agriculture. Food and Nutrition Service. FY 2014 Strategic Priorities. Available at http://www.fns.usda.gov/sites/default/files/FNSStrategicPriorities_021913.pdf, accessed February 15, 2015.

US Department of Agriculture. Food and Nutrition Service. National School Lunch Program Fact Sheet. Available at http://www.fns.usda.gov/sites/default/files/NSLPFactSheet.pdf, accessed February 15, 2015.

US Department of Agriculture. Food and Nutrition Service. National School Lunch Program National Level Monthly Data: FY 2012 through November 2014. Available at http://www.fns.usda.gov/pd/36slmonthly.htm, accessed February 15, 2015.

US Department of Agriculture. Food and Nutrition Service. Nutrition Program Facts: WIC—The Special Supplemental Nutrition Program for Women, Infants and Children. Available at http://www.fns.usda.gov/sites/default/files/wic/wic-fact-sheet.pdf, accessed January 9, 2015.

US Department of Agriculture. Food and Nutrition Service. Nutrition Services Incentive Program. About NSIP. Available at http://www.fns.usda.gov/fdd/programs/nsip/about_nsip.htm, accessed January 10, 2015.

US Department of Agriculture. Food and Nutrition Service. Nutrition Services Incentive Program. Eligibility Requirements. Available at http://www.fns.usda.gov/fdd/programs/nsip/nsip_eligibility.htm, accessed February 15, 2015.

US Department of Agriculture, Food and Nutrition Service, Office of Research and Analysis. *Building a Healthy America: A Profile of the Supplemental Nutrition Assistance Program*, 2012. Available at http://www.fns.usda.gov/sites/default/files/BuildingHealthyAmerica.pdf, accessed February 15, 2015.

US Department of Agriculture, Food and Nutrition Service. School Breakfast Program (SBP) Fact Sheet. Available at http://www.fns.usda.gov/sites/default/files/SBPfactsheet.pdf, accessed August 21, 2015.

US Department of Agriculture. Food and Nutrition Service. School Meals. An Opportunity for Schools. Available at http://www.fns.usda.gov/cnd/seamless_summer.htm, accessed January 8, 2015.

US Department of Agriculture. Food and Nutrition Service. School Meals. Rates of Reimbursement. Correction to SY 2014–2015 Notice. Available at http://www.fns.usda.gov/school-meals/rates-reimbursement, accessed February 15, 2015.

US Department of Agriculture. Food and Nutrition Service. Senior Farmers' Market Nutrition Program Overview. Available at http://www.fns.usda.gov/sfmnp/overview, accessed February 15, 2015.

US Department of Agriculture. Food and Nutrition Service. SNAP-Ed Connection. FY 2015 SNAP Education Plan Guidance. Available at http://snap.nal.usda.gov/snap/Guidance/FinalFY2015SNAP-EdGuidance.pdf, accessed February 15, 2015.

US Department of Agriculture. Food and Nutrition Service. Special Milk Program Fact Sheet. Available at http://www.fns.usda.gov/cnd/milk/AboutMilk/SMPFactSheet.pdf, accessed February 15, 2015.

US Department of Agriculture, Food and Nutrition Service. Special Supplemental Nutrition Program for Women, Infants and Children (WIC): Implementation of the Electronic Benefit Transfer-Related Provisions of Public Law 111-296, Proposed Rule. *Fed Reg.* 2013;78(40):13549–13563. Available at http://www.fns.usda.gov/sites/default/files/FR-022813_WIC.pdf.

US Department of Agriculture. Food and Nutrition Service. Summer Food Average Daily Attendance. Available at http://www.fns.usda.gov/pd/04sffypart.htm. Accessed July 8, 2013.

US Department of Agriculture. Food and Nutrition Service. Summer Food Service Annual Summary. Available at http://www.fns.usda.gov/sites/default/files/pd/sfsummar.pdf, accessed February 15, 2015.

US Department of Agriculture. Food and Nutrition Service. Summer Food Service Program: Frequently Asked Questions. Available at http://www.fns.usda.gov/cnd/summer/FAQs.htm, accessed February 15, 2015.

US Department of Agriculture. Food and Nutrition Service. Supplemental Nutrition Assistance Program Annual State Level Data FY 2009–2014: Average Monthly Benefit per Household. Available at http://www.fns.usda.gov/sites/default/files/pd/19SNAPavg$HH.pdf, accessed February 15, 2015.

US Department of Agriculture. Food and Nutrition Service. Supplemental Nutrition Assistance Program Annual State Level Data FY 2009–2014: Average Monthly Benefit per Person. Available at http://www.fns.usda.gov/sites/default/files/pd/18SNAPavg$PP.pdf, accessed February 15, 2015.

US Department of Agriculture. Food and Nutrition Service. Supplemental Nutrition Assistance Program. Benefit Redemption Division 2011 Annual Report. Available at http://www.fns.usda.gov/sites/default /files/2011-annual-report-revised.pdf, accessed February 15, 2015.

US Department of Agriculture. Food and Nutrition Service. Supplemental Nutrition Assistance Program Eligibility. Available at http://www.fns.usda.gov/snap/applicant_recipients/eligibility.htm, accessed January 20, 2015.

US Department of Agriculture. Food and Nutrition Service. Supplemental Nutrition Assistance Program Eligibility. Available at http://www.fns.usda.gov/snap/eligibility, accessed February 15, 2015.

US Department of Agriculture. Food and Nutrition Service. Supplemental Nutrition Assistance Program. From Food Stamps to SNAP: State Name Change Tracking Chart. Available at http://www.fns.usda.gov/sites /default/files/state-chart.pdf, accessed January 19, 2015.

US Department of Agriculture, Food and Nutrition Service. Supplemental Nutrition Assistance Program. Quality Control, January 6, 2015. Available at http://www.fns.usda.gov/snap/quality-control, accessed February 15, 2015.

US Department of Agriculture. Food and Nutrition Service. The Business Case for Increasing Supplemental Nutrition Assistance Program (SNAP) Participation. Available at http://www.fns.usda.gov/snap/outreach/business -case.htm, accessed February 15, 2015.

US Department of Agriculture, Food and Nutrition Service. The Emergency Food Assistance Program Fact Sheet, July 2014a. Available at http://www.fns.usda.gov/sites/default/files/pfs-tefap.pdf, accessed February 15, 2015.

US Department of Agriculture. Food and Nutrition Service. WIC Breastfeeding Data Local Agency Report, FY 2012. Available at http://www.fns.usda.gov/sites/default/files/WIC%20BFDLA%20Report%20FY%20 2012.pdf, accessed February 15, 2015.

US Department of Agriculture. Food and Nutrition Service. WIC Eligibility Priority System. Available at http:// www.fns.usda.gov/wic/howtoapply/eligibilityprioritysystem.htm, accessed February 15, 2015.

US Department of Agriculture. Food and Nutrition Service. WIC Fact Sheet, April 2014. Available at http:// www.fns.usda.gov/sites/default/files/WIC-Fact-Sheet.pdf, accessed February 15, 2015.

US Department of Agriculture. Food and Nutrition Service. WIC Farmers' Market Nutrition Program Fact Sheet. Available at http://www.fns.usda.gov/sites/default/files/WIC-FMNP-Fact-Sheet.pdf, accessed February 15, 2015.

US Department of Agriculture. Food and Nutrition Service. WIC Program Annual Summary. Available at http://www.fns.usda.gov/pd/wisummary.htm, accessed February 15, 2015.

US Department of Agriculture. Food and Nutrition Service. WIC Program Monthly Data. Available at http:// www.fns.usda.gov/pd/37WIC_Monthly.htm, accessed February 15, 2015.

US Department of Agriculture. Food and Nutrition Service. Women, Infants, and Children. Annual State Level Data. Available at http://www.fns.usda.gov/pd/wic-program, accessed February 15, 2015.

US Department of Agriculture. Food and Nutrition Service. Women, Infants, and Children Frequently Asked Questions About WIC. Available at http://www.fns.usda.gov/wic/frequently-asked-questions-about -wic#7, accessed February 15, 2015.

US Department of Agriculture. Food and Nutrition Services. Supplemental Nutrition Assistance Program Research. Available at http://www.fns.usda.gov/ORA/menu/Published/SNAP/SNAP.htm#Building, accessed January 19, 2015.

US Department of Agriculture, Food and Nutrition Services. Supplemental Nutrition Assistance Program (SNAP) State Outreach Plan Guidance, 2009. Available at http://www.fns.usda.gov/sites/default/files /Outreach_Plan_Guidance.pdf, accessed February 15, 2015.

US Department of Agriculture. FY 2015 Budget Summary and Annual Performance Plan. Available at http:// www.obpa.usda.gov/budsum/FY15budsum.pdf, accessed February 15, 2015.

US Department of Agriculture. SNAP-ED Strategies & Interventions: An Obesity Toolkit for States. Update May 2014. Available at http://snap.nal.usda.gov/snap/SNAP-EdInterventionsToolkit.pdf, accessed January 24, 2015.

US Department of Agriculture. Supplemental Nutrition Assistance Program. Short History. Available at http:// www.fns.usda.gov/snap/short-history-snap, accessed February 15, 2015.

US Department of Agriculture. Strategic Plan FY 2010–2015. Available at http://www.ocfo.usda.gov/usdasp /sp2010/sp2010.pdf, accessed February 15, 2015.

US Department of Agriculture. Strategic Plan FY 2010–2015: Update Addendum. Available at http://www .ocfo.usda.gov/usdasp/sp2010/StrategicPlanUpdate.pdf, accessed February 15, 2015.

US Department of Agriculture. Strategic Plan FY 2014–2018. Available at http://www.usda.gov/documents /usda-strategic-plan-fy-2014-2018.pdf, accessed February 15, 2015.

WhyHunger. Farm to Cafeteria: An Introduction. Available at http://www.whyhunger.org/getinfo/showArticle /articleId/92, accessed January 24, 2015.

Worthington V. Nutritional quality of organic versus conventional fruits, vegetables, and grains. *J Altern Complement Med.* 2001;7(2):161–173.

Yanyuan Wu A. *Why Do So Few Elderly Use Food Stamps?* Chicago, IL: University of Chicago, Harris School of Public Policy Studies, 2009. Available at http://www.ifigr.org/workshop/fall09/wu.pdf, accessed January 20, 2015.

12 Social Marketing and Other Mass Communication Techniques

What is in a name?*

William Shakespeare

INTRODUCTION

Health communication is the study and use of communication strategies to inform and influence individual and community decisions around health (Health.gov, http://www.health.gov/communication/resources/). Health communication contributes to improving the public's health through public education campaigns that create awareness, alter the social climate, change attitudes, and motivate individuals to adopt recommended behaviors. Campaigns traditionally have relied on mass communication (such as public service announcements on billboards, radio, and television) and in the form of printed educational materials such as pamphlets and fact sheets. Social marketing has become a valuable tool in promoting health behavior change. Increasingly, health promotion activities take advantage of digital technologies to use multiple channels to target audiences, tailor messages, and engage people in interactive, ongoing exchanges about health.

We describe social marketing, examine the use of social marketing in food and nutrition public health campaigns, and briefly introduce the use of tailored health communication messaging and social media.

SOCIAL MARKETING

Many health campaigns have turned to social marketing techniques to effect change. Coined in 1971 (Kotler and Zaltman 1971), the term *social marketing* describes the application and adaptation of commercial marketing concepts to the design, implementation, and control of programs designed to increase the acceptability of a social idea or bring about behavior change to improve the welfare of targeted individuals or their society. It is, in essence, marketing for societal benefit rather than commercial profit.

At the heart of health promotion is the need to influence consumers, program developers, policymakers, and others. Our ability to change people's lifestyles through improved diets and increased physical activity is intimately connected to our ability to influence behavior supporting good nutrition.

Communication experts posit a conceptual framework for approaching public health and social behaviors, a continuum of options through which to pursue goals of population-based behavior change. This framework assumes that a recommended behavior is a freely available option (an assumption that may only be partly true, as for example, in the case of access to fresh fruits and vegetables and other healthy foods or to opportunities for physical activity). Table 12.1 presents a behavior-change continuum. At one end of the continuum, we find people who are motivated to act

---

* William Shakespeare. (Paraphrased) Romeo and Juliet (Act II, Scene II).

TABLE 12.1
Continuum of Activities to Promote Desirable Changes in Food Handling, Nutrient Intake, and Diet

Desirable Consumer Behavior	Information *Use Education if Knowing Is Enough*	Social Marketing *Use Social Marketing When People Need to Be Convinced*	Policy or Law *Use the Law When People Refuse to Change*
Increase physical activity	*Dietary Guidelines for Americans*[1]	VERB[2] We Can![3]	School district policies
Practice safe food handling	Dietary Guidelines	Fight BAC!® Like a Produce Pro[4]	HAACP
Consume adequate calcium	Dietary Guidelines	Best Bones Forever[5]	Child Nutrition Program milk requirements
Consume adequate folic acid	Folic Acid Awareness Week[6]	Folic Acid. Every Body Needs It. The Folic Acid Community Campaign[7]	Folic acid added to the standard of identify recipe for enriched grains[8]
Consume less total fat	Dietary Guidelines	1% or Less Campaign[9]	Milk offered in child nutrition programs is limited to fat-free and low-fat[10]
Prevent, or manage, diabetes	National Diabetes Education Program[11]	Small Steps. Big Rewards. Prevent Type 2 Diabetes[12]	Type 2 diabetes screening under the Affordable Care Act of 2010[13]
Breastfeed	CDC Guide To Breastfeeding Interventions[14]	WIC Breastfeeding Promotion and Support[15]	Breastfeeding legislation[16]

Source:

[1] US Department of Agriculture, US Department of Health and Human Services. *Dietary Guidelines for Americans*, 2010, 7th ed. Washington, DC: US Government Printing Office, December 2010. Available at http://www.health.gov/dietaryguidelines /dga2010/dietaryguidelines2010.pdf, accessed February 14, 2015.

[2] Wong F, Huhman M, Heitzler C et al. VERB™—A social marketing campaign to increase physical activity among youth. Prev Chronic Dis. 2004a. Available at http://www.cdc.gov/pcd/issues/2004/jul/04_0043.htm, accessed January 20, 2015.

[3] National Institutes of Health. National Heart, Lung, and Blood Institute. We Can! Available at http://www.nhlbi.nih.gov /health/public/heart/obesity/wecan/, accessed January 20, 2015.

[4] Partnership for Food Safety Education. Fight Bac! Availbale at www.fightbac.org, accessed June 29, 2015.

[5] US Department of Health and Human Services. Office on Women's Health. Best Bones Forever. Available at http://www .bestbonesforever.org, part of http://www.girlshealth.gov, accessed January 20, 2015.

[6] National Birth Defects Prevention Network. Folic Acid Awareness Week 2015. Available at http://www.nbdpn.org/faaw2015. php, accessed January 20, 2015.

[7] The Folic Acid Community Campaign. Available at http://cchealth.org/folic-acid/, accessed January 20, 2015.

[8] Bentley TG et al., *Public Health Nutr.* 2009;12(04):455–467.

[9] Reger B et al., *Public Health Rep.* 1998 Sep–Oct;113(5):410–419.

[10] Federal Register. Nutrition Standards in the National School Lunch and Breakfast Programs; Final Rule. Vol. 11, No. 17. Thursday, January 26, 2012. Available at http://www.gpo.gov/fdsys/pkg/FR-2012-01-26/pdf/2012-1010.pdf, accessed January 20, 2015.

[11] National Diabetes Education Program: Available at http://ndep.nih.gov/, accessed January 20, 2015.

[12] Small Steps. Big Rewards. Prevent Type 2 Diabetes. Available at http://ndep.nih.gov/partners-community-organization /campaigns/SmallStepsBigRewards.aspx, accessed January 20, 2015.

[13] US Department of Health and Human Services. Preventive Services Covered Under the Affordable Care Act. Available at http://www.hhs.gov/healthcare/facts/factsheets/2010/07/preventive-services-list.html, accessed January 20, 2015.

[14] CDC Guide to Breastfeeding Interventions. Available at http://www.cdc.gov/breastfeeding/resources/guide.htm, accessed January 20, 2015.

[15] United States Department of Agriculture. Food and Nutrition Services. Breastfeeding Promotion and Support in WIC. Available at http://www.fns.usda.gov/wic/breastfeeding-promotion-and-support-wic, accessed January 20, 2015.

[16] National Conference of State Legislatures. Breastfeeding State Laws. Available at http://www.ncsl.org/research/health /breastfeeding-state-laws.aspx, accessed January 20, 2015.

BOX 12.1 FOCUS GROUPS

A focus group is a gathering of individuals who have been chosen as representatives of a target audience to discuss a specific topic, usually for several hours and in great detail. A focus group generally consists of 6–12 participants, with the focus provided by a trained moderator. A focus group study is often used in the development of product concepts or in the first phase of an exploratory investigation of a problem. Qualitative data collected in focus groups provide in-depth information necessary to understanding attitudes and motivations that influence consumers' decisions and behavior. Focus groups give participants an opportunity to describe their experiences and preferences without the limitation of preset response categories.

Source: Burroughs, E. et al. Using focus groups in the consumer research phase of a social marketing program to promote moderate-intensity physical activity and walking trail use in Sumter County, SC. Prev Chronic Dis. 3(1), A08, January 2006.

on the basis of information. Those people are likely to adopt a recommended behavior because they are able to see it as in their best interest. Educational campaigns alone may suffice to create behavior change among populations at this end of the continuum. On the other hand, populations at the opposite end of the continuum are resistant to the recommended behavior. They may not see a change in behavior as in their self-interest or making the change may be too much trouble. Law- or policy-based approaches such as the fortification of milk with vitamin D in the 1930s and with vitamin A in the 1940s (Murphy et al. 2001) may be required to assure these people receive the nutrition they need (Maibach 2002; Rothschild 1999).

In the middle of the continuum are populations who are neither inclined nor resistant to the recommended behavior. Social marketing may be used to bring about behavior change in this population by increasing the perceived benefits, reducing the perceived barriers, or in other ways improving opportunities and thus enhancing the perceived value of adopting the recommended behavior.

Through market research techniques, such as the use of focus groups, social marketers seek to identify and understand the intended audience and discover the factors that prevent them from adopting a healthy behavior (Box 12.1).

People are more likely to adopt a desired behavior if we first assess and then attempt to change attitudes toward the behavior, perceptions of the benefits of the new behavior, and perceptions of how their peers will view that behavior. Social marketers develop, monitor, and constantly adjust a program to stimulate appropriate behavior change. Social marketing programs can address any or all of the traditional marketing mix variables: product, price, place, or promotion (Montazeri 1997).

WHAT SOCIAL MARKETING CAN DO FOR PUBLIC HEALTH

A strong communications program will both target a specific audience with a prevention message and increase the general public's awareness of prevention-related issues. Raising public awareness can also frequently result in a change in social policies and practices. In addition, effective social marketing and communications can increase knowledge; influence attitudes; show benefits of behavior change; reinforce the desired knowledge, attitudes, and behavior; demonstrate skills; increase demand for services; refute myths and misconceptions; and influence norms.

Every year, new public health mass media campaigns attempting to change health behavior and improve health outcomes are launched. These campaigns enter a crowded media arena flooded with messages from competing sources. Public health practitioners must not only capture the attention of the public amid this competition but also motivate communities to change entrenched health behaviors or initiate habits that may be new or difficult.

TABLE 12.2

Low-Fat Milk Consumption Campaign Illustrates Types of Social Change, by Time and Level of Society

	Micro Level (Individual Consumer)	Group Level (Group or Organization)	Macro Level (Society)
Short-term change	*Behavior change* Example: Switch to low-fat milk at school	*Change in norms; administrative change* Example: Voluntarily provide low-fat and fat-free milk as part of the school breakfast and school lunch programs	*Policy change* Example: Provide price supports for low-fat and fat-free dairy products so they cost the consumer less than their full-fat counterparts
Long-term change	*Lifestyle change* Example: All dairy products consumed are either low fat or fat free	*Organizational change* Example: Require that all schools provide low-fat and fat-free milk	*Sociocultural evolution* Example: Eradication of nutrition-related diseases, such as heart disease

The public health approach to prevention acknowledges that problems arise through the interaction of a host(s), an agent, and the environment. Prevention programs that focus exclusively on the host may overlook influences in the environment or community such as advertisements for foods of high energy but low nutritional value, which promote nutrition-related problems including obesity, type 2 diabetes, heart disease, osteoporosis, and eating disorders. Effective programs take a comprehensive, ecological approach, addressing individual risk factors, but also community norms, local policies, the built environment, mass media, and other factors. The ecological model of public health emphasizes the linkages and relationships among multiple factors (or determinants) affecting health (Public Health Foundation, http://www.phf.org//resourcestools /Pages/ecological_Model_publichealth.aspx).

Encouraging people to take greater responsibility of their health decisions is facilitated by empowering individuals and communities, such as through the use of positive opinion leaders, social support, and empowerment, while also manifesting environmental and policy changes (Lindridge et al. 2013). Table 12.2 describes a sample low-fat milk consumption campaign to illustrate types of social change by time and level of society.

HOW SOCIAL MARKETING WORKS

Every social marketing campaign starts with an extensive formative evaluation process that includes focus groups. The content, tone, and execution of a campaign is determined by formative research, which includes reviews of existing and new research; discussions with expert consultants who conducted similar projects in nongovernmental and state, local, and national organizations; and primary audience research with a small group of representatives from the target audiences in order to understand their interests, attributes, and needs. Formative research occurs before a program is designed and implemented. It can help define and understand target populations, help in the creation of programs that are specific to the needs of the target populations, ensure that programs and materials are acceptable and feasible to clients before launching the program, and even improve relationships between clients and agencies. Formative research should be an integral part of developing programs or adapting programs (Gittelsohn et al. 2006).

For example, the formative research that was conducted prior to the development of VERB included primary audience research with *tweens*, parents, and other influencers (educators and youth leaders) (Centers for Disease Control and Prevention, http://www.health.gov/communication/db /report_detail.asp?ID=20&page=1&z_26=on&sp=2); expert consultants; local, state, and national organizations; and lessons learned from other large-scale national media campaigns (Centers for Disease Control and Prevention, http://www.cdc.gov//youthcampaign/research/PDF/Formative ResearchProcess.pdf).

The fundamental elements of every social marketing program, examples of which are detailed in the sections that follow, are the *product* being promoted; its *price* to the target audience; the strategy to *promote* the product; and the *place* or channel through which the product is communicated to the intended audience. These factors—product, price, promotion, and place—are often referred to as *the four P's* of social marketing.

Additional P's included in the social marketing mix are the *public*, or intended audience for the product promotion; *partners*, or alliances in the campaign; *purse* strings or budget; and *policy* (Weinreich 1999) and *politics*, or the rules, systems, and environmental change factors that influence voluntary behavior change, not policies that punish undesired behavior (Social Marketing National Excellence Collaborative 2002).

Product (Social Proposition)

Product refers to the knowledge, attitudes, or behavior social marketers want the target audience to adopt. In addition to a desired behavior change, such as drinking low-fat milk, the product may be an actual commodity, such as flavored low-fat milk varieties. A continuum of products exists, ranging from tangible, physical products (low-fat milk), to services (a nutrition education module that promotes low-fat milk), and to practices (eating low-fat dairy products). The social marketing product may also be a policy (a regulation addressing the types of milk served in a school district). Framing the desired behavior change in a positive manner is one way to sell the *product*. For example, the Special Supplemental Nutrition Program for Women, Infants, and Children (WIC) Breastfeeding Promotion Project promotes breastfeeding as a means toward mother–child bonding rather than as a way to confer passive immunity on the infant (Lindenberger and Bryant 2000). Similarly, the VERB campaign (Wong et al. 2004) presents physical activity as a way to have fun, spend time with friends, and gain recognition from peers and adults rather than to prevent obesity or chronic disease later in life.

Whatever the product, the marketer must develop an enticing package with which it is associated. A viable product helps the target audience first understand that they have a genuine problem, and then recognize the product being offered as a good solution to that problem. One role of social market research is to discover the audience's perceptions of the problem and the product and to determine how important they feel it is to resolve the problem.

In contrast to commercial exchanges where consumers receive a product or service in exchange for a cash outlay, public health markets rarely exchange an immediate, explicit payback for adoption of healthy behavior. Social marketers distinguish between the *core product* (what people will gain when they perform the behavior) and the *actual product* (the desired behavior). To succeed, the product must provide a solution to problems that consumers consider important and/or that offers them a benefit they truly value.

For this reason, social marketers conduct research to help them understand the target audience's aspirations, preferences, and other desires (in addition to their health needs) and to identify the benefits most appealing to consumers. The marketing objective is to discover which benefits have the greatest appeal to the target audience and design a product that provides those benefits. In some cases, public health professionals must change their recommendations or modify their programs to provide benefits valued by consumers (Grier and Bryant 2005).

Price (Cost)

Price describes what the consumer must do or pay to obtain the social marketing product. Specifically, it refers to the money or, more often, intangibles such as time, effort, social approval, lost opportunities, or embarrassment involved in a person's changing his or her behavior. In social marketing, price might be the perceived cost of giving up the rich taste of whole milk or the discomfort associated with behaving differently from one's peers. If the costs outweigh the benefits for an individual, the perceived value of the offering will be low, and it is unlikely that it will be adopted. However, if the benefits are perceived as greater than their costs, the chance of trial and adoption of the product is much greater. Price, therefore, represents a balance of the product's benefits with its cost to members of the target audience.

To reduce the perceived costs of behavior change and make the change easy to adopt, social marketers recommend removing social and environmental obstacles. Enacting policy change can help address these barriers by minimizing the price the target audience believes it must pay in the exchange. There are many issues to consider in setting the price: if the product is priced too low or provided free of charge, the consumer may perceive it as being low in quality; if the price is too high, some will be unable to afford it. Social marketers must balance these considerations, while also conferring a sense of dignity on the transaction. Perceptions of costs and benefits can be determined through research and used in positioning the product.

What is the price to the target audience for changing their behavior? The VERB campaign proposes a voluntary exchange: tweens who take up physical activity, presumably in place of watching television or just sitting around, will derive the benefits of fun and social engagement (Bauman 2004).

Place (Accessibility)

Place is where the target audience either performs the desired behavior or accesses programs and services. Place also describes how the product reaches the intended audience. For a tangible product, place refers to the distribution system—including the warehouse, trucks, sales force, and retail outlets where it is sold—or locations where it is distributed for free. For an intangible product, place is less clear-cut but refers to the channels through which consumers are provided with information or training. These may include doctors' offices, shopping malls, mass media outlets, schools, houses of worship, or in-home demonstrations.

Place affects price. For instance, if the message to drink more low-fat milk is promoted through the school lunch program, the price of peer pressure may be reduced. The exchange and its opportunities should be made available in places that reach the audience and fit its lifestyles. Another consideration of place is deciding how to ensure accessibility of the offering and quality of the service delivery. Place should be readily available.

By determining the activities and habits of the target audience, as well as their experience and satisfaction with the present delivery system, researchers can pinpoint the most ideal means of distribution for the offering, such as where the behaviors should or should not occur or what barriers or opportunities exist for the behavior's occurrence. To ease access, social marketers should be prepared to move programs or products to places that the intended audience frequents. According to the VERB campaign, a VERB place is where tweens can be physically active in a safe environment.

Promotion (Communication)

Because of its visibility, promotion is often mistakenly assumed to comprise the whole of social marketing, although it is only one component. Promotion focuses on creating and sustaining demand for a product through the integrated use of advertising, public relations, media advocacy, personal selling, and entertainment vehicles to convince the target audience that the product is worth its price. It may include publicity campaigns through the mass media, such as news stories and advertisements on television, radio, and in newspapers; public service advertisements and paid advertising; coupons; editorials; food demonstrations and taste tests at a variety of community sites; and supermarket shelf labeling initiatives to draw attention to the program's message.

Research is crucial to determine the most effective and efficient vehicles to reach the target audience and increase demand. Research helps determine the communications that should occur, from what sources to whom, and through what channels of influence. For example, trusted healthcare providers and clergy from communities of various faiths can deliver messages in person about the benefits of physical activity, changing one's diet, and screening for diabetes. The exchange should be promoted creatively and through channels and tactics that maximize desired responses. Promotion includes multiple ways to reach the target audience to advocate the benefits of the behavior change, including product, price, and place components. Some of the promotion strategies and tactics employed by the VERB campaign include paid media advertising, community-based events, contests and sweepstakes, community and corporate partnerships, and websites.

Public (Target Audiences)

To be successful, the programs that social marketers promote must often reach multiple audiences. These publics include external and internal groups involved in or affected by the program. External publics encompass the target audience, as well as secondary and tertiary audiences, policymakers, and gatekeepers. The primary audience might be children ages 9 through 13, with a secondary audience of the people who influence their decisions—such as parents, teachers, clergy, and physicians—and a tertiary audience of policymakers and directors at local radio stations. Internal publics encompass those involved in some capacity with approval or implementation of the program, such as board of directors and office staff.

The VERB program initially segmented its target population by age (youth aged 9–13 and parents/influencers). It then conducted research that identified important differences among specific segments within the tween audience on the basis of activity level, receptivity to physical activity, ethnicity, and gender (Grier and Bryant 2005).

Policy (Environmental Supports)

Social marketing programs can inspire individual behavior change, but sustaining that change is difficult unless it is supported in the long run by environmental components. Often, policy change is needed to bring about lasting behavior change. For example, a campaign to encourage the consumption of low-fat milk might include a policy component of changing the milk choices available in the school cafeteria to include a greater number of options, or conversely, to limit choices by removing the high-fat option. Similarly, the policy component of the VERB campaign might focus on increasing the number of bicycle paths in a community and increasing the availability of after-school programs that appeal to the targeted age group.

Partnerships (Alliances)

Health issues are often so complex that one agency cannot make a dent by itself. Partnerships or alliances should be cultivated with local or national groups, corporate sponsors, medical organizations, service clubs, or media outlets that have goals similar to those of the social marketing campaign. Partnerships can increase the likelihood for success by creating buy-in throughout the community, enhancing credibility of the program through connections with well-known partners, increasing available financial and human resources, and gaining access to a greater area of expertise in health, social service, and business fields. Keeping VERB a "cool brand for tweens" is a critically important goal for partners (parks, schools, youth-serving organizations) as they collaborate on the campaign.

Strategic alliances with for-profit partners may offer many important benefits to the social organization, including improved delivery of their message, heightened influence, and broader reach. However, there are risks involved in the strategic alliance process, such as conflicts of interest (Box 12.2).

Purse Strings (Budget)

Purse strings refer to the funding component of strategy development. Most organizations that develop social marketing programs operate with funds provided by foundations, government grants, or donations. When planning and allocating funds, consider how long the funding will last, how strategic partnerships can foster more resources, and whether products or services must be offered for a cost.

BOX 12.2   WORKING WITH FOR-PROFIT PARTNERS

Consider these guidelines when contemplating working with for-profit partners:

- Carefully review each partnership proposal and do not enter into any collaboration that endorses a specific commercial product, service, or enterprise. Only allow your program's logo to be used in conjunction with approved projects and only with your written permission. Retain the right to review all copy such as advertising or publicity prior to the partner's using your program's name or logo.
- Prior to partnership negotiations, confirm that a partnership with this company will not create tensions or conflicts with another partner for your program. Ensure that the company has no unresolved disputes with or is not currently in negotiation for a grant or contract from your organization; that it conforms to standards of health, medical care, and labor practices; and that its products, services, or promotional messages do not conflict with your organization's policies or programs.

Source: Adapted from US Department of Health and Human Services. National Institutes of Health. National Cancer Institute. *Making Health Communication Programs Work*, 1989, rev. 2001. Available at http://www.cancer .gov/cancertopics/cancerlibrary/pinkbook/pink-book.pdf, accessed January 20, 2015.

THE SOCIAL MARKETING CAMPAIGN

A social marketing campaign consists of six stages: planning the approach, defining the program's messages and channels, developing and pretesting program materials, implementing the program, evaluating the program, and using feedback to refine the program. Each of these components of a health communication campaign can be viewed as a self-contained project of its own and is further defined in the following sections.

Step 1: Plan the Approach

Planning establishes the foundation for the entire campaign. Before moving ahead, an assessment of the problem is undertaken and available resources are identified. During this stage, the target audience is identified and should become increasingly segmented, for example, into groups with common risk behaviors, motivations, or information channel preferences to aid in developing appropriate messages. Goals and objectives are developed during planning. Formative evaluation also begins during the planning stage and continues through the development of materials to be used in the program.

The following should be undertaken during the planning stage:

1. *Perform literature review.* This defines the scope of the problem and identifies the types of programs that have already been developed to address the situation.
2. *Define the audience.* A social marketing program may need to address more than one audience to accomplish its objectives (Box 12.3).

   Planners often differentiate among primary, secondary, and tertiary audiences to pinpoint whom they are trying to reach. The *primary audience* is the specific group or groups that the program is designed to influence. A primary audience may consist of one subgroup (adolescent males) or a combination of groups (adolescent males and their parents). A *secondary audience* includes individuals who influence the primary audience, such as peers, parents, teachers, clergy, and role models. The *tertiary audience* comprises community decision makers who influence policy and offer financial and logistical support to community-based prevention programs. The support of this group is critical to any prevention program. These individuals may actually comprise the primary audience in some social marketing programs.

> **BOX 12.3   DEFINING THE AUDIENCE**
>
> A social marketing program may need to address more than one audience to accomplish its objectives. Even small, apparently homogeneous communities contain various subgroups within their populations, with personal, environmental, and geographic differences. Personal factors include age, gender, ethnicity and cultural background, socioeconomic level, literacy or educational level, occupation, or gang membership. Environmental factors include stress, social support, access and barriers, and exposure to harmful agents. The geographic area is where people live.

3. *Analyze the community.* A community analysis helps identify its driving (positive) and restraining (negative) forces. Your action plan should build on the driving forces and diminish the restraining forces to strengthen a community's prevention efforts. *Social asset mapping* creates an in-depth understanding of a community by identifying local resources, networks, places of importance, prevalent issues, current connections, and where potential new connections might be made. Such an understanding creates numerous possibilities for new and innovative approaches to community empowerment that are compatible with maintaining healthy environments. All communities have assets that can be used as building blocks for economic and social development. Geographic information systems may be used to literally map these assets.

4. *Develop the concept.* State the issue or broad goal the campaign is trying to address, for example, to promote physical activity.

5. *Set goals and objectives.* Determine what you are trying to achieve and what behaviors, if changed, would have the greatest difference. State the desired attributes and expected benefits of each targeted behavior. For example, for physical activity, the desired attributes and anticipated benefits might include burning fat to lose weight, look better, and be sexier; producing endorphins to reduce stress and feel more energy; and building muscle strength to become stronger and thus more independent in daily activities. Describe the specific behaviors the campaign intends to change, how much change is anticipated, who is expected to change, and by when. For example, by July 2017, the percentage of adults in Peoria who engage in regular physical activity will increase by 30%.

6. *Identify core components or strategies.* This includes deciding how to communicate challenging messages about the desired behaviors, making the desired behaviors more rewarding or attractive, making the desired behaviors easier to achieve or of lower cost, improving peoples' abilities to adopt the behavior change, and decreasing the attractiveness of competing behaviors.

7. *Outline basic principles.* As previously discussed, the principles of a social marketing campaign include product, price, public, place, promotion, policies, and the development of a budget.

Step 2: Define the Message and Select Channels and Materials

The second step in a social marketing campaign is to identify the message or messages to be delivered and choose appropriate and effective channels of communications. It is also important to identify the environments, situations, or settings in which the targeted behavior should (or should not) occur, such as at home or while using transportation, at schools, parks, or other public places.

Typical communication channels include television, radio, newspapers and other print media, and bulletin boards in supermarkets, churches, neighborhood centers, and other places where people congregate, as well as Internet, email, texting, and social media platforms. Using multiple channels ensures greater coverage of the issues and improved reach of the target population. A multiple-outlet or a limited-outlet approach may be used.

- A *multiple outlet approach* uses as many available resources as possible including television and radio stations, newspapers, and billboards. The community is inundated with information from these outlets.
- A *limited-outlet approach* concentrates a significant commitment of time and resources on one or two outlets only, resulting in a campaign that becomes very closely tied to the chosen outlet.

When choosing communications channels, consider the channel's credibility, cost, reach (the number of people or households exposed to a specific message during a set period of time), and the average number of times an audience is exposed to the message.

The messages the program sends must be meaningful and appealing to the target audience. An effective message stimulates the target audience to think about and discuss the issues. The message should be based on facts and tied to the present, because Americans value instant gratification. The campaign should develop and convey clear, concrete suggestions and model alternative behaviors or ways of doing things without resorting to scare tactics and negativism. The threat of osteoporosis in 30 or 40 years poses little incentive to a 15-year-old to drink milk. Consider, instead, stressing the convenience of a single-serve milk bottle, cheese stick, or yogurt drink that fits easily into a backpack, book bag, or bicycle rack.

The program's ultimate outcome should be to establish social norms that promote and sustain healthy, safe behaviors. The message should minimize the psychological or physical cost of the product to the target audience.

Step 3: Develop and Pretest Materials and Methods

Develop a draft of all marketing materials for pretesting with an audience similar to or a subset of your target audience. Ask this group if these materials produce the intended results, and revise if needed based on their criticism and suggestions. Repeat this process until all stakeholders are satisfied with the end product. A focus group can greatly facilitate the process of preparing materials that appeal to your audience. The use of a logic model is highly recommended (Box 12.4).

Step 4: Implement the Program

Before launching the campaign, all communication materials should be ready and available in sufficient quantities. A method to track and evaluate the program must already also be in place. Tracking allows the program planners to determine where the program is succeeding and identify areas

---

BOX 12.4   LOGIC MODELS

Logic models are often developed for public health programs and campaigns. A logic model links campaign inputs and activities with campaign outcomes. It describes the sequence of events for bringing about behavior change and presents the relationship among campaign inputs (research and consultation), campaign activities (marketing and partnership tactics), the impact on outputs (number of people exposed), and outcomes (knowledge, attitude, and behavior change).

A logic model can be used as a tool to

1. Identify the short-term, intermediate, and long-term outcomes for the campaign.
2. Link those outcomes to each other and to campaign activities.
3. Select outcomes to measure depending on the stage of the campaign's development.
4. Demonstrate how it may take time before long-term outcomes can be associated with the campaign.

where changes are needed. The most successful programs are constantly being updated with current information about the program and the target audience. The process evaluation, which essentially reviews those tasks involved in implementing the program, is appropriate for use during the implementation phase of the program.

Step 5: Program Evaluation

Assessing a program's effectiveness goes beyond the process evaluation of the planning, defining, and development stages of a campaign. Program evaluation measures if and how much the program affects beliefs, attitudes, and behaviors of the target audience. While outcome and impact evaluation should be designed during the planning stage, it is not conducted until the evaluation stage. When designing a program evaluation, include key questions such as what are our success indicators and how will we know if we have achieved them.

The type of evaluation conducted depends upon several factors, including money, time, policies affecting the ability to gather information, the level of support for evaluation, and the overall design of the program.

- *Outcome evaluation* is used to gather descriptive information about knowledge and attitude changes, expressed intentions of the target audience, and the initiation of policy changes.
- *Impact evaluation*, the most comprehensive evaluation, focuses on the long-term outcomes of the program. It measures factors such as changes in morbidity and mortality, long-term maintenance of behavior change, and changes in absenteeism from work or school. Impact evaluation is most often used in multifaceted health education programs that include awareness, education, training, and communication components.

The evaluation should involve all stakeholders including members of the target audience, program implementers, and grant makers. It must identify indicators of success, document evidence of success, and determine how overall improvement may be made.

Step 6: Refine the Program and Plan for Sustainability

Use evaluation feedback to make adjustments in campaign components as needed. If, for instance, no change in behavior is seen with a particular subgroup, evaluation is needed to determine if campaign components should be modified or if increased exposure to the campaign is necessary.

Strategies to sustain the effort long enough to make a difference are vital, such as

- Using process evaluation information to help secure sustained support from grant makers and other funding sources.
- Securing media coverage of the issue or goal and successful implementation of relevant components. Hold a news conference and pitch feature stories as part of a media advocacy campaign to promote continued awareness and enhance public support for attempts to address it.
- Promoting adoption of effective campaign components or advocating for changes that contribute to improvement.
- Promoting ongoing implementation through collaborating partners.

ETHICS IN SOCIAL MARKETING

Social marketers must pay careful attention to ethical standards and practices if the field is to mature as a profession. Most social marketing and health communications projects give rise to ethical dilemmas related to either the ends being pursued or the strategies and tactics used to achieve them. During the course of a project, issues might be raised by managers, colleagues, audience

---

BOX 12.5   EXAMPLE OF INTENDED AUDIENCE ISSUE

Consider the use of a website designed to provide health information to parents in a specific targeted low socioeconomic group. Will your intended audience actually be accessing the website, whether once or on an ongoing basis? A case study of a children's oral health program in Scotland (Childsmile) cites research that text used in websites often becomes increasingly complex and prohibitive for those with low health literacy, and further notes that the use of a website may be less relevant to the target audience of parents while actually more relevant to increasing visibility of the initiative and addressing wider political concerns such as being seen to involve parents.

Source: Lindridge A et al., *European Journal of Marketing* 47(9) pp. 1399–1420. Available at http://oro.open.ac .uk/35900/2/991AF55F.pdf, accessed February 14, 2015.

BOX 12.6   CELEBRATE!

Always be sure to celebrate successes. Group celebrations of accomplishments, such as successfully establishing a supportive policy change, help maintain morale and enthusiasm for the program. Focus attention on improvements in desired behavior and outcomes and honor the individuals who have contributed to those improvements. This may be a simple awards ceremony to acknowledge community champions.

---

members, community groups, partners, or the media, or from critics. During the planning stages, one might ask if the goals of the program are truly in the public's interest and whether the primary beneficiaries of the program are the targeted groups and subgroups—not the change agents (Box 12.5).

Social alliances—in other words, partnerships between for-profit and nonprofit organizations—can present ethical challenges for one or both partners. It is thus incumbent upon both companies and nonprofits to give considerable attention to developing ethical standards and procedures for addressing ethical issues (Andreasen and Drumwright 2000).

During the evaluation phase, one might want to determine if the strategies and components of the program were implemented responsibly, if potential negative side effects were avoided or minimized, and if the benefits of the program outweighed the risks. Complex ethical challenges may arise, such as the following:

- Is it acceptable to exaggerate risk and heighten fear if doing so saves more lives or at least reduces morbidity?
- When is it acceptable to improve the lives of people in one group at the expense of another?
- Does a marketing campaign respect a group's culture if it calls for fundamental change within it?
- Celebrate successes (Box 12.6).

FOOD AND NUTRITION SOCIAL MARKETING CAMPAIGNS

Since the genesis of the term *social marketing* in 1971, the concepts have been widely adopted in public health as a tool to *sell behavior*, whether encouraging a new behavior, rejecting initiation of an undesirable behavior, modifying a current behavior, or abandoning an undesirable one

---

BOX 12.7   HOW EASY IS THAT?

The Iowa Nutrition Network's social marketing campaign, Pick a Better Snack™, encourages fruit and vegetable choices for snacks. The catchy tagline is of note as it also incorporates food safety into the message: "Wash. Bite. How easy is that?"

In-class lessons and community-based social marketing materials are available at http://www.idph.state.ia.us/inn/PickABetterSnack.aspx.

(Kotler and Lee 2008). Social marketing ideas can be used even when not conducting an extensive campaign, as researchers have found that students were more likely to eat vegetables when they were *sold* to the kids as "X-Ray Vision Carrots" instead of as unnamed or "food of the day" (Wansink et al. 2012).

Although food and nutrition social marketing campaigns are also used at the state and local level, such as Iowa's "Pick a Better Snack™" campaign (Iowa Department of Public Health, http://www.idph.state.ia.us/inn/PickABetterSnack.aspx), the most extensive nutrition-related social marketing campaigns in the United States are national campaigns operated by the US Department of Agriculture (USDA) and by the Department of Health and Human Services (HHS). Food- and nutrition-related issues addressed by federal social marketing campaigns include campaigns to promote health as well as prevent disease (Box 12.7).

We introduce below a number of social marketing campaigns that have been implemented to address issues of public health concern, such as obesity, diabetes, osteoporosis, cardiovascular disease (CVD), and others. Some campaigns of note are examined more closely than others.

Campaigns to Prevent Overweight and Obesity

Data indicate that the prevalence of obesity has significantly increased among the US population since the 1960s (Flegal et al. 1998). Recent studies in the United States have found high levels of obesity among adults and children, with one-third of adults and 17% of children obese; however, the rate appears to have leveled off between 2003–2004 and 2009–2010 (Ogden et al. 2014). Obesity among young people aged 2–19 is about 17% as of 2011–2012 and has not changed significantly since 2003–2004 (Centers for Disease Control and Prevention, http://www.cdc.gov/obesity/data/childhood.html).

Overweight and obesity are defined in relation to body mass index (BMI), which is weight in kilograms divided by the square of height in meters. In adults, a BMI of 25.0–29.9 is overweight, of 30.0–39.9 is obese, and over 40.0 is extremely obese (Hedley et al. 2004). Children are considered overweight if their BMI is between the 85th and 95th percentiles for age and gender and are considered obese with a BMI above the 95th percentile (Ogden 2010).

Overweight and obesity are known risk factors for CVD, diabetes, metabolic syndrome, high blood pressure, high cholesterol levels, asthma, arthritis, and poor health status as well as physiological ailments such as orthopedic abnormalities and premature menarche (Eckel et al. 2005; Hardy et al. 2004; Mokdad et al. 2003). Because of the strong correlation between overweight/obesity and the risk factors for morbidity and mortality, confronting the obesity epidemic is an urgent public health priority.

VERB: It's What You Do

Lack of physical activity is a contributing factor to the increase in childhood overweight as well as the emergence of type 2 diabetes among youth. In 2001, physical education had been cut back or eliminated in many US schools and many youth lead sedentary home lives as well, spending hours of their free time watching television or playing computer games. Youth also tend to participate in risky activities such as smoking, drinking, and violence. In response to these unhealthy behaviors, in 2001 Congress appropriated $125 million to the Centers for Disease Control and Prevention (CDC) for 5 years to change children's health behaviors. The CDC's response to this sweeping mandate was to focus on the sedentary lifestyle of young adolescents.

The VERB Youth Media Campaign, launched in 2002, was a 5-year, multiethnic, demonstration media campaign designed to increase and maintain physical activity among tweens, children aged 9–13 years (Bauman 2004). VERB's secondary audience includes parents and influencers such as educators and youth leaders. The campaign's goals were to increase knowledge and improve attitudes and beliefs about tweens' regular participation in physical activity; increase parental and influencer support for and encouragement of their participation; heighten awareness of options and opportunities for participation; facilitate opportunities for participation; and increase and maintain the number of tweens who regularly participate in physical activity.

VERB's social marketing included websites, paid traditional media such as television, radio, print, outdoor advertising, and advertorials, targeted distribution of posters, book covers, murals, and school materials and marketing promotions, such as contests, events, and sweepstakes.

VERB's Logic Model

The VERB logic model (Figure 12.1) illustrates the campaign's vision—all youth leading healthy lifestyles—and mission: to increase and maintain physical activity among tweens (Wong et al. 2004). The *inputs* of the campaign are its consultants, staff, contractors, partnerships, the community infrastructure, and the program's research and evaluation. All of these inputs contribute to the campaign activities, which include advertising, promotions, websites, public relations, and outreach nationally and into particular communities.

The short-term outcome for the campaign is tween and parent awareness as well as *buzz* about the campaign brand and its messages. Awareness and buzz lead to *midterm outcomes* that include changes in subjective norms, beliefs, self-efficacy, and perceived behavioral control. The logic model indicates that if these changes occur, there will be a positive *buzz* among tweens about physical activity, and these responses will lead to tweens enlisting support from their parents to participate in physical activity. Awareness and understanding of the campaign and brand messages by parents lead to changes for parents in knowledge, beliefs, and expectations.

Campaign planners hypothesized that as parents internalize changes in knowledge, beliefs, and expectations, they will support tween participation in physical activity, reciprocally enhanced by tweens requesting support from them. As depicted in the model, planners also expect that as parents prioritize their child's physical activity needs, the parents, as well as other influencers of tweens, will mobilize to advocate for physical activity. This mobilization as well as national and community outreach will lead to the availability of and access to organized and non-organized settings for physical activity. Tweens' behavioral intentions as well as available and accessible settings are likely to encourage them to engage in physical activity.

The campaign's *long-term outcomes* include tweens engaging in and maintaining physical activity, thereby reducing chronic diseases. The model indicates that there is a possible displacement strategy that tweens who participate in physical activity may also have fewer unhealthy, risky behaviors.

Evaluating VERB

Rigorous multiyear evaluation of the campaign is designed to determine its effectiveness in motivating young adolescents to be more active. Specifically, VERB's outcome evaluation assesses changes in the target audiences' awareness, knowledge, attitudes, and behaviors related to physical activity and measures how these changes can be attributed to campaign exposure. Campaign effects are assessed in two ways: through a longitudinal survey at the national level (6000 youth and their parents) and through surveys of the high-dose markets of Los Angeles, California; Miami, Florida; Columbus, Ohio; Greenville, South Carolina; Houston, Texas; and Green Bay, Wisconsin, where

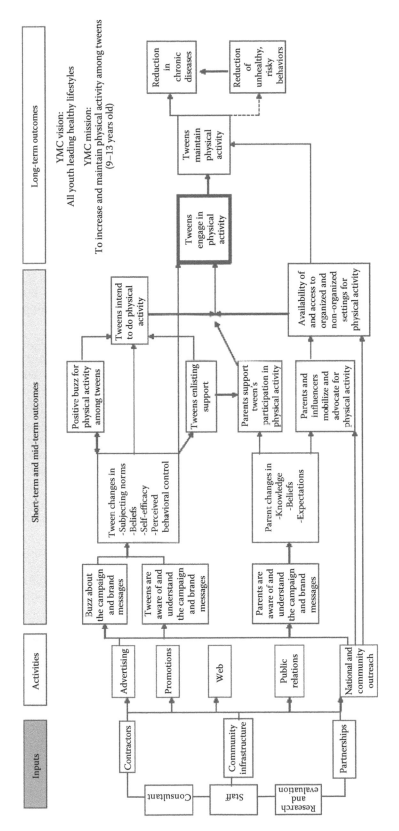

FIGURE 12.1 VERB logic model. (From Huhman, M et al., *Prev Chronic Dis.* [serial online] July 2004. Available at http://www.cdc.gov/pcd/issues/2004/jul/04_0033 .htm, accessed August 28, 2005.)

campaign activities such as community-level partnership development, increased media buys, and local events were concentrated.

A telephone survey was conducted in 2002 and repeated among the same families prior to launching the VERB campaign in 2003, and again in 2004. Evaluation results show that after 1 year of the campaign, three-quarters (74%) of the children surveyed were aware of VERB, and levels of reported sessions of free-time physical activity increased for subgroups of children aged 9–13 years (Huhman et al. 2005).

We Can!

Analysis of the National Heart, Lung, and Blood Institute (NHLBI)-supported Dietary Intervention Study in Children (DISC) data indicates that children and their parents can be taught to make lifestyle changes that result in a diet low in saturated fat and dietary cholesterol (Van Horn et al. 2005). DISC demonstrates that children and their families can learn to enjoy healthy foods, be selective in their food choices, and maintain these healthy habits for up to 3 years. The children in the DISC experimental group reported consuming more servings per day of *go* grains, dairy, meats, and vegetables compared with children in the usual-care group, although intake of fruits and vegetables remained below recommended levels in both groups. The DISC study also suggests that children and their families need the right tools to help them make positive lifestyle changes. To date, however, no longitudinal studies demonstrate that healthy eating habits engendered in childhood carry over to adolescence or adulthood.

Nevertheless, emboldened by the positive results of the DISC analysis, in 2005, the DHHS launched *We Can!* (Ways to Enhance Children's Activity and Nutrition), a national education program from the National Institutes of Health (NIH) to help prevent overweight and obesity among youth ages 8–13 years (National Institutes of Health, http://www.nhlbi.nih.gov/health/public/heart/obesity /wecan/). We Can! provides resources for parents, caregivers, and communities to help youth stay at a healthy weight by encouraging healthy eating, increased physical activity, and reduced screen time (National Heart, Lung, and Blood Institute, National Institutes of Health, US Department of Health and Human Services, http://www.nhlbi.nih.gov/health/educational/wecan/about-wecan/index.htm). Because achieving and maintaining a healthy weight is a universal chronic disease prevention goal, the program is promoted by the NHLBI in collaboration with three other NIH Institutes: the National Institute for Diabetes and Digestive and Kidney Disease (NIDDK), the National Cancer Institute (NCI), and the National Institute of Child Health and Human Development (NICHD) as well as several national private sector organizations (see Chapter 5).

Sisters Together: Move More, Eat Better

The *Sisters Together: Move More, Eat Better* pilot campaign (1995–1998) was designed to increase awareness of the importance of healthy eating and physical activity among young African American women aged 18–35 in three Boston-area, predominantly black communities. The program's "Move More, Eat Better" message was promoted through educational materials and planned activities such as walking groups, dance classes, and cooking demonstrations; distribution of materials promoting healthy eating and regular exercise; and media outreach. The program combined social marketing strategies with a community development focus. The experience resulted in guidelines for communicators using the expanded campaign model for a community campaign. These guidelines are summarized in Table 12.3: strategies for an expanded campaign model developed for *Sisters Together: Move More, Eat Better* (Goldberg et al. 1999). After the success of the pilot program, Sisters Together became a national program of the Weight-Control Information Network (WIN), a national information service of NIDDK (Box 12.8).

An updated program guide is available at the website to download to start one's own Sisters Together program with tip sheets for participants, advice on planning meetings, and using Facebook and other websites (WIN, http://win.niddk.nih.gov/sisters/).

TABLE 12.3

Strategies for an Expanded Campaign Model Developed for *Sisters Together: Move More, Eat Better*

Stage in the Campaign	Activity
Formative research	Include members of the target population in the planning component of the program
Campaign design	Build a campaign that supports community development
Promotion	Highlight action steps for key public health messages; promote existing community resources
Demonstration	Design activities that can be adapted for existing community groups
Transfer	Share evaluation findings, skills, and materials with existing community organizations
Sustainability	Work with local groups to integrate the campaign message with their program focus

---

BOX 12.8   MOVE MORE, EAT BETTER

A manual prepared by NIDDK based on *Sisters Together: Move More, Eat Better* outlines the social marketing approach used to develop the program. It is available online at http://win .niddk.nih.gov/publications/sisterstogether.htm.

CAMPAIGNS TO PREVENT OSTEOPOROSIS

Osteoporosis is defined as a bone mineral density (BMD) value of more than 2.5 standard deviations below the mean for normal young white women. Based on this definition, it is estimated that in the United States, roughly 10 million individuals over age 50 have osteoporosis of the hip, and an additional 33.6 million individuals over age 50 have low bone mass (sometimes referred to as *osteopenia*) of the hip. As such, they are at risk of osteoporosis later in life. The low bone mass and architectural abnormalities that characterize osteoporosis contribute to bone fragility and increased fracture risk. Although osteoporosis is the underlying cause of most fractures in older people, the condition is silent and undetected in the majority of cases until a fracture occurs. A fracture is not a benign event, particularly in older people. The major fracture sites associated with osteoporosis are the hip, the spine, and the wrist. Of all the injury sites, hip fractures have the greatest morbidity and socioeconomic impact. During the first 6 months following a hip fracture, there is a 10–20% mortality rate. Fifty percent of those people experiencing a hip fracture will be unable to walk without assistance, and 25% will require long-term care (US Department of Health and Human Services 2004).

Osteoporosis does not need to be a consequence of aging. As it is largely preventable, public and private organizations have mounted campaigns to promote bone health through increased intake of calcium and increased physical activity.

The National Bone Health Campaign

The Office on Women's Health (OWH) of HHS focuses on the overall health of all women throughout their lifespan. Adolescence represents a dynamic developmental period when young women make important choices about lifestyle behaviors, including diets, physical activity, sexual activity, and use of tobacco, alcohol, and other drugs that can influence their health and well-being throughout adulthood.

OWH along with the CDC and the National Osteoporosis Foundation partnered to promote the National Bone Health Campaign, a multiyear (2001–2005) initiative using social marketing to promote optimal bone health in girls 9–12 years old and thus reduce their risk of osteoporosis later in life. The goal of this public/nonprofit partnership was to educate and encourage young girls to establish lifelong healthy habits, especially increased calcium consumption and physical activity to build and maintain strong bones. The campaign targets adult influencers, including parents, teachers, coaches, youth group leaders, and healthcare professionals.

Six main messages were developed, held together by the campaign tag line: Powerful Bones. Powerful Girls. The six messages are as follows: (1) bone health is an important part of fitness, strength, and power; (2) calcium-rich foods and regular physical activity build strong bones; (3) calcium can be obtained from a variety of tasty and easily accessible foods; (4) there are a variety of easy and fun ways to get physical activity every day; (5) being more physically active is fun, and provides energy, fitness, health, and social interaction; (6) good nutrition helps you stay fit and active. In addition to a website, the campaign ran paid advertisements in children and youth magazines, radio ads, a radio media tour (with 200 interviews), and print materials such as calendars, stickers, presentations, and fact sheets (US Department of Health and Human Services 2004).

To help extend the reach and impact of its messages, partnerships with a broad range of organizations were developed. For example, The Girl Scouts developed troop activity cards, a videotape, and a bone health patch, and Girls Inc. created activity guides and facilitator manuals. The National Association of School Nurses developed materials for use in schools. As of spring 2004, the campaign had more than 122 million print media mentions and more than 3.1 million website visits (US Department of Health and Human Services 2004).

In 2010, Best Bones Forever! (Girls health.gov, http://www.bestbonesforever.org/) was launched as an update to Powerful Bones and was designed to appeal to girls as they mature. Thus, the earlier campaign's cartoon character was replaced with an *exskullmation* point, brighter, edgier colors, and a focus on friendship and fun. Formative research about tweens was conducted and further informed by the evaluations conducted for VERB (Sawatzki 2011).

Campaigns to Prevent Diabetes, Heart Disease, and Cancer

CVD, diabetes, and cancer account for nearly two-thirds of all deaths in the United States. Campaigns to reduce the incidence and prevalence of these diseases target their shared risk factors—tobacco use, insufficient physical activity, and poor diet (Box 12.9).

Excess body weight is an independent risk factor for CVDs as well as causing other risk factors such as hypertension, dyslipidemia, and type 2 diabetes. An estimated 70% of type 2 diabetes risk in the United States is attributable to overweight and obesity. Modest weight loss of 10% of initial body weight and increases in physical activity result in reduced cardiovascular risk factors such as hypertension, dyslipidemia, and type 2 diabetes. Weight reduction decreases insulin resistance and improves measures of glycemia and dyslipidemia in diabetics.

Epidemiologic and animal studies indicate that overweight and obesity are associated with increased risk for cancers at numerous sites, including breast (among postmenopausal women), colon, endometrium, esophagus, gallbladder, liver, prostate, ovarian, pancreas, and kidney (World Cancer Research Fund and American Institute for Cancer Research 2007). Obesity may account for 14% of cancers in men and 20% of cancers in women (Calle et al. 2003).

BOX 12.9   CDC SOCIAL MARKETING RESOURCES

CDC's Division of Nutrition, Physical Activity and Obesity (DNPAO) provides numerous social marketing resources, including a training course, at http://www.cdc.gov/nccdphp /dnpao/socialmarketing/index.html. Additionally, the division provides technical assistance in social marketing for nutrition and physical activity. Several case studies providing real-life examples of how states have used social marketing are available at http://www.cdc.gov /nccdphp/dnpao/socialmarketing/casestudies.html.

BOX 12.10   NATIONAL DIABETES EDUCATION PROGRAM MATERIALS

Online access is available to all NDEP's campaign tools, including public service announcements (PSAs), fact sheets, press releases, and feature articles that can be customized, distributed, and promoted in local markets. These materials are available at http://ndep.nih.gov/resources/index.aspx.

National Diabetes Education Program

The National Diabetes Education Program (NDEP) (US Department of Health and Human Services, http://www.cdc.gov/diabetes/ndep/about.htm) was launched in 1997 to improve diabetes management and reduce the morbidity and mortality from diabetes and its complications. NDEP is sponsored by the CDC and NIH, and also partners with more than 200 other entities at the federal, state, and local levels. The NDEP message is that diabetes is serious, common, costly, and controllable. NDEP aims to change the way diabetes is treated—by the media, by the public, and by the healthcare system.

To help fulfill its mission of changing the way diabetes is treated, NDEP has developed awareness campaigns to disseminate information about diabetes prevention and control. Partners who work with NDEP can adopt the program's messages and tailor them for their members, disseminate information to the media, coordinate education activities, and share resources with other partner organizations. The campaign has developed tools for local organizations to provide motivational messages to members of the community. Clinical practice tools and patient education materials are also available for use by professionals (Box 12.10).

1% or Less*

The 1% or Less campaign is an example of a short-term social marketing campaign. Developed in the mid-1990s by the Center for Science in the Public Interest (CSPI), a nonprofit organization dedicated to improving the nation's health through better nutrition, this 1-month campaign encouraged adults and children over age 2 to switch from whole and 2% milk to low-fat or fat-free milk as a way to reduce consumption of saturated fat. The campaign included news stories and advertisements on television, radio, billboards, and newspapers; milk taste tests at a variety of community sites; supermarket shelf labeling to draw attention to low-fat milk; and school activities.

Results of 1% or Less campaigns conducted in Wheeling, West Virginia (Reger et al. 1998) (population 34,882) and East Los Angeles, California (*Connection* 2000) (population 124,283) suggest that this type of social marketing campaign can be effective. Milk sales data were collected from supermarkets in Wheeling and from comparison communities for three 1-month time periods (at baseline, immediately following the campaign, and 6 months after its completion). In addition, pre- and post-intervention telephone surveys were conducted. Results showed that low-fat milk's market share increased from 18% of overall milk sales at baseline to 41% of overall milk sales in the month following the end of the campaign, an increase that was sustained at the 6-month follow-up. In the post-intervention telephone survey, 38% of those respondents who reported drinking high-fat milk at baseline reported having switched to low-fat milk. Although it was not a program goal, overall milk sales increased by 16% in the intervention cities following the campaign and remained high at follow-up. Similarly, the bilingual (Spanish/English) *Adelante con Leche Semi-descremada 1% Campaign*, implemented by California Adolescent Nutrition and Fitness Program (CAN Fit) in East Los Angeles in 2000, resulted in a doubling of 1% milk sales in Latino communities and a 30%

---

* Health, Nutrition and Diet. 1 1% of less School Kit. Available at https://www.cspinet.org/nutrition/schoolkit.html, accessed February 14, 2015.

increase in milk purchases overall. The 1% Or Less School Kit is available at https://www.cspinet
.org/nutrition/schoolkit.html.

5 A Day for Better Health/Fruits & Veggies—More Matters®

The 5 A Day for Better Health program was a national initiative to increase consumption of fruits
and vegetables by all Americans to 5–9 servings a day (Centers for Disease Control and Prevention
2005). Eating 5–9 servings of fruits and vegetables a day promotes good health and reduces the risk
of many cancers, high blood pressure, heart disease, diabetes, stroke, and other chronic diseases.
The program sought to increase public awareness of the importance of eating 5–9 servings of fruits
and vegetables every day, providing consumers with specific information about how to include more
servings of fruits and vegetables in their daily routines, and to increase the availability of fruits and
vegetables at home, school, work, and other places where food is served. The program provides
a simple, positive message: eat 5 or more servings of fruits and vegetables every day for better
health. Program components included state, regional, and community interventions; media communications; environmental and policy change advocacy; point-of-sale advertising; and behavioral
research (National Cancer Institute 2001).

The program has been extensively evaluated. People are more aware now of the need to consume
fruits and vegetables, but data from the Behavioral Risk Factor Surveillance System (BRFSS) indicate that there has been little change in fruit and vegetable consumption between 1994 and 2000
(Serdula et al. 2004). However, the 5 A Day program has been instrumental in effecting environmental change, which in turn is expected to increase consumption of fruits and vegetables.

An example of the environmental change produced by 5 A Day advocacy is the Fruit and
Vegetable Pilot Program passed as part of the 2002 Farm Bill. The pilot allocated $6 million to
25 schools in Iowa, Indiana, Michigan, and Ohio, and 6 schools on an Indian reservation in New
Mexico for purchase of fruit and vegetable snacks to be offered free to children throughout the
school day. High schools, middle schools, and elementary schools all participated and distributed
fruits and vegetables using a combination of kiosks, vending machines, and in-class methods.

The Fruit and Vegetable Pilot Program was an unqualified success (Buzby et al. 2003); in 2004,
the Child Nutrition and WIC Reauthorization Act made the Fruit and Vegetable Pilot Program
permanent. The act also provides for expanding the program to three other states (Washington,
North Carolina, and Pennsylvania) and two Indian reservations (one or more tribes belonging to the
Intertribal Council of Arizona and the Ogallala Sioux Tribe of the Pine Ridge Reservation in South
Dakota). Effective October 1, 2004, $9 million became available to participating schools to operate
the program during the 2004–2005 school year. The USDA and the National 5 A Day Partnership
also provide educational materials to participating schools. The program has been nationwide since
2008, and $174.5 million in funds were available to schools for FY 2014–2015.

Evaluation of the Fruit & Veggies More Matters campaign found that it raised mothers' awareness and behavioral intent, but consumption of fruit and vegetables was hindered by cost, different
family preferences, and limited restaurant choices, which reflects the need for policy and environmental changes to support behavior-based interventions (Kraak et al. 2013).

In late 2006, *Fruits & Veggies—More Matters*® replaced 5 A Day as the brand promoted by
PBH. During focus groups, PBH discovered that women preferred the term *veggies*. The message
also needed to be refreshed for consistency with the 2005 Dietary Guidelines as the number of recommended servings had increased.

CAMPAIGNS TO PREVENT FOODBORNE ILLNESS

The CDC estimates that 3000 people die annually from foodborne disease, and 128,000 are hospitalized (United States Department of Health and Human Services, Centers for Disease Control
and Prevention, http://www.cdc.gov/foodborneburden/2011-foodborne-estimates.html). Known
pathogens account for an estimated 14 million illnesses, 60,000 hospitalizations, and 1800 deaths.

Three pathogens—*Salmonella, Listeria, Toxoplasma*—are responsible for 1500 deaths annually or more than 75% of those caused by known pathogens. Unknown agents account for the remaining 62 million illnesses, 265,000 hospitalizations, and 3200 deaths. Overall, foodborne diseases appear to cause more illnesses (but fewer deaths) than previously estimated (Mead et al. 1999; Nestle 2003). Several factors explain why the incidence of foodborne illnesses has increased: fewer meals are prepared at home; one quarter of the US population is composed of people with weakened immune systems—the elderly, pregnant women, the very young, and people with HIV/AIDS; and diets include more fresh, often imported, produce (McCabe-Sellers and Beattie 2004). The number of documented outbreaks of human infections associated with the consumption of raw fruits, vegetables, and unpasteurized fruit juices has increased in recent years. In the United States, the number of reported produce-related outbreaks per year doubled between the periods 1973–1987 and 1988–1992 (Buck et al. 2003; US Food and Drug Administration and Center for Food Safety and Applied Nutrition 2001).

Food safety educators, food microbiologists, food safety policy specialists, and epidemiologists were asked to rank food-handling and consumption behaviors associated with 13 foodborne illnesses. Assessment of their collective opinions indicates the extent to which various foodborne illnesses could be prevented by such behaviors as keeping foods at safe temperatures, using a thermometer to cook foods adequately, protecting food and equipment from cross-contamination, hand washing, and avoiding high-risk foods (Hillers et al. 2003). The results of this study are summarized in Table 12.4.

Food Safety Education

Food-handling observations show that food-handling errors are made by consumers during home food preparation (Anderson et al. 2004), by food service employees at the retail level, and to a lesser extent in hospitals and schools (US Department of Health and Human Services et al. 2000). Four broad categories of risk factors contributing to foodborne illness were identified in consumers' homes. These include improper cleaning (inadequately washing hands and food preparation

TABLE 12.4
Food-Handling Behaviors and Prevention of Foodborne Illness

	Relative Importance in Preventing Foodborne Illness	
Behavior	**First-Degree Importance**	**Second-Degree Importance**
Keeping foods at safe temperatures	*Bacillus cereus*	*Staphylococcus aureus*
	Clostridium perfingens	
The use of a thermometer to cook foods adequately	*Campylobacter jejuni*	
	Salmonella species	
	E. coli O157:H7	
	Toxoplasma gondii	
	Yersinia enterocolitica	
Avoiding cross-contamination		*Campylobacter jejuni*
		Salmonella species
		E. coli O157:H7
		Toxoplasma gondii
		Yersinia enterocolitica
Hand-washing	Shigellosis	
Avoiding specific contaminated foods	*Listeria monocytogenes*	
	Noroviruses	
	Vibrio species	

Source: Hillers, VN et al., *J Food Prot.* 66, 1893–1899, 2003.

surfaces), cross-contamination, improper refrigeration, and cooking foods to less than the proper temperature. Similarly, five broad categories of risk factors contributing to foodborne illness were identified in institutional food service establishments, restaurants, retail food stores, schools, and hospitals: food from unsafe sources, inadequate cooking, improper holding temperatures, contaminated equipment, and poor personal hygiene.

The Food Safety Inspection Service (FSIS) is the public health agency within the USDA responsible for ensuring that the nation's commercial supply of meat, poultry, and egg products is safe, wholesome, and correctly labeled and packaged. FSIS works with the Food and Drug Administration (FDA) and state and local authorities to improve food safety practices at the retail level. It also works with other government agencies, the food industry, and others to educate consumers on safe food handling practices. FSIS consumer education programs are modeled on the concept of integrated marketing, a management concept designed to make all aspects of marketing communication such as advertising, sales promotion, public relations, and direct marketing work together as a unified force, rather than permitting each to work in isolation. The three components of the FSIS integrated marketing model each support the other:

- Mass media—reaching out to the broad public.
- *Cluster targeting*—using demographic, geographic, and sociodemographic information to target communications to segmented audiences.
- *One-on-one interactions* such as through the USDA's Food Safety Discovery Zone, which expands outreach programs to places like county and state fairs (US Department of Agriculture, http://www.fsis.usda.gov/wps/portal/fsis/topics/food-safety-education/get-answers/usda-food-safety-discovery-zone-mobile/event-schedule-by-date).

Each component of the integrated marketing program is developed based on risk research, delivered via social marketing concepts, and assessed through evaluative research. Ongoing nationwide surveys and consumer focus group studies are used to evaluate and ensure the continuing effectiveness of the initiative and to continue to track the documented changes in consumer behavior.

FSIS is committed to communicating with all food handlers, especially those who serve others in large-scale food operations or are personally at risk for foodborne illness. The agency has made great strides in reaching out to citizens who may not speak English. Food safety publications for both industry and consumers have been translated into several languages including Spanish, Korean, and Mandarin Chinese. The agency employs national television, cable networks, educational television, radio, magazines, newspapers, and websites to enhance public education efforts.

As did the 2005 *Dietary Guidelines*, the 2010 *Dietary Guidelines for Americans* contains recommendations for food safety. In sum, the advice is to

- *Clean* hands, food contact surfaces, and vegetables and fruits.
- *Separate* raw, cooked, and ready-to-eat foods while shopping, storing, and preparing foods.
- *Cook* foods to a safe temperature.
- *Chill* (refrigerate) perishable foods promptly.

The 2010 *Dietary Guidelines* also advises that some foods pose high risk of foodborne illness and should be avoided, namely, raw (unpasteurized) milk, cheeses, and juices; raw or undercooked animal foods, such as seafood, meat, poultry, and eggs; and raw sprouts (US Department of Agriculture and US Department of Health and Human Services 2010).

Fight BAC!

The public/private Partnership for Food Safety Education (PFSE) is a nonprofit organization dedicated to educating the public about safe food handling to help reduce foodborne illness. PFSE was formed as a direct response to a 1996 independent panel report, *Putting the Food Handling Issue on the Table: The Pressing Need for Food Safety Education* (US Department of Agriculture and Food Safety and Inspection Service 1996), which specifically called for a public–private partnership to educate the public about safe food handling and preparation.

PFSE uses a social marketing model to decrease foodborne illness by educating consumers on simple steps they can take to reduce or eliminate foodborne pathogens. Scientific and technical experts reviewed extant public opinion research to develop campaign concepts, messages, and graphics materials that are accurate, understandable, and persuasive. The PFSE campaign is named Fight BAC! Its key message is the same as that of the *2010 Dietary Guidelines*: *clean, separate, chill,* and *cook.*

Fight BAC! combines the resources of the federal government, industry, and several consumer organizations to implement a broad-based food safety education campaign designed to reach men, women, and children of all ages (Box 12.11).

The Fight BAC! campaign uses multiple information channels, such as the mass media, public service announcements, the Internet, point-of-purchase materials, and school and community outreach to a broad constituency of educators, media groups, and consumers to bring Americans face to face with the problem of foodborne illness and to motivate them to take action. The campaign enlists a national network of public health, nutrition, food science, education, and special constituency groups to support the campaign and greatly extend its reach. Initially, the campaign was funded by the contributions of industry trade associations with technical assistance and in-kind support provided by government agencies and consumer organizations. To date, Fight BAC! has reached millions of consumers through government outreach, private industry initiatives, school education programs, and media placements.

PFSE was charged with keeping the Fight BAC! campaign fresh and providing ongoing value-added products to keep the target audiences engaged and advance the four basic safe food handling messages. Encouraged by the success of Fight BAC!, in 2004, PFSE launched the Produce Handling Education Campaign, which focuses on safe handling of fresh fruits and vegetables. As part of the produce education campaign, additional recommendations highlight the consumer's need to *check* produce for bruising or damage and to make sure that the products have been refrigerated if fresh cut and to *throw away* fresh produce under certain conditions that render them unsafe (Box 12.12) (Partnership for Food Safety Education, http://www.fightbac.org/campaigns /produce-handling).

BOX 12.11   MOBILE FOOD SAFETY VAN

From 2003 through 2005, FSIS sponsored a Food Safety Mobile, a grassroots education campaign designed to reach millions of consumers with food safety messages. The mobile was a 35-ft., recreational-type vehicle emblazoned with bold, eye-catching graphics and prominent food safety messages, including PFSE's four Fight BAC!® messages. It served as a *rolling billboard* for food safety messages and as an attention-getting backdrop for educational exhibits and events appealing to adults and children alike. The graphic nature of the mobile was designed to attract diverse groups including children, parents, seniors, and various ethnic, low-literacy, and non-English-speaking audiences. It was stocked with materials for general audiences, for specific audiences just listed, and for food service personnel and included materials in Spanish.

Source: US Department of Health and Human Services. Food and Drug Administration, Food Safety and Inspection Service, Centers for Disease Control and Prevention. *Healthy People 2010* Food Safety Data Progress Review. Food Safety Education Examples. May 11, 2004.

BOX 12.12   FIGHT BAC!® FOOD SAFETY GUIDELINES

- *Clean* hands often by washing them thoroughly with soap and water; air dry or use a clean towel. Be sure there are plenty of clean utensils and platters for food preparation and serving. Clean food thermometer after use.
- *Separate* raw and cooked/ready-to-eat food to prevent cross-contamination.
- *Cook* to a safe internal temperature. Ground beef should be cooked to 160°F.
- *Chill* leftovers in the refrigerator or freezer within 2 hours of taking food off the grill. On hot days above 90°F, refrigerate or freeze within 1 hour. Make sure the temperature is 40°F or below and 0°F or below in the freezer. Check the temperature occasionally with a refrigerator/freezer thermometer.
- *Check* fresh fruits and vegetables for bruising and damage, and appropriate refrigeration temperature, if cut.
- *Throw away* fresh fruits and vegetables under certain conditions that may render them unsafe.

National Food Thermometer Education Campaign

Prior to 1997, consumers who did not use a food thermometer had been advised by FSIS to cook ground beef patties until the center and the cooked-out juices were no longer pink. In 1998, the USDA concluded that the internal temperature and therefore the safety of cooked hamburgers could not be judged by visual inspection. Data showing that nearly 25% of the hamburgers judged to be thoroughly cooked according to color could still be contaminated with *Salmonella* and *Escherichia coli* O157:H7 (USDA-ARS/FSIS 1998) demonstrated the need for a meat thermometer. The temperature at which most pathogens are killed, 160°F, is considered the threshold for safe consumption of ground beef (US Department of Agriculture, Food Safety and Inspection Service, http://www.fsis .usda.gov/wps/portal/fsis/topics/food-safety-education/get-answers/food-safety-fact-sheets/meat -preparation/ground -beef-and-food-safety/CT_Index).

For this reason, the Food Safety Education Staff (FSES) of FSIS undertook a campaign to promote the use of food thermometers. Initial focus groups found that consumer food safety knowledge was lacking, particularly with regard to thermometer use to gauge doneness of cooked meat. Key recommendations from these groups suggested that the FSES promote food thermometer use for everyday meals and as a means to improve taste as well as safety. They further suggested that FSES should target parents of young children.

In 2000, FSIS launched a national food safety education campaign, employing the best of social marketing concepts, to promote the use of food thermometers. The campaign theme "It's safe to bite when the temperature is right!" (US Department of Agriculture et al. 2001) was delivered by Thermy™, a cartoon food thermometer, and was designed to encourage consumers to use a food thermometer when cooking meat, poultry, and egg products. PFSE, the Food Temperature Indicator Association, and a number of grocery chains and thermometer companies around the country cooperated in the Thermy™ campaign (Box 12.13) (US Department of Agriculture et al. 2001).

A social marketing approach was developed to increase the impact of the national food thermometer education program. Goals of the social marketing project were to refine and define appropriate audience segments; identify appropriate desired behaviors of those segments; identify barriers to behavior change and ways to overcome them; identify opportunities and strategies for education;

BOX 12.13   THERMY

You can find information about Thermy's campaign at http://www.fsis.usda.gov/thermy.

BOX 12.14   IS IT DONE YET?

In 2004, FSIS partnered with Michigan State University's National Food Safety and Toxicology Center, Department of Food Science and Human Nutrition, and Extension service in an effort to increase consumers' use of food thermometers. The "Is It DONE Yet?" initiative again used social marketing principles to promote positive behavior change among parents of children under 10 years of age, chosen as those most likely to change behavior. The campaign included carnival games, a full media and advertising plan, construction of a pretest/posttest survey technique, and development of strategies to attract target audiences. Researchers studied how to field test social-marketing tactics, develop skills in determining target audiences, identify strategies that can change consumers' behavior, and recognize styles for communicating with different audiences.

Source: MSUToday Food-Safety Campaign Stresses Thermometer Use. August 3, 2004. Available at http://msutoday.msu.edu/news/2004/food-safety-campaign-stresses-thermometer-use/, accessed February 14, 2015.

---

identify setting, time, and delivery systems for implementation; and recommend evaluation techniques for the campaign (Box 12.14) (US Department of Agriculture et al. 2001).

National Food Safety Education Month

The National Restaurant Association Educational Foundation's International Food Safety Council designated September as the National Food Safety Education Month[SM] (NFSEM) to heighten awareness of the importance of food safety education throughout the restaurant and food service industry. Goals of NFSEM are to reinforce food safety education and training among restaurant and foodservice workers, and to educate the public on how to handle and prepare food properly at home, whether cooking from scratch or serving take-out meals and restaurant leftovers. Restaurants and food service operations; hospitality associations; colleges and universities; federal, state, and local government agencies; and consumer organizations across the country participate in NFSEM in a variety of ways each year. The FDA and FSIS have developed kits of consumer education materials for NFSEM in support of the four key food safety practices. These kits reach more than 40,000 health educators, including FDA and USDA field staff. State and local health department personnel, school food service directors, and school nurses are involved in a variety of local educational activities (Boyle 2003; Food and Drug Administration et al. 2004). Each year, a new theme and training activities are created for the restaurant and food service industry to reinforce proper food safety practices and procedures. Themes for previous NFSEM are summarized in Table 12.5.

CAMPAIGNS TO PROMOTE HEALTH THROUGH NUTRITION

In addition to preventing disease, nationwide efforts are made to actively promote health through nutrition, beginning with conception. These efforts provide target audiences such as women of child-bearing age, nursing mothers, and low-income individuals with the supportive environment needed to make healthy choices that will circumvent the onset of disease. A supportive environment model can include the nature of food available for purchase (folate fortification), emotional support (WIC peer counseling, as discussed in Chapter 6), financial assistance, and/or enhanced nutrition knowledge through education and outreach, such as from the Supplemental Nutrition Assistance Program (SNAP).

National Folic Acid Education Campaign

According to the CDC, 3000 pregnancies are affected by spina bifida or anencephaly annually (Centers for Disease Control and Prevention, http://www.cdc.gov/ncbddd/folicacid/data.html).

TABLE 12.5
Themes Used for National Food Safety Education Month:
1998–2014

1998	Keep It Clean—The First Step to Food Safety
1999	Cook it Safely—It's a Matter of Degrees
2000	Be Smart. Keep Foods Apart—Don't Cross Contaminate
2001	Be Cool. Chill Out. Refrigerate Promptly
2002 (retail)	CHECK IT OUT before You Check It In
2002 (consumer)	Four Steps to Food Safety
2003	Store It. Don't Ignore It
2004	Be Aware When You Prepare
2005	Keep Hands Clean with Good Hygiene
2006	Don't Compromise—Clean and Sanitize
2007	Viruses: They're in Your Hands
2008	Take Action to Prevent an Allergic Reaction
2009	Food Safety Thrives When You Focus on Five
2010 (retail)	High-Risk Customers: Serve Your Fare with Extra Care
2011 (retail)	Lessons Learned from the Health Inspection
2012	Be Safe, Don't Cross-Contaminate
2013	Allergens: Avoid a Reaction by Taking Action!
2014	20 Tips for 20 Years of National Food Safety Month

These conditions in which the neural tube fails to close properly are known as neural tube defects (NTDs). The neural tube closes early in embryonic development, within 17–30 days of gestation. As 50% of pregnancies in the United States are unplanned, and as NTDs can occur even when there is no family history of the disorder, NTDs can occur before a woman has access to prenatal care or takes supplements. The medical costs for treating US children with NTDs are estimated to exceed $200 million per year (Backstrand 2002).

Studies have shown that folate supplements taken around the time of conception significantly reduce the occurrence of NTDs in infants. To lower the risk of NTDs, the US Public Health Service and the CDC recommend that all women of childbearing age consume 400 µg of folic acid daily (Centers for Disease Control and Prevention, http://www.cdc.gov/ncbddd/folicacid/recommendations .html). The true target of NTD prevention is the population of women who actually become pregnant. However, reaching this population through primary and prenatal care is difficult due to numerous reasons, including the early manifestation of NTDs in gestation, the fact that many pregnancies are unplanned, and the lack of consistent, universal access to primary healthcare. Women may not have access to prenatal care and counseling until it is too late to address NTDs. Furthermore, it was felt that many women of childbearing age would not adhere to these recommendations (Crider et al. 2011).

Accordingly, in 1996, the FDA introduced mandatory fortification of all enriched cereal-grain products with folic acid (US Department of Health and Human Services and US Food and Drug Administration 1996). Any such product marketed as *enriched* was required to be fortified with folic acid. The CDC reports that post folic acid fortification, the prevalence of spina bifida declined 31%, and the prevalence of anencephaly declined 16%. An estimated 1000 more babies are born without NTDs since fortification (Centers for Disease Control and Prevention, http://www.cdc.gov /ncbddd/folicacid/data.html).

Fortification was also supported by the social marketing efforts of the National Folic Acid Campaign launched in 1999. In 1998, the March of Dimes conducted an informal study of obstetrics and gynecology grand rounds attendees and found that 30% did not know the recommended daily amount of folic acid and 36% reported that they rarely or only sometimes recommended folic acid to their patients. (This serves as a good reminder that social marketing and education campaigns are not limited to consumer education.) The March of Dimes then invested $10 million in a 3-year national folic acid education campaign, and with the CFC, co-convened the National Council on Folic Acid (Centers for Disease Control and Prevention 1999). Formative research was conducted, including a focus group that found that different communication strategies would be required to reach and influence women trying to become pregnant or planning pregnancy in the next year (contemplators) and women *not* intending pregnancy (noncontemplators). Noncontemplators tend to be uninterested in or resistant to the folic acid message unless it is couched in terms of nonpregnancy-related health benefits. Accordingly, the CDC developed two public service announcements (and related campaign materials): "Before You Know It" aimed at pregnancy contemplators and "Ready...Not" aimed at noncontemplators (Treiman et al. 2000).

Although no longer formally described as a campaign, CDC is engaging in ongoing folic acid education, prevention, and research. Educational material is available at http://www.cdc.gov/ncbddd/folicacid/freematerials.html. The National Birth Defects Prevention Study is the largest population-based US study looking at potential risk factors and causes of birth defects. Current folic acid research activities include

- Looking at how a woman's intake of micronutrients, including folic acid, may affect the risk for specific birth defects.
- Studying why Hispanics appear to be at higher risk for NTDs.
- Learning about women's behaviors related to preventing birth defects, including folic acid use and alcohol use (Centers for Disease Control and Prevention, http://www.cdc.gov/ncbddd/folicacid/aboutus.html).

Racial-ethnic disparities in the rates of NTDs remain (Dowd and Aiello 2008). The prevalence of NTD-affected pregnancies had been higher among Hispanic women than women in other racial/ethnic populations before fortification and remained higher post fortification (Centers for Disease Control and Prevention, http://www.cdc.gov/features/dsSpinaBifidaTrends/). Folic acid intake from fortified foods and supplements has been found to be lower among Hispanic women (Hamner et al. 2009). Additionally, Hispanic women are less likely to have heard about folic acid, to know it can prevent birth defects, or to take vitamins containing folic acid before pregnancy (Centers for Disease Control and Prevention. Folic Acid. Data and Statistics. Last reviewed July 7, 2010. Available at http://www.cdc.gov/ncbddd/folicacid/data.html, accessed September 26, 2014). The CDC is evaluating whether using promotoras (lay health outreach workers) is effective in communicating to Latinas that taking folic acid before and during pregnancy can help prevent NTDs (Centers for Disease Control and Prevention, http://www.cdc.gov/ncbddd/folicacid/aboutus.html).

SNAC and SNAP

In 1995 and 1996, the USDA stimulated the development of 22 state-based nutrition education social marketing networks. Housed principally in land grant universities, cooperative extensions, and state health departments, the networks moved ahead independently to develop an array of innovative interventions for low-income population groups ranging from preschoolers to senior citizens, based on state priorities. Programs varied widely in focus, scope, complexity, and funding levels.

In 2003, the USDA conducted a series of networking sessions with state representatives from the various nutrition assistance programs to strengthen collaboration on nutrition education and promotion efforts. Over 300 representatives from programs in 49 states met to identify a common nutrition goal and begin formulating a plan for working together to achieve that goal. Over 90% of the states identified their common goal—for example, Iowa's goal is to promote fruit and vegetable consumption, whereas that for Texas is to promote healthy eating and active lifestyles—and began developing a statewide nutrition plan with objectives, strategies, and tactics for achieving that single goal. As of 2007, 48 states had adopted a State Nutrition Action Plan, which has since been renamed to the State Nutrition Action Coalition (SNAC) in order to reduce confusion with the SNAP benefit program (US Department of Agriculture and Food and Nutrition Service 2010).

SNAP offers nutrition assistance that enables low-income families to buy food with Electronic Benefits Transfer (EBT), purchases that in turn can provide economic benefits to communities (US Department of Agriculture, Food and Nutrition Service, http://www.fns.usda.gov/snap /supplemental-nutrition-assistance-program-snap).

Currently, SNAP Nutrition Education (SNAP-ED) is the largest adult-oriented nutrition promotion effort in the United States. As such, the lessons being learned from the program may inform the development of other initiatives to prevent chronic diseases, including those aimed at eliminating health disparities and reversing the nation's obesity epidemic. SNAP-ED Connection, available at http://snap.nal.usda.gov, is an online resource center.

As part of the SNAP-ED connection, the USDA provides professional development resources, including social marketing information and links to many interesting social campaigns that we are not able to profile here at http://snap.nal.usda.gov/professional-development-tools/social-marketing.

TAILORED HEALTH COMMUNICATION AND SOCIAL MEDIA

Tailored health communication has emerged as a promising, innovative approach to addressing public health issues. Defined as "any combination of information and behavior change strategies intended to reach one specific person, based on characteristics that are unique to that person, related to the outcome of interest, and derived from an individual assessment" (Kreuter et al. 2000), tailored communications are created especially for an individual based on knowledge of that person. This information may be gathered through a survey, a brief personal interview with a professional, or potentially through the use of alternative data sources. The results of these questions are entered into a computer, which draws from a *library* of possible messages to create materials that directly address the individual's needs, interests, or concerns. Once a program has been developed for a certain health issue, it can be used to produce tailored print materials with the potential to reach large populations. Thus, tailored communications are a promising and innovative approach that can be used to address a variety of public health issues.

A subset of the larger field of health communications, tailored communications are distinct from more familiar, but less personalized, methods of developing *targeted* materials—messages prepared using information about population segments. A population segment, or subgroup, may be very small and quite specifically defined, such as African American women in the specific age bracket 50–65 who belong to a particular neighborhood health center (Kreuter and Skinner 2000).

When a subgroup is small, targeting may be easily confused with tailoring. Tailoring is individualized, which affords the opportunity to address cognitive and behavioral patterns of specific individuals.

According to the first scientific review of tailoring research, "tailored print communications have demonstrated an enhanced ability to attract notice and readership ... are more effective than non-tailored communications for influencing health behavior change ... (and) can be an important adjunct to other intervention components" (Skinner et al. 1999). Although the field is still emerging, empirical research shows that tailored print materials are more effective than nontailored ones in helping people change health behaviors, such as physical activity and diet (Patrick et al. 2001), although tailored materials have not been equally effective for all individuals (Holt et al. 2000). Tailored weight loss materials are more effective in bringing about more positive thoughts about the materials, personal connections to the materials, self-assessment thoughts, and thoughts indicating behavioral intention than nontailored materials (Kreuter et al. 1999). Thus, the tailoring of health information can significantly improve the chances that the information will be considered and can stimulate prebehavioral changes such as self-assessment and intention.

NCI maintains an online guide that coaches the user to create a simple tailored letter (US Department of Health and Human Services, National Institutes of Health, National Cancer Institute. Cancer Control and Population Sciences. Health Communication and Informatics Research. Health Message Tailoring. Available at http://cancercontrol.cancer.gov/messagetailoring/guide.html, accessed January 20, 2015). The topics covered in the demonstration program include creating a sample database, creating a master letter, linking the main document to the database, inserting merge fields and word fields into the master document, adding a tailored illustration, and performing the merge. A study of NCI's tailored print materials to increase fruit and vegetable consumption found a significant mean serving difference between those receiving untailored and tailored materials (Heimendinger et al. 2005).

Text Messaging

Text messaging provides a seemingly excellent opportunity to disseminate tailored health messages and has been implemented and tested in numerous areas of public health interest. Tailored text messaging has been found to be helpful as an adjunct to multidisciplinary obesity treatment for adolescents (Woolford et al. 2010), but not as part of a worksite weight loss program for obese men in Korea (Kim et al. 2015). A 2-year pilot project using both an automated message-tailoring algorithm and bidirectional text messaging showed success in improving self-management of HIV/AIDS, reducing risky behaviors, and increasing overall well-being (AHRQ Health Information Technology Accelerating Change and Transformation in Organizations and Networks (ACTION), http://healthit.ahrq.gov/sites/default/files/docs/page/uhrigsuccessstory.pdf). A randomized controlled trial, Connecting Health and Technology (CHAT), is testing the use of mobile devices to assess dietary intake and provide tailored dietary feedback and text messages to motivate young adults to make dietary improvements in fruit, vegetable, and junk food consumption (Kerr et al. 2012).

Social Media in Social Marketing

The use of social media and technology (as noted above in the brief discussion on texting) is a quickly advancing component of social marketing campaigns. (The use of social media as a marketing tool is not, in and of itself, social marketing). Because of the breadth of adoption of social media, we anticipate that you are not only familiar with social media but that you may have already experienced the use of social media to convey messages around food and nutrition, if not an actual social marketing campaign. We briefly introduce this topic by describing the 4 Day Throw Away study below.

The 4 Day Throw Away study evaluated and compared the use of traditional and social media in a food safety social marketing campaign. The goal was to examine whether the campaign reached the intended audience and also initiated behavior change for appropriate food safety practices related to leftovers. The target audience was the primary food preparer in families with children aged 10 and under. The study found that both methods (tradition and social media) were valid methods of reaching the target audience of young parents/guardians regarding food safety information. A total of 4984 unique users visited the initiative's website; 60% of the website users were referred by traditional media methods, whereas 40% were referred from social media methods (YouTube, Facebook, and Twitter).

However, the study notes that because of the popularity of social media with younger audiences, messages that are appealing to individuals using social networking have a high probability of being spread to others in a short period of time. In general, although more research is needed on evaluation and efficacy, the researchers concluded that interventions using a mix of media channels broaden the reach and potential for intended behavior change (James et al. 2013).

CONCLUSION

Health communication can be used to influence the public health agenda, advocate for policies and programs, promote desirable changes in the socioeconomic and physical environment, and encourage social norms that benefit health and quality of life (Piotrow et al. 1997). Although health communication techniques can be tailored to offer individual's health information and behavior change tips based on their unique characteristics, health communication generally supports community-centered prevention, which shifts attention from individual- to group-level change and emphasizes the ability of communities and the individuals comprising those communities to effect change on multiple levels.

Social marketing is a highly adopted tool used to promote behavior change related to food and nutrition. Techniques such as *rebranding* boring vegetables with fun names can be used even if a full-scale social marketing campaign cannot be implemented. Furthermore, the escalating adaptation of Internet-based technologies for communications presents an increasing number of opportunities to expand social marketing and influence health behavior change. The use of social media as part of a social marketing campaign can greatly increase the reach of a message. Examining campaign successes from the past as well as incorporating lessons learned from new research in methods and technologies can lead to effective health communication programs and sustainable behavior change.

ACRONYMS

BMD	Bone mineral density
BMI	Body mass index
BRFSS	Behavioral Risk Factor Surveillance System
CDC	Centers for Disease Control and Prevention
CSPI	Center for Science in the Public Interest
CVD	Cardiovascular disease
DISC	Dietary Intervention Study in Children
DNPAO	Division of Nutrition, Physical Activity and Obesity
EBT	Electronic benefits transfer
FDA	Food and Drug Administration
FSES	Food Safety Education Staff
FSIS	Food Safety Inspection Service
HHS	Department of Health and Human Services
NCI	National Cancer Institute
NDEP	National Diabetes Education Program
NFSEM	National Food Safety Education Month
NHLBI	National Heart, Lung, and Blood Institute
NICHD	National Institute of Child Health and Human Development
NIDDK	National Institute for Diabetes and Digestive and Kidney Disease
NIH	National Institutes of Health
NTD	Neural tube defect
OWH	Office of Women's Health
PBH	Produce for Better Health Foundation
PFSE	Partnership for Food Safety Education
PSA	Public Service Announcement
SNAC	State Nutrition Action Coalition
SNAP	Supplemental Nutrition Assistance Program
SNAP-ED	SNAP Education

USDA   United States Department of Agriculture
WIC   Special Supplemental Nutrition Program for Women, Infants, and Children
WIN   Weight-Control Information Network

STUDENT ASSIGNMENTS AND ACTIVITIES DESIGNED TO ENHANCE LEARNING AND STIMULATE CRITICAL THINKING

1. Identify a current social marketing campaign (other than any mentioned in the book) that seeks to address a nutritional issue. For your campaign, answer the following questions:
   a. When was the campaign launched? Who funds the campaign? How much money is it funded for? How long will it be funded? Who are the secondary sources of funds (if there are any)?
   b. Who will implement the campaign? Which other organizations (if any) will the campaign partner with?
   c. Who is the campaign's target audience? Secondary audience? Other audiences? How many people (families, communities, etc.) are expected to be reached by the campaign?
   d. What are the campaign's vision, mission, goals, and objectives?
   e. Why was the campaign launched? Which *Healthy People* objectives are addressed by the campaign?
   f. Summarize the methods being used to implement the campaign.
   g. Summarize the qualitative and/or quantitative research that was used in the design of the campaign.
   h. How will the campaign be evaluated?
   i. What provisions exist for continuation after the campaign's funding runs out?
   j. If there are additional comments you care to make about the campaign or additional information about the campaign you would like to share, please provide it here.
      Reference all the information you provide.
2. Choose a nutritional issue prevalent in your community and answer the following questions:
   a. Using the steps identified in the chapter, plan the approach for a social marketing campaign that will address the nutritional issue. Be sure to include a description of each step.
   b. Based on your planning in the previous question, what channel and materials would you use for this social marketing campaign? Justify your choices.
   c. Develop a logic model for your social marketing campaign. For additional information and examples of logic models, refer to the W.K. Kellogg Foundation's Logic Model Development Guide at http://www.wkkf.org/Pubs/Tools/Evaluation/Pub3669.pdf.
   d. Describe how you would evaluate your social marketing campaign.
3. Answer the questions below with regard to the following scenario:
      "When the Ad Council proposed a campaign that focused on 'the risks associated with not breastfeeding' and included statistics from studies that have found that babies fed formula have a higher risk of developing asthma, diabetes, leukemia, and other illnesses, federal officials pulled the ads after two formula companies complained that claims made in the government's campaign were not based on solid science and that the overall approach was like a scare tactic."
      Is it acceptable to exaggerate risk and heighten fear if doing so saves more lives or at least reduces morbidity?
   a. When is it acceptable to improve the lives of people in one group at the expense of another?
   b. Does a marketing campaign respect a group's culture if it calls for fundamental change within it?

4. Breastfeeding has many health benefits. Infants who are breastfed are less likely to develop a wide range of infectious diseases or become overweight. Breastfeeding also lowers the mother's risk of breast and ovarian cancer, as well as helps the mother return to her pre-pregnancy weight. While breastfeeding rates in the United States have increased over time, many states have not reached the Healthy People 2020 objectives of 75% of mothers initiating breastfeeding, 50% of mothers breastfeeding at 6 months, and 25% of mothers breastfeeding at 12 months.

   a. Write a 15-, 30-, and 45-second Public Service Announcement (PSA) for the radio to encourage new mothers in your community to breastfeed their children. Also, design a 60-second PSA for television. Make sure the PSAs are engaging and interesting for new mothers. Also, specify the station(s)/channel(s), time(s), and day(s) you recommend broadcasting each PSA.

   b. Write an opinion-editorial (op-ed) for your local newspaper about breastfeeding promotion. For more information about breastfeeding, see

      i. *Department of Health and Human Services* at http://www.4woman.gov/Breastfeeding/index.cfm?page=home

      ii. *Centers for Disease Control and Prevention* at http://www.cdc.gov/breastfeeding/index.htm

      iii. *La Leche League* at http://www.lalecheleague.org/ab.html?m=1

   For information on how to write an op-ed, go to

      i. *Physicians for a National Health Program* at http://www.pnhp.org/action/how_to_write_an_oped_and_letter_to_the_editor.php

      ii. *National Association of County and City Health Officials* at http://www.naccho.org/advocacy/MarketingPublicHealth_guide_op_ed.cfm

      iii. *Advocates for Youth* at http://www.advocatesforyouth.org/media/oped.htm

REFERENCES

Anderson JB, Shuster TA, Hansen KE, Levy AS, Volk A. A camera's view of consumer food-handling behaviors. *J Am Diet Assoc.* 2004;104:186–191.

Andreasen AR, Drumwright ME. Alliances and ethics in social marketing. In Andreasen AR, ed. *Ethics in Social Marketing.* Washington, DC: Georgetown University Press, 2000, Chap. 5.

Backstrand JR. The history and future of food fortification in the United States: A public health perspective. *Nutr Rev.* 2002;60(1):15–26.

Bauman A. Commentary on the VERB™ campaign—Perspectives on social marketing to encourage physical activity among youth. *Prev Chronic Dis.* 2004. Available at http://www.cdc.gov/pcd/issues/2004/jul/04_0054.htm, accessed January 20, 2015.

Boyle MA. *Community Nutrition in Action: An Entrepreneurial Approach*, 3rd ed. Belmont, CA: Thomson Wadsworth, 2003.

Buck JW, Walcott RR, Beuchat LR. Recent trends in microbiological safety of fruits and vegetables. *Plant Health Progr.* 2003;10:1094.

Buzby JC, Guthrie JF, Kantor LS. Evaluation of the USDA Fruit and Vegetable Pilot Program: Report to Congress. Food Assistance and Nutrition Research Program, Food and Rural Economics Division, Economic Research Service, US Department of Agriculture. E-FAN No. (03-006), April 2003.

Calle EE, Rodriguez C, Walker-Thurmond K, Thun MJ. Overweight, obesity, and mortality from cancer in a prospectively studied cohort of US adults. *N Engl J Med.* 2003;348:1625–1638.

Centers for Disease Control and Prevention. Childhood Obesity Facts. Prevalence of Childhood Obesity in the United States, 2011–2012. Available at http://www.cdc.gov/obesity/data/childhood.html, accessed January 20, 2015.

Centers for Disease Control and Prevention. Folic Acid. Data and Statistics. Last reviewed July 7, 2010. Available at http://www.cdc.gov/ncbddd/folicacid/data.html, accessed September 26, 2014.

Centers for Disease Control and Prevention. Folic Acid Recommendations. Last updated December 18, 2014. Available at http://www.cdc.gov/ncbddd/folicacid/recommendations.html, accessed February 14, 2015.

Centers for Disease Control and Prevention. Knowledge and use of folic acid by women of childbearing age, United States, 1995 and 1998. *MMWR*. 1999:48(16):325.

Centers for Disease Control and Prevention. Message Strategy Research to Support Development of the Youth Media Campaign (YMC). Revealing Target Audience Receptiveness to Potential YMC Message Concepts. Available at http://www.health.gov/communication/db/report_detail.asp?ID=20&page=1&z_26=on &sp=2, accessed January 20, 2015.

Centers for Disease Control and Prevention, National Center on Birth Defects and Developmental Disabilities. Folic Acid. About Us. Available at http://www.cdc.gov/ncbddd/folicacid/aboutus.html, accessed February 14, 2015.

Centers for Disease Control and Prevention. Trends in Spina Bifida by Race/Ethnicity, United States. Reviewed May 15, 2012. Available at http://www.cdc.gov/features/dsSpinaBifidaTrends/, accessed September 26, 2014.

Centers for Disease Control and Prevention. VERB's Formative Research Process. Available at http://www.cdc.gov/youthcampaign/research/PDF/FormativeResearchProcess.pdf, accessed January 20, 2015.

Centers for Disease Control and Prevention. *5 A Day Works!* Atlanta, GA: US Department of Health and Human Services, 2005. Available at http://www.cdc.gov/nccdphp/dnpa/nutrition/health_professionals /programs/5aday_works.pdf, accessed February 14, 2015.

Crider KS, Bailey LB, Berry RJ. Folic acid food fortification—Its history, effect, concerns, and future directions. *Nutrients*. 2011;3:370–384.

Dowd JB, Aiello AE. Did national folic acid fortification reduce socioeconomic and racial disparities in folate status in the US? *Int J Fam Med*. 2008;37(5):1059–1066.

Eckel RH, Grundy SM, Zimmet PZ. The metabolic syndrome. *Lancet*. 2005;365:1415–1428.

Flegal KM, Carroll MD, Kuczmarski RJ, Johnson CL. Overweight and obesity in the United States: Prevalence and trends, 1960–1994. *Int J Obes Relat Metab Disord*. 1998;22(1):39–47.

Food and Drug Administration, Food Safety and Inspection Service, Centers for Disease Control and Prevention. *Healthy People 2010 Food Safety Data Progress Review*. Food Safety Education Examples, May 11, 2004.

Girls health.gov. Best Bones Forever! Available at http://www.bestbonesforever.org/, accessed February 14, 2015.

Gittelsohn J, Steckler A, Johnson CC et al. Formative Research in School and Community-Based Health Programs and Studies: "State of the Art" and the TAAG Approach. *Health Educ Behav*. 2006;33(1):25–39.

Goldberg J, Rudd RE, Dietz W. Using 3 data sources and methods to shape a nutrition campaign. *J Am Diet Assoc*. 1999;99:717–722.

Grier S, Bryant CA. Social marketing in public health. *Ann Rev Public Health*. 2005;26:319–339.

Hamner HC, Mulinare J, Cogswell ME et al. Predicted contribution of folic acid fortification of corn masa flour to the usual folic acid intake for the US population: National Health and Nutrition Examination Survey 2001–2004. *Am J Clin Nutr*. 2009;89(1):305–315.

Hardy LR, Harrell JS, Bell RA. Overweight in children: Definitions, measurements, confounding factors, and health consequences. *J Pediatr Nurs*. 2004;19(6):376–384.

Health.gov. Home of the Office of Disease Prevention and Health Promotion. Health Communication. Available at http://www.health.gov/communication/resources/, accessed January 20, 2015.

Hedley AA, Ogden CL, Johnson CL, Carroll MD, Curtin LR, Flegal KM. Prevalence of overweight and obesity among US children, adolescents, and adults, 1999–2002. *JAMA*. 2004;291(23):2847–2850.

Heimendinger J, O'Neill C, Marcus AC et al. Multiple tailored messages are effective in increasing fruit and vegetable consumption among callers to the Cancer Information Service. *J Health Commun*. 2005;10(Suppl 1):65–82.

Hillers VN, Medeiros L, Kendall P, Chen G, DiMascola S. Consumer food-handling behaviors associated with prevention of 13 foodborne illnesses. *J Food Prot*. 2003;66:1893–1899.

Hinkle AJ, Boykin N, Hernandez EM. CANFIT *Connection* (The Quarterly Newsletter of the California Adolescent Nutrition and Fitness Program), Fall 2000. Available at http://www.canfit.org/pdf/newsletter_fall_2000.pdf, accessed February 14, 2015.

Holt CL, Clark EM, Kreuter MW, Scharff DP. Does locus of control moderate the effects of tailored health education materials? *Health Educ Res*. 2000;15:393–403.

Huhman M, Potter LD, Wong FL, Banspach SW, Duke JC, Heitzler CD. Effects of a media campaign to increase physical activity among children: Year-1 results of the VERB campaign. *Pediatrics*. 2005;116:e277–e284.

Iowa Department of Public Health. Iowa Nutrition Network. Pick a Better Snack. Available at http://www .idph.state.ia.us/inn/PickABetterSnack.aspx, accessed February 14, 2015.

James K, Albrecht JA, Litchfield RE, Weishaar CA. A summative evaluation of a food safety social marketing campaign "4-Day Throw-Away" using traditional and social media. *Journal of Food Science Education.* 2013;12(3):48–55.

Kerr DA, Pollard CM, Howat P et al. Connecting Health and Technology (CHAT): Protocol of a randomized controlled trial to improve nutrition behaviours using mobile devices and tailored text messaging in young adults. *BMC Public Health.* 2012;12:477.

Kim JY, Oh S, Steinhubl S et al. Effectiveness of 6 months of tailored text message reminders for obese male participants in a worksite weight loss program: Randomized controlled trial. *JMIR Mhealth Uhealth.* 2015;3(1):e14.

Kotler P, Zaltman G. Social marketing: An approach to planned social change. *J Mark.* 1971;35:3–12.

Kotler P, Lee N. *Social Marketing: Influencing Behaviors for Good,* 3rd ed. Thousand Oaks, CA: Sage Publications, 2008.

Kraak VI, Story M, Swinburn B. Addressing barriers to improve children's fruit and vegetable intake. *Am J Clin Nutr.* 2013;97(3):653–655.

Kreuter MW, Skinner CS. Tailoring: What's in a name? *Health Educ Res.* 2000;15(1):1–4.

Kreuter MW, Bull FC, Clark EM, Oswald DL. Understanding how people process health information: A comparison of tailored and nontailored weight-loss materials. *Health Psychol.* 1999;18:487–494.

Kreuter M, Farrell D, Olevitch L, Brennan L. *Tailored Health Messages: Customizing Communication with Computer Technology.* Mahwah, NJ: Lawrence Erlbaum Associates, 2000.

Lindenberger JH, Bryant CA. Promoting breastfeeding in the WIC Program: A social marketing case study. *Am J Health Behav.* 2000;24:53–60.

Lindridge A, MacAskill S, Gnich W, Eadie D, Holme I. Applying an ecological mode to social marketing communications. *Eur J Mark.* 2013;47(9):1399–1420. Available at http://oro.open.ac.uk/35900/2/991AF55F .pdf, accessed February 14, 2015.

Maibach EW, Rothschild ML, Novelli WD. Social marketing. In Glanz K, Rimer BK, Lewis FM, eds. *Health Behavior and Health Education: Theory, Research, and Practice,* 3rd ed. San Francisco: Jossey-Bass, 2002, Chap. 19.

McCabe-Sellers BJ, Beattie SE. Food safety: Emerging trends in foodborne illness surveillance and prevention. *J Am Diet Assoc.* 2004;104:1708–1717.

Mead PS, Slutsker L, Dietz V. et al. Food-related illness and death in the United States. *Emerg Infect Dis.* 1999;5:607. Available at http://www.cdc.gov/ncidod/EID/vol5no5/mead.htm, accessed January 20, 2015.

Mokdad AH, Ford ES, Bowman BA, Dietz WH, Vinicor F, Bales VS, Marks JS. Prevalence of obesity, diabetes, and obesity-related health risk factors, 2001. *JAMA.* 2003;289(1):76–79.

Montazeri A. Social marketing: A tool not a solution. *J R Soc Health.* 1997;117:115–118.

Murphy SC, Whited LJ, Rosenberry LC, Hammond BH, Bandler DK, Boor KJ. Fluid milk vitamin fortification compliance in New York State. *J Dairy Sci.* 2001;84:2113–2820.

National Cancer Institute. Monograph. Five-a-Day for Better Health Program. National Institutes of Health. NIH Publication 01-5019, September 2001.

National Heart, Lung, and Blood Institute, National Institutes of Health, US Department of Health and Human Services. About We Can! Available at http://www.nhlbi.nih.gov/health/educational/wecan/about-wecan /index.htm, accessed January 20, 2015.

National Institutes of Health. National Heart, Lung, and Blood Institute. We Can! Available at http://www .nhlbi.nih.gov/health/public/heart/obesity/wecan/, accessed January 20, 2015.

Nestle M. *Safe Food: Bacteria, Biotechnology, and Bioterrorism.* Berkeley, CA: University of California Press, 2003.

Ogden CL. Changes in terminology for childhood overweight and obesity. *Natl Health Stat Rep.* 2010;(25). Available at http://www.cdc.gov/nchs/data/nhsr/nhsr025.pdf, accessed February 14, 2015.

Ogden CL, Carroll MD, Kit BK, Flegal KM. Prevalence of childhood and adult obesity in the United States, 2011–2012. *JAMA.* 2014;311(8):806–814.

Partnership for Food Safety Education. Safe Produce Handling Education Campaign. Available at http://www .fightbac.org/campaigns/produce-handling, accessed February 14, 2015.

Patrick K, Sallis JF, Prochaska JJ et al. A multicomponent program for nutrition and physical activity change in primary care: PACE+ for adolescents. *Arch Pediatr Adolesc Med.* 2001;155:940–946.

Piotrow PT, Kincaid DL, Rimon JG, II et al. *Health Communication.* Westport, CT: Praeger, 1997.

Public Health Foundation. Council on Linkages: Ecological Model of Public Health. Available at http://www .phf.org/resourcestools/Pages/ecological_Model_publichealth.aspx, accessed January 20, 2015.

Reger B, Wootan MG, Booth-Butterfield S, Smith H. 1% or less: A community-based nutrition campaign. *Public Health Rep.* 1998;113:410–419.

Rothschild M. Carrots, sticks, and promises: A conceptual framework for the management of public health and social behaviors. *J Mark.* 1999;63:24–37.

Sawatzki D. Rebranding: A Look in the Rear-View Mirror. *Social Marketing Quarterly,* November 6, 2011. Available at http://www.socialmarketingquarterly.com/rebranding-look-rear-view-mirror, accessed February 14, 2015.

Serdula MK, Gillespie C, Kettel-Khan L, Farris R, Seymour J, Denny C. Trends in fruit and vegetable consumption among adults in the United States: Behavioral risk factor surveillance system, 1994–2000. *Am J Pub Health.* 2004;94:1014–1918.

Skinner CS, Campbell MK, Rimer BK, Curry S, Prochaska JO. How effective is tailored print communication? *Ann Behav Med.* 1999;21:290–298.

Social Marketing National Excellence Collaborative. *Social Marketing: A Resource Guide,* 2002. Available at http://socialmarketingcollaborative.org/smc/pdf/social_marketing_101.pdf, accessed January 20, 2015.

Text Message for Managing Chronic Disease: A Model for Tailored Health Communication. AHRQ Health Information Technology Accelerating Change and Transformation in Organizations and Networks (ACTION). Available at http:// healthit.ahrq.gov/sites/default/files/docs/page/uhrigsuccessstory.pdf, accessed February 15, 2015.

Treiman KA, Volansky M, Hammond SL, Prue C, Daniel KL. Promoting folic acid to reduce the risk of birth defect: Targeting contemplators in the National Folic Acid Campaign. Presentation at APHA Conference, 2000. Available at https://apha.confex.com/apha/128am/techprogram/paper_13623.htm, accessed February 14, 2015.

US Department of Agriculture, Food Safety and Inspection Service, Consumer Education and Information/ Consumer Research and Focus Group Testing. Final Research Report: A Project to Apply Theories of Social Marketing to the Challenge of Food Thermometer Education in the United States. Report Provided by the Baldwin Group, Inc., December 21, 2001. Updated 2002.

US Department of Agriculture. Food Safety and Inspection Service. Food Safety Discovery Zone Event Schedule. Available at http://www.fsis.usda.gov/wps/portal/fsis/topics/food-safety-education/get-answers /usda-food-safety-discovery-zone-mobile/event-schedule-by-date, accessed February 14, 2015.

US Department of Agriculture, Food Safety and Inspection Service. The Final Rule on Pathogen Reduction and Hazard Analysis and Critical Control Point (HACCP) Systems, July 1996. Available at http://www .fsis.usda.gov/OA/background/finalrul.htm, accessed January 20, 2015.

US Department of Agriculture, Food and Nutrition Service. Nutrition Education and Promotion. The Role of FNS in Helping Low-Income Families Make Healthier Eating and Lifestyle Choices. A Report to Congress, March 2010. Available at http://www.fns.usda.gov/sites/default/files/NutritionEdRTC.pdf, accessed February 14, 2015.

US Department of Agriculture, Food and Nutrition Service. Supplemental Nutrition Assistance Program. Available at http://www.fns.usda.gov/snap/supplemental-nutrition-assistance-program-snap, accessed February 14, 2015.

US Department of Agriculture, U.S. Department of Health and Human Services. *Dietary Guidelines for Americans, 2010,* 7th ed. Washington, DC: U.S. Government Printing Office, December 2010. Available at http://www.health.gov/dietaryguidelines/dga2010/dietaryguidelines2010.pdf, accessed February 14, 2015.

US Department of Health and Human Services. *Bone Health and Osteoporosis: A Report of the Surgeon General.* Rockville, MD: U.S. Department of Health and Human Services, Office of the Surgeon General, 2004.

US Department of Health and Human Services, Centers for Disease Control and Prevention. Estimates of Foodborne Illness in the United States. Available at http://www.cdc.gov/foodborneburden/2011-foodborne -estimates.html, updated January 8, 2014, accessed December 30, 2014.

US Department of Health and Human Services. Centers for Disease Control and Prevention. National Center for Chronic Disease Prevention and Health Promotion. National Diabetes Education Program. Available at http://www.cdc .gov/diabetes/ndep/about.htm, accessed January 20, 2015.

US Department of Health and Human Services, National Institutes of Health, National Cancer Institute. Cancer Control and Population Sciences. Health Communication and Informatics Research. Health Message Tailoring. Available at http://cancercontrol.cancer.gov/messagetailoring/guide.html, accessed January 20, 2015.

US Department of Health and Human Services, U.S. Food and Drug Administration. Food standards: Amendment of standards of identity for enriched grain products to require addition of folic acid. *Fed Reg.* 1996;61:8781–8797. Available at http://www.gpo.gov/fdsys/pkg/FR-1996-03-05/pdf/96-5014.pdf #page=1, accessed January 25, 2015.

US Department of Health and Human Services, U.S. Food and Drug Administration, Center for Food Safety and Applied Nutrition. Report of the FDA Retail Food Program Database of Foodborne Illness Risk Factors. Prepared by the FDA Retail Food Program Steering Committee, August 10, 2000.

US Food and Drug Administration, Center for Food Safety and Applied Nutrition. Analysis and Evaluation of Preventive Control Measures for the Control and Reduction/Elimination of Microbial Hazards on Fresh and Fresh-Cut Produce. A Report of the Institute of Food Technologists for the Food and Drug Administration of the United States Department of Health and Human Services, September 21, 2001.

USDA-ARS/FSIS. Premature Browning of Cooked Ground Beef. Food Safety and Inspection Service Public Meeting on Premature Browning of Ground Beef. Washington, DC: USDA, May 27, 1998.

Van Horn L, Obarzanek E, Friedman LA, Gernhofer N, Barton B. Children's adaptations to a fat-reduced diet: The Dietary Intervention Study in Children (DISC). *Pediatrics.* 2005;115:1723–1733. Available at http://pediatrics.aappublications.org/cgi/content/full/115/6/1723, accessed January 20, 2015.

Wansink B, Just DR, Collin R, Klinger M. Attractive names sustain increased vegetable intake in schools. *Prev Med.* 2012;55(4):330–332.

Weinreich NK. Hands-on Social Marketing: *A Step-by-Step Guide.* Thousand Oaks, CA: Sage Publishing, 1999.

WIN. Sisters Together. Move More, Eat Better. Updated December 12, 2014. Available at http://win.niddk.nih.gov/sisters/, accessed February 14, 2015.

Wong F, Huhman M, Heitzler C et al. VERB™—A social marketing campaign to increase physical activity among youth. *Prev Chronic Dis.* 2004. Available at http://www.cdc.gov/pcd/issues/2004/jul/04_0043.htm, accessed January 20, 2015.

Woolford SJ, Clark SJ, Strecher VJ, Resnicow K. Tailored mobile phone text messages as an adjunct to obesity treatment for adolescents. Tailored mobile phone text messages as an adjunct to obesity treatment for adolescents. *J Telemed Telecare.* 2010;16(8):458–461.

World Cancer Research Fund, American Institute for Cancer Research. *Food, Nutrition, Physical Activity, and the Prevention of Cancer: A Global Perspective.* Washington DC: AICR, 2007.

13 Food Safety and Defense

I prefer butter to margarine, because I trust cows more than chemists.

Joan Dye Gussow (2001)

INTRODUCTION*

Food safety refers to protecting food from biological and other sources of contamination. *Food security* refers to access to food and issues of hunger as discussed in Chapter 11. Food supplies in the United States are generally maintained at high levels of safety—protected from accidental or deliberate contamination—so that citizens seldom give much thought to the subject. For the most part, food safety becomes a public issue only on occasions when outbreaks of foodborne illness or malicious threats make headline news. We may tend to think of food safety issues as primarily pathogens, but in general, food safety is concerned with making sure that food has not accidentally become unsafe to consume from *any* cause. Thus, in addition to illness-causing pathogens, pesticides, chemicals used in food production, reactions between the food and packaging, or other possible hazards, such as food additives or food allergens, are all items covered under the umbrella of food safety. Intentional contamination is also a food safety issue, although a better term in that case might be *food defense*.

We introduce the federal agencies involved in food safety, examine issues of food safety and labeling, discuss foodborne pathogens and surveillance, and conclude with food defense, the intersection of food safety, public health nutrition, and disaster response.

FEDERAL ROLE IN FOOD SAFETY

The website http://www.FoodSafety.gov is self-described as the *gateway* to food safety information from the federal government and clearly assigns responsibility between industry and government, maintaining that industry is responsible for producing safe food while government is responsible for setting food safety standards, conducting inspections, ensuring that standards are met, and maintaining a strong enforcement program (Keep Food Safe: What Government Does, http://www.food safety.gov). The website also provides educational resources for consumers.

The safety and quality of the US food supply are governed by a complex system administered by the 15 agencies listed in Table 13.1, with the Food and Drug Administration (FDA) and the Food Safety and Inspective Service (FSIS) of the United States Department of Agriculture (USDA) having primary oversight (Federal Food Safety Oversight 2014).

The FSIS is the self-described "public health agency in the US Department of Agriculture" (United States Department of Agriculture, http://www.fsis.usda.gov/About_FSIS/index.asp) and ensures that the commercial supply of meat, poultry, eggs, poultry-based foods, and some egg-based products are safe, wholesome, correctly packaged, and accurately labeled. Much of this responsibility is during the slaughter and processing of animal food sources.

The FDA is charged with protecting consumers from impure, unsafe, and fraudulently labeled domestic and imported foods, other than those regulated by the FSIS. As the federal agency responsible for overseeing the safety and security of most of the nation's food supply, the FDA sets and

TABLE 13.1
US Federal Agencies' Food Safety Responsibilities

Agency		Responsible for
US Department of Agriculture	Food Safety and Inspection Service (FSIS)	All domestic and imported meat, poultry, and egg products, safe, wholesome, and correctly labeled (and catfish pending)
	Animal and Plant Health Inspection Service	Preventing the introduction or dissemination of (1) plant pests and (2) livestock pests or diseases
	Grain Inspection, Packers, and Stockyards Administration	Establishing quality standards, inspection procedures, and marketing of grain and other related products
	Agricultural Marketing Service (AMS)	Establishing quality and condition standards for, among other things, dairy, fruit, vegetables, and livestock
	Agricultural Research Service	Providing the scientific research to help ensure that the food supply is safe and secure and that foods meet foreign and domestic regulatory requirements
	Economic Research Service	Providing analyses of the economic issues affecting the safety of the US food supply
	National Agricultural Statistics Service	Providing statistical data, including agricultural chemical usage data, related to the safety of the food supply
Department of Health and Human Services	Food and Drug Administration	All domestic and imported food products, except meat, poultry, and processed egg products, *are safe, wholesome, and properly labeled*
	Centers for Disease Control and Prevention	Preventing the transmission, dissemination and spread of foodborne illness to protect the public health
Department of Commerce	National Marine Fisheries Service	Voluntary, fee-for-service examinations of seafood for safety and quality
Environmental Protection Agency		Regulating the use of certain chemicals and substances that present an unreasonable risk of injury to health or the environment; issuing regulations to establish, modify, or revoke tolerances for pesticide chemical residues; setting national drinking water standard of quality and consulting with the FDA before FDA promulgates regulations for standard of quality for bottled water
Department of the Treasury	Alcohol and Tobacco Tax and Trade Bureau	Regulation, enforcing, and issuing permits for the production, labeling, and distribution of alcoholic beverages
Department of Homeland Security	Customs and Border Protection	Inspecting imports, including food products, plants, and live animals, for compliance with US law and assisting all federal agencies in enforcing their regulations at the border
Federal Trade Commission		Enforcing prohibitions against false advertising, for, among other things, food products

Source: Federal Food Safety Oversight: Additional Actions Needed to Improve Planning and Collaboration. December 2014; GAO: GAO-15-180.

enforces standards regarding food safety; such safety standards address food additives, the prevention of foodborne illness, the safety of animal feed and drugs, including any residue of such in human foods, and truthful, reliable food labels (United States Food and Drug Administration, http://www.fda.gov/AboutFDA/Transparency/Basics/ucm242648.htm).

Two other agencies have important, broad food safety responsibilities: the Centers for Disease Control and Prevention (CDC) and the Environmental Protection Agency (EPA). We will briefly introduce the responsibilities of these two agencies, then turn to focus on the FDA.

Centers for Disease Control and Prevention

The CDC provides the critical connection between illness in people and our food system. The information gathered by the CDC during research and outbreak surveillance informs new food safety regulation and guidance (Centers for Disease Control and Prevention, http://www.cdc.gov/food safety/cdc-and-food-safety.html). The CDC's role includes investigating outbreaks and establishing both short-term control measures and long-term improvements to prevent similar outbreaks in the future. The CDC works with state and local health departments to investigate foodborne outbreaks and make information available to the public.

Environmental Protection Agency

The establishment of the EPA in 1970 fostered developments in pesticide regulation. The EPA approves which pesticides may be used on food and sets acceptable tolerances of pesticide residue that are then enforced by the FDA (United States Environmental Protection Agency, http://www.epa.gov/pesticides/factsheets/securty.htm); by the FSIS for meat, poultry, and some egg products; and also by the USDA's Office of Pest Management Policy. Laboratory studies show that pesticides can cause health problems, such as birth defects, nerve damage, cancer, and other effects, that might develop over a long period of time. These effects depend on the pesticide's toxicity and how much of it is consumed. Some pesticides also pose unique health risks to children. For these reasons, the EPA, in cooperation with the individual states, regulates pesticides to ensure that their use does not pose unreasonable risks to infants, children, and adults, or the environment.

The EPA regulates pesticides under two major federal statutes, the Federal Food, Drug and Cosmetic Act of 1938 (FDCA) and the Federal Insecticide, Fungicide, and Rodenticide Act of 1947 (FIFRA). Under the FDCA, EPA establishes tolerances (maximum legally permissible levels) for pesticide residues in food (United States Environmental Protection Agency, http://www.epa.gov /pesticides/regulating/laws/fqpa/backgrnd.htm). When FIFRA was passed in 1947, it established procedures for registering pesticides with the USDA and established labeling provisions. The law was still, however, primarily concerned with the *efficacy* of pesticides rather than regulating the safe use of pesticides. FIFRA provides EPA with the authority to oversee the sale and use of pesticides, and authorizes the EPA to register pesticides for use in the United States and prescribe labeling and other regulatory requirements to prevent unreasonable adverse effects on health or the environment. FIFRA does not fully preempt state/tribal or local law, however; thus each state/ tribe and local government may also regulate pesticide use (United States Environmental Protection Agency, http://www.epa.gov/agriculture/lfra.html).

In 1996, Congress passed the Food Quality Protection Act (FQPA), which amended both laws to establish a more consistent, protective regulatory scheme. The FQPA mandates a single, health-based standard for all pesticides in all foods; provides special protection for infants and children; expedites approval of safer pesticides; creates incentives for the development and maintenance of effective crop protection tools for farmers; and requires periodic reevaluation of pesticide registrations and tolerances to ensure that the scientific data supporting pesticide registrations will remain current in the future (United States Environmental Protection Agency, http://www.epa.gov/pesti cides/regulating/laws/fqpa/backgrnd.htm).

The FQPA also set a herculean task for the EPA by requiring the completion of a review and reassessment of the tolerances (maximum permitted residues) for all food use pesticides (close to 10,000) within a decade. The EPA recommended revoking 3200 tolerances and modifying 1200. In some cases, rather than develop new data to address questions about safety, registrants voluntarily withdrew tolerances and registrations for crop uses. This, in turn, spurred companies to develop and growers to pursue reduced-risk alternatives (United States Environmental Protection Agency, http:// www.epa.gov/pesticides/regulating/laws/fqpa/fqpa_accomplishments.htm).

Focus on the FDA

Although as noted above, numerous agencies play a role in food safety, we are focusing on the FDA in this chapter. The FDA is coming to prominence in US food safety policy with the Food Safety Modernization Act of 2011 (FSMA), the largest expansion of FDA's food safety authority since the 1930s (Johnson 2014). The FSMA reflects the division of responsibility between industry for safety

---

BOX 13.1 HAZARD ANALYSIS AND CRITICAL CONTROL POINT

In the early 1980s, the Government Accountability Office (GAO) had recommended that the USDA reform meat inspection and institute Hazard Analysis and Critical Control Point (HACCP). Developed by Pillsbury in 1959 to create a food system for NASA to provide critically necessary safe food for astronauts, HACCP is aimed at preventing contamination at every stage of food production and processing.[1]

HACCP is a preventive process control system designed to identify and prevent microbial and other hazards in food production. HACCP systems are based on seven principles: (1) hazard analysis, (2) critical control point identification, (3) establishment of critical limits, (4) monitoring procedures, (5) corrective actions, (6) record keeping, and (7) verification procedures.[2]

The idea is to use a systematic approach to the identification and assessment of the risk of biological, chemical, and physical hazards from a particular food production process or practice and then control those hazards. Science-based analyses of food production processes allow manufacturers to locate where the hazards can occur, take steps to prevent problems, and respond rapidly to problems.

HACCP places the responsibility for identifying safety problems with the manufacturer. Although inspectors may do spot-checks to ensure that the processors' HACCP systems are working, the use of the HACCP system means that a firm is engaged in continuous problem prevention and problem solving, rather than relying on facility inspections by regulatory agencies or consumer complaints.[3]

Although HACCP was recommended in the 1980s, just as in 1906 and in 1938, government action happened after a public health crisis. In the case of HACCP, implementation by the USDA was prompted by a 1992 *Escherichia coli* outbreak transmitted through fast food chain Jack in the Box hamburgers that turned deadly as the specific strain of *E. coli* (O157:H7) had acquired the ability to produce the shigella toxin. In 1994, the USDA announced the proposal of rules requiring HACCP systems in all ground beef and poultry processing plants.[4]

Meanwhile, the FDA's leisurely rollout of HACCP controls, starting with foods considered most hazardous—seafood in 1995, with raw sprouts and eggs to follow effective 1999 and fresh juice in 2001—was interrupted in the fall of 1996 by an outbreak of *E. coli* O157:H7 in unpasteurized apple juice.[1] It had become clear that all foods should be produced under a HACCP system. HACCP was a significant change in regulatory philosophy, shifting the burden of responsibility from government to industry.[5]

Source:
[1]Data from Nestle, M. *Safe Food: The Politics of Food Safety.* California: University of California, 2010.
[2]Data from United States Department of Agriculture. Food Safety and Inspection Service. Key Facts: HACCP Final Rule, Revised January 1998. Available at http://www.fsis.usda.gov/Oa/background/keyhaccp.htm, accessed January 20, 2015.
[3]Data from US Food and Drug Administration. Hazard Analysis & Critical Control Points (HACCP). Available at http://www.fda.gov/Food/GuidanceRegulation/HACCP/default.htm, accessed January 20, 2015.
[4]Data from Morris, Jr., J.G. and Potter, M.E., eds. Foodborne infections and intoxications. Waltham, MA: Academic Press, 2013, 501.
[5]Data from United States Department of Agriculture, Food Safety and Inspection Service, FSIS history. Available at http://www.fsis.usda.gov/wps/portal/informational/aboutfsis/history, updated May 25, 2013, accessed December 30, 2014.

and the government only as the enforcer, as it emphasizes government review of HACCP or similar systems designed to identify critical food safety hazard points rather than inspections (Box 13.1).

Within the FDA, four directorates oversee the core functions of the agency: medical products and tobacco, foods, global regulatory operations and policy, and operations. The Office of Foods was created in 2009 with the goal to lead a "functionally unified FDA Foods Program," and in 2012 renamed "Office of Foods and Veterinary Medicine." It houses the Center for Food Safety and Applied Nutrition (CFSAN) and the Center for Veterinary Medicine.

Historically, the FDA has always been underfunded in comparison to the USDA. In fiscal year (FY) 2012, the FDA's food safety program activities were funded at $866 million, while the USDA FSIS were funded at $1.004 billion. In other words, the FSIS covers 10–20% of the US food supply with 60% of the funds available allotted to the two agencies; the FDA covers 80–90% of the food supply with 40% of the funds, though slowly the FDA is being allocated more funds.

Staffing levels also vary considerably, with around 9400 full-time employees at FSIS and about 3400 full-time food-related employees at FDA (Johnson 2014). Although the law authorized appropriations when FSMA was enacted, it did not provide the actual funding needed for FDA to perform these activities. The Congressional Budget Office (CBO) estimated at the time that FSMA could increase net federal spending subject to appropriation by about $1.4 billion over a 5-year period (FY2011–FY2015) (Johnson 2014).

Food Safety: Federal Authority

Federal responsibility for food safety began in 1906, with the passage of the Pure Food and Drug Act and the Meat Inspection Act, prompted by public outrage over *The Jungle*, Upton Sinclair's exposé of insanitary and inhumane working conditions in meatpacking plants.

Oversight of the 1906 Pure Food and Drug Act and the Meat Inspection Act was given entirely to the USDA as the prevailing pressure concerned meat inspections and keeping sick animals out of the food supply. Internally, the USDA split this new responsibility over food safety between two bureaus, giving enforcement of the Meat Inspection Act to the Bureau of Animal Industry and enforcement of the Food and Drugs Act to the Bureau of Chemistry (Nestle 2010). The Bureau of Chemistry was later renamed the Food and Drug Administration (1931) and transferred out of the USDA (1940), (United States Food and Drug Administration, http://www.fda.gov/AboutFDA/WhatWeDo/History/Overviews/ucm056044.htm), resulting in a division in authority and responsibilities over the nation's food safety that continues today.

The 1906 Meat Inspection Act (Meat Act) required every animal and carcass produced for interstate commerce to be inspected. Meat "found to be not adulterated shall be marked, stamped, tagged, or labeled as 'Inspected and passed'" (21 U.S.C. § 604, United States Food and Drug Administration, http://www.fda.gov/RegulatoryInformation/Legislation/ucm148693.htm). Meat found to be adulterated could not legally be sold in interstate commerce. The inspection of slaughterhouses that only produced meat for sale within its state borders was left under state authority. The Meat Act and subsequent amendments set inspection standards to determine adulteration and thus remove unsafe food from the market. These standards made sense in 1906, but much later the USDA's authority regarding deadly pathogens in food would be greatly circumscribed.

Under the Meat Act, slaughterhouses could only be operated while the inspector was present. Through the inspection stamp, the inspector passed approval of the safety of the meat, and the packer and producer had no further safety requirements. In effect, under the Meat Act, the government was responsible for the safety of meat inspected and stamped as approved, even though authority of safety was limited to the slaughterhouse premises exactly, as the inspector had no ability to recall meat.

The 1906 Pure Food and Drug Act (Pure Food Act) also defined what would cause a food to be considered adulterated, (Federal Food and Drugs Act of 1906 (The "Wiley Act"), http://www.fda.gov/RegulatoryInformation/Legislation/ucm148690.htm), but the Pure Food Act required sampling, not continuous inspection, and made the producers responsible for safety. The government was only the enforcer (Nestle 2010). Thus, the two originating laws, although each passed in 1906, manifested two different policy approaches, one in which the government was responsible for food safety, and one in which industry was responsible.

Unfortunately, the Pure Food Act lacked the provision of a means of enforcement, and accelerating new technologies and production methods for food and drugs quickly outpaced the law. By 1933, it was clear that a complete overhaul was needed. Nonetheless, the revisions languished for another 5 years, until a medical drug disaster occurred, which prompted the passage of the Federal Food, Drug and Cosmetic Act (FDCA) in 1938 (Box 13.2).

Under the authority of the 1938 FDCA, the FDA has established guidance and regulatory requirements for manufacturers to assure that food is safe and unadulterated. The FDCA prohibits the entry into interstate commerce of adulterated or misbranded foods (United States Food and Drug Administration, http://www.fda.gov/AboutFDA/WhatWeDo/History/ProductRegulation/Sul fanilamideDisaster/default.htm). The FDCA, in conjunction with the FSMA, provides the basis of FDA's authority in food safety today.

Other important legislation includes the following:

- Fair Packaging and Labeling Act (1965) regulates appropriate labeling of consumer products in interstate commerce.
- Food Additives Amendment of the FDCA (1958) gives the authority to the FDA to establish the conditions of usage for food additives (to ensure safety) including labeling. Any food additive shown to cause cancer in animals or humans was prohibited.
- The Infant Formula Act of 1980, as amended (Box 13.3).
- The Nutrition Labeling and Education Act of 1990 preempts state requirements and standardized the food ingredient panel, serving size, and some important descriptive terms

---

BOX 13.2   SULFANILAMIDE DISASTER

Congress had been lagging on passing updated food and drug safety laws until a precipitating event in the form of a medical drug disaster occurred in 1937. Sulfanilamide, in tablet and powder form, had been successfully and safely used for some time to treat streptococcal infections. A new liquid formulation had been devised and distributed by a pharmaceutical company, and, in absence of any required regulatory toxicity testing for new products, the new formula turned out to be lethal. The dissolving agent used was diethylene glycol, a deadly poisonous chemical normally used as antifreeze. The drug caused over 100 deaths in 2 months, including the chemist by suicide upon learning of his error. Although upon realizing the error, the pharmaceutical firm had already sent out telegrams requesting the product be returned, the telegrams failed to describe the urgency or advise of the lethality of the drug, and the FDA began an intensive campaign to retrieve the drug, recovering 234 gallons and 1 pint out of a total of 240 gallons distributed. Under the 1906 Pure Food and Drugs law, the only legal authority the FDA had to recover the product was through misbranding, and luckily the product happened to be *misbranded*—because it coincidentally happened to be labeled an elixir when it was actually technically a solution. If this had not been the cause, the FDA would have had no legal authority to demand the recall. Thus, not coincidentally, the languishing Federal Food, Drug and Cosmetic Act became law a year later in 1938.

Source: Ballentine, C. Taste of Raspberries, Taste of Death. The 1937 Sulfanilamide Incident. FDA Consumer, June 1981. Available at http://www.fda.gov/aboutfda/whatwedo/history/productregulation/sulfanilamidedisaster /default.htm, accessed January 20, 2015.

BOX 13.3   INFANT FORMULA

Prior to 1980, infant formula was regulated under 21 Code of Federal Regulations (CFR) 105.65, Infant Foods. This regulation specified minimum levels of certain nutrients for infant formulas, including protein, fat, and some vitamins and minerals, but a level for chloride was not specified.

In 1978, a major manufacturer of infant formula reformulated two of its soy products by discontinuing the addition of salt. This resulted in infant formula products containing an inadequate amount of chloride, an essential nutrient for infant growth and development. By mid-1979, a cluster of infants had been diagnosed with hypochloremic metabolic alkalosis, a syndrome associated with chloride deficiency, which was eventually associated with prolonged and exclusive use of the chloride-deficient soy formulas. Chloride deficiency can result in growth retardation or manifest central nervous system effects such as cerebral dysfunction or impaired cognitive function. This outbreak highlights two critically important elements of public health practice: First, developing and using appropriate case definitions for both surveillance and for the investigation of outbreaks of both infectious and noninfectious origin enables local and state health departments and the Public Health Service to respond rapidly. Second, clinicians play a significant role in identifying and resolving public health emergencies.[1]

After reviewing the matter, Congress determined that to improve protection of infants using infant formula products, greater regulatory control over the formulation and production of infant formula was needed, including modification of industry and the FDA's recall procedures. Thus, the Infant Formula Act of 1980 (P.L. 96-359) was born. The FDA, in turn, adopted regulations implementing the act, including regulations on recall procedures, quality control procedures, labeling, and nutrient requirements.[2]

The Infant Formula Act was designed to ensure the safety and nutrition of infant formulas, including minimum and, in some cases, maximum levels of specified nutrients. One of the most specific and detailed acts ever passed by Congress, the act gives the FDA authority to regulate the labeling of infant formula and to establish quality control rules and regulations governing formula manufacturing. The act establishes minimum nutrient requirements, defines adulteration, provides for establishing nutrient and quality control procedures, prescribes recall procedures, and specifies inspection requirements. It addresses three related requirements for the manufacturer of the formula: (1) notifying the FDA before processing an infant formula, (2) notifying the FDA after a change in formulation or processing, and (3) meeting testing requirements based on regulations with regard to major and minor changes in the formula. In 1985, the act was revised to include minimum concentrations of 29 nutrients and maximum concentrations of 9 nutrients in infant formula. In 2005, the FDA requested more explicit guidelines for assessing safety of new ingredients added to infant formula.[3] A key limitation of the current approach is the lack of explicit guidelines to help formula manufacturers and outside expert reviewers determine what safety data are needed on a proposed ingredient, and how they should be gathered.

In passing the 1980 Infant Formula Act and its amendments, Congress recognized infant formulas as a special category of foods that requires more regulation than other types of foods, simply because there is no margin for error in ensuring the healthy growth and development of infants. Regulation of infant formulas involves both general safety provisions of the act and additional requirements specific to infant formulas (e.g., CGMPs, quality control procedures, nutrient levels and analysis, and quality factors). For most of the requirements specific to infant formula, manufacturers must provide assurances that the requirements have been met for each new product (including marketed products in which a major change has occurred) prior to marketing.

Source:
[1]Data from Infant metabolic acidosis and soy-based formula—United States. *MMWR.* 28, 358–359, 1979. Republished with 1996 editorial in Landmark articles from the *MMWR* 1961–1996. *MMWR.* 45, 985–988, 1996.
[2]Data from Kleinman, R.E., ed. Pediatric Nutrition Handbook, 5th ed. American Academy of Pediatrics, 2004.
[3]Data from Committee on the Evaluation of the Addition of Ingredients New to Infant Formula. *Infant Formula: Evaluating the Safety of New Ingredients.* Washington, D.C.: National Academies Press, 2004.

such as *low fat* and *light* (Significant Dates in US Food and Drug Law History, http://www .fda.gov/AboutFDA/WhatWeDo/History/Milestones/ucm128305.htm).
• Food Allergen Labeling and Consumer Protection Act of 2004 requires labels to clearly identify if any of the ingredients are sourced from the eight most common allergens. The 2013 regulation issued by the FDA concerning *gluten-free* is made under the authority of this Act.

FOOD SAFETY AT THE STATE LEVEL AND THE FOOD MODEL CODE

The roles and responsibilities of the states, however, are not completely subsumed. The federal government needs help from the states in inspecting and enforcing, and may provide financial assistance to the states to do so. In addition to inspections conducted by the federal government, states and territories also oversee inspection and regulation activities that help ensure the safety of foods produced, processed, or sold within their jurisdictions.

State and local agencies are involved in outbreak response and recalls, surveillance through collaboration with the CDC, and using tools such as FoodNet, PulseNet, and Outbreak Net; laboratory testing; technical training and assistance; education; and retail, processing, and farm inspections. In fact, states have primary jurisdiction over enforcement pesticide regulations, and they conduct the majority of *FDA* inspections, under contract with the FDA (David et al., http://www.thefsrc.org /State_Local/StateLocal_June17_background.pdf).

State and local authorities—not federal agencies—are responsible for licensing and inspecting food retailers and institutional food service establishments operating in the United States, such as supermarkets, grocery stores, restaurants, nursing homes, child care agencies, and other food establishments.

To help increase uniformity throughout the states regarding regulation of the retail and restaurant sectors of food provision, the FDA has created advisory guidance in the form of a model Food Code. Published from 1993 to 2005 in a 2-year cycle, full updates are now scheduled for every 4 years, with supplements being published between cycles. The most recent full Code was published in 2013 (US Food and Drug Administration, http://www.fda.gov/food/guidanceregulation/retailfood protection/foodcode/default.htm).

Although the goal of uniformity among the states is laudable, the feasible extent of uniformity is modified by several factors. For example, the states have used various versions of the Food Code as models for regulation, so inherent differences between the versions will remain as differences among the states, particularly if the states lack automatic means to update their regulations as the model code changes. Also, the regulations that states adopt may be based on the Code, but not exactly the same as the Code.

Nonetheless, the Code provides practical, science-based guidance and manageable, enforceable provisions for mitigating risk factors known to cause foodborne illness. The code is a reference document for regulatory agencies that oversee food safety in food service establishments, retail food stores, other food establishments at the retail level, and institutions such as nursing homes and child care centers. Adoption of the code is endorsed by the Department of Health and Human Services (HHS) and the USDA as a strategy for the local jurisdictions to attain at least minimum national food safety standards and to enhance the overall efficiency and effectiveness of the nation's food safety system. As of 2013, versions of the Model Code have been adopted by all 50 states, 54 of the 564 federally recognized tribes, and three of the six territories of the United States (US Food and Drug Administration, http://www.fda.gov/Food/GuidanceRegulation/RetailFoodProtection/FoodCode/ucm 108156.htm).

FOOD SAFETY THROUGH LABELING

The FDA is in charge of regulating food product labeling. Labeling may not seem directly connected to food safety, as the label itself cannot make the food inherently safe or unsafe when it comes to pathogens, a very much currently emphasized issue of food safety (Nestle 2010). However, the idea of safe food and the original mandate for the FDA was grounded in what we value as to the nature of food, namely, food as *pure and wholesome*. In order for any consumer to be confidant in the purity or wholesomeness of a purchased food product, some basic information must be provided to the consumer. Although this may sound obvious to us today as we read ingredient and nutrition information on labels, this level of regulation and access to this much information is comparatively recent. With standardized label requirements followed by regulations regarding ingredients, nutritional information, and allergens, food labeling began to act more concertedly as protection for the consumer. The following highlights three areas in which food safety is a concern of labeling, namely, food additives, allergens, and GMOs.

1958 FOOD ADDITIVE AMENDMENT

The 1958 Food Additive Amendment of the FDCA provides a legal definition of food additives for the purpose of imposing a premarket approval requirement by the FDA. Food additives are defined as "all substances, the intended use of which results or may reasonably be expected to result, directly or indirectly, either in their becoming a component of food, or otherwise affecting the characteristics of food." The definition specifically excludes items whose use is "generally recognized as safe" (GRAS); manufacturers can add such items to foods without seeking government approval (Code of Federal Regulations, http://www.gpo.gov/fdsys/pkg/CFR-2012-title21-vol3/xml/CFR-2012-title21-vol3 -sec170-3.xml). Pesticide chemicals, pesticide chemical residue, and color additives are subject to different legal regulations for premarket approval.

Determining Safety: GRAS

If an additive is determined to be unsafe, the food containing the additive is considered adulterated under the FDCA and cannot be sold in interstate commerce. Additives have two routes to being considered safe.

- If a substance was used in food prior to January 1, 1958, an additive can be considered "generally recognized as safe" (GRAS) "through experience based on common use in food," defined as a history of consumption by a substantial number of users.
- The other option is to have qualified scientific experts evaluate the safety of the item (US Food and Drug Administration, http://www.fda.gov/food/ingredientspackaginglabeling /gras/default.htm).

The FDA developed an initial list of food substances considered to be GRAS; however, much of what industry considered as GRAS was not on this list and manufacturers asked for opinion letters. In the late 1960s, the FDA banned an artificial sweetener, cyclamate, and President Nixon ordered the FDA to review the GRAS list. Accordingly, the authority of the opinion letters was revoked, and the FDA contracted a scientific review of presumed GRAS substances and established rulemaking procedures to affirm the GRAS status of substances that were either on the GRAS list or the subject of a petition from manufacturers (United States Food and Drug Administration, http://www.fda.gov /AboutFDA/WhatWeDo/History/Milestones/ucm128305.htm).

In 1997, to eliminate the resource-intensive rulemaking procedures, the FDA proposed to replace the GRAS affirmation petition process with a notification procedure (United States Food and Drug Administration, http://www.fda.gov/Food/IngredientsPackagingLabeling/GRAS/ucm094040.htm). FDA started accepting GRAS notices in 1998 as if the proposed rule was final, although, as of the end of 2014, the FDA has not yet finalized the rule.

Under the GRAS notification program, the FDA is simply notified by a manufacturer of a determination that the use of a substance is GRAS, rather than the manufacturer petitioning the FDA to affirm that the use of a substance is GRAS (US Food and Drug Administration 2006). After receiving a GRAS notice, the FDA responds with one of three letters:

1. The FDA does not question the basis for the GRAS determination.
2. The FDA concludes that the notice does not provide a sufficient basis for a GRAS determination, either because information is lacking or because the information available raises safety questions.
3. The FDA has, at the request of the notifying party, ceased to evaluate the GRAS notice (US Food and Drug Administration 2006).

The notification process is voluntary. The FDA makes it clear that if a manufacturer determines a substance to be GRAS, the product can be marketed without notifying the FDA. Furthermore, if the manufacturer does decide to notify the FDA, the product can still be marketed while waiting for a response.

This process means that there is no all-inclusive list of substances considered to be GRAS. The FDA has several lists of GRAS substances but also states that a substance is not required to be on these lists in order to be considered GRAS, as "the use of a substance is GRAS because of widespread knowledge among the community of qualified experts, not because of a listing or other administrative activity." The FDA notes in the proposed-but-never-finalized rule that publication in a peer-reviewed scientific journal may be supplemented by secondary scientific literature, including the opinion of an *expert panel* specifically convened for this purpose, and that consensus does not mean unanimity (Box 13.4) (Food and Drug Administration 1997).

Voluntary notification is a policy that favors corporate interest. An April 2014 report from the National Resources Defense Council spells GRAS out as "Generally Recognized as Secret" and comments that one problem with a voluntary notification program is in fact that it is voluntary. The NRDC report identified 275 chemicals from 56 companies that appear to have been marketed in the United States for use in food since 1997 by companies that made their own GRAS safety determinations without, in fact, notifying the FDA, which means that a chemical's identity, chemical composition, and safety determination are not publicly disclosed. And, as noted above, a manufacturer may continue to sell a product even if the GRAS notification is voluntarily withdrawn (Neltner and Maffini 2014).

BOX 13.4   GRAS NOTICES

GRAS notices, along with FDA's response, can be searched from this link: http://www .accessdata.fda.gov/scripts/fdcc/?set=GRASNotices. As of August 31, 2014, 539 notices have been submitted to the FDA. The very first notice on this list is for soy isoflavone extract. The FDA closed this notice on November 3, 1998, ceasing evaluation at the request of the notifying company, Archer Daniels Midland (ADM) (US Food and Drug Administration 2004).

Safety of Intended Conditions of Use

Although the intent of the law in 1958 may have been to ensure that common food ingredients or items were not subject to food additive regulations, the change in 1997 to a notification process allows the GRAS carve-out to cover new or innovative ingredients, not just ones already commonly consumed.

The criteria of "common use in food" leading to GRAS includes the amount of an additive commonly used and consumed, described by the FDA as "intended conditions of use of the substance" and "in consideration of the population that will consume the substance." This point is manifesting in controversies, such as caffeine. Caffeine has been considered GRAS since the initial FDA list in 1958, but rising volumes in energy drinks and the use of caffeine in alcohol have raised concerns. In 2010, the FDA declared that caffeine mixed with alcohol is not GRAS, citing in part the lack of scientific data to support the idea that it would be safe for young adults, the intended market (United States Food and Drug Administration 2010).

2004 Food Allergen Labeling and Consumer Protection Act

Some foods can cause severe illness and, in extreme cases, a life-threatening allergic reaction. A food allergy is caused when your immune system overreacts to a particular protein found in that food. Proteins that are major allergens in foods include casein and whey in cow's milk, ovomucoid in egg whites, and tropomycin in shellfish. Eight foods account for 90% of allergic reactions: milk, eggs, peanuts, tree nuts, soy, wheat, fish, and shellfish (Boyce et al. 2010).

The CDC estimated in 2008 that 4–6% of children in the United States are affected by food allergies (Branum and Lukacs 2008). Research suggests that the prevalence of food allergies is on the rise, and indeed, a 2014 study of 516 inner-city children followed from birth to 5 years reports that almost 10% were categorized as having a food allergy based on sensitization tests and clinical history over the 5-year period (McGowan et al. 2015).

In 2004, Congress passed the Food Allergen Labeling and Consumer Protection Act (FALCPA; (Public Law 108–282), http://www.fda.gov/Food/GuidanceRegulation/GuidanceDocumentsRegulatory Information/Allergens/ucm106187.htm), which is applicable to all food regulated by the FDA. Under FALCPA, the label must clearly identify if any of the ingredients are sourced from the eight most common allergens (milk, eggs, peanuts, tree nuts, soy, wheat, fish, and shellfish). The label can either make a *contains* statement (contains soy, wheat, eggs) or list the source in parentheses next to the ingredient, e.g., *lecithin (soy), whey (milk)* (United States Food and Drug Administration, http://www.fda.gov/Food/ResourcesForYou/Consumers/ucm079311.htm).

Nonetheless, consumers with allergies should still read the ingredient list on the label. Being allergic to a food may also mean being allergic to a similar protein found in a different food. This reaction, known as cross-reactivity, occurs when your immune system thinks one protein is very much like another. For example, if you are allergic to ragweed, you may also develop reactions to bananas or melons (American Academy of Asthma, Allergy, and Immunology, http://www.aaaai .org/conditions-and-treatments/allergies/food-allergies.aspx). Some people who are allergic to peanuts are also allergic to sweet lupin, a legume in the same family as peanuts. Lupin flour and protein are becoming more commonly used in the United States, such as in gluten-free products. Lupin is not a FALCPA allergen and thus will not be highlighted as an allergen. Individuals who are allergic to peanuts will also need to carefully read the list of ingredients, as lupin must be declared in the list of ingredients (United States Food and Drug Administration, http://www.fda.gov/Food/Ingredients PackagingLabeling/FoodAdditivesIngredients/ucm410111.htm).

Even more problematically, fenugreek is also an emerging cross-sensitive allergen for people allergic to peanuts (Vinje et al. 2012) and, as a spice, may be present in a food product without being specifically called out by name. Food products made in the United States can have potential food allergens masked by nonspecific terms, such as natural flavors, seasonings, and spices, in the

---

BOX 13.5   CFR CODE OF FEDERAL REGULATIONS TITLE 21, VOLUME 2

Revised as of April 1, 2014
2CFR101.22
Part 101—Food Labeling
Subpart B—Specific Food Labeling Requirements
Sec. 101.33 Foods; labeling of spices, flavorings, colorings and chemical preservatives

(a) (2) The term spice means any aromatic vegetable substance in the whole, broken, or ground form, except for those substances which have been traditionally regarded as foods, such as onions, garlic and celery; whose significant function in food is seasoning rather than nutritional; that is true to name; and from which no portion of any volatile oil or other flavoring principle has been removed. Spices include the spices listed in 182.10 and part 184 of this chapter, such as the following: Allspice; Anise; Basil; Bay leaves; Caraway seed; Cardamon; Celery seed; Chervil; Cinnamon; Cloves; Coriander; Cumin seed; Dill seed; Fennel seed; Fenugreek; Ginger; Horseradish; Mace; Marjoram; Mustard flour; Nutmeg; Oregano; Paprika; Parsley; Pepper, black; Pepper, red; Pepper, white; Rosemary; Saffron; Sage; Savory; Star aniseed; Tarragon; Thyme; Turmeric. Paprika, turmeric, and saffron or other spices which are also colors, shall be declared as "spice and coloring" unless declared by their common or usual name.

---

ingredients list. Currently, the FDA defines spice in a manner that allows manufacturers to use the term *spice* in the ingredient list without requiring that the spice be named. The declaration *spices* can be used (as can *flavor, natural flavor*, or *artificial flavor*; Box 13.5) (US Food and Drug Administration 2013a).

Furthermore, although the FDA requires food processors to label foods with all ingredients, business practices, such as shared manufacturing equipment, for example, could lead to potential contamination of food products by items not intended to be ingredients. Advisory label statements that indicate a food product "may contain" allergens or may be "cross-contaminated" with allergens are not required under FALCPA. This means that a manufacturer who uses tree nuts in one product on a manufacturing line is not required by law to make a statement on the label of a different product that does not contain nuts but is produced on the same equipment. Manufacturers, however, may choose to add these advisory statements for their own business reasons. The FDA states that such precautionary statements as "may contain" or "produced in facilities that also process tree nuts," must be truthful, not misleading, and not a substitute for good manufacturing practices (United States Food and Drug Administration, http://www.fda.gov/Food/ResourcesForYou/Consumers/ucm079311.htm).

GENETIC MODIFICATION OF FOODS

Although many characteristics of food products are required to be identified on the label, as of the end of 2014, the fact that a food product is genetically modified is not one of those characteristics. As of 2014, 80–89% of corn (depending on variety) and 94% of all soybeans grown in the United States were genetically engineered varieties (United States Department of Agriculture, http://www.ers.usda.gov/data-products/adoption-of-genetically-engineered-crops-in-the-us/recent-trends-in-ge-adoption.aspx). Even if consumers do not choose to eat soy in a recognizable whole form, such as tofu or soy beverage, soy is present in many processed foods in the United States. Thus, most Americans have been exposed to some amount of genetically modified soy.

The FDA first approved genetically modified crops in 1994, having earlier decided in 1992 that labeling items as genetically modified was not required. The FDA did not see a distinction between the normal practices of hybridization as conducted by farmers and genetic modification, and felt the important issue was the end result. The 1992 policy statement pointed out that food product labeling is required to "reveal all facts that are material in light of representations made or suggested by labeling or with respect to consequences which may result from use." Thus, the FDA concluded that consumers must be appropriately informed through labeling only if an engineered food product differed from a traditional food counterpart such that the common name was no longer applicable or if there was a safety or usage issue (United States Food and Drug Administration, http://www.fda.gov/food/guidanceregulation /guidancedocumentsregulatoryinformation/biotechnology/ucm096095.htm).

However, even in this case, the label would refer to the consequential difference between the products, not necessarily to the genetic engineering process that caused the difference. For example, in December of 1996 when DuPont's genetically modified soybean oil turned out to have a much higher level of oleic acid than do conventional soybeans, DuPont's oil no longer met the FDA's standard of composition of soybean oil. DuPont proposed it be labeled accordingly as "high oleic soybean oil" to which the FDA agreed (United States Food and Drug Administration, http://www.fda.gov/food/food scienceresearch/biotechnology/submissions/ucm161157.htm), not labeled as "oil genetically engineered to be higher in oleic acid."

One specific concern regarding genetic engineering/modification and food safety is the potential of creating unrecognized new food allergens. All food allergens are proteins, and the technology of introducing a gene into another plant can carry along an allergenic protein (United States Food and Drug Administration, http://www.fda.gov/food/guidanceregulation/guidancedocumentsregulatoryinfor mation/biotechnology/ucm096095.htm). Thus, under the FDA's 1992 policy, labeling of a genetically engineered food would be required if known food allergy issues existed, if for example, a peanut protein was introduced to a tomato. A peanut-protein-modified tomato, even if it looked and tasted like a regular tomato, would require an informative label as to the peanut protein, but not necessarily to the genetic engineering process that introduced the protein (United States Department of Agriculture, http://www.fda.gov/food/guidanceregulation/guidancedocumentsregulatoryinformation/labelingnutri tion/ucm059098.htm). Known allergens can be tested for. For example, one company used a Brazil nut gene to improve the nutritional quality of soybeans, but then had to pull the soybean from the market after testing revealed that people who were allergic to Brazil nuts were also now allergic to the genetically engineered soybean (Nordlee et al. 1996). To this extent, the risks of allergies can be mitigated through testing. However, the allergic potentiality of a new protein cannot be tested (Box 13.6).

In 2001, the FDA issued draft guidance for industry regarding labeling bioengineered foods, which reaffirmed its decision to not require special labeling of all bioengineered foods, noting that there was still no basis for concluding that the use of bioengineering is a material fact that must be disclosed under sections 403(a) and 201(n) of the Federal Food Drug and Cosmetic Act (United States Department of Agriculture, http://www.fda.gov/food/guidanceregulation/guidancedocumentsregulatoryinformation /labelingnutrition/ucm059098.htm).

Conversely, in the draft guidance, the FDA also curtailed label descriptions from food makers who do not use genetically modified or engineered ingredients and wish to promote their product accordingly. Since the FDA has concluded that the use or absence of bioengineering does not in and of itself mean there is a material difference in the food, the label must not somehow suggest to the consumer that genetically modified food is inferior to nonmodified foods, or less safe, and thus falsely alarm consumers, as that would be misleading (United States Department of Agriculture, http://www.fda.gov/food /guidanceregulation/guidancedocumentsregulatoryinformation/labelingnutrition/ucm059098.htm). In the meantime, many food manufacturers who wish to promote their non-GMO products have used a *Non-GMO Project* association stamp (Non GMO Project, http://www.nongmoproject.org).

Publishing final guidance for manufacturers who wish to voluntarily label their foods as being made with or without the use of bioengineered ingredients is on CFAN's agenda of program priorities for 2013 (United States Food and Drug Administration, http://www.fda.gov/AboutFDA /CentersOffices/OfficeofFoods/CFSAN/WhatWeDo/ucm366279.htm?source=govdelivery&utm _medium=email&utm_source=govdelivery). Significantly, final guidance by the FDA on GMO labeling could preempt laws made by states, such as the GMO labeling law passed by Vermont in 2014. The Vermont law requires that food produced entirely or in part from genetic engineering

BOX 13.6   ARGUMENTS FOR AND AGAINST GENETICALLY MODIFIED ORGANISMS (GMOs)

Arguments for:
- Reduces pesticide use.[1,2]
- Improves crop yield.[1–3]
- Reduces famine due to crop failure.[4]
- Improves weed control and reduces fuel use and soil erosion.[2]
- Enhances nutritional quality,[1,3,5] for example, in rice enhanced with vitamin A.
- Eliminates allergens, for example, the P34 gene in soy.[6]
- Incorporates vaccines that can eliminate disease.[5]
- Expands agriculture to inhospitable land, for example, in sub-Saharan Africa[1,4,5] and to resource-poor farmers.[4,5]

Arguments against:
- Introduces new allergens into the food supply.[3,7–9]
- Antibiotic resistance to marker genes.[10]
- Reduces nutrient quality such as loss of phytoestrogens.[7,9]
- Reduces usefulness of Bt as an insecticide[3,8,9] and harms nontarget organisms.[5,7]
- Introduces superweeds through gene flow from herbicide-resistant crops to wild relatives.[7,8]
- Impacts animals, such as the medaka fish, where genetic manipulation for size affected reproductive fitness.[8]
- Possible long-term side effects of ingesting genetically modified foods.[6]
- Lack of the promised yields in GM crops,[7] possibly from conflict with other selection criteria.[8,11]
- Contaminates due to cross-pollination (inevitable and hard to detect).[2]
- Lack of adequate testing for environmental and human impact before release.[7]

Source:
[1]Data from Timmer, C.P., *J Nutr.* 133: 3319–3322, 2003.
[2]Data from Harlander, S.K., *Toxicol Pathol.* 30(1): 132–134, 2002.
[3]Data from Atherton, K.T., *Toxicology.* 181–182, 421–426, 2002.
[4]Data from Borlaug, N.E., *Plant Physiol.* 124: 487–490, 2000.
[5]Data from McGloughin, M., *AgBioForum.* 2(3&4): 163–174, 1999.
[6]Data from Bren, L. Genetic engineering: The future of foods? FDA Consumer Magazine. November–December 2003. Available at http://permanent.access.gpo.gov/lps1609/www.fda.gov/fdac/features/2003/603_food.html, accessed February 12, 2015.
[7]Data from Altieri, M.A. and Rosset, P., *AgBioForum.* 2(3&4): 155–162, 1999.
[8]Data from McCullum, C., *J Am Diet Assoc.* 100(11): 1311–1315, 2000.
[9]Data from Fagan, J.B. Assessing the safety and nutritional quality of genetically engineered foods. Available at http://www.psrast.org/jfassess.htm, accessed January 13, 2015.
[10]Data from Bakshi, A., *J Toxicol Environ Health.* 6(3): 211–225, 2003.
[11]Data from Babcock, B.C. and Francis, C.A., *J Am Diet Assoc.* 100(11): 1308–1311, 2000.

include the phrase "Produced with Genetic Engineering" on the label (The Vermont Legislative Bill Tracking System, http://www.leg.state.vt.us/database/status/summary.cfm?Bill=H.0112). Vermont's law becomes effective in 2016, unless the lawsuit filed against it by the Grocery Manufacturers Association, Snack Food Association, International Dairy Foods Association, and the National Association of Manufacturers prevails. Table 13.2 provides a timeline regarding GMO labeling.

TABLE 13.2
GMOs and Labeling: A Timeline

Year	Events (Still in Progress) Leading to GMO Labeling
1953	Watson and Crick discover the structure of DNA.
1968	Gellert discovers DNA ligase, the enzyme used to join DNA fragments together.[1]
1972	Paul Berg creates the first genetically modified DNA molecule.[2,3]
1973	Stanley Cohen, Annie Chang, Herbert Boyer, and Bob Helling created the first recombinant DNA organism (i.e., DNA segments containing a desirable gene are inserted [recombined] into the DNA of a distinct organism).[4,5]
1974	Stanford University files the first patent applications to cover rDNA technology.[6] NIH convenes an rDNA Advisory Committee (RAC) to oversee genetic research.
1975	At the Asilomar Conference in California, scientists agree to draft and abide by a set of research guidelines for the safe use of the technology.[7]
1976	NIH releases a comprehensive set of rules governing the practice of rDNA technology and banning the release of GMOs into the environment.[8]
1980s	The emergence of innovations in plant genetic engineering in the early 1980s results in an upsurge of takeovers and mergers within the plant seed industry. Chemical and pharmaceutical industries were the major purchasers of independent seed companies.[9]
1980	The US Supreme Court rules on the landmark case, Diamond v. Chakrabarty,[10] allowing for the first patent on a living organism, a crude-oil-spill-eating bacterium. Congress enacted the Bayh–Dole Act allowing universities and government laboratories such as those within NIH to hold patents on federally funded research.
1981	Over 80 new biotechnology firms formed by the end of the year.[11]
1983	Four independent groups of scientists working on transgenic plants announce successful results. Three have inserted bacterial genes into plants; the fourth has inserted a bean gene into a sunflower plant.
1986	The USDA issues a policy statement: The Coordinated Framework for Regulation of Biotechnology.[12] It becomes the cornerstone of US biotechnology policy but does not establish any new regulatory or legal requirements.
1989	AquAdvantage Salmon created.[13]
1992	The FDA issues official Statement of Policy on Foods Derived from New Plant Varieties,[14] described by Vice President Quayle to mean that "biotech products will receive the same oversight as other products, instead of being hampered by unnecessary regulation."[15] In its statement, the FDA embraces the substantial equivalence doctrine (focus on product rather than process; a food product that is substantially equivalent to an existing food need not be put through further regulatory requirements) developed by an OECD Working Group earlier that year.[16] Most of the remaining countries, including the European Union countries and Japan, adopt instead the precautionary principle (government may impose restrictions on activities that pose potential risks to human health or to the environment without scientific proof pertaining to the nature and seriousness of those risks).
1993	Pioneer Hi-Bred voluntarily removes from market a GE soybean, intended for poultry feed, containing a sulfur gene from a Brazil nut that when tested induced allergic reactions in humans having Brazil nut allergies.[17]

(Continued)

TABLE 13.2 (CONTINUED)
GMOs and Labeling: A Timeline

Year	Events (Still in Progress) Leading to GMO Labeling
1994–1995	The FDA approves sale of Monsanto's controversial recombinant bovine growth hormone (rBGH) that increases levels of insulin-like growth factor-I (IGF-I) in cow's milk, a possible cancer stimulant in adults.[18] The FDA also approves the Flavr Savr tomato, the first genetically engineered crop to be commercialized. The Flavr Savr had a longer shelf life than conventional tomatoes as it would not soften as quickly, and thus could be picked ripe, providing the vine-ripened array of aroma and flavors. Calgene's GE canola and Monsanto's first Roundup Ready soybean approved by the USDA. Monsanto's pest protected potato plant (the first pest protected plan) is approved by the EPA and FDA. Genetically modified foods appear in grocery stores. Incidences of food allergies rise significantly in the ensuing decade.[19] However, the FDA's position that GE foods are no different from traditional foods and the lack of labeling leaves no practical way to learn if increase in food allergies is associated with GE foods.[20]
1996	Monsanto's first GE insect-resistant corn variety approved by USDA. Dairy manufacturers challenge the constitutionality of a Vermont statute requiring identification of products that were, or might have been, derived from dairy cows treated with rBST.[21] The Vermont Court of Appeals agrees with the dairy manufacturers that such labeling infringes on their constitutional right not to speak, which is not outweighed by the state's interest in informing its citizens; the legislation is based on the public's right to know rather than on any health or safety concerns. The court notes that it is unaware of any case where consumer interest alone is sufficient to justify a requirement that is the functional equivalent of a warning.
1997	The European Union rules in favor of mandatory labeling on all GMO food products, including animal feed.
1998	The Alliance for Bio-Integrity leads a coalition of scientists, health professionals, religious leaders, and consumers in filing a lawsuit against the FDA, alleging that the agency's policy permitting GE foods to be marketed without testing and labels violates the agency's mandate to protect the national food supply. The judge rules against the plaintiffs on every claim in the complaint, holding that the FDA's right to set policy trumps consumers' right to know. However, a major result of the discovery phase of the lawsuit was the revelation of the FDA internal documents that indicated that their own scientists had safety concerns about GM foods.[22]
1992–2000	Under the Clinton Administration, the FDA holds public hearings on GE foods in response to public criticism of regulatory policies. In May 2000, the FDA proposes a rule to make premarket consultation with the agency mandatory.[23]
1999	Rep. Dennis Kucinich (D-OH) introduces HR 3377, Genetically Engineered Food Right-to-Know Act, which would require mandatory labeling for all foods containing at least 0.1% ingredients of GMOs. It was subsequently introduced to the House a number of times, most recently in 2006.
2000	StarLink, a GE corn developed by Aventis Corp. but not approved by the EPA for human consumption, is detected in Taco Bell's taco shells distributed by Kraft Foods Inc., and voluntarily recalled. StarLink is subsequently detected in a plethora of corn products. Although only 1% of the year's corn crop, StarLink may have contaminated up to 50% of the year's total corn harvest. After testing only 18–20 people, the CDC and the FDA conclude that there is insufficient evidence that sensitivity to the inserted protein caused an allergic reaction.[24]
2001	In 2001, the FDA issued draft guidance for industry regarding labeling bioengineered foods, which reaffirmed its decision to not require special labeling of all bioengineered foods, noting that the comments received had been mainly expressions of concern about the unknown, and that there was still no basis for concluding that the fact that a food or its ingredients were produced using bioengineering is a material fact that must be disclosed under sections 403(a) and 201(n) of the Federal Food Drug and Cosmetic Act.[25]
2003	The Cartagena Protocol on Biosafety (Protocol) was entered into force on September 11, 2003. As of the end of 2014, 168 parties have signed on to the Protocol, which is an international treaty governing the movements of living modified organisms (LMOs) resulting from modern biotechnology from one country to another, allowing parties to ban imports or require labeling.[26]

(Continued)

TABLE 13.2 (CONTINUED)
GMOs and Labeling: A Timeline

Year	Events (Still in Progress) Leading to GMO Labeling
2013	Publishing final guidance for manufacturers who wish to voluntarily label their foods as being made with or without the use of bioengineered ingredients is on the FDA's Center for Food Safety and Applied Nutrition's agenda of program priorities for 2013.[27]
2014	GMO labeling law passed by Vermont in 2014. The Vermont law requires that food produced entirely or in part from genetic engineering include the phrase "Produced with Genetic Engineering" on the label. Connecticut and Maine passed labeling laws as well over the summer of 2013, but the laws will take effect only if additional states sign up.[28]

Source: [1]Alberts, B. et al. *Molecular Biology of the Cell.* 4th edition. New York: Garland Science, 2002. [2]Genome News Network. Genetics and Genomics Timeline. 1972. Available at http://www.genomenewsnetwork.org/resources/timeline/1972_Berg.php, accessed January 20, 2015. [3]Wageningen Bioinformatics Webportal. History of Molecular Biology and Bioinformatics. Available at http://www.bioinformatics.nl/webportal/background/history.html, accessed January 20, 2015. [4]Cornell University Department of Animal Science. Genetics for a New Generation. Genetics Timeline. Available at http://www.ansci.cornell.edu/usdagen/timeline_print.html, accessed January 20, 2015. [5]Clinical Microbiology at the University of Pennsylvania. Developments in Microbiology. Available at http://www.sas.upenn.edu/hss/microbio/devts.html, accessed January 20, 2015. [6]Wright, S. *Molecular Politics: Developing American and British Regulatory Policy for Genetic Engineering, 1972–1982.* University of Chicago Press, 1994, pp. 73–78. [7]Barkstrom, J.E. Recombinant DNA and the Regulation of Biotechnology: Reflections on the Asilomar Conference, Ten Years Later. Available at http://www.uakron.edu/dotAsset/01da5583-1ad4-46e3-9632-fdf3e743a5a6.pdf, accessed January 20, 2015. [8]Kysar D.A., Preferences for processes: The process/product distinction and the regulation of consumer choice, *Harv. L. Rev.* 2004;118:525, 559. [9]Cowan, T. Agricultural Biotechnology: Background and Recent Issues. *Congressional Research Service.* June 18, 2011. [10]447 US 303 (1980). [11]US Congress, Office of Technology Assessment. *Biotechnology in a Global Economy OTA-BA-494.* Washington, DC: US Government Printing Office, October 1991. [12]51 Fed. Reg. 23,302 (June 26, 1986). [13]Environmental Assessment for AquAdvantage Salmon, Aqua Bounty Technologies, Inc., August 25, 2010. Available at http://www.fda.gov/downloads/AdvisoryCommittees/CommitteesMeetingMaterials/VeterinaryMedicineAdvisoryCommittee/UCM224760.pdf, accessed January 20, 2015. [14]57 Fed. Reg. 22, 984 (May 29, 1992). [15]Smith, J.M. *Seeds of Deception: Exposing Industry and Government Lies about the Safety of the Genetically Engineered Foods You're Eating.* Fairfield, IA: Yes! Books, 2003. [16]McGarity, T.O. and Hansen, P.I. Breeding Distrust: An Assessment and Recommendations for Improving the Regulation of Plant Derived Genetically Modified Foods. Prepared for the Food Policy Institute of the Consumer Federation of America, January 11, 2001. Available at http://www.mindfully.org/GE/Breeding-Distrust-2.htm, accessed January 20, 2015. [17]Schmidt, C.W, *Environmental Health Perspectives* 2005;113(8):A526–A533. [18]Nestle, M. *Safe Food: Bacteria, Biotechnology and Bioterrorism.* Berkeley, CA: University of California Press, 2003. [19]Huffman, W. Consumer Acceptance of Genetically Modified Foods: Traits, Labels and Diverse Information. Department of Economics, Iowa State University, Working Paper No. 10029. August 2010. Available at http://ageconsearch.umn.edu/bitstream/93168/2/p11835-2010-08-10.pdf, accessed January 20, 2015. [20]Van Tassel, K. The introduction of biotech foods to the tort system: Creating a new duty to identify. *U Cin L Rev* 2004;72:1645, 1662. [21]International Dairy Foods Assn v. Amestoy, 92 F. 3d 67 (1996). [22]Alliance for Bio-Integrity v. Shalala, 116 F. Supp. 2d 166, D.D.C., September 29, 2000. [23]66 FR 4706 Proposed Rule. [24]Bratspies, R.M. Myths of voluntary compliance: Lessons from the Starlink corn fiasco. *William and Mary Environmental Law and Policy Review.* 27:593. [25]US Food and Drug Administration. DRAFT Guidance for Industry: Voluntary Labeling. January 2001. Available at http://www.fda.gov/Food/GuidanceRegulation/GuidanceDocuments RegulatoryInformation/LabelingNutrition/ucm059098.htm, accessed January 20, 2015. [26]Convention on Biological Diversity. The Cartagena Protocol on Biosafety. Available at http://bch.cbd.int/protocol, accessed January 20, 2015. [27]United States Food and Drug Administration; Center for Food Safety and Applied Nutrition Plan for Program Priorities, 2013–2014, updated September 4, 2013. Available at http://www.fda.gov/AboutFDA/CentersOffices/OfficeofFoods/CFSAN/WhatWeDo/ucm366279.htm?source=govdelivery&utm_medium=email&utm_source=govdelivery, accessed January 30, 2015. [28]Kaste, M., "So what happens if the movement to label GMOs succeeds?" *npr,* October 16, 2013. Available at http://www.npr.org/blogs/thesalt/2013/10/16/235525984/so-what-happens-if-the-movement-to-label-gmos-succeeds, accessed January 15, 2015.

FOODBORNE PATHOGENS AND SURVEILLANCE

Although most experts agree that the US food supply is among the safest in the world, foodborne illness is nevertheless a significant public health problem. Almost 48 million cases of illness are estimated to occur each year in the United States. It is also likely that this number of illnesses, which entail 1 of every 6 Americans, is an underestimate, as many people do not seek medical help; thus occurrences are not officially reported. The CDC estimates that 3000 people die annually from foodborne disease, and 128,000 are hospitalized (United States Department of Health and Human Services, Centers for Disease Control and Prevention, http://www.cdc.gov/foodborneburden/2011-foodborne-estimates .html).

Furthermore, the consequences of foodborne disease can be far-reaching, and health statistics that speak only to mortality miss the impact of a less than full recovery. Cases of certain *E. coli* strains can result in kidney disease and hemolytic uremic syndrome. Salmonella and shigella infections can induce long-term effects such as reactive arthritis, urinary tract problems, and damage to the eye. Campylobacter infection can lead to Guillain–Barré syndrome and ulcerative colitis (a chronic bowel inflammation) (McKenna 2012). Most vulnerable to foodborne diseases are children, pregnant women, the elderly, and people who are immune-compromised (Mead et al. 1999). As a large proportion of prisoners are HIV positive, they are also a particularly vulnerable population (Cieslak et al. 1996).

PATHOGENS OF INTEREST TO PUBLIC HEALTH

Thirty-one pathogens are known to cause foodborne illness in humans. *Norovirus* is the most common cause of foodborne disease outbreaks in the United States and is the leading cause of diarrhea in the country. The CDC estimates that *Norovirus* causes 19–21 million illnesses and contributes to 56,000–71,000 hospitalizations and 570–800 deaths each year. Any food can be contaminated with norovirus if handled by someone who is infected with this virus. Although outbreaks can happen at any time, 80% of norovirus cases occur from November to April (Centers for Disease Control and Prevention, http://www.cdc.gov/norovirus/).

However, our overarching public health policy, as manifested through *Healthy People* 2020 (HP2020), is not concerned with norovirus, but instead focused on the following six pathogens: salmonella, shiga toxin producing *E. coli* (STEC), campylobacter, vibrio, yersinia, and listeria monocytogenes.

- *Salmonella.* Salmonella is the most common source of death from foodborne illness. Sources of infection include raw and undercooked eggs, undercooked poultry and meat, dairy products, seafood, fruits, and vegetables. Salmonella bacteria are often found on poultry and pork. It exists environmentally, such as in chicken feed and bedding (Jones 2011). One strain has been found that penetrates the egg shell. However, it can be controlled. Some countries and/or producers have gone to great lengths to control salmonella, and chicken flocks have become salmonella free (Scandi Standard, http://www.scandistandard .com/en/About-us/Why-Scandinavian-chickenisk-kyckling/). Fresh produce outbreaks have occurred as well, notably in sprouts, cantaloupe, papayas, and tomatoes. Cantaloupes are problematic, as low acidity (pH 5.2–6.7) and high water activity (0.97–0.99) support the growth of pathogens. Salmonella and other pathogens can exist on seed sprouts through the process of seed-to-sprout, multiplying to high levels during the sprouting process due to favorable conditions and then survive the typical shelf life of refrigeration (United States Food and Drug Administration, http://www.fda.gov/Food/FoodScienceResearch/Safe PracticesforFoodProcesses/ucm091265.htm). Generally, symptoms of diarrhea, fever, and cramps occur 12–72 hours after consumption, lasting 4–7 days. Most people do not need treatment, but severe diarrhea symptoms may need to be treated in the hospital. About 42,000 cases are reported yearly, but many milder cases are not reported, perhaps as many as 29 times more. The CDC estimates that salmonella is responsible for 1.2 million cases of foodborne illness annually, 19,000 hospitalizations, and 380 deaths (Centers for Disease Control and Prevention, http://www.cdc.gov/salmonella/general/index.html).

- *Escherichia coli.* Known as *E. coli*, most strains are harmless and can contribute to a healthy human digestive tract. Other strains cause a variety of illnesses, including, perhaps surprisingly, pneumonia. The form of *E. coli* that is associated with *travelers' diarrhea* is usually found on raw vegetables and garden salads. Strains that produce the shigella toxin, such as *E. coli* O157:H7, can be very dangerous, including bloody diarrhea and hemolytic uremic syndrome. CDC estimates that about 265,000 infections occur yearly by shigella-producing *E. coli*, and about 36% of these are *E. coli* O157:H7 (Centers for Disease Control and Prevention, http://www.cdc.gov/ecoli/general/index.html). The infectious dose is very low, can develop acid resistance, and can grow rapidly in some types of raw fruit and vegetables. The vast majority of outbreaks have been associated with consuming undercooked beef and dairy products, but outbreaks have also been linked to lettuce, unpasteurized apple cider, cantaloupe, and sprouts (US Food and Drug Administration, http://www.fda.gov/Food/FoodScienceResearch/SafePracticesforFoodProcesses/ucm091265.htm).
- *Campylobacter.* Campylobacter is a leading bacterial cause of diarrhea in the United States. Most human illness is caused by one species, *Campylobacter jejuni*, which can be carried by birds without the birds themselves becoming ill. Although sources can include raw milk and untreated water, most cases are from eating undercooked poultry. Generally, these bacteria are not hardy and can be killed by drying or oxygen, and freezing can reduce the number of bacteria on raw meat; however, it can take very little (less than 500 bacteria) to infect a person. That could be just a drop of raw chicken *juice*, which could then easily cross-contaminate produce and other items. An estimated 1.3 million persons are affected yearly. Most people recover within 5 days, but there are more seriously, albeit rare, consequences, including arthritis, Guillain–Barré syndrome, and death (Centers for Disease Control and Prevention, http://www.cdc.gov/nczved/divisions/dfbmd/diseases/campylobacter/). Campylobacter enteritis has also been associated with lettuce or salads (US Food and Drug Administration, http://www.fda.gov/Food/FoodScienceResearch/SafePracticesforFoodProcesses/ucm091265.htm).
- *Yersinia enterocolitica.* Animals, usually swine, are the natural reservoir, but it can also be found on raw vegetables, tending toward root and leafy produce (US Food and Drug Administration, http://www.fda.gov/Food/FoodScienceResearch/SafePracticesforFoodProcesses/ucm091265.htm). Preparing raw chitterlings (pork intestine) can cause cross-contamination when handling infants or their toys, bottles, or pacifiers, which can result in transmission and infection of the infant (Centers for Disease Control and Prevention, http://www.cdc.gov/ncidod/dbmd/diseaseinfo/yersinia_g.htm).
- *Listeria monocytogenes.* For the most part, listeria induces only mild symptoms in healthy adults but poses a significant problem to elderly, immunocompromised, and pregnant women. Outbreaks can be small in number, with only about 1600 cases a year, but with high mortality, with about 1 in 5 deaths. It is the third leading cause of deaths from foodborne illness in the United States (Centers for Disease Control and Prevention, http://www.cdc.gov/vitalSigns/listeria/index.html). Sources include unpasteurized dairy products and soft cheeses, but it can grow on fresh produce in the refrigerator (US Food and Drug Administration, http://www.fda.gov/Food/FoodScienceResearch/SafePracticesforFoodProcesses/ucm091265.htm).
- *Vibrio.* *Vibrio vulnificus* bacteria live in warm seawater. It can be contracted from eating contaminated seafood or from the seawater itself through open wounds. If healthy, a person could suffer gastrointestinal symptoms, but if immunocompromised, it can infect the bloodstream with a 50% likelihood of fatality. It is rare but underreported, with as many as 95 nationally reported cases annually, and an average of 50 culture-confirmed cases reported from the Gulf Coast region, with most occurring between May and October (Box 13.7; Centers for Disease Control and Prevention, http://www.cdc.gov/vibrio/vibriov.html).

BOX 13.7   *CLOSTRIDIUM BOTULINUM, STAPHLYOCOCCUS AUREUS, TAXOPLASMA GONDII*

Three other pathogens, although not on Healthy People's hit list, are nonetheless significant food safety issues.

- *Clostridium botulinum* produces a toxin that causes botulism, a life-threatening illness that can prevent the breathing muscles from moving air in and out of the lungs. In the United States, an average of 145 cases are reported each year; 15% are foodborne cases (toxin already in the food), and 65% are infant botulism, in which the bacteria spores are consumed and grow in the intestine, then releasing the toxin. Outbreaks of foodborne botulism involving two or more persons occur most years and are usually caused by home-canned foods with low acid content, such as asparagus, green beans, beets, and corn, which is caused by failure to follow proper canning methods. As high temperatures will destroy the botulinum toxin, persons who eat home-canned foods should consider boiling the food for 10 minutes before eating. Oils infused with garlic or herbs should be refrigerated. Honey can contain the bacteria that causes infant botulism, so children less than 12 months old should not be fed with honey.[1]
- *Staphylococcus aureus* is a common bacterium found on the skin and noses of about 25% of healthy people and animals. Although it has the ability to produce several types of toxins, it usually does not cause illness in healthy people unless transmitted to food products, where the bacterium multiplies and produces toxins. Food workers who carry *Staphylococcus* and then handle food without washing their hands can contaminate foods by direct contact. The bacterium can also be found in unpasteurized milk and cheese products. *Staphylococcus* is salt-tolerant and can grow in salty foods like ham. Staphylococcal toxins are resistant to heat and cannot be destroyed by cooking, but even more problematic, the foods at highest risk of producing toxins from *S. aureus* are those that are made by hand and require no cooking, such as sliced meat, puddings, pastries, and sandwiches.[2]
- *Toxoplasma gondii* are parasites that cause toxoplasmosis, a disease that can produce central nervous system disorders, particularly mental retardation and visual impairment in children. Pregnant women and people with weakened immune systems are at higher risk. Although many people may be infected (more than 60 million in the United States), the parasite is usually kept at bay by the immune system. Toxoplasma infection can be acquired through eating undercooked, contaminated meat (pork, lamb, and venison), eating food that was contaminated through contact with raw, contaminated meat, drinking contaminated water, or accidentally swallowing the parasite through contact with cat feces that contain *T. gondii*.[3]

Source:

[1]Data from Centers for Disease Control and Prevention. Botulism. Available at http://www.cdc.gov/nczved/divisions/dfbmd/diseases/botulism/, updated April 25, 2014, accessed January 20, 2015.

[2]Data from Centers for Disease Control and Prevention. Staphylococcal Food Poisoning. Available at http://www.cdc.gov/nczved/divisions/dfbmd/diseases/staphylococcal/, updated June 7, 2010, accessed January 20, 2015.

[3]Data from Centers for Disease Control and Prevention. Parasites–Toxoplasmosis (*Toxoplasma* infection). Available at http://www.cdc.gov/parasites/toxoplasmosis/gen_info/faqs.html, updated January 10, 2013, accessed January 20, 2015.

EPIDEMIOLOGY OF FOODBORNE ILLNESS

The epidemiology of foodborne illness has changed (Tauxe 1997). In the early twentieth century, contaminated food, milk, and water caused many foodborne infections, including typhoid fever, tuberculosis, botulism, and scarlet fever. Prior to vaccines or antibiotics, such disease transmissions were greatly reduced through hand-washing, sanitation, refrigeration, and pasteurization (Centers for Disease Control and Prevention 1999). Typhoid fever has now been almost completely eradicated by the disinfection of drinking water, milk pasteurization, and shellfish bed sanitation.

However, since the mid-1970s, more than a dozen microorganisms have been newly identified as human pathogens associated with foodborne transmission, including the ones of greatest public health concern as targeted by Healthy People (Tauxe 1997). No doubt there are still pathogens or agents causing foodborne illnesses that have not yet been identified (Mead et al. 1999).

Factors contributing to the emergence of foodborne diseases include changes in human demographics, changes in our food processing, distribution and consumption habits, industry and technology, microbial adaptation, economic development and land use, and the breakdown of the public health infrastructure (Altekruse et al. 1997; Global Microbial Threats in the 1990s, http://clinton1.nara.gov/White_House/EOP/OSTP/CISET/html/toc.html). The impact of our demographics and changing relationship with food is described in more detail in the following (Box 13.8).

Human Demographics

The proportion of the US population with heightened susceptibility to foodborne disease has increased both due to the increased proportion of the population with the human immunodeficiency

---

BOX 13.8   INDUSTRIAL FOOD PROCESSING *E. COLI*

The Jack in the Box *E. coli* outbreak that started in December 1992 and caused the death of four children alerted Americans to the industrialized shift in our food production system. Economies of scale meant numerous small processing plants turned into fewer, larger ones, with a greater number of cattle crowded together in feedlots for fattening prior to slaughter—standing on their own feces—increasing the likelihood of spreading pathogens. Post-slaughter commingling ground beef can then spread contamination widely through the beef processed that day.[1] Because bacteria multiply rapidly, food that started out only lightly contaminated can become highly dangerous.[2] This is why commingling of ground beef from many cows can become highly problematic. The slaughtering process can cause bacteria from the animal's stomach or manure to spread. Further processing of meat, such as grinding or mechanical tenderizing, can also be risky. Mechanical tenderizing is done at the processor with a machine that presses blades or needles into the meat, increasing the risk of cross-contamination of fecal matter entering below the surface of the meat, and thus becoming less likely to be destroyed in the cooking process.[3] Even prior to the slaughter process, larger farms, holding facilities, and markets bring together many animals in close contact with each other—and with humans—and our food production itself becomes a fertile ground for disease.[4]

Source:
[1]Data from Drexler, M. *Secret Agents: The Menace of Emerging Infections.* Washington, DC: The National Academies Press, 2002.
[2]Data from Ackerman, J. "Food, how safe?" *National Geographic*, May 2002. Available at http://science.nationalgeographic.com/science/article/food-how-safe.html, accessed August 30, 2014.
[3]Data from McGraw, M. "Beef's raw edges," *The Kansas City Star*, December 8, 2012.
[4]Data from World Health Organization. 10 facts on food safety. Available at http://www.who.int/features/factfiles/food_safety/facts/en/index3.html, accessed August 30, 2014.

virus (HIV) and to the increasing median age of the population. Similarly, advances in medical technology have extended the life expectancy of people with organ transplants and those who are undergoing cancer therapy, heightening their susceptibility to severe foodborne illness.

Changing Relationship with Food

Our increased appetite for international travel and international exports raises the risk of food-borne illness; the centralization of the food industry has increased dispersion of outbreaks, which affect large numbers of people; and the increase in the number of meals eaten away from home has increased exposure to outbreaks. Although norovirus is not one of the six pathogens targeted for reduction in HP2020, noroviruses are the leading cause of illness from contaminated food in the United States, causing about 50% of all food-related illness outbreaks (Centers for Disease Control and Prevention, http://www.cdc.gov/norovirus/trends-outbreaks.html), and new strains tend to appear every 2 to 3 years (Centers for Disease Control and Prevention 2013). Most norovirus food outbreaks are caused through transmission from food workers. Noroviruses are transmitted through food by people who are infected with the virus, most commonly leafy greens, fresh fruits, and shellfish that are handled raw and then served raw for consumption. However, any food served raw, or handled after being cooked, can become contaminated with norovirus (Centers for Disease Control and Prevention, http://www.cdc.gov/norovirus/trends-outbreaks.html). Norovirus is highly contagious and can persist on surfaces due to resistance to many disinfectants. This is a particular problem for cruise ships, schools, and other institutional settings (Box 13.8; Centers for Disease Control and Prevention, http://www.cdc.gov/norovirus/about/transmission.html).

Foodborne Outbreak Incidence

Incidences for the foodborne illnesses tracked by the CDC from 1996 to 2011 have generally been on the decline or flat since 1996, with the exception of a salmonella uptick in 2010 and an overall increase over time in vibrio (United States Department of Health and Human Services, Centers for Disease Control and Prevention, http://www.cdc.gov/foodnet/data/trends/trends-2011.html). The vibrio increase may be attributable in part simply to our increased appetite for seafood and global imports.

The perception that foodborne illness outbreaks have been increasing may have contributed to the adoption of the FSMA. However, there has not in fact been such an increase in total numbers of outbreaks. Instead, outbreaks have increased among foods previously considered unlikely culprits, such as produce. Between 2006 and 2008, the CDC identified produce as either the first or second leading source of foodborne illness outbreaks in the United States. Produce items viewed as healthy, whole, nonprocessed foods—spinach, lettuce, cantaloupe—have become significant potential carriers of pathogens. Commodity produce as a group—fruits, nuts, and five vegetables—is the leading cause of foodborne illness in the United States, and of all items, more illnesses were attributed to leafy greens than any other item (Painter et al. 2013). We have now learned that fast-food hamburgers are not the only risky food—foods that are also *positive* markers of health and socioeconomic status can now also be risky (Box 13.9).

BOX 13.9   CONTAMINATION OF PRODUCE

Contamination of produce can occur through various means, but one particular concern is animal waste. Animal waste is often used as a fertilizer, and without any required treatment for reduction of pathogens, there is a risk of contamination if time between manure application and harvest is too short. The recent outbreaks have in fact caused leafy green producers to create more stringent requirements regarding manure than those promulgated by the USDA's National Organic Program. And, as part of the FSMA, the FDA will include a produce safety rule addressing the application of manure (Erickson and Doyle 2012).

Food Safety and Public Health: Promotion of Fruit and Vegetable Consumption

Government public health messages promote the increased consumption of fruit and vegetables. Promoting the consumption of fruit and vegetables in the face of increasing foodborne illnesses related to produce is a balance of risk.

HP2020's food safety objectives are as follows:

- FS-1. Reduce infections caused by (six) key pathogens transmitted through food (which includes an objective to reduce postdiarrheal hemolytic uremic syndrome [HUS] in children under 5 years of age).
- FS-2. To reduce the number of outbreak-associated infections caused by Shiga-toxin producing *E. coli* O157, *Campylobacter*, *Listeria*, or *Salmonella* associated with the commodity food groups of beef, dairy, fruits and nuts, leafy vegetables, and poultry.
- FS-3. To prevent increases in the proportions of nontyphoidal *Salmonella* and *C. jejuni* isolates found in humans that are resistant to certain antimicrobial treatments.
- FS-4. To reduce severe allergic reactions to food among adults with diagnosed food allergies.
- FS-5. To increase the number of consumers who follow governmental food safety guidance.
- FS-6. A developmental objective (as there is no means yet to track data) is to improve food safety practices associated with foodborne illness preparation in the retail and food service sectors (Healthy People 2020, https://www.healthypeople.gov/2020/topics-objectives /topic/food-safety/objectives).

HP2020's nutrition goals include increasing consumption of total vegetables to the diets of the population aged 2 years and older. The importance of increasing vegetable intake is underscored by the identification of the objective as a Leading Health Indicator, a subset of HP 2020 objectives selected to communicate high-priority health issues (Healthy People 2020, https://www.healthypeo ple.gov/2020/leading-health-indicators/2020-lhi-topics/Nutrition-Physical-Activity-and-Obesity). Increasing the variety of vegetables consumed is also an HP2020 objective: with an initial specific focus on "dark green vegetables, orange vegetables, and legumes," which was later revised to "dark green vegetables, red and orange vegetables, and beans and peas" (Box 13.10; Healthy People 2020, https://www.healthypeople.gov/node/4940/data_details#revision_history_header).

The HP2020 objectives do not prescribe the means of increasing fruit and vegetable consumption; and the objective is to generally increase the consumption of vegetables and other produce in any form—cooked, canned, processed, fresh, or raw. However, promoting the convenience of having raw fruit and vegetables available as snacks is an oft-used tool to encourage consumption of produce and is suggested by the 2010 Dietary Guidelines (US Department of Agriculture and US Department of Health and Human Services 2010b).

The last paragraph of Appendix 3 of the 2010 *Dietary Guidelines for Americans*, entitled "Risky Eating Behaviors," emphasizes the dangers of consuming raw or undercooked animal products and the risk of foodborne illness. The recommendation to avoid raw sprouts is repeated, specifically for

---

BOX 13.10   CONTAMINATION OF SPROUTS

Sprouts are often sprouted legumes. People who turn to sprouts as part of their vegetable and legume consumption must be wary, as sprouts are germinated seeds that are at high risk for contamination due to the conditions required for germination. The 2010 *Dietary Guidelines for Americans* specifically recommend avoiding raw sprouts due to the high risk of contamination (US Department of Agriculture and US Department of Health and Human Services 2010a).

populations at high risk, but there is no other mention of risk in relation to consuming any other type of raw produce (US Department of Agriculture and US Department of Health and Human Services 2010c).

Yet, as noted above, recently more foodborne illnesses have been attributed to leafy greens than any other item, in part because leafy greens are often consumed raw, and in part to norovirus being a likely culprit. We make the consumption of vegetables more convenient through incorporation into mixed dishes, often prepared for us, and the high risk attributed to leafy greens is attributed in part by the CDC to this dietary pattern (Painter et al. 2013).

Norovirus is not one of the six key pathogens targeted in food safety objectives of HP2020. In the *social determinants* section of the food safety overview, however, it is noted that the processing and retail food industries continue to be challenged by two issues related to food-service workers, namely, a large employee population with high rates of turnover and a need for appropriate training (Healthy People 2020, http://www.healthypeople.gov/2020/topics-objectives/topic/food-safety). Although Healthy People recognizes that a living wage is a social determinant of health for individuals receiving the wage (Healthy People 2020, http://www.healthypeople.gov/2020/about/foundation-health-measures/Determinants-of-Health), it fails to take the next step of recognizing that in the case of foodborne disease outbreaks transmitted by people who cannot afford to stay home when ill, a living wage might actually be a social determinant of health not just for the worker but also for those who receive the services of the food worker.

In the case of food-service and food production workers, a living wage and appropriate work conditions could potentially reduce employee turnover and allow for better food safety training and education as part of an employee participating in an overall food safety culture. Upton Sinclair's intended message of *The Jungle* is still lost on us. He had not meant to singlehandedly launch a food safety movement. His goal had been to stir public outrage over the condition and plight of the workers (Arthur A. Upton Sinclair, http://www.nytimes.com/ref/timestopics/topics_uptonsinclair.html).

CRITIQUE OF THE FOOD SAFETY REGULATORY APPARATUS

For many years, analysts in the GAO have questioned the organizational efficiency and jurisdictional responsibilities of the current food safety regulatory structure. It is their unequivocal position that enhancing the safety of the nation's food supply will remain spotty until the department and the other agencies that share this responsibility are brought together in a single food safety focus (Food Safety 1996, 1997, 1998; Food Safety and Quality 1990, 1992).

GAO proponents of a streamlined federal food inspection system claim that the current system is ill-equipped to meet the challenges of emerging pathogens, an aging population, an increasing number of food imports, and potential terrorist threats to our food supply. GAO representatives have testified many times that oversight and inspection resources, as well as differences in state and local laws and regulations, leave the US system fragmented, inconsistent, and lacking in a strategic design intended to protect the public.

The GAO has recommended that the several different federal agencies currently responsible for food safety be consolidated into a single entity (Food Safety and Security 2001). In 2004, GAO suggested that Congress consider enacting a comprehensive, uniform, and risk-based food safety legislation and establish a single food safety agency or consider modifying existing laws to designate a lead agency for food safety inspection matters (Federal Food Safety and Security System 2005). Indeed, in January of 2007, the GAO added the federal oversight of food safety to their list of high-risk areas because of risks to the economy, public health, and safety (Federal Food Safety Oversight 2014). Bills have been introduced at each Congress starting with the 107th Congress (2001–2002) to the 111th (2009–2010) that have called for a consolidated food safety agency.* According to the GAO, the 2011 FSMA strengthens a major part of the food safety

---

* Key word search conducted at http://www.congress.gov, January 20, 2015.

system, and it does require some interagency collaboration but still does not apply to the federal system as a whole (US Government Accountability Office, http://www.gao.gov/key_issues/food_safety/issue_summary).

THE FOOD SAFETY MODERNIZATION ACT OF 2011

The Food Safety Modernization Act of 2011 (FSMA) focuses on the FDA and the areas of regulations under the FDA's control, with no direct change to food safety efforts in other agencies, such as the USDA. FSMA amended the FDA's existing structure and statutory authorities (Johnson 2014). The new law is aimed at emphasizing prevention versus outbreak response (Robert Wood Johnson Foundation 2011).

The FSMA's policy of prevention versus outbreak management is implemented through the idea that improved process and oversight of food production and processing is a better prevention tool than increasing inspection. Early twentieth century food safety law, as manifested in the 1906 Acts, naturally focused on the then current industrial management practice. Early twenty-first century food safety law, heralded by the 1996 HACCP regulatory efforts and manifested in the 2011 FSMA, broadens the perspective up and down the supply chain. Although the FSMA does expand government powers, in turn, it may provide for more flexibility within industry to reach safety goals through systematic review of process and performance goals rather than through inspection standards (Hoffman 2010).

Some very critical and expanded powers were available immediately to the FDA upon the signing of the FSMA:

- Access to documents at food companies tied to outbreak causing illness/death.
- Increased frequency of inspection.
- Power to order a mandatory recall and the ability to suspend operations (Box 13.11; United States Food and Drug Administration, http://www.fda.gov/Food/GuidanceRegulation/FSMA/ucm257978.htm).

BOX 13.11   RECALLING CONTAMINATED FOOD

Prior to the FSMA, the FDA did not have the power to do a mandatory recall. Even though from a consumer perspective, recalls may have appeared authoritative, they were in fact voluntary.

The FDA has not been aggressive with this new power, instead continuing to seek voluntary compliance. In November 2012, the FDA suspended operation of a business for the first time,[1] following a nationwide salmonella outbreak that sickened at least 42 people, and suspended a second business in March 2014, after a multistate listerosis outbreak.[2]

As of December 2013, only one mandatory recall process had been initiated with a notification to a pet-food manufacturer that had been slow to do a full voluntary recall, but the manufacturer complied voluntarily post the notification.[3] Up-to-date information about recalls and other food safety issues is available daily from Food Safety News. For a free subscription, go to http://www.foodsafetynews.com/subscribe/#.VZG_ipuDSDQ.

Source:
[1]Data from Satran J. Sunland: FDA didn't warn of peanut butter recall-related suspension. *Huffington Post*. Available at http://www.huffingtonpost.com/2012/11/28/sunland-fda-peanut-butter_n_2206353.html, November 28, 2012.
[2]Data from Schnirring L. FDA shutters cheese facility in wake of Listeria findings. *CIDRAP*. Available at http://www.cidrap.umn.edu/news-perspective/2014/03/fda-shutters-cheese-facility-wake-listeria-findings, accessed March 12, 2014.
[3]Data from US Food and Drug Administration. Annual Report to Congress on the Use of Mandatory Recall Authority, December 2013. Last updated August 5, 2014. Available at http://www.fda.gov/Food/GuidanceRegulation/FSMA/ucm382490.htm.

Although Congress mandated deadlines for the FDA, the complexity has given some pause to implementation, and the Congressional Research Service also found that Congress did not provide enough funding (Johnson 2014). In early January 2013, a year behind schedule, the FDA released two proposed rules (United States Food and Drug Administration, http://www.fda.gov/Food/Guidance Regulation/FSMA/ucm255893.htm#progress_oct_dec). Some of the delay was due to the fact that the rules go through the Office of Management and Budget (OMB) before they can even be released for public review, and the delays at OMB have stretched beyond the normal 90-day limit (Bottemiller 2012). The FDA had been sued in 2012 by the Center of Food Safety for failure to meet several deadlines, and the lawsuit sought not only that the FDA met the deadlines but also to prevent the OMB from delaying the FDA's compliance with the deadlines. In February 2014, a settlement was reached that extends and staggers the final rule deadlines out to 2016 (Center for Food Safety 2014).

As these rules are not finalized at the time of writing this chapter, our intent is to take a look at the first two rules proposed by the FDA to highlight some of the changes in thoughts and trends regarding food safety. The two proposed rules published in January 2013 concerned preventive controls for human food (hazard analysis and risk-based preventative controls, similar to HAACP plans) and standards for the growing, harvesting, packing, and holding of produce for human consumption (United States Food and Drug Administration, http://www.fda.gov/Food/GuidanceRegulation /FSMA/ucm334120.htm).

Domestic and foreign firms that manufacture, process, pack, or hold human food (with some exceptions) will be required to have written plans that identify hazards, specify the steps to minimize or prevent those hazards, identify monitoring procedures and record monitoring results, and specify what actions will be taken to correct problems that arise. The FDA is in charge of evaluating plans and inspecting facilities for plan implementation (United States Food and Drug Administration, http://www.fda.gov/food/guidanceregulation/fsma/ucm334115.htm). The original proposed rule was published on January 16, 2013, and the comment period closed on November 22, 2013. In September of 2014, the FDA proposed some revisions and reopened the comment period until December 15, 2014 (only for the revisions) (United States Food and Drug Administration, http://www.fda.gov/food/guidanceregulation/fsma/ucm334115.htm).

The burden on industry could be significant one-time and recurring costs, as this would include not only adopting new plans but also training workers, implementing new equipment and techniques, auditing suppliers, and documenting the process. The cost to industry is balanced against avoiding the economic cost of an estimated 1 million illnesses, costing $2 billion a year (United States Food and Drug Administration, http://www.fda.gov/food/guidanceregulation/fsma/ucm334115.htm). This calculation assumes each illness costs about $2000 a year. Of course, ideally, the very costly cases would be the ones prevented, such as the *E. coli* infections that cause hemolytic uremic syndrome and put children on lifetime dialysis.

The second rule involves more stringent safety guidelines for growing and harvesting fresh produce that is commonly eaten raw. Section 105 of the FSMA directs FDA to set science-based standards for the safe production and harvesting of fruits and vegetables. The proposed standards cover known means of microbial contamination of product, namely, (1) agricultural water; (2) biological soil amendments of animal origin; (3) health and hygiene; (4) animals in the growing area; and (5) equipment, tools, and buildings, with additional provisions related to sprouts. It would not apply to produce rarely consumed raw, those produced for personal or on-farm consumption, and produce with a documented commercial processing destination (US Food and Drug Administration, http:// www.fda.gov/Food/GuidanceRegulation/FSMA/ucm304045.htm).

Regulating foods through the defining characteristic of whether or not eaten raw might have some unexpected results. Under the proposed rule, kale is on the exemption list as a vegetable almost always consumed only after cooking. Apparently, the recent raw kale salad and smoothie trend was not common enough to get kale on the "commonly eaten raw" short list.

Furthermore, farms under certain criteria are exempted, including size and local nature of sales (such as within state). The exemptions, due to a concern that the new regulations could be too costly for smaller farmers, mean that about 8 in 10 growers will be exempt from the rule. Even with these exemptions, the FDA believes that 90% of acreage used to grow US produce will either be covered by the regulations or the regulations will not be applicable due to the produce being processed or cooked. The estimated number of prevented illnesses is 1.75 million at a savings of $1.04 billion (Regulations.gov 2013).

Unaccountably, the diseases prevented by the produce safety rule appear on average to cost less than those prevented by the production hazard analysis rule. The original proposed rule was published on January 16, 2013, and the comment period closed on November 22, 2013. In September of 2014, the FDA proposed some revisions and reopened the comment period until December 2014 (only for the revisions).

FSMA Cost

A significant cost of the FSMA will be borne by farmers and producers, with small farms chipping in about $13,000 a year and large ones about $30,000. For producers, the total cost is expected to be $320–475 million (United States Food and Drug Administration, http://www.fda.gov/downloads /Food/FoodSafety/FSMA/UCM334117.pdf). As of FY2012, the HHS secretary reported that the FDA needed an increase of $400–450 million over the existing FY2012 food safety budget, and a request to implement user fees was proposed (United States Food and Drug Administration, http:// www.fda.gov/NewsEvents/Testimony/ucm384687.htm).

Recall the paragraph above regarding the estimates by the FDA as to the number of illnesses the new rules should prevent—almost 2 million. Two million is a lot of cases—but not very many of the total estimated cases of 48 million a year. We can only hope that these new rules will be highly cost-effective by preventing the worst possible 2 million cases.

Surveillance Systems

Enhanced surveillance and investigation are integral to developing and evaluating new prevention and control strategies, which can improve the safety of our food and the public's health. By monitoring the number and extent of foodborne illness outbreaks, ongoing surveillance helps determine whether food safety control measures are effective, helps determine the causes of outbreaks, and aids in developing intervention and prevention efforts. This section introduces the primary surveillance systems that monitor the incidence of foodborne illness in the United States.

Case-based surveillance relies on the collection of reports of cases of illness, reported to the CDC by state and territorial public health departments. These case reports include information such as the symptoms of illness, demographic information about the ill person, and key risk factor information (e.g., travel, activities, foods consumed). CDC conducts case-based surveillance for botulism, cholera, vibrio, listeria, and typhoid infections by collecting case report forms for each person who is diagnosed with a case of one of these illnesses.

Laboratory-based surveillance relies on the collection of information about bacteria that have been identified by laboratory testing of ill persons. Bacteria are isolated and identified from patient specimens by clinical laboratories, and the isolates are then submitted to state public health laboratories for further characterization or are reported to them. CDC conducts laboratory-based surveillance for infections caused by *Salmonella, Shigella,* Shiga toxin-producing *E. coli,* and *Campylobacter* using reports from state and territorial public health laboratories (Centers for Disease Control and Prevention, http://cdc.gov/foodborneburden/surveillance-systems.html).

Surveillance data help identify

- Common and rare foods associated with outbreaks.
- New and emerging pathogens as well as ongoing problems.
- Food preparation and consumption setting where outbreaks occur.
- Points of contamination needing prevention and control measures.

- Trends in foodborne disease outbreaks (Centers for Disease Control and Prevention, http://www.cdc.gov/foodsafety/fdoss/surveillance/index.html).

CDC maintains a surveillance program, the Foodborne Disease Outbreak Surveillance System, for collection and periodic reporting of data on the occurrence and causes of foodborne disease outbreaks in the United States. This surveillance system is the primary source of national data describing the numbers of illnesses, hospitalizations, and deaths; etiologic agents; implicated foods; contributing factors; and settings of food preparation and consumption associated with recognized foodborne disease outbreaks in the United States (Gould et al. 2013).

For surveillance efforts in general, state, local, and territorial public health agencies are on the frontline. These agencies identify and investigate outbreaks, then voluntarily report to the CDC through the National Outbreak Reporting System (NORS). If the outbreak concerns food, NORS interfaces with the Foodborne Disease Outbreak Surveillance System to collect relevant information. The Foodborne Disease Outbreak Surveillance System has been operating since 1973, when reports came in on paper forms (Centers for Disease Control and Prevention, http://www.cdc.gov/food safety/fdoss/overview/index.html). In 2009, the Foodborne System was integrated with the system for waterborne diseases and began using NORS. In 2010, foodborne disease outbreaks became a nationally notifiable disease (Box 13.12).

CDC's surveillance team analyzes the outbreak data and makes them available online via the Food Outbreak Online Database (FOOD). FOOD provides the public direct access to information on foodborne outbreaks reported to CDC. Most outbreaks are reported to the system by the state, local, territorial, or tribal health department that conducted the outbreak investigation. Data from the surveillance system informs Healthy People's measures and objectives (Centers for Disease Control and Prevention, http://www.cdc.gov/foodsafety/fdoss/overview/index.html).

CDC has multiple foodborne illness surveillance, response, and data systems, most of which rely on data from state and local health agencies. Some systems focus on specific pathogens and have been used extensively for decades. Newer systems, such as sentinel national laboratory networks, have focused on improving the quality, quantity, and timeliness of data. Sentinel surveillance involves the collection of case data from a sample of providers to learn something about the larger population. Each surveillance system plays a role in detecting and preventing foodborne disease and outbreaks. The systems are briefly described next and even more briefly summarized in Table 13.3.

FoodNet (CDC)

Established in 1995, the Foodborne Diseases Active Surveillance Network (FoodNet) is a sentinel network that collects information from sites in 10 states (Connecticut, Georgia, Maryland, Minnesota, New Mexico, Oregon, Tennessee, and selected counties in California, Colorado, and New York), which represent 15% of the US population (Centers for Disease Control and Prevention 2006), and accordingly produces national estimates of the burden and sources of foodborne diseases in the United States. FoodNet quantifies and monitors the incidence of nine pathogens (*Campylobacter, Cryptosporidium, Cyclospora, Listeria, Salmonella,* STEC O157 and non-O157, *Shigella, Vibrio,* and *Yersinia*) by conducting active surveillance for laboratory-diagnosed illness. The network augments long-standing activities at the CDC, the USDA, the FDA, and at the state level, identifies, controls, and prevents foodborne disease hazards (Centers for Disease Control and Prevention, http://www.cdc.gov/foodnet/).

National Antibiotic Resistance Monitoring System (FDA, CDC, and USDA)

Established in 1995, the National Antibiotic Resistance Monitoring System (NARMS), a cooperative enterprise of the CDC, the FDA, and the USDA, monitors emerging resistance in foodborne pathogens. CDC's primary role is to track and report antibiotic resistance in enteric bacteria isolated from people who have infections caused by *Salmonella, Campylobacter,*

BOX 13.12   NATIONAL NOTIFIABLE DISEASES SURVEILLANCE SYSTEM

The National Notifiable Diseases Surveillance System (NNDSS) is a nationwide collaboration that enables all levels of public health (local, state, territorial, federal, and international) to share health information to monitor, control, and prevent the occurrence and spread of state-reportable and nationally notifiable infectious and some noninfectious diseases and conditions.

NNDSS is a multifaceted program that includes the surveillance system for collection, analysis, and sharing of health data and also policies, laws, electronic messaging standards, people, partners, information systems, processes, and resources at the local, state, and national levels.[1]

Each state has laws requiring certain diseases be reported at the state level, but it is voluntary for states to provide information or notifications to CDC at the federal level. There are several important distinctions between a reportable disease and a notifiable disease.

- *Reportable*: It is mandatory that reportable disease cases be reported to state and territorial jurisdictions when identified by a health provider, hospital, or laboratory. This type of required reporting uses personal identifiers and enables the states to identify cases where immediate disease control and prevention is needed. Each state has its own laws and regulations defining what diseases are reportable. The list of reportable diseases varies among states and over time.
- *Notifiable*: It is voluntary that notifiable disease cases be reported to CDC by state and territorial jurisdictions (without direct personal identifiers) for nationwide aggregation and monitoring of disease data. Regular, frequent, timely information on individual cases is considered necessary to monitor disease trends, identify populations or geographic areas at high risk, formulate and assess prevention and control strategies, and formulate public health policies. The list of notifiable diseases varies over time and by state. The list of nationally notifiable diseases is reviewed and modified annually by the CSTE and CDC. Every nationally notifiable disease is not necessarily reportable in each state.[2]

Source:
[1]Data from Centers for Disease Control and Prevention. National Notifiable Diseases Surveillance System (NNDSS). Available at http://wwwn.cdc.gov/nndss/document/NNDSS_Fact_Sheet_FINAL_3_13_2014.pdf, accessed January 20, 2015.
[2]Data from Centers for Disease Control and Prevention. National Notifiable Diseases Surveillance System (NNDSS). Data Collection and Reporting. Available at http://wwwn.cdc.gov/nndss/script/DataCollection.aspx, accessed January 20, 2015.

E. coli O157, *Shigella*, or *Vibrio* species other than *V. cholerae*. Participating health departments forward certain isolates received at their public health departments to the CDC for testing; the FoodNet sites send one *Campylobacter* isolate each week (Centers for Disease Control and Prevention, http://www.cdc.gov/foodborneburden/surveillance-systems.html). NARMS facilitated the recognition of *Salmonella typhimurium* DT 104 as highly resistant to antibiotics and prompted the CDC to alert state health departments, provide preventive steps, and minimize its spread (US Food and Drug Administration 2001).

CaliciNet

Surveillance of noroviruses is important, as noroviruses cause the majority of foodborne illness in the United States. The CDC developed CaliciNet to fingerprint strains of calicivirus, which includes noroviruses (Centers for Disease Control and Prevention, http://www.cdc

TABLE 13.3

CDC Foodborne Illness Surveillance Systems

Surveillance System	Brief Description
Foodborne Disease Active Surveillance Network (FoodNet)	Reports trends in foodborne infections and tracks the impact of food safety policies nationally
National Antimicrobial Resistance Monitoring Systems—enteric bacteria (NARMS)	Tracks trends in antimicrobial resistance and food
National Electronic Norovirus Outbreak Network (CaliciNet)	Rapidly links clusters of illness and identifies emerging norovirus strains
National Molecular Subtyping Network for Foodborne Disease Surveillance (PulseNet)	Connects cases of illness nationwide to quickly identify outbreaks
National Surveillance for Enteric Disease	Provides a national picture of the occurrence of infections and their impact on human health
Foodborne Disease Outbreak Surveillance System (FDOSS)	Captures outbreak data on agents, foods, and settings responsible for illness
Environmental Health Specialist Network (EHS-Net)	Links environmental health specialist to epidemiologists and laboratories to identify and prevent environmental factors of illnesses and outbreaks
Laboratory Identification of Parasites of Public Health Concern (DPDx)	Strengthens diagnosis of parasitic disease in the United States and around the world through interactive technology and distance-based education
National Notifiable Diseases Surveillance System (NNDSS)	Tracks notifiable infectious diseases across the United States

Source: Centers for Disease Control and Prevention. CDC Estimates of Foodborne Illness in the United States. Foodborne Illness Surveillance, Response, and Data Systems. Available at http://www.cdc.gov/foodborneburden/surveillance -systems.html, accessed January 20, 2015; Centers for Disease Control and Prevention. Foodborne Outbreak Tracking and Reporting. FAQs about the Foodborne Disease Outbreak Surveillance System (FDOSS). Available at http://www.cdc.gov/foodsafety/fdoss/faq/faq-food-tool.html, accessed January 20, 2015.

.gov/norovirus/reporting/calicinet/). The National Electronic Norovirus Outbreak Network (CaliciNet) identifies emerging norovirus strains and rapidly links norovirus clusters to outbreaks with a common food source. The network allows public health agencies to determine if the samples are part of the same outbreak. CaliciNet went live in March 2009. As of April 2014, 33 laboratories in 28 states and the District of Columbia have been certified for participation (Centers for Disease Control and Prevention, http://www.cdc.gov/norovirus/reporting/calicinet /participants.html).

PulseNet (CDC)

PulseNet, the National Molecular Subtyping Network for Foodborne Disease Surveillance, is the CDC's network of public health laboratories, established in 1996, which perform a DNA *fingerprinting* method known as *pulsed field gel electrophoresis* (PFGE) on bacteria. The network permits rapid comparison of these fingerprint patterns through an electronic database, making it possible to identify pathogen strains quickly and remove contaminated food from the market before more people become ill (Centers for Disease Control and Prevention, http://www.cdc.gov/pulsenet/). PulseNet connects cases of illnesses to potential outbreaks and revolutionized the detection and investigation of foodborne disease outbreaks, especially those occurring in multiple sites across the country, which, before PulseNet, often went undetected or were detected only after they grew very large (Centers for Disease Control and Prevention, http://www.cdc.gov/foodborneburden/sur veillance-systems.html). The network currently consists of 87 laboratories, at least one in each state. Each year, PulseNet identifies about 1500 clusters of foodborne disease at local or state levels, about

BOX 13.13   PULSENET

The genesis of PulseNet was the 1993 Jack in the Box outbreak. Prompted by the need to be able to address such emergencies faster, CDC reasoned that decentralizing the use of molecular sub-typing methodology would speed up investigation outbreak, and partnered with the Association of Public Health Laboratories to develop PulseNet in 1995. PulseNet almost immediately proved a worthwhile investment, as in 1996 it assisted epidemiologists in Washington State health departments in tracing an outbreak of *E. coli* O157:H7 infections in four states and one Canadian province to commercial unpasteurized apple juice. Of 70 persons identified as part of this outbreak, 25 required hospitalizations, 14 had hemolytic uremic syndrome, and 1 died. DNA fingerprinting by PFGE at the Washington State Public Health Laboratory, a PulseNet area laboratory, showed that isolates from patients and the apple juice were the same strain. Prompt recognition of the apple juice as the source of this outbreak resulted in rapid recall of the widely distributed product. Furthermore, the understanding of the culprit behind this severe outbreak helped foster the promotion of HACCP and other food safety improvements.

Source: Centers for Disease Control and Prevention. PulseNet. Frequently Asked Questions. PulseNet Explained. Available at http://www.cdc.gov/pulsenet/about/faq.html, accessed January 20, 2015.

250 clusters that span multiple states, and 10–15 multistate outbreaks that are widely dispersed (Box 13.13; Centers for Disease Control and Prevention, http://www.cdc.gov/pulsenet/).

National Surveillance for Enteric Disease

CDC collects and analyzes data from all states on infections due to enteric bacterial pathogens (*Listeria, Salmonella, Shigella, Vibrio*, and STEC, and case reports of botulism) in order to track and improve understanding of the human health impact of these infections in particular populations. Many states also voluntarily submit data on *Campylobacter* infections to CDC. Information is gathered from both *case-based* and *laboratory-based* surveillance systems.

Foodborne Disease Outbreak Surveillance System

Since 1973, the CDC has collected reports of foodborne outbreaks due to enteric bacterial, viral, parasitic, and chemical agents through the Foodborne Disease Outbreak Surveillance System (FDOSS). State, local, and territorial public health agencies report these outbreaks to FDOSS through the NORS. The CDC surveillance team conducts analyses of these data to improve understanding of the human health impact of foodborne outbreaks and the pathogens, foods, settings, and contributing factors (for example, food not kept at the right temperature) involved in these outbreaks, which can identify microbes and their associated foods. Since 2009, the system has also included modules for reporting enteric disease outbreaks transmitted through water, person-to-person contact, or direct contact with animals.

Foodborne Diseases Centers for Outbreak Response Enhancement (FoodCORE) (CDC)

FoodCORE began in 2009 as a pilot project to improve state and local responses to foodborne disease outbreaks. Launched in three centers, it was so successful that it was expanded in 2010 and named FoodCORE in 2011. As of 2014, 10 centers participate. FoodCORE centers work together to develop new and better methods to detect, investigate, respond to, and control multistate outbreaks of foodborne diseases. Efforts are primarily focused on outbreaks caused by bacteria, including *Salmonella*, STEC, and *Listeria*.

FoodCORE's key areas are enhancement of public health laboratory surveillance, epidemiologic interviews and investigations, environmental health assessments, and best practices and replicable models for detection, investigation, response, and control (Centers for Disease Control and Prevention, http://www.cdc.gov/foodcore/partners-resources.html).

eLEXNET

The FDA's electronic Laboratory Exchange Network (eLEXNET) is a network of food test data from federal, state, and local food safety laboratories. eLEXNET facilitates the sharing of real-time food safety sample and analysis data among multiple government agencies and food testing laboratories, thus providing an early warning system for potentially hazardous food. eLEXNET deals with numerous food safety issues, such as pesticides, naturally occurring toxins, mycotoxins, and toxic/ radioactive elements. As part of the FDA's priority shift under FSMA to early detection and prevention (rather than post-outbreak reaction), eLEXNET has become the central food testing repository.

The goal of eLEXNET is to improve food safety analyses by

- Streamlining and improving food safety testing efforts through increased data sharing and collaboration.
- Enhancing communication and collaboration among food safety agencies so that they can more easily perform risk assessment analysis and locate problem products.
- Involving federal, state, and local food safety partners in forming standards, food safety data elements, test methods, data sharing, and electronic data submission.
- Disseminating information on the effectiveness of food-related test methods (eLEXNET, https://www.elexnet.com/elex/).

Food Safety Survey

And last, but not least, the federal government also conducts surveillance as to consumer's food safety knowledge and practices through the Food Safety Survey (FSS), a joint FDA/USDA production. The FSS is a periodically conducted random-digit, dial survey of a nationally representative sample of American consumers. The survey is of self-reported behaviors, knowledge, attitudes, and beliefs about food safety. The information obtained by the FSS is used for risk assessments, regulatory and policy matters, and consumer education purposes. The questionnaires are designed to measure trends in consumer food safety practices, such as hand and cutting board washing; preparing and consuming risky foods; and using food thermometers. Data are used to inform Healthy People initiatives as well as to target education outreach (US Food and Drug Administration, http:// www.fda.gov/Food/FoodScienceResearch/ConsumerBehaviorResearch/default.htm). Surveys have been conducted in 1988, 1993, 1998, 2001, 2006, and 2010 with sample sizes of 3200, 1620, 2001, 4482, 4539, and 4568, respectively. The two agencies have agreed to conduct another survey in 2014, with the results available in 2015 (2016 Budget Explanatory Notes, http://www.obpa.usda .gov/23fsis2016notes.pdf).

The 2010 survey reports a substantial improvement in safe food handling and consumption practices and an increase in perceived risk from 1993 to 1998, which was maintained or declined until 2006. Between 2006 and 2010, safe food handling increased, but safe consumption declined—i.e., there was an increase in raw fish and raw egg consumption. The changes in safety practices were found to be consistent with media attention. One very interesting note: the oldest and the youngest respondents—and those with the highest education—had the least safe food handling behavior (Box 13.14) (US Food and Drug Administration 2011).

BOX 13.14   FOOD SAFETY SURVEY

The 2006 FSS questionnaire with response percentages is available at http://www.fda.gov /downloads/Food/FoodScienceResearch/ConsumerBehaviorResearch/UCM407007.pdf.

In each survey conducted through 2001, the key factor influencing consumer behavior was individual perception of risk. Survey questions regarding behavior and risk were the most likely to yield a strong link to good food safety practices (US Department of Health and Human Services et al. 2002).

FOOD DEFENSE

Food safety includes food defense, namely, the protection of our food supply from intentional tampering or contamination. Food terrorism is an act or threat of deliberate contamination of food for human consumption with chemical, biological, or radioactive agents for the purpose of causing injury or death to civilian populations and/or disrupting social, economic, or political stability. Theoretically, terrorists could attack livestock, crops, or processed food at any stage of the food supply cycle: production, processing, harvesting, storage, manufacturing, transport, storage, distribution, or service. For example, food terrorism targeted at livestock and crops during the food cycle could consist of deliberately introducing disease intended to generate fear, cause economic losses, and/or undermine stability.

Is the threat of a terrorist event compromising our food supply real or exaggerated? On the one hand, the FDA has concluded that there is a possibility for a terrorist event that might affect a large number of people (US Food and Drug Administration 2003), and WHO has warned that "the malicious contamination of food for terrorist purposes is a real and current threat." However, although a widespread act of political nature is a deeply held concern in post-9/11 United States, to date, only one instance of food terrorism in the United States has occurred: in 1984, a religious cult in Oregon sprayed salad bars with salmonella; the goal was to sicken people to keep them from voting in a local election; 751 people were sickened.

However, it took a year for an investigation to determine that the salmonella illnesses in Oregon was not an *ordinary* outbreak but instead a deliberate contamination (Torok et al. 1997), which raises the question as to whether we would even be able to discern intentional contamination of our food supply.

Not all public health practitioners consider widespread food terrorism a realistic scenario (Box 13.15).

Our surveillance methods have advanced significantly since the 1984 Oregon incident, however; and we have greater access to population level data than ever before. The term *syndromic surveillance* applies to surveillance using health-related data that precede diagnosis and signal a sufficient probability of a case or an outbreak to warrant further public health response. Though historically syndromic surveillance has been utilized to target investigation of potential cases, its utility for detecting outbreaks associated with bioterrorism is increasingly being explored by public health officials. Syndromic surveillance focuses on the early symptoms that arise prior to clinical or laboratory diagnoses, and uses both clinical and alternative or surrogate data sources (Henning 2004). For example, examining restaurant review postings online can provide an alternative data source to food poisoning (Box 13.16) (Harrison et al. 2014).

Farm animals and livestock, plant crops, and the food processing, distribution, and retailing system could all provide potential terrorist targets (Goodrich Schneider et al. 2005). As urban growth has occurred, agricultural operations, including farms, packinghouses, and processing plants, have become larger, more centralized, and more intensive. With such consolidation, a targeted agroterrorism event could have a serious, adverse impact.

A poison or contaminant introduced directly into our food supply may be our first concern over food-related terrorism. However, a livestock epidemic could also be disastrous. For example, foot-and-mouth disease (FMD) confined to a very small geographically distinct herd is a vastly different situation than FMD spreading through a large cattle operation (Olson 2012). Although FMD does not infect humans, it is highly transmissible among animals. A 2002 estimate calculated the costs of even a 10-farm outbreak in the United States at $2 billion (Monke 2007). Furthermore, the

BOX 13.15   IS PREPARING FOR A BIOTERRORIST ATTACK A MISAPPROPRIATION OF OUR LIMITED PUBLIC HEALTH RESOURCES?

Infectious disease epidemiologist and colleague Philip Alcabes asks if the *bio* in *biosecurity* means that we should turn our public health into a matter of civil defense? He wants to know if it is prudent public policy to rush to protect the country against the threat of attack with germs that could cause an epidemic. Sometimes epidemics have come from foreign enemies. For example, although it is unlikely that the Spaniards deliberately infected the Aztecs with smallpox, the disease so diminished the American natives that Cortés had only to finish the debacle the disease started. However, in the French and Indian War in the early 1760s, smallpox does seem to have been spread deliberately. Lord Jeffrey Amherst, the British commanding general, approved a plan to distribute smallpox-contaminated blankets "to inoculate the Indians" besieging Fort Pitt. Later, during World War I, the German biological warfare program sought to create animal epidemics that would diminish their enemies' ability to fight. More than 200 Argentine mules intended as dray animals for Allied forces died after being inoculated with both glanders (principally an equine disease) and anthrax. During World War II, one report holds that Colorado beetles were dropped by German airplanes on potato crops in southern England.

The best documented, and most successful, deliberately caused human epidemic was set by the infamous Unit 731 of the Japanese Imperial Army, stationed in conquered China during World War II. The unit dropped plague-carrying fleas on 11 Chinese towns. The number of Chinese who died of plague was probably about 700.

There is little evidence that terrorists are more likely, or better able, to use microbes as part of their armamentarium than ever before. In the creation of epidemics, the gap between intention and deed itself is a wide one. Just four communicable diseases—malaria, smallpox, AIDS, and tuberculosis—killed well over half a billion people in the twentieth century, or about 10 times the combined tolls of World Wars I and II, history's bloodiest conflicts. The Black Death killed a third of Europe's population in just 4 years in the mid-1300s. The Spanish flu killed between 20 and 40 million in 16 months in 1918–1919. Pre-vision is of little help against epidemic disasters but neither is pre-science necessary. Each epidemic, even the ones that turned out to be the most terrible, began slowly, percolated a while, and could have been stopped with conventional public health responses had anyone acted in time. It is usually social circumstances that make epidemics possible and public health funding that stops them. If we worry about the germ-bearing foreign enemy, we forgo the upkeep of a workaday public health apparatus.

Federal grant money, such as the multimillion-dollar Project BioShield program, has been allocated to technologic innovation for bioterrorism prevention. The NIH has funded two new National Biocontainment Laboratories and new facilities at Regional Biocontainment Laboratories, most at major universities, to the tune of $360 million in start-up costs.

The core issue here is that bioterrorism is not a public health problem and will not become one. The biopreparedness campaign discredits the simple logic of public health: lose the distinction between the miniscule risk of dying in an intentional outbreak and the millionfold higher chance of dying in a natural pandemic, it says; ignore the hundredfold higher still chance of dying of cancer or heart disease; defund the prenatal care clinics, the chest clinics, the exercise and cancer screening, and lead abatement programs; ignore the lessons of history, forget that human attempts to create epidemics have almost always failed; and dismiss the repeated ability of a well-funded public health apparatus to control epidemic disease with time-tested measures. The lesson of history that we ignore at our peril is this: nobody can tell us how the next epidemic will happen. Anyone who promises certain protection from the next plague is selling us a bill of goods.

Source: Adapted from Alcabes, P. *American Scholar.* 73(2): 35–45, 2004.

BOX 13.16   POTENTIAL DATA SOURCES FOR SYNDROMIC SURVEILLANCE

Clinical
- Emergency department (ED) or clinic total patient volume.
- Total hospital or intensive-care-unit admissions.
- ED triage log of chief complaints.
- ED visit outcome (diagnosis).
- Ambulatory-care clinic/HMO outcome diagnosis.
- Emergency medical system (911) call type.
- Provider hotline volume, chief complaint.
- Poison control center calls.
- Unexplained deaths.
- Medical examiner case volume, syndromes.
- Insurance claims or billing data
- Clinical laboratory or radiology ordering volume.

Alternative data source
- School absenteeism.
- Work absenteeism.
- Over-the-counter medication sales.
- Healthcare provider database searches.
- Volume of Internet-based health inquiries by the public.
- Internet-based illness reporting (including social media).
- Animal illnesses or deaths.

Source: Henning, K.J. "Overview of Syndromic Surveillance. What Is Syndromic Surveillance?" *MMWR* September 24, 2004 / 53(Suppl);5–11. Available at http://www.cdc.gov/MMWR/preview/mmwrhtml/su5301a3.htm#box, accessed January 20, 2015.

---

biological agents that could inflict damage to livestock may be more readily available than those that could harm humans (Yeh et al. 2012).

Deliberate food contamination most often is not political or widespread, but instead simply the act of a disgruntled employee. Technology can provide solutions, such as the creation of zones in factories in which entry by a staff member not wearing the appropriate authorized radio tag would set off security alerts (Watson 2012). However, HACCP plans regarding food safety could also include critical checkpoints that are relevant to employees—not just employee training, but employee satisfaction, with living wage and humane working conditions.

INDUSTRY VULNERABILITY

The agricultural industry consists of both consolidated and highly fragmented sectors. Food safety is an issue across the entire food supply chain. However, vulnerability to agroterrorism is greatest in locations where food storage or processing is centralized, and therefore more susceptible to tampering or contamination. For example, fresh produce is low risk because its production and distribution is highly fragmented among local and regional growers. Meatpacking, on the other hand, tends to be dominated by a few large companies with concentrated centers and thus is far more vulnerable to contamination, intentional or otherwise. This is particularly true with distribution and transportation companies, which employ centralized facilities. However, tampering at food production centers is a lower risk, because there are thousands of widely dispersed facilities. Additionally, the intentional contamination of animal feed to reduce the availability of animal-derived food or to infect human populations could be a target for bioterrorists (van Bredow 1999).

The Public Health Security and Bioterrorism Preparedness and Response Act of 2002 (2002) (the Bioterrorism Act), which became fully operational in 2006, was enacted to improve the ability of the United States to prevent, prepare for, and respond to bioterrorism and other public health emergencies, and among other things, includes provisions to help protect our food supply from intentional contamination.

For purposes of food safety, the FDA is responsible for developing and implementing regulations on the following major provisions of the Bioterrorism Act: Registration of Food Facilities, Prior Notice of Imported Food, Establishment and Maintenance of Records, and Administrative Detention. The definition of food used in these regulations includes food and beverages for human and animal consumption, including dietary supplements, infant formula, and food additives. It does not, however, cover food products such as meat and poultry that are regulated by the USDA-FSIS.

In general, these provisions aim to improve the process by which imported food is inspected in order to decrease the likelihood that imported food can become a vehicle for bioterrorism through tampering. The act requires (1) all food facilities—domestic and foreign—to register with the FDA; (2) the FDA to maintain records on the sources and recipients of foods; (3) the FDA to receive notice in advance of food shipments being imported into the United States with details about the type of food, country of origin, and so on; and (4) businesses involved in the nation's human and animal food supply to maintain records showing where they received food from and where they shipped it. This fourth rule applies to any firms that manufacture, process, pack, transport, distribute, receive, hold, or import food and will help investigators determine the source of contamination after the fact. The FDA is permitted to detain any foods thought to cause harm to humans or animals without court hearings or a specified time frame. The FDA established regulations effective December 12, 2003.

Nonetheless, it seems that the combination of inexpensive food from overseas and the consolidation of domestic production may compromise America's ability to feed itself safely and sustainably. There are many points along the globalized farm-to-table continuum during which infectious agents can arise from or be introduced into the food supply. Food is a major item of trade for many countries; furthermore, most countries, including developing countries, are both importers and exporters of food (Knobler et al. 2002).* A food system where control of critical elements is concentrated in a few hands is prone to accidents and is vulnerable to terrorism (Box 13.17). Is it possible that any vulnerability to terrorism could be reduced by decentralization of our food supply and relying more on locally produced products?

The term *food system* is another way to describe the food supply chain that all of us, unless completely self-sufficient, engage with in order to eat. The *chain* diverges in numerous places as food is harvested (or sometimes not) and processed and packaged in differing ways for different uses and different markets. A large-scale production model may emphasize maximum efficiency to boost overall production, and consequentially, consumer costs may be lower. Other models of food production emphasize other values, such as fair labor practices, humane animal treatment, or local production, which in turn may result in higher costs to the consumer. In general, food production methods with the end goal of maximum efficiency tend toward fewer touch points (fewer but larger farms, cattle feed lots, meat packing plants, etc.).

Reinventing community-based food systems to include numerous small farmers raising a diversity of products would make it impossible to intentionally contaminate the food supply on a large scale. Decentralizing the nation's processing, production, and distribution systems, and placing greater reliance on small family farms—potentially key factors in the ability of the United States to protect its food supply—are summed up with the maxim "Think globally, eat locally" (Wilkins 2004).

---

* Schlunt, J. Terrorist Threats to Food: WHO Activities and Guidance for Prevention and Response (abstract).

> **BOX 13.17 NATIONAL CENTER FOR FOOD PROTECTION AND DEFENSE**
>
> The National Center for Food Protection and Defense (NCFPD) is a university-based Homeland Security Center established in 2004. NCFPD addresses the vulnerability of the nation's food system to attack through intentional contamination with biological or chemical agents at any point along the food supply chain and mitigating potentially catastrophic public health and economic effects of such attacks.
>
> *Source:* National Center for Food Protection and Defense. Center of Excellence. Available at https://www.ncfpd .umn.edu, accessed January 20, 2015.

PUBLIC NUTRITION: DISASTER RESPONSE

In light of the critical role that public nutrition plays in emergency situations, which incorporates food security (but not just food security) and which incorporates food safety (but not just food safety), we are also reviewing the intersection of public nutrition with disaster response in this chapter on food safety. Responding to a disaster is a complex multipronged effort; depending on the nature of the disaster, responders provide basics such as food, water, and shelter, as well as medical care for both acute and chronic conditions, security services, and damage control. An effective response demands advanced planning and a high level of organization.

FEDERAL AUTHORITY

The governing authorities directing federal activities related to public health emergencies are principally found in the Public Health Service Act (PHS) administered by the Secretary of Health and Human Services (HHS). Core laws include the Bioterrorism Preparedness and Response Act of 2002 (Bioterrorism Act) passed in the aftermath of the 2001 terror attacks. The Bioterrorism Act reauthorized several existing programs of the Public Health Threats and Emergencies Act of 2000 and established new ones, including grants to states to build hospital and health system preparedness. Project BioShield Act of 2004 encouraged the development of specific bioterrorism countermeasures (drugs and vaccines for bioterrorism agents) that would not otherwise have a commercial market (The Pandemic and All-Hazards Preparedness Act (P.L. 109-417): Provisions and Changes to Preexisting Law, http://congressionalresearch.com/RL33589/document.php?study=The+Pandemic+and+All-Hazards+Preparedness +Act+P.L.+109-417+Provisions+and+Changes+to+Preexisting+Law).

The Pandemic and All-Hazards Preparedness Act of 2006, which established Biomedical Advanced Research and Development Authority (BARDA) within the HHS, was reauthorized in 2013 (PAHPRA). PAHPRA establishes and reauthorizes certain programs under the PHS as well as the FDCA to deal with public health security and emergency preparedness and response (US Food and Drug Administration, http://www.fda.gov/AboutFDA/WhatWeDo/History/Milestones/ucm 128305.htm).

The creation of the Department of Homeland Security (DHS) and the passage of the Robert T. Stafford Disaster Relief and Emergency Assistance Act (the Stafford Act, administered by DHS), which authorizes federal assistance and other activities in response to presidentially declared emergencies and major disasters, are also relevant (The Pandemic and All-Hazards Preparedness Act (P.L. 109-417): Provisions and Changes to Preexisting Law, http://congressionalresearch.com/RL 33589/document.php?study=The+Pandemic+and+All-Hazards+Preparedness+Act+P.L.+109-417 +Provisions+and+Changes+to+Preexisting+Law). The DHS's mission as of the end of 2014 consists of five parts: prevent terrorism and enhance security; secure and manage our borders; enforce and administer our immigration laws; safeguard and secure cyberspace; ensure resilience to disasters (Homeland Security, http://www.dhs.gov/our-mission).

National Response Framework

The Bioterrorism Act additionally directed HHS to develop a national preparedness strategy (National Plan) designed to improve communications between state and local governments, and federal agencies. The National Response Framework (NRF) has superseded the initial National Plan. The NRF, updated in 2013, is the current operating procedure guiding a national response to an emergency. The NRF described the principles, roles and responsibilities, and coordinating structures for responding to emergencies (Federal Emergency Management Agency 2013), including those of the *whole community*, which includes roles of individuals, families, and households.

The NRF incorporates best practices and procedures from multiple public entities, including homeland security, emergency management, law enforcement, firefighting, public works, public health, responder and recovery, worker health and safety, emergency medical services, as well as the private sector, integrating them into a unified structure. It forms the basis of how the federal government coordinates with the state, local, and tribal governments and the private sector during incidents. The NRP establishes processes, protocols, and best practices for these entities to work in concert to identify standardized training, organization, and communication procedures for an incident involving multiple jurisdictions. It also identifies local jurisdictions and first responders as the primary entities for handling incidents. The plan provides a comprehensive framework for private and nonprofit institutions to plan and integrate their own preparedness and response activities, nationally and within their own communities. This comprehensive approach to disaster response clarifies the role of the federal government, reinforces its partnerships with state governments and local communities, and continues to expand the concept of citizen preparedness.

USDA AND FOOD AND NUTRITION SERVICE: DISASTER MANAGEMENT

Under the NRP, Food and Nutrition Service (FNS) has primary responsibility for supplying food to disaster relief organizations, such as the Red Cross and the Salvation Army, for both mass feeding and household distribution. The USDA supports a multiagency response to domestic incidents through provision of nutrition assistance and assurance of food safety and security in accordance with other responsible federal agencies. HHS, in coordination with state health agencies, enhances existing surveillance systems to monitor the health of the general population and special high-risk populations.

Disaster response in which food and water are most heavily involved includes mass care, housing, and human services and public health and medical services. Mass care involves coordinating nonmedical mass care services such as feeding operations. Feeding may be provided to victims through a combination of fixed sites, mobile feeding units, and bulk distribution of food. Feeding operations are based on current dietary guidelines that include meeting requirements of those with special dietary needs. Bulk distribution includes providing relief items to meet the needs of victims through sites established within the affected area. These sites are used to coordinate food, water, and ice requirements and distribution systems with federal, state, local, and tribal governmental entities and nongovernmental organizations (NGOs), such as the Red Cross.

When a disaster strikes and food assistance is needed, the USDA has three disaster feeding options through FNS: mass feeding, also known as *congregate feeding sites*, distribution of commodity foods directly to households in need, and the Disaster Food Stamp Program (DFSP).

The USDA coordinator directs all of the department's emergency activities. FNS's National Disaster Coordinator is the point person who coordinates FNS's nutrition assistance response activities with other agencies on behalf of FNS's disaster task force. However, the FSIS assumes primary responsibility for any incident involving food safety. Assurance of the safety and security of the commercial food supply includes the inspection and verification of food safety aspects of slaughter and processing plants, products, distribution and retail sites, and import facilities at ports of entry; lab analysis of food samples; control of products suspected of being adulterated; plant closures; and foodborne disease surveillance. The district and field offices nationwide coordinate the field response activities for food supply and safety according to internal policies and procedures. These activities include assessing the operating status of inspected meat, poultry, and egg product processing, distribution, import, and retail facilities in the affected area, and evaluating the adequacy of available inspectors, program investigators, and laboratory services relative to the emergency on a geographical basis.

Once the teams are activated at the National Response Coordination Center in Washington, DC, activities are coordinated through the USDA. USDA officials coordinate with and support agencies responsible for mass care, housing, and human services that are involved in mass feeding. The coordinator convenes a conference call with appropriate support agencies and NGO partners to assess the situation and determine appropriate actions. The agency then alerts supporting organizations and requests that they provide representation. Disaster organizations request food and nutrition assistance through state agencies that run the USDA's nutrition assistance programs. These agencies notify the USDA of the types and quantities of food that relief organizations need for emergency feeding operations (United States Department of Agriculture, Food and Nutrition Service, http://www.fns.usda.gov/fdd/programs/fd-disasters).

FNS Disaster Response

The provision of nutrition assistance by FNS includes determining nutrition assistance needs, obtaining appropriate food supplies, arranging for delivery of the supplies, and authorizing the use of disaster SNAP benefits (Disaster SNAP Program [D-SNAP]). The FNS

- Determines the availability of the USDA foods, including raw agricultural commodities such as wheat, corn, oats, and rice that can be used for human consumption, and assesses damage to food supplies.
- With state, local, and tribal officials, determines the nutritional needs of the population in the affected area, based on the following categories: acutely deficient, deficient, self-sufficient, and surplus supplies. Priority is given to moving critical supplies of food into areas of acute need and then to areas of moderate need.
- At the discretion of the FNS administrator and upon request of the state, approves emergency issuance of D-SNAP to qualifying households within the affected area.
- At the discretion of the FNS administrator, makes emergency food supplies available to households for take-home consumption in lieu of providing food stamp benefits for qualifying households.
- Works with state and voluntary agencies to develop a plan of operation that ensures timely distribution of food in good condition to the proper location, once the need has been determined. Transportation and distribution of food supplies within the affected area will be arranged by federal, state, local, and voluntary organizations.

The regional FNS disaster coordinator is the point person for nutrition assistance. The regional coordinator

- Determines the critical needs of the affected population in terms of numbers of people, their location, and usable food preparation facilities for congregate feeding, and then establishes logistical links with organizations involved in long-term congregate meal services.
- Catalogs available resources of food, transportation, equipment, storage, and distribution facilities, and locates these resources geographically.
- Ensures that all identified USDA food is fit for human consumption; determines if suitable for household distribution or for congregate meal service.
- Coordinates shipment of the USDA food to staging areas within the affected area.
- Initiates direct market procurement of critical food supplies that are unavailable from existing inventories.

- If necessary, authorizes the Disaster SNAP Program (D-SNAP) and expedites requests for emergency issuance of D-SNAP benefits after access to commercial food channels is restored (the D-SNAP is described next).
- Establishes the need for an effects replacement of food products transferred from existing FNS nutrition assistance program inventories (see the section "Commodity Donations").

Disaster SNAP Program

Each year, disasters damage and destroy personal property, cut access to financial resources, disrupt links to human services programs, interrupt employment, or result in sudden medical expenses. Any of these misfortunes may precipitate a crisis for low-income communities. The cornerstone of federal nutrition assistance in a disaster scenario is the D-SNAP, because it is less complex to provide food stamps in areas where retail food stores are still operating than it is to identify and arrange for the transportation of commodity foods (United States Department of Agriculture, Food and Nutrition Service, http://www.fns.usda.gov/fdd/programs/fd-disasters).

The Food and Nutrition Act of 2008 and the Robert T. Stafford Disaster Relief and Emergency Assistance Act grant the president and the USDA FNS broad authority to provide emergency food relief after disasters, including emergency food stamps. The D-SNAP provides timely food assistance to households who lose food or have limited access to food as a result of a declared state of emergency. The D-SNAP operates under a different set of eligibility and benefit delivery requirements than SNAP. People who might not ordinarily qualify for food stamps may be eligible under the D-SNAP if they have had damage to their homes, expenses related to protecting their homes, and lost income as a result of the disaster, or have no access to bank accounts or other resources.

Commodity Donations

Commodities may be taken from local, state, and federal inventories. Every state and US territory has on-hand stocks of commodity foods used for the USDA-sponsored food programs, such as the National School Lunch Program, the Emergency Food Assistance Program, and the Food Distribution Program on Indian reservations. Local inventories from school kitchens and school district warehouses located close to the emergency are usually the first sources disaster organizations turn to when they want donations of the USDA commodities.

State inventories from within the state, and sometimes from another state, are tapped when local inventories do not contain sufficient resources. In an emergency, the USDA can authorize states to release these food stocks to disaster relief agencies to feed people at shelters and mass feeding sites. If the president declares a disaster, states can also, with the USDA approval, distribute commodity foods directly to households that are in need as a result of an emergency. Such direct distribution takes place when normal commercial food supply channels, such as grocery stores, have been disrupted, damaged, or destroyed, or cannot function for some reason, such as lack of electricity. If a state does not have enough food on hand to meet emergency needs, the USDA makes arrangements for food to be shipped from other states or from the USDA's own food inventories (United States Department of Agriculture, Food and Nutrition Service, http://www.fns.usda.gov/disaster /food-assistance-disaster-situations).

The Rapid Food Response System was established to supplement existing disaster feeding efforts by making a nutritionally balanced commodity offering available for congregate feeding during presidentially declared disasters. The commodity offering contains five basic categories of the USDA commodity foods that can be used to supplement existing disaster feeding efforts.

Under the aegis of the regional FNS offices, seven states (New York, Pennsylvania, North Carolina, Ohio, Oklahoma, Colorado, and California) will make their currently existing inventory available to any state nationwide when local inventories are not adequate (US Department of Agriculture 2014).

The events of September 11, 2001, gave rise to concerns about unconventional terrorist attacks, including the threat of attacks on the US food supply. Those events also heightened international awareness that nations could be targets for biological or chemical terrorism, a threat that had long concerned military and public health officials. According to the United Nations' World Health Organization (WHO), plans to mitigate the effects of sabotage of the food supply should be incorporated within existing emergency response systems. Nevertheless, a system for responding to food sabotage possesses some unique aspects. For example, national emergency plans should incorporate laboratory capacity for analyzing uncommon agents in food. It should also have closer links with food tracing and recall systems. In general, national needs and priorities with respect to food terrorism should be considered in order to ensure that the measures are proportional to other public health priorities (Schlundt 2003).

CONCLUSION

Protecting our food supply from accidental or deliberate contamination, ensuring accurate labeling on packaging, and avoiding potentially deadly nutrient deficiencies are a complex enterprise requiring coordination within and between every level of government. A wide array of individuals—from politicians to emergency and healthcare personnel to scientists—must be trained to respond rapidly and appropriately to any number of possible events, whether food poisoning at a local restaurant or providing safe food to thousands of displaced persons. Individual citizens must also be educated to read food labels to avoid allergic reactions, to maintain stores of safe food, and to seek help from the appropriate sources should the need arise.

ACRONYMS

AMS	Agricultural Marketing Service (USDA)
APC	America Prepared Campaign, Inc.
BSE	Bovine spongiform encephalopathy
CDC	Centers for Disease Control and Prevention
CFR	Code of Federal Regulations
CFSAN	Center for Food Safety and Applied Nutrition (FDA)
CGMPs	Current Good Manufacturing Practices
CSPI	Center for Science in the Public Interest
CVM	Center for Veterinary Medicine
DFSBP	Disaster Food Stamp Benefit Program
DSHEA	Dietary Supplement Health and Education Act
EPA	Environmental Protection Agency
ESF	Emergency Support Function
FAO	Food and Agriculture Organization (United Nations)
FDA	Food and Drug Administration (HHS)
FDCA	Federal Food Drug and Cosmetic Act (1906)
FEMA	Federal Emergency Management Agency
FIFRA	Federal Insecticide, Fungicide, and Rodenticide Act
FNS	Food and Nutrition Service (USDA)
FSIS	Food Safety Inspection Service (USDA)
FSS	Food Safety Survey
GAO	Government Accountability Office
GAPs	Good Agricultural Practices
HACCP	Hazard Analysis and Critical Control Point
HHS	Department of Health and Human Services
NARMS	National Antibiotic Resistance Monitoring System
NCFPD	National Center for Food Protection and Defense
NGO	Nongovernmental organization

NIH	National Institutes of Health
NIMS	National Incident Management System
NRP	National Response Plan
PFGE	Pulse-field gel electrophoresis
TSE	Transmissible spongiform encephalopathy
USDA	US Department of Agriculture
WHO	World Health Organization

STUDENT ASSIGNMENTS AND ACTIVITIES DESIGNED TO ENHANCE LEARNING AND STIMULATE CRITICAL THINKING

1. Research the agency that licenses and inspects the restaurants in your community. Is the agency on the state or local level? Describe the agency's process for restaurant licensing and inspection.
2. Has your state adopted a version of the model food code? Are there specific temperature cooking requirements or a warning requirement on restaurant menus for certain foods?
3. Visit the FoodNet website (http://www.cdc.gov/foodnet/reports.htm). Based on the most recent report available
   - What is the most common foodborne illness?
   - How have the rates of this illness changed over time?
   - What are the most common sources and symptoms of contracting this illness?
   - How could future illness from this foodborne pathogen be prevented?
4. Visit the http://foodsafety.gov website. Describe "Check Your Steps." Review "Food Safety Myths Exposed." Were you surprised by any of the myths?
5. What is HACCP? Describe the HACCP process for three different food items.
6. Research the FDA final rule on gluten labeling. When was the rule proposed? When was it finalized? When did it take effect? What is the maximum amount of gluten a food may have in order to be labeled "gluten-free"? What reasoning does the FDA provide?
7. The FDA issued draft guidance in 2001 regarding labeling bioengineered foods. Has this guidance been finalized? Research the GMO labeling law passed in Vermont in 2014. Describe the requirements of the Vermont law. If the FDA guidance has been finalized, describe any difference between the two. What are the arguments for and against GMO labeling?
8. You have been appointed to be the Nutrition and Food Security Emergency Advisor to the Governor of your state. Research the current emergency plan (including response, recovery, mitigation, prevention, and preparedness) through your state's Health Department or Emergency Management Office website.
   - Briefly describe your state's emergency plan.
   - What are the different disasters that you need to plan for?
   - What are the food security and food safety issues that should be considered?
   - Name the different state and local organizations that you would collaborate with, both prior to and in the event of an emergency.
9. Research a natural disaster that occurred in the United States within the past 10 years.
   - Briefly describe the disaster: What type of disaster was it? When did it happen? Where did it take place? Who was affected?
   - What was the emergency food response?
   - Based on what you read, was the emergency food response adequate? Why or why not?
10. Describe the disaster response plan at your workplace or school, including the provisions for food and water. Is this plan adequate? Why or why not?

REFERENCES

2016 Budget Explanatory Notes. Food Safety and Inspection Service. Available at http://www.obpa.usda .gov/23fsis2016notes.pdf, accessed February 14, 2015.

21 U.S.C. § 604, United States Food and Drug Administration, Regulatory Information. Updated May 25, 2009. Available at http://www.fda.gov/RegulatoryInformation/Legislation/ucm148693.htm, accessed January 15, 2015.

Altekruse SF, Cohen MI, Swerdlow DL. Emerging foodborne diseases. *Emerg Infect Dis.* 1997;3:285–293.

American Academy of Asthma, Allergy, and Immunology. Food Allergy Overview. Available at http://www .aaaai.org/conditions-and-treatments/allergies/food-allergies.aspx, accessed January 12, 2015.

Arthur A. Upton Sinclair. *The New York Times.* Available at http://www.nytimes.com/ref/timestopics/topics _uptonsinclair.html, accessed August 30, 2014.

Bottemiller H. Key FSMA rules continue to languish at OMB, months after deadline. *Food Safety News*, April 23, 2012. Available at http://www.foodsafetynews.com/2012/04/key-fsma-rules-continue-to-languish -at-omb-months-after-deadline/#.Ul4QWr9Ry1s, accessed December 30, 2014.

Boyce JA, Assa'ad A, Burks AW et al. Guidelines for the diagnosis and management of food allergy in the United States: Report of the NIAID-sponsored expert panel. *J Allergy Clin Immunol.* 2010;126(Suppl 6):S1–S58.

Branum AM, Lukacs SL. Food allergy among US children: Trends in prevalence and hospitalizations. *NCHS Data Brief.* 2008;10:1–8.

Center for Food Safety, February 20, 2014. Available at http://www.centerforfoodsafety.org/files/2014-2-20 -dkt-82-1--joint--consent-decree_31089.pdf, accessed December 30, 2014.

Centers for Disease Control and Prevention. About Norovirus. Transmission. Updated June 3, 2014. Available at http://www.cdc.gov/norovirus/about/transmission.html, accessed January 20, 2015.

Centers for Disease Control and Prevention. Achievements in public health, 1900–1999: Safer and healthier- foods. *MMWR.* 1999;48(40):905–913. Available at http://www.cdc.gov/mmwr/preview/mmwrhtml/mm 4840a1.htm, accessed February 12, 2015.

Centers for Disease Control and Prevention. CDC and Food Safety, What is CDC's Role in Food Safety? Updated April 19, 2014. Available at http://www.cdc.gov/foodsafety/cdc-and-food-safety.html, accessed December 30, 2014.

Centers for Disease Control and Prevention. CDC Estimates of Foodborne Illness in the United States. Foodborne Illness Surveillance, Response, and Data Systems. Available at http://www.cdc.gov/food borneburden/surveillance-systems.html, accessed January 20, 2015.

Centers for Disease Control and Prevention. CDC Vital Signs, Recipe for Food Safety. Updated October 29, 2013. Available at http://www.cdc.gov/vitalSigns/listeria/index.html, accessed December 2, 2014.

Centers for Disease Control and Prevention. *E. coli.* Updated December 1, 2014. Available at http://www.cdc .gov/ecoli/general/index.html, accessed December 2, 2014.

Centers for Disease Control and Prevention. Foodborne Diseases Active Surveillance Network (FoodNet). Available at http://www.cdc.gov/foodnet/, accessed January 20, 2015.

Centers for Disease Control and Prevention. Foodborne Diseases Centers for Outbreak Response Enhancement. Available at http://www.cdc.gov/foodcore/partners-resources.html, accessed January 20, 2015.

Centers for Disease Control and Prevention. Foodborne Outbreak Tracking and Reporting. Overview. Available at http://www.cdc.gov/foodsafety/fdoss/overview/index.html, accessed January 20, 2015.

Centers for Disease Control and Prevention. Foodborne Outbreak Tracking and Reporting. Surveillance for Foodborne Disease Outbreaks. Available at http://www.cdc.gov/foodsafety/fdoss/surveillance/index .html, accessed January 20, 2015.

Centers for Disease Control and Prevention. Norovirus. Updated December 30, 2014. Available at http://www .cdc.gov/norovirus/, accessed January 20, 2015.

Centers for Disease Control and Prevention. Norovirus Trends and Outbreaks. Updated December 30, 2014. Available at http://www.cdc.gov/norovirus/trends-outbreaks.html, accessed December 30, 2014.

Centers for Disease Control and Prevention. Notes from the field: Emergence of new norovirus strain gii.4 Sydney, United States 2010. *MMWR.* 2013;63(03):55. Updated January 25, 2013. Available at http:// www.cdc.gov/mmwr/preview/mmwrhtml/mm6203a4.htm?s_cid=mm6203a4_x, accessed December 30, 2014.

Centers for Disease Control and Prevention. Preliminary FoodNet Data on the Incidence of Infection with Pathogens Transmitted Commonly Through Food—10 States, United States, 2005. *MMWR.* 2006;55(14):392–395.

Centers for Disease Control and Prevention. Public Health Laboratories Participating in CaliciNet and Support Centers. Available at http://www.cdc.gov/norovirus/reporting/calicinet/participants.html, accessed January 20, 2015.

Centers for Disease Control and Prevention. PulseNet. National Molecular Subtyping Network for Foodborne Disease Surveillance. Available at http://www.cdc.gov/pulsenet/, accessed January 12, 2015.

Centers for Disease Control and Prevention. Reporting and Surveillance for Norovirus: CaliciNet. Available at http://www.cdc.gov/norovirus/reporting/calicinet/, accessed January 12, 2015.

Centers for Disease Control and Prevention. Salmonella. Updated April 5, 2012. Available at http://www.cdc.gov/salmonella/general/index.html, accessed December 2, 2014.

Centers for Disease Control and Prevention. Vibrio Illness. Updated October 21, 2013. Available at http://www.cdc.gov/vibrio/vibriov.html, accessed December 2, 2014.

Centers for Disease Control and Prevention, Disease Listing, Yersinia enterocolitica. Updated October 25, 2005. Available at http://www.cdc.gov/ncidod/dbmd/diseaseinfo/yersinia_g.htm, accessed December 2, 2014.

Centers for Disease Control and Prevention, National Center for Emerging and Zoonotic Infectious Diseases. Campylobacter. Updated June 3, 2014. Available at http://www.cdc.gov/nczved/divisions/dfbmd/diseases/campylobacter/, accessed December 2, 2014.

Cieslak, PR, Curtis MB, Coulombier DM, Hathcock AL, Bean NH, Tauxe RV. Preventable disease in correctional facilities: Desmoteric foodborne outbreaks in the United States, 1974–1991. *Arch Intern Med.* 1996;156:1883–1888.

Code of Federal Regulations, 21 CFR 170.3. Available at http://www.gpo.gov/fdsys/pkg/CFR-2012-title21-vol3/xml/CFR-2012-title21-vol3-sec170-3.xml, accessed January 15, 2015.

David S, Austin J, Batz M et al. The Essential Role of State and Local Agencies in Food Safety and Reform. The Food Safety Resource Consortium. Available at http://www.thefsrc.org/State_Local/StateLocal_June17_background.pdf, accessed October 15, 2013, no longer available online as of August 30, 2014.

eLEXNET. Available at https://www.elexnet.com/elex/, accessed January 20, 2015.

Erickson MC, Doyle MP. Plant Food Safety Issues: Linking Production Agriculture with One Health. Improving Food Safety through a One Health Approach, Workshop Summary, Institute of Medicine, 2012. Available at http://www.ncbi.nlm.nih.gov/books/NBK114507/, accessed December 30, 2014.

Federal Emergency Management Agency. National Response Framework. Updated July 31, 2014. Available at https://www.fema.gov/national-response-framework, accessed January 20, 2015.

Federal Emergency Management Agency. *National Response Framework*, 2nd ed., Department of Homeland Security, May 2013. Available at http://www.fema.gov/media-library-data/20130726-1914-25045-1246/final_national_response_framework_20130501.pdf, accessed June 29, 2015.

Federal Food and Drugs Act of 1906 (The "Wiley Act") P.L. Number 59-384, 34 Stat. 786 (1906). Available at http://www.fda.gov/RegulatoryInformation/Legislation/ucm148690.htm, accessed January 15, 2015. Federal Food Safety and Security System: Fundamental Restructuring Is Needed to Address Fragmentation and Overlap. GAO: GAO-04-588T, March 30, 2005.

Federal Food Safety Oversight: Additional Actions Needed to Improve Planning and Collaboration. GAO: GAO-15-180, December 2014.

Food Allergen Labeling and Consumer Protection (Public Law 108–282). Available at http://www.fda.gov/Food/GuidanceRegulation/GuidanceDocumentsRegulatoryInformation/Allergens/ucm106187.htm, accessed January 15, 2015.

Food and Drug Administration. HHS. Substances generally recognized as safe. Proposed rule. *Fed Reg.* 1997;62(74):18938–18964. Available at http://www.gpo.gov/fdsys/pkg/FR-1997-04-17/html/97-9706.htm, accessed June 29, 2015.

Food Safety: Fundamental Changes Needed to Improve Food Safety. GAO/RCED-97-249R, September 9, 1997.

Food Safety: New Initiatives Would Fundamentally Alter the Existing System. GAO/RCED-96-81, March 27, 1996.

Food Safety: Opportunities to Redirect Federal Resources and Funds Can Enhance Effectiveness. GAO/RCED-98-224, August 6, 1998.

Food Safety and Quality: Uniform, Risk-Based Inspection System Needed to Ensure Safe Food Supply. GAO/RCED-92-152, June 26, 1992.

Food Safety and Quality: Who Does What in the Federal Government. GAO/RCED-90-19A & B, December 21, 1990.

Food Safety and Security: Fundamental Changes Needed to Ensure Safe Food. Statement of Robert A. Robinson, Managing Director, Natural Resources and Environment. GAO: GAO-02-47T, October 10, 2001.

Global Microbial Threats in the 1990s. Report of the NSTC Committee on International Science, Engineering, and Technology (CISET) Working Group on Emerging and Re-emerging Infectious Diseases. Available at http://clinton1.nara.gov/White_House/EOP/OSTP/CISET/html/toc.html, accessed January 12, 2015.

Goodrich Schneider R, Schneider KR, Webb CD, Hubbard M, Archer DL. Agroterrorism in the U.S.: An Overview. Institute of Food and Agricultural Sciences, University of Florida, August 2005. Available at http://edis.ifas.ufl.edu/fs126, accessed December 2, 2014.

Gould LH, Walsh KA, Vieira AR, Herman K, Williams IT, Hall AJ, Cole D. Surveillance for Foodborne Disease Outbreaks—United States, 1998–2008. *Surveill Summ.* 2013;62(SS02):1–34. Available at http://www.cdc.gov/mmwr/preview/mmwrhtml/ss6202a1.htm?s_cid=ss6202a1_w, accessed January 20, 2015.

Gussow JD. *This Organic Life: Confessions of a Suburban Homesteader.* New York: Chelsea Green Publishing Co., 2001.

Harrison C, Jorder M, Stern H et al. Using online reviews by restaurant patrons to identify unreported cases of foodborne illness—New York City, 2012–2013. *MMWR.* 2014;63(20):441–445. Available at http://www.cdc.gov/mmwr/preview/mmwrhtml/mm6320a1.htm, accessed February 12, 2015.

Healthy People 2020. About Healthy People. Available at http://www.healthypeople.gov/2020/about/foundation-health-measures/Determinants-of-Health, accessed January 20, 2015.

Healthy People 2020. Food Safety. Available at http://www.healthypeople.gov/2020/topics-objectives/topic/food-safety, accessed January 20, 2015.

Healthy People 2020. Food Safety. Available at https://www.healthypeople.gov/2020/topics-objectives/topic/food-safety/objectives, accessed January 20, 2015.

Healthy People 2020. Nutrition, Physical Activity, and Obesity Leading Health Indicators. Available at https://www.healthypeople.gov/2020/leading-health-indicators/2020-lhi-topics/Nutrition-Physical-Activity-and-Obesity, accessed January 20, 2015.

Healthy People 2020. Nutrition and Weight Status, Revision History. Available at https://www.gov/node/4940/data_details#revision_history_header, accessed January 20, 2015.

Henning KJ. Overview of syndromic surveillance. What is syndromic surveillance? *MMWR.* 2004;53(Suppl):5–11. Available at http://www.cdc.gov/MMWR/preview/mmwrhtml/su5301a3.htm#box, accessed January 20, 2015.

Hoffman S. Food Safety Policy and Economics: A Review of the Literature. Resources for the Future, July 2010. Available at http://www.rff.org/RFF/Documents/RFF-DP-10-36.pdf, accessed December 30, 2014.

Homeland Security. Our Mission. Available at http://www.dhs.gov/our-mission, accessed January 20, 2015. Johnson R. The Federal Food Safety System: A Primer. Congressional Research Service, January 17, 2014. Available at https://www.fas.org/sgp/crs/misc/RS22600.pdf, accessed January 15, 2015.

Jones FT. A review of practical Salmonella control measures in animal feed. *J Appl Poult Res.* 2011; 20(1):102–113.

Keep Food Safe: What Government Does. Available at http://www.foodsafety.gov, accessed January 15, 2015.

Knobler SL, Mahmoud AAF, Pray LA, eds. Biological Threats and Terrorism: Assessing the Science and Response Capabilities. Workshop Summary. Based on a Workshop of the Forum on Emerging Infections. Washington, DC: National Academy Press, 2002. McGowan EC, Bloomberg GR, Gergen PJ et al. Influence of early-life exposures on food sensitization and food allergy in an inner-city birth cohort. *J Allergy Clin Immunol.* 2015;135(1):171–178.e4.

McKenna M. Food poisoning's hidden legacy. *Sci Am.* 2012;306(April 4). Available at http://www.scientificamerican.com/article.cfm?id=food-poisonings-hidden-legacy, accessed December 30, 2014.

Mead PS, Slutsker L, Dietz V et al. Food-related illness and death in the United States. *Emerg Infect Dis.* 1999;5:607–625. Available at http://www.nc.cdc.gov/eid/article/5/5/99-0502, accessed February 12, 2015.

Monke J. Agroterrorism: Threats and Preparedness. Congressional Research Service Report for Congress, March 12, 2007.

Neltner T, Maffini M. Generally Recognized as Secret: Chemicals Added to Food in the United States. NRDC Report. National Resources Defense Council, April 2014. Available at http://www.nrdc.org/food/files/safety-loophole-for-chemicals-in-food-report.pdf, accessed September 20, 2014.

Nestle M. *Safe Food: The Politics of Food Safety.* Berkeley, CA: University of California, 2010.

Non GMO Project. Available at http://www.nongmoproject.org, accessed November 20, 2014.

Nordlee JA, Taylor SL, Townsend JA, Thomas LA, Bush RK. Identification of a brazil-nut allergen in transgenic soybeans. *New Engl J Med.* 1996;334:688–692.

Olson D. Threats to America's Economy and Food Supply. The Federal Bureau of Investigation, Agroterrorism, February 2012. Available at http://leb.fbi.gov/2012/february/agroterrorism-threats-to-americas-economy-and-food-supply, accessed January 20, 2015.

Painter JA, Hoekstra RM, Ayers T, Tauxe RV, Braden CR, Angulo FJ, Griffin PM. Attribution of foodborne illnesses, hospitalizations, and deaths to food commodities by using outbreak data, United Sates, 1998–2008. *Emerg Infect Dis.* 2013;19:3. Updated February 25, 2013. Available at http://wwwnc.cdc.gov/eid/article /19/3/11-1866_article.htm, accessed December 30, 2014.

Regulations.gov. Proposed Rule, February 12, 2013. Available at http://www.regulations.gov/#!document Detail;D=FDA-2011-N-0921-0001, accessed December 30, 2014.

Robert Wood Johnson Foundation. How Does Federal Food Safety Legislation Protect the Nation's Food Supply? Health Policy Snapshot Series, September 2011. Available at http://www.rwjf.org/en/research -publications/find-rwjf-research/2011/09/how-does-federal-food-safety-legislation-protect-the-nation -s-fo.html, accessed January 15, 2015.

Scandi Standard. Why Scandinavian Chicken? Available at http://www.scandistandard.com/en/About-us/Why -Scandinavian-chickenisk-kyckling/, accessed December 2, 2014.

Schlundt J. *Terrorist Threats to Food: WHO Activities and Guidance for Prevention and Response.* World Health Organization, Geneva, Switzerland, October 2003.

Significant Dates in US Food and Drug Law History. US Food and Drug Administration. Last updated December 19, 2014. Available at http://www.fda.gov/AboutFDA/WhatWeDo/History/Milestones/ucm 128305.htm, accessed January 15, 2015.

Tauxe RV. Emerging foodborne diseases: An evolving public health challenge. *Emerg Infect Dis.* 1997;3:425–434.

The Pandemic and All-Hazards Preparedness Act (P.L. 109-417): Provisions and Changes to Preexisting Law. Available at http://congressionalresearch.com/RL33589/document.php?study=The+Pandemic+and+All -Hazards+Preparedness+Act+P.L.+109-417+Provisions+and+Changes+to+Preexisting+Law, accessed January 20, 2015.

The Public Health Security and Bioterrorism Preparedness and Response Act of 2002. PL 10–188, June 12, 2002. Available at http://www.gpo.gov/fdsys/pkg/PLAW-107publ188/pdf/PLAW-107publ188.pdf, accessed January 12, 2015.

The Vermont Legislative Bill Tracking System, Current Status, 2013–2014, Legislative Session. Available at http://www.leg.state.vt.us/database/status/summary.cfm?Bill=H.0112, accessed August 30, 2014.

Torok TJ, Tauxe RV, Wise RP et al. A large community outbreak of salmonellosis caused by intentional contamination of restaurant salad bars. *JAMA.* 1997;278:389–395.

US Department of Agriculture, Food and Nutrition Service. USDA Foods Program Disaster Manual, June 2014. Available at http://www.fns.usda.gov/sites/default/files/FDDDisasterManual.pdf, accessed January 20, 2015.

US Department of Agriculture, US Department of Health and Human Services. *Dietary Guidelines for Americans, 2010,* 7th ed. Washington, DC: U.S: Government Printing Office, 2010a, p. 48. Available at http://www.health.gov/dietaryguidelines/2010.asp, accessed December 30, 2014.

US Department of Agriculture, US Department of Health and Human Services. *Dietary Guidelines for Americans, 2010,* 7th ed. Appendix 2 Key Consumer Behaviors and Potential Strategies for Professionals, Table A2 1, 65. Washington, DC: US Government Printing Office, 2010b. Available at http://www.health.gov/dietaryguidelines/2010.asp, accessed December 30, 2014.

US Department of Agriculture, US Department of Health and Human Services. *Dietary Guidelines for Americans, 2010,* 7th ed. Washington, DC: US Government Printing Office, 2010c, p. 72. Available at http://www.health.gov/dietaryguidelines/2010.asp, accessed December 30, 2014.

US Department of Health and Human Services, Food and Drug Administration, Center for Food Safety and Applied Nutrition, Consumer Studies Branch. Food Safety Survey: Summary of Major Trends in Food Handling Practices and Consumption of Potentially Risky Foods, August 27, 2002.

US Food and Drug Administration. 2010 Food Safety Survey: Key Findings and Topline Frequency Report, September 2011. Available at http://www.fda.gov/Food/FoodScienceResearch/ConsumerBehaviorRe search /ucm259074.htm, accessed February 17, 2015.

US Food and Drug Administration. Annual Report to Congress on the Use of Mandatory Recall Authority, December 2013b. Last updated August 5, 2014. Available at http://www.fda.gov/Food/Guidance Regulation/FSMA/ucm382490.htm.

US Food and Drug Administration. Chapter IV. Outbreaks Associated with Fresh and Fresh-Cut Produce. Incidence, Growth, and Survival of Pathogens in Fresh and Fresh-Cut Produce. Updated April 24, 2013. Available at http://www.fda .gov/Food/FoodScienceResearch/SafePracticesforFoodProcesses/ucm 091265.htm, accessed December 2, 2014.

US Food and Drug Administration. Consumer Behavior Research. Food Safety Surveys. Available at http://www .fda.gov/Food/FoodScienceResearch/ConsumerBehaviorResearch/default.htm, accessed February 17, 2015.

US Food and Drug Administration. FDA Food Code. Updated October 27, 2014. Available at http://www.fda.gov/food/guidanceregulation/retailfoodprotection/foodcode/default.htm, accessed January 15, 2015.

US Food and Drug Administration. Federal Food Safety System, October 10, 2001. Available at http://www.fda.gov/NewsEvents/Testimony/ucm114861.htm, accessed January 20, 2015.

US Food and Drug Administration. Generally Recognized as Safe (GRAS). Last updated November 26, 2014. Available at http://www.fda.gov/food/ingredientspackaginglabeling/gras/default.htm, accessed January 15, 2015.

US Food and Drug Administration. Guidance for Industry: A Food Labeling Guide (6. Ingredient List), January 2013a. Available at http://www.fda.gov/Food/GuidanceRegulation/GuidanceDocuments RegulatoryInformation/LabelingNutrition/ucm064880.htm, accessed January 15, 2015.

US Food and Drug Administration. Guidance for Industry: Frequently Asked Questions about GRAS. Last updated July 7, 2014, December 2004. Available at http://www.fda.gov/Food/GuidanceRegulation /GuidanceDocumentsRegulatoryInformation/IngredientsAdditivesGRASPackaging/ucm061846 .htm#Q16, accessed January 15, 2015.

US Food and Drug Administration. How US FDA's GRAS Notification Program Works, January 2006. Available at http://www.fda.gov/Food/IngredientsPackagingLabeling/GRAS/ucm083022.htm, accessed January 15, 2015.

US Food and Drug Administration. Produce Safety Standards. Last updated September 19, 2014. Available at http://www.fda.gov/Food/GuidanceRegulation/FSMA/ucm304045.htm, accessed January 20, 2015.

US Food and Drug Administration. Real Progress in Food Code Adoptions. Updated October 24, 2013. Available at http://www.fda.gov/Food/GuidanceRegulation/RetailFoodProtection/FoodCode/ucm108156 .htm, accessed January 15, 2015.

US Food and Drug Administration. Significant Dates in US Food and Drug Law History. Available at http://www.fda.gov/AboutFDA/WhatWeDo/History/Milestones/ucm128305.htm, accessed January 20, 2015.

US Food and Drug Administration, Center for Food Safety and Applied Nutrition/Office of Regulations and Policy. Risk Assessment for Food Terrorism and Other Food Safety Concerns, October 7, 2003.

US Government Accountability Office. Food Safety. Issue Summary. Available at http://www.gao.gov/key _issues/food_safety/issue_summary, accessed January 20, 2015.

United States Department of Agriculture. Economic Research Service. Updated July 14, 2014. Available at http://www.ers.usda.gov/data-products/adoption-of-genetically-engineered-crops-in-the-us/recent-trends -in-ge-adoption.aspx, accessed December 30, 2014.

United States Department of Agriculture. Food Safety and Inspection Service. Updated April 29, 2014. Available at http://www.fsis.usda.gov/About_FSIS/index.asp, accessed August 30, 2014.

United States Department of Agriculture. Guidance and Regulation, DRAFT Guidance for Industry: VoluntaryLabeling Indicating Whether Foods Have or Have Not Been Developed using Bioengineering; Draft Guidance, Updated December 26, 2014. Available at http://www.fda.gov/food/guidanceregulation /guidancedocumentsregulatoryinformation/labelingnutrition/ucm059098.htm, accessed December 30, 2014.

United States Department of Agriculture, Food and Nutrition Service. Disaster Assistance, Available at http://www.fns.usda.gov/disaster/food-assistance-disaster-situations, accessed January 20, 2015.

United States Department of Agriculture, Food and Nutrition Service. Food Distribution Programs. Available at http://www.fns.usda.gov/fdd/programs/fd-disasters, accessed January 12, 2015.

United States Department of Health and Human Services, Centers for Disease Control and Prevention. Estimates of Foodborne Illness in the United States. Updated January 8, 2014. Available at http://www.cdc.gov/foodborneburden/2011-foodborne-estimates.html, accessed December 30, 2014.

United States Department of Health and Human Services, Centers for Disease Control and Prevention. Foodborne Diseases Active Surveillance Network (FoodNet). Updated January 30, 2013. Available at http://www.cdc.gov/foodnet/data/trends/trends-2011.html, accessed December 30, 2014.

United States Environmental Protection Agency. Accomplishments under the Food Quality Protection Act(FQPRA). Available at http://www.epa.gov/pesticides/regulating/laws/fqpa/fqpa_accomplishments .htm, accessed January 15, 2015.

United States Environmental Protection Agency. Federal Insecticide, Fungicide, and Rodenticide Act (FIFRA). Available at http://www.epa.gov/agriculture/lfra.html, accessed January 15, 2015.

United States Environmental Protection Agency. The EPA and Food Security. Updated August 1, 2014. Available at http://www.epa.gov/pesticides/factsheets/securty.htm, accessed August 30, 2014.

United States Environmental Protection Agency. The Food Quality Protection Act (FQPA) Background. Last updated February 4, 2014. Available at http://www.epa.gov/pesticides/regulating/laws/fqpa/backgrnd .htm, accessed January 15, 2015.

United States Food and Drug Administration. About FDA. Updated April 10, 2014. Available at http://www
.fda.gov/AboutFDA/Transparency/Basics/ucm242648.htm, accessed December 30, 2014.

United States Food and Drug Administration. About FDA. Updated March 11, 2014. Available at http://www
.fda.gov/AboutFDA/WhatWeDo/History/Overviews/ucm056044.htm, accessed January 15, 2015.

United States Food and Drug Administration, About FDA. Updated October 7, 2010. Available at http://
www.fda.gov/AboutFDA/WhatWeDo/History/ProductRegulation/SulfanilamideDisaster/default.htm,
accessed January 15, 2015.

United States Food and Drug Administration. Biotechnology Consultation Note. Updated December 5, 2014.
Available at http://www.fda.gov/food/foodscienceresearch/biotechnology/submissions/ucm161157.htm,
accessed December 30, 2014.

United States Food and Drug Administration. Center for Food Safety and Applied Nutrition Plan forProgram
Priorities, 2013–2014. Updated September 4, 2013. Available at http://www.fda.gov/AboutFDA/Centers
Offices/OfficeofFoods/CFSAN/WhatWeDo/ucm366279.htm?source=govdelivery&utm_medium
=email&utm_source=govdelivery, accessed December 30, 2014.

United States Food and Drug Administration. FDA's approach to the GRAS Provision: A History of Processes.
Last updated April 23, 2013. Available at http://www.fda.gov/Food/IngredientsPackagingLabeling/GRAS
/ucm094040.htm, accessed January 15, 2015.

United States Food and Drug Administration. Food Allergies: What You Need to Know. Updated October 23,
2014. Available at http://www.fda.gov/Food/ResourcesForYou/Consumers/ucm079311.htm, accessed
December 30, 2014.

United States Food and Drug Administration. Food Safety Modernization Act. Updated September 15, 2014.
Available at http://www.fda.gov/Food/GuidanceRegulation/FSMA/ucm257978.htm.

United States Food and Drug Administration. Frequently Asked Questions on Lupin and Allergenicity. Last
updated August 15, 2014. Available at http://www.fda.gov/Food/IngredientsPackagingLabeling/Food
AdditivesIngredients/ucm410111.htm, accessed December 21, 2014.

United States Food and Drug Administration. FSMA Preliminary Regulatory Impact Analysis. Available
at http://www.fda.gov/downloads/Food/FoodSafety/FSMA/UCM334117.pdf, accessed December 30,
2014.

United States Food and Drug Administration. FSMA Progress Reports. Available at http://www.fda.gov
/Food/GuidanceRegulation/FSMA/ucm255893.htm#progress_oct_dec, accessed December 30, 2014.

United States Food and Drug Administration. FSMA Proposed Rule for Preventative Controls for Human
Food. Updated December 15, 2014. Available at http://www.fda.gov/food/guidanceregulation/fsma
/ucm334115.htm, accessed December 30, 2014.

United States Food and Drug Administration. FSMA. Updated September 15, 2014. Available at http://www
.fda.gov/Food/GuidanceRegulation/FSMA/ucm334120.htm, accessed December 30, 2014.

United States Food and Drug Administration. Guidance & Regulation. Updated August 15, 2013. Available at
http://www.fda.gov/food/guidanceregulation/guidancedocumentsregulatoryinformation/biotechnology
/ucm096095.htm, accessed December 30, 2014.

United States Food and Drug Administration. Guidance to Industry for Foods Derived from New Plant
Varieties. Updated August 15, 2013. Available at http://www.fda.gov/food/guidanceregulation/guidance
documentsregulatoryinformation/biotechnology/ucm096095.htm, accessed December 30, 2014.

United States Food and Drug Administration. Implementing the FDA Food Safety Modernization Act,
February 5, 2014. Available at http://www.fda.gov/NewsEvents/Testimony/ucm384687.htm, accessed
January 20, 2015.

United States Food and Drug Administration. Inspections, Compliance, Enforcement, and Criminal
Investigations. Warning Letter, Phusion Projects Inc., November 17, 2010. Available at http://www.fda
.gov/ICECI/EnforcementActions/WarningLetters/ucm234023.htm, accessed January 15, 2015.

United States Food and Drug Administration. Safe Practices for Food Processes. Updated April 24, 2013.
Available at http://www.fda.gov/Food/FoodScienceResearch/SafePracticesforFoodProcesses/ucm091265.
htm, accessed December 2, 2014.

United States Food and Drug Administration. Significant Dates in US Food and Drug Law History. Last
updated December 19, 2014. Available at http://www.fda.gov/AboutFDA/WhatWeDo/History/Mile
stones/ucm128305.htm, accessed January 15, 2015.

van Bredow J, Myers M, Wagner D, Valdes JJ, Loomis L, Zamani K. Agroterrorism: Agricultural infrastructure vulnerability. *Ann N Y Acad Sci.* 1999;894:168–180.

Vinje NE, Namork E, Løvik M. Cross-allergic reactions to legumes in Lupin and Fenugreek-Sensitized mice.
Scand J Immunol. 2012;76:387–397.

Watson E. How Vulnerable Is Your Supply Chain? Food Defense, FSMA, Big Brother and Virtual "Hot Zones." Food Navigator-USA.com, December 18, 2012. Available at http://www.foodnavigator-usa .com/Markets/How-vulnerable-is-your-supply-chain-Food-defense-FSMA-Big-Brother-and-virtual -hot-zones, accessed January 20, 2015.

Wilkins J. Think globally, eat locally. *New York Times*, December 18, 2004. Available at http://www.nytimes .com/2004/12/18/opinion/18wilkins.html?_r=0, accessed January 20, 2015.

Yeh JY, Seo HJ, Park JY et al. Livestock agroterrorism: The deliberate introduction of a highly infectious animal pathogen. *Foodborne Pathog Dis.* 2012;9(10):869–877. Available at http://www.ncbi.nlm.nih .gov/pubmed/23035724, accessed December 2, 2014.

14 Grants to Support Initiatives in Public Health Nutrition

Fundraising is an extreme sport!

Pitman (2008)

INTRODUCTION

Community-based nonprofit organizations fill the gap that is created when the for-profit sector and government systems do not adequately address community needs, often with the help of grants. A grant is an award made to an organization. The grant is earmarked to carry out a specific project proposed by one or more of the organization's members. The grant may be in the form of goods and services as well as money. Occasionally, an award is made to an individual, but most grantors prefer to make awards to the organization itself because the life span of the organization is greater than the expected tenure of an individual employee. Thus, the applicant for a grant is the organization submitting the proposal, not the employee writing the grant application.

Grants are important to the welfare of many communities. Grants made to community-based organizations help these agencies improve the overall health, education, work skills, and earning power of people in the neighborhood. With greater purchasing power of its citizens, community-based commerce is strengthened. Thus, local businesses as well as individuals profit from funds awarded to organizations charged with improving the community's health, education, and welfare. However, as the number of community-based organizations increases, there is an increase in competition to secure the grant money needed to stimulate and support their work.

It is not surprising, then, that people who have developed grant-writing skills are among the most coveted professionals in the public health workforce. Public health agencies, including community-based organizations, have an insatiable appetite for external support to start new projects and to expand existing ones. Fundraising is integral to the functioning of these organizations and is particularly important for nonprofit community-based entities that rely heavily on grants.

The information in this chapter applies to all seekers of funds to support public health nutrition programs. The chapter's particular focus is on obtaining external funding for nonprofit organizations. *Nonprofit organization* is the legal term that indicates that an organization is exempt from federal income tax under Section 501(c)(3) of the Internal Revenue Code. Private sector grantors rely on this determination to claim a tax deduction for contributions they make, and government relies on this determination when defining eligibility for certain programs (Box 14.1).

All the references in this chapter are available online. This is consistent with the current practice of grantors providing information about their funding opportunities online and with their requirement that applicants submit grant applications electronically. In the following sections, we describe the public sector and public funding sources, the private sector and funding sources, and how to apply for funds.

BOX 14.1 NONPROFIT ORGANIZATIONS EXEMPT FROM TAXATION: SECTION 501(C)(3) OF THE INTERNAL REVENUE CODE

"Corporations, and any community chest, fund, or foundation, organized and operated exclusively for religious, charitable, scientific, testing for public safety, literary, or educational purposes, or to foster national or international amateur sports competition (but only if no part of its activities involve the provision of athletic facilities or equipment), or for the prevention of cruelty to children or animals, no part of the net earnings of which inures to the benefit of any private shareholder or individual, no substantial part of the activities of which is carrying on propaganda, or otherwise attempting, to influence legislation (except as otherwise provided in subsection (h)), and which does not participate in, or intervene in (including the publishing or distributing of statements), any political campaign on behalf of (or in opposition to) any candidate for public office."

Source: 26 USC § 501(c)(3). Available at http://www.law.cornell.edu/uscode/text/26/501, accessed February 13, 2015.

PUBLIC FUNDING SOURCES

This section describes the public sector, presents an overview of the two major federal departments that support programs in public health nutrition, and provides examples of the kinds of projects that government supports.

Grants in support of public health initiatives are available from the government and from the private sector. In 2012, it is estimated that the annual total dollar value of assistance from public and private sources was over half a trillion dollars ($1 trillion is $1 billion multiplied by 1000). Government supplied $542 billion in the form of grants to nonfederal entities for a defined public or private purpose (Office of Management and Budget, http://www.usaspending.gov). Foundations, corporations, and individuals contributed over $51 billion in grant support (The Foundation Center, http://data.foundationcenter.org/).

PROGRAMS IN THE PUBLIC SECTOR (TAX-SUPPORTED PROGRAMS)

The US government is divided into three branches—executive, judicial, and legislative (also referred to as Congress, which is composed of the US House of Representatives and the US Senate). The executive branch of the federal government is composed of the White House offices and agencies. These offices include the cabinet, which helps develop and implement the policies and programs of the president. The cabinet is made up of the vice president and, by law, the heads of 15 executive departments—the secretaries of the US Departments of Agriculture (USDA), Commerce, Defense, Education, Energy, Health and Human Services (HHS), Homeland Security, Housing and Urban Development, Interior Justice, Labor, State, Transportation, Treasury, and Veterans Affairs. Seven additional officials have cabinet-level rank: the White House chief of staff, administrator of the Environmental Protection Agency, director of the Office of Management and Budget, US trade representative, US ambassador to the United Nations, chairman of the Council of Economic Advisers, and administrator of the Small Business Administration (The White House, http://www.whitehouse .gov/administration/cabinet). Congress appropriates funds to each of these departments every year. In other words, agencies in the public sector are supported by taxes paid to the government.

The executive branch of the US government has 26 grant-making agencies that together award more than $500 billion annually to state and local governments, academia, nonprofit, and other organizations. The government's support is awarded through over 1000 grant programs in 21 categories (Grants.gov, http://www.grants.gov/web/grants/about.html).

Through its grants website, the federal government provides a unified electronic "storefront" for its agencies to announce their grant opportunities and for potential applicants to find and apply for grants. Grants.gov (http://www.grants.gov) is a single, comprehensive website that contains information about finding and applying for all federal grant programs.

HHS and the USDA are the major federal sources of funding for nutrition programs at the state and local levels. The majority of government support for domestic, nutrition-related research and training is supplied by these two departments, the vast proportion by USDA (General Services Administration, https://www.cfda.gov/; Office of Management and Budget, http://www.usaspend ing.gov/search?form_fields={%22search_term%22%3A%22nutrition%22%2C%22spending_cat %22%3A[%22g%22]}&sort_by=dollars&per_page=25). A large percentage of funds from HHS and the USDA are distributed by the states to local governments and community-based organizations to address local public health problems. Some funds are awarded directly from the federal government to community organizations (Box 14.2).

BOX 14.2 IDENTIFYING SOURCES OF PUBLIC SECTOR FUNDING

US Government: http://www.grants.gov

- Department of Health and Human Services: http://www.hhs.gov.
  - Administration for Children and Families: http://www.acf.hhs.gov.
    - Grants: http://www.acf.hhs.gov/grants.
  - Administration on Aging: http://www.aoa.gov.
    - Grant opportunities: http://www.acl.gov/Funding_Opportunities/Index.aspx.
  - Centers for Disease Control and Prevention: http://www.cdc.gov.
    - Budget, grants, and funding: http://www.cdc.gov/stltpublichealth/GrantsFunding /index.html.
    - Funding opportunities: http://www.cdc.gov/stltpublichealth/GrantsFunding /opportunities.html.
  - Food and Drug Administration: http://www.fda.gov.
    - Grant opportunities: http://www.fda.gov/AboutFDA/business/ucm119348.htm
  - Indian Health Service: http://www.ihs.gov.
    - Funding opportunities: http://www.ihs.gov/dgm/index.cfm?module=dsp_dgm _funding.
  - National Institutes of Health: http://www.nih.gov.
    - Grants and funding: http://grants.nih.gov/grants/oer.htm.
    - Funding opportunities and notices: http://grants.nih.gov/grants/guide/index .html.
  - US Department of Agriculture: http://www.usda.gov.
    - Food and Nutrition Service: http://www.fns.usda.gov/.
      - Discretionary grant application process: http://www.fns.usda.gov/fm /Documents/GrantsProc.htm.
    - Food Safety and Inspection Service: http://www.fsis.usda.gov.
    - National Institute of Food and Agriculture: http://www.csrees.usda.gov.
      - Grant openings and closings: http://www.csrees.usda.gov/fo/recentReleased Grants.cfm.

DEPARTMENT OF HEALTH AND HUMAN SERVICES

HHS is the cabinet-level department of the federal executive branch most involved with the nation's human concerns. It was created as the Department of Health, Education, and Welfare in 1953 and became the HHS in 1980 (http://www.hhs.gov/about/hhshist.html). In one way or another, HHS touches the lives of more Americans than any other federal agency because of the wide spectrum of activities it covers, including the health promotion and disease prevention objectives of *Healthy People 2020*. The department is sectioned into more than 300 programs that include such activities as the following:

- Gathering national health and other data.
- Health and social science research.
- Preventing disease, including immunization services.
- Assuring food and drug safety.
- Medicare (health insurance for elderly and disabled Americans) and Medicaid (health insurance for low-income people). Medicaid is the nation's largest health insurer, covering over 68 million (more than one in every five) Americans (Kaiser Family Foundation 2015).
- Financial assistance and services for low-income families.
- Improving maternal and infant health.
- Head Start (preschool education and services for low-income families).
- Services for older Americans, including home-delivered meals.
- Comprehensive health services for Native Americans.

In fiscal year (FY) 2014, the HHS budget was authorized at $974.0 billion (US Department of Health and Human Services, http://www.hhs.gov/budget/fy2014/fy-2014-budget-in-brief.pdf). HHS represents almost a quarter of all federal outlays and administers more grant dollars than all other federal agencies combined. The department works closely with state and local governments because many HHS-funded services are provided at the local level by state or county agencies, or through private sector grantees. In addition, HHS maintains regional offices throughout the United States. You can locate the one nearest you at http://www.hhs.gov/iea/regional/index.html.

One of the agencies in HHS is the Office of the Assistant Secretary for Health (OASH) (US Department of Health and Human Services, http://www.hhs.gov/ash/). The functions of this office are to provide assistance in implementing and coordinating secretarial decisions for the Public Health Service and coordination of population-based health clinical divisions; provide oversight of research conducted or supported by HHS; implement programs that provide population-based public health services; and provide direction and policy oversight, through the Office of the Surgeon General, for the Public Health Service Commissioned Corps (Office of the Federal Register, http://www.usgovernmentmanual.gov/). The corps is a uniformed service of more than 6500 health professionals, including about 100 registered dietitians, who serve in HHS and other federal agencies, such as the USDA and the Department of Justice (US Department of Health and Human Services, http://dcp.psc.gov/osg/dietitian).

HHS programs are administered by operating divisions:

- Administration for Children and Families (ACF).
- Administration for Community Living (ACL).
- Agency for Healthcare Research and Quality (AHRQ).
- Agency for Toxic Substances and Disease Registry (ATSDR).
- Centers for Disease Control and Prevention (CDC).
- Centers for Medicare & Medicaid Services (CMS).
- Food and Drug Administration (FDA).

- Health Resources and Services Administration (HRSA).
- Indian Health Service (IHS).
- National Institutes of Health (NIH).
- Substance Abuse and Mental Health Services Administration (SAMHSA).

Highlights are provided in the following text for those HHS agencies most likely to fund programs and research concerned with nutrition in public health, namely, ACF, ACL, CDC, FDA, and NIH.

Administration for Children and Families
ACF is responsible for some 60 programs that promote the economic and social well-being of children, families, and communities (http://www.acf.hhs.gov/). ACF administers the state and federal welfare programs and the Temporary Assistance for Needy Families (TANF) program, providing assistance to an estimated 4.5 million persons, including 3.4 million children. ACF administers the Head Start program to increase school readiness, annually serving over a million low-income children from birth to age 5. It also provides funds to assist low-income working families in paying for childcare and supports state programs for foster care. ACF was established in 1991 by bringing together several already existing programs. In FY 2015, its budget was more than $51 billion, making it the second largest agency in HHS. A directory of ACF program services can be found at https://www.acf.hhs.gov/sites/default/files/assets/acf_directory.pdf.

Community Services Block Grant
The Community Services Block Grant (CSBG) is administered by the Division of State Assistance in the Office of Community Services (OCS) within ACF. The CSBG provides federal funds to states, territories, and federally recognized and state-recognized Indian tribes and tribal organizations for distribution to local agencies in support of antipoverty activities (http://www.acf.hhs.gov/programs/ocs/programs/csbg). CSBG funds are used to provide a range of services to ameliorate the causes and conditions of poverty, such as helping low-income Americans obtain employment, increase their education, access vital early childhood programs, and maintain their independence. Actual services are provided by state, county, city, and tribal governments, and public and private local agencies; a minimum of 90% of the grants must be passed from the states to local grantees. ACF assists these organizations through funding, policy direction, and information services. In FY 2013, $635 million was provided for the CSBG (Spar 2013). More than 1000 CSGB networked entities serve 99% of US counties. These local entities provided services to 15.7 million low-income individuals in 6.7 million families and reported spending CSBG funds for a wide variety of activities, including emergency services (19%), activities to promote self-sufficiency (17%), activities to promote linkages (13%), employment-related activities (12%), education-related activities (12%), housing-related services (8%), nutrition services (6%), income management (6%), health services (4%), and other services and activities (3%) (National Association for State Community Services Programs 2014). CSBG legislation and appropriations by state are available on the CSBG website at http://www.acf.hhs.gov/programs/ocs/programs/csbg.

Community Economic Development
The Community Economic Development (CED) program is a federal grant program administered by ACF that helps support local community development corporations to create sustainable business development and employment opportunities for low-income residents (http://www.acf.hhs.gov/programs/ocs/programs/ced). Community development corporations are private, nonprofit organizations that are governed by a board of directors consisting of residents of the community served and local business and civic leaders, and have as their principle purpose planning, developing, or managing low-income housing or community development projects. Grants are awarded for project

costs for start-up or expansion of business, physical, or commercial activities; capital expenditures (such as the purchase of equipment or real property); allowable operating expenses; and loans or equity investments. A variety of projects are funded, including business incubators, shopping centers, manufacturing businesses, agricultural initiatives, and the Healthy Food Financing Initiative (HFFI).

Administration for Community Living

Established in 2012, ACL brings together the Administration on Aging (AoA), the Office on Disability, and the Administration on Developmental Disabilities into a single agency that focuses on the unique needs of older adults and individuals with disabilities (http://www.acl.gov). Of relevance to nutrition in public health are the services offered by AoA (http://www.aoa.gov), which supports a nationwide Aging Network (a national coalition of 56 state units on aging, 629 area agencies on aging, and 246 tribal and native organizations, plus thousands of service providers, adult-care centers, caregivers, and volunteers [US Department of Health and Human Services, http://www.aoa.gov/AoA_Programs/OAA/Aging_Network/Index.aspx]) and provides services to older adults so that they may remain independent and involved in their communities. AoA helps provide home-delivered meals, congregate meals, nutrition education, transportation, adult day care, and in-home services, such as personal care and homemaker assistance. It offers ombudsman services for the elderly and provides policy leadership on aging issues. In FY 2013, AoA's budget was just over $2.0 billion.

The Older Americans Act (OAA, http://www.aoa.gov/AoA_programs/OAA/) created the AoA in 1965 and authorized grants to states for community planning and service programs, as well as for research, demonstration, and training projects in the field of aging. Later amendments to the OAA added grants to area agencies on aging for local needs identification, planning, and funding of services, including nutrition programs in the community as well as for those who are homebound, programs which serve Native American elders, services targeted at low-income minority elders, health promotion and disease prevention activities, in-home services for frail elders, and services to protect the rights of older persons. Each year, AoA provides grant funding to states and territories, recognizes Native American tribes and Hawaiian Americans, as well as nonprofit organizations, including faith-based and academic institutions. Individuals are not eligible to apply for AoA funding. Through grants and cooperative agreements, AoA transfers its appropriated funding resources to the AoA's National Aging Network. Grants are used when AoA has no substantial involvement in the administration of a project, and there is no direct benefit to AoA. If, however, AoA expects to have substantial involvement in the direction and implementation of a project, it often uses cooperative agreements.

Centers for Disease Control and Prevention

CDC works with states and other partners to provide a system of health surveillance to monitor and prevent disease outbreaks (including bioterrorism); implements disease prevention strategies; maintains national health statistics; and provides for immunization services, workplace safety, and environmental disease prevention (http://www.cdc.gov/). Working with the World Health Organization, CDC also guards against international disease transmission, with personnel stationed in more than 25 foreign countries. CDC was established in Atlanta in 1946 as the Communicable Disease Center. Each year, CDC awards approximately 4200 grants and cooperative agreements, obligating approximately $5.0 billion in federal funds (http://www.cdc.gov/grants/index.html).

The CDC administers the Preventive Health and Health Services Block Grant (PHHSBG) program (US Department of Health and Human Services, http://www.cdc.gov/phhsblockgrant). Block grants are the primary source of funding giving states the latitude to fund any of the 600 national health objectives in Healthy People 2020. The PHHSBG supports clinical services, preventive screenings, essential health services, outbreak control, workforce training, public education, data surveillance, and program evaluation. A strong emphasis is placed on programs for adolescents, communities with little or poor healthcare services, and disadvantaged populations. The states depend on the block grant to support public health funding where no other adequate resources are available. The PHHSBG is a major source of funding for health promotion and disease prevention in communities across the nation, and it funds health programs in heart disease and stroke, physical activity and nutrition, oral health and fluoridation, diabetes, cancer, and arthritis. Beginning with FY 2014, funding for the PHHSBG is through the Prevention and Public Health Fund under the Affordable Care Act provisions. In FY 2014, appropriations for PHHSBG were $160 million (US Department of Health and Human Services, http://www.cdc.gov/phhsblockgrant/history.htm).

Food and Drug Administration

FDA (http://www.fda.gov/) assures the safety of foods and cosmetics, and the safety and efficacy of pharmaceuticals, biological products, and medical devices—products that represent one-quarter of US consumer spending. The FDA was established in 1906, when the Pure Food and Drugs Act gave regulatory authority to the Bureau of Chemistry, then part of the USDA. In FY 2014, its budget was $4.3 billion. FDA's Center for Food Safety and Applied Nutrition (CFSAN) supports research that aims to reduce the incidence of food-borne illness and protect the integrity of the nation's foods and the food supply, including additives and dietary supplements. Food safety guidance and policy making are other areas of research interest.

Indian Health Service

IHS (http://www.ihs.gov/) provides federal health services to 2 million American Indians and Alaska Natives representing more than 560 federally recognized tribes. The Indian health system includes 44 hospitals, 296 health centers, 108 health stations, 164 Alaska Native village clinics, and 33 urban Indian health centers. The IHS clinical staff includes about 2640 nurses, 820 physicians, 670 pharmacists, 640 engineers/sanitarians, 340 physician assistants/nurse practitioners, and 310 dentists, as well as nutritionists, health administrators, and medical records administrators. The IHS was established in 1921, and its mission was transferred from the Interior Department in 1955. In FY 2014, the IHS budget was $4.58 billion.

The IHS's Special Diabetes Program for Indians was created by Congress in 1998 and provided $150 million from 2003 to 2008 to support the prevention and treatment of diabetes among American Indians and Alaska Natives, especially children and teenagers. Funds have been reauthorized at $150 million per year through FY 2015. Since the inception of the program, diabetes health outcomes have improved significantly in American Indian and Alaska Native communities. One of the most important improvements is a 10% reduction in the mean blood sugar level (A1c) of diabetics between 1996 and 2012 (US Department of Health and Human Services, http://www.ihs.gov/newsroom/factsheets/diabetes).

National Institutes of Health

NIH (http://www.nih.gov) is the largest source of funding for medical research in the world, supporting nearly 50,000 competitive grants to more than 300,000 researchers at more than 2500 universities, medical schools, and other research institutions in the United States and globally. Funds are spent in over 200 research and disease areas, including Alzheimer's disease, arthritis, cancer, diabetes, heart ailments, and human immunodeficiency virus/acquired immunodeficiency syndrome (HIV/AIDS). NIH includes 27 separate health institutes and centers. It was established in 1887 as the Hygienic Laboratory in Staten Island, New York. The goal of all the research supported by NIH is to advance scientific knowledge in order to improve public health. In FY 2015, the NIH budget was about $30 billion. NIH funds researchers to undertake a wide spectrum of basic, clinical, and epidemiologic training and other programs in universities, medical schools, and academic health centers (known as *extramural* research). They also employ nearly 6000 scientists who conduct research in laboratories on the NIH campus (known as *intramural* research).

The Research Portfolio Online Reporting Tools (RePORT, http://report.nih.gov) is a searchable database of reports, data, and analyses of NIH research activities, including information on NIH expenditures and the results of NIH-funded research. RePORT replaces the former Computer Retrieval of Information on Scientific Projects (CRISP) database. RePORT is maintained by the Office of Extramural Research at the NIH and includes projects supported by the NIH, AHRQ, CDC, HRSA, SAMHSA, and US Department of Veterans Affairs. Users can use the RePORT interface to search for specific areas of research, conditions, or diseases; funding to specific organizations or geographical regions; and application success rates.

Introduced here are the institutes within the NIH that fund most studies in areas related to nutrition in public health.

National Heart, Lung, and Blood Institute

The National Heart, Lung, and Blood Institute (NHLBI, http://www.nhlbi.nih.gov/) provides leadership for a national program in diseases of the heart, blood vessels, lung, and blood; blood resources; and sleep disorders. It plans, conducts, fosters, and supports integrated and coordinated programs of basic research, clinical investigations and trials, observational studies, and demonstration and education projects. Research related to the causes, prevention, diagnosis, and treatment of the diseases and disorders mentioned earlier is conducted in the institute's own laboratories and by institutions supported by research grants and contracts. NHLBI also has administrative responsibility for the NIH Women's Health Initiative (US Department of Health and Human Services, https://www.nhlbi .nih.gov/whi/), a 15-year national health study focused on the prevention of heart disease, breast and colorectal cancer, and osteoporotic fractures in postmenopausal women.

National Institute on Aging

The National Institute on Aging (NIA, http://www.nia.nih.gov) sponsors research on aging through extramural and intramural programs. The extramural program funds research and training at universities, hospitals, medical centers, and other public and private organizations nationwide; the intramural program conducts basic and clinical research in NIA's own facilities by institutions supported by research grants and contracts.

National Institute of Diabetes and Digestive and Kidney Diseases

The National Institute of Diabetes and Digestive and Kidney Diseases (NIDDK, http://www.niddk .nih.gov) supports research programs in the areas of diabetes and other endocrine and metabolic diseases, digestive diseases, nutritional disorders, obesity, and kidney diseases. Located across the country are 7 centers for diabetes translation research, 16 diabetes research centers (US Department of Health and Human Services, http://www.niddk.nih.gov/research-funding/research-programs /Pages/diabetes-centers.aspx) and 12 nutrition and obesity research centers (NORCs, http://www .norccentral.org/home.do) supported by the institute. NIDDK supports research on the causes and consequences of obesity and potential prevention and treatment strategies, including behavioral and environmental approaches, and provides an evidence base to inform policy decisions. The institute's Weight-control Information Network (WIN, http://win.niddk.nih.gov) provides up-to-date, science-based information on weight control, obesity, physical activity, and related nutritional issues.

Trans-NIH Research

Frequently, a request for applications (RFA) or program announcement (PA) will be posted by a consortium of NIH agencies. For example, in 2012, seven NIH divisions jointly offered grants of up to $650,000 for the purposes of promoting substantive improvements in the assessment of diet and physical activity through the development of better instruments, innovative technologies, and/or applications of advanced statistical or analytic techniques (US Department of Health and Human Services, http://grants.nih.gov/grants/guide/pa-files/PAR-12-198.html). The aim of this research initiative is to improve the current state of dietary and physical activity assessment methods, since self-report instruments are prone to varying degrees of measurement error and may be cognitively difficult for respondents.

UNITED STATES DEPARTMENT OF AGRICULTURE

The USDA was founded by President Abraham Lincoln in 1862, when almost half of the nation's population produced at least some of their own food. Today, the USDA's services focus on all aspects of the US food supply and the effects of diet and nutrition on health. Seven agencies along with their affiliated offices are located within the department: Farm and Foreign Agricultural Services; Food, Nutrition, and Consumer Services; Food Safety; Marketing and Regulatory Programs; Natural Resources and Environment; Research, Education, and Economics; and Rural Development. In FY 2015, the USDA's budget was about $140 billion (US Department of Agriculture, http://www.obpa .usda.gov/budsum/FY15budsum.pdf).

The USDA offices most likely to fund programs and research concerned with nutrition in public health include the Food and Nutrition Service (FNS), the Food Safety and Inspection Service (FSIS), and the National Institute of Food and Agriculture (NIFA).

Food and Nutrition Service

FNS (http://www.fns.usda.gov/programs-and-services) administers USDA's nutrition assistance programs:

- Child and Adult Care Food Program (CACFP).
- Commodity Supplemental Food Program (CSFP).
- Farmers' Market Nutrition Program (FMNP).
- Food Assistance for Disaster Relief (FADR).
- Food Distribution Program on Indian Reservations (FDPIR).
- Fresh Fruit and Vegetable Program (FFVP).
- National School Lunch Program (NSLP).
- Nutrition Assistance Block Grants (NABG).
- School Breakfast Program (SBP).
- Senior Farmers' Market Nutrition Program (SFMNP).
- Special Milk Program (SMP).
- Special Supplemental Nutrition Program for Women, Infants, and Children (WIC).
- Summer Food Service Program (SFSP).
- Supplemental Nutrition Assistance Program (SNAP, formerly the Food Stamp Program).
- The Emergency Food Assistance Program (TEFAP).

FNS provides children and low-income families better access to food and a more healthful diet through its food assistance programs and nutrition education efforts. FNS works in partnership with the states in all its programs, serving one in four Americans during the course of a year. States determine most administrative details regarding distribution of food benefits and participants' eligibility, whereas FNS provides funding to cover most of the states' administrative costs. In FY 2015, the FNS budget totaled $112.2 billion.

Food Safety and Inspection Service

Research plays an important role in the ability of the FSIS (http://www.fsis.usda.gov/wps/portal/fsis /topics/science/food-safety-research-priorities) to assure that the foods it regulates—meat, poultry, and processed egg products—continue to be safe, wholesome, and correctly labeled and packaged. As FSIS does not carry out its own research, nor does it fund research, it depends on both the public and private research communities to conduct the research vital to its mission, and provides a list of research areas that may be useful to researchers preparing grants to other agencies that fund food safety research. As of November 2014, several FSIS public health nutrition research priorities included the following:

*   Conduct ex post evaluation of regulatory initiatives.
*   Determine retail use statistics/practices that could contribute chemicals (insecticide, rodenticide, fungicide, antimicrobial) or pathogens to FSIS-regulated products.
*   Develop or refine cooking and cooling methods.
*   Identify consumer practices that compromise the safety of FSIS-regulated products and/or generate data to develop public education and outreach to improve food-handling practices.

In FY 2015, the FSIS budget was just over $1.0 billion.

National Institute of Food and Agriculture

NIFA (http://www.nifa.usda.gov/) (formerly the Cooperative State Research, Education, and Extension Service [CSREES]) focuses on critical issues affecting people's daily lives and the nation's future. Nutrition and health research supported by NIFA empowers people and communities to solve problems and improve their lives at the local level. NIFA maintains an extensive network of state, regional, and county extension offices in every US state and territory. These offices have educators and other staff who respond to public inquiries and conduct informal, noncredit workshops and other educational events. NIFA supports the base programs of state agricultural experiment stations and the cooperative extension system nationwide at land-grant universities (Box 14.3). In FY 2015, the NIFA budget totaled $1.49 billion.

As the USDA's primary extramural research agency, NIFA provides working funds to researchers at institutions of higher education throughout the United States. These research programs benefit all Americans. NIFA helps ensure that a high-quality higher-education infrastructure will be available at the nation's land-grant universities to address national needs. It uses the scientific expertise from these and other colleges, universities, and public and private laboratories to address national priorities.

BOX 14.3   LAND-GRANT UNIVERSITY SYSTEM

The National Institute of Food and Agriculture (NIFA) supports the nation's land-grant university system, comprised of 109 colleges and universities that have been designated by the states or Congress to receive unique federal support in return for extension services. Land-grant institutions extend their resources to local communities through nonformal, noncredit programs. Each state and territory of the United States, as well as the District of Columbia, has a land-grant institution originating from the Morrill Act of 1862. In addition, most Southern states have a second land-grant institution as a result of the Second Morrill Act of 1890, which requires each state to show that race is not an admissions criterion, or else designate a separate land-grant institution for persons of color. Likewise, several Western and Plains states have one or more of the land-grant tribal colleges named in the Equity in Education Land-Grant Status Act of 1994. A list and map of the land-grant colleges and universities can be found at http://nifa.usda.gov/qlinks/partners/state_partners.html. Legislation related to the land-grant university system is available at http://www.csrees.usda.gov/about/offices/legis/legis_statutes .html.

In 2012, NIFA supported five priority science areas (US Department of Agriculture, http://www
.nifa.usda.gov/newsroom/factsheet.pdf) four of which address issues of food and nutrition:

- Food security and hunger: boost domestic agricultural production, improve capacity to
  meet growing global food demand, and foster innovation in fighting hunger and food
  insecurity.
- Climate change: help producers adapt to changing weather patterns and sustain economic vitality, while also reducing greenhouse gas emissions and increasing carbon
  sequestration.
- Sustainable energy: develop optimum biomass, forests, and crops for bioenergy production, and produce value-added, bio-based industrial products.
- Childhood obesity: ensure that nutritious foods are affordable and available, and that
  individuals and families are able to make informed, science-based decisions about
  health.
- Food safety: address the causes of microbial contamination and antimicrobial resistance,
  educate consumers and food safety professionals, and develop enhanced food processing
  technologies.

NIFA administers federal appropriations through three basic funding mechanisms: competitive
grants, formula grants, and noncompetitive grants.

- *Competitive grants.* Competitive programs enable NIFA to attract a large pool of applicants to work on agricultural issues of national interest, and to select the highest-quality
  proposals submitted by highly qualified individuals, institutions, or organizations.
  Awards are made following a rigorous peer-review process, and eligibility, administrative
  rules, and procedures vary for each specific program according to authorizing statutes.
  NIFA's competitive programs include the Community Food Projects Competitive Grant
  (CFPCG), which funds projects to meet the food needs of low-income people; increase
  the self-reliance of communities in providing for their own food need; and promote comprehensive responses to local food, farm, and nutrition issues. For all but training and
  capacity-building projects, these grants require a dollar-for-dollar match in resources,
  meaning that the agency applying for the grant must be able to demonstrate in-kind or
  other support from nonfederal sources (in-kind support is described in more detail later
  in the chapter).
- *Formula grants.* NIFA provides support for research and extension activities at land-grant
  institutions through programs that distribute federal appropriations on the basis of statutory formulas that may include variables such as the rural population, farm population,
  and poverty. NIFA's formula-funded programs include the cooperative extension system
  and the Expanded Food and Nutrition Education Program (EFNEP), designed to assist
  low-income groups in acquiring the knowledge, skills, attitudes, and behavior changes
  necessary for nutritionally sound diets.
- *Noncompetitive grants.* Each year, Congress directs NIFA to fund and administer certain
  state or commodity-specific programs through the special research or federal administration appropriation accounts. These funds are awarded to a designated institution or set of
  institutions for particular research, education, or extension topics of importance to a state
  or region. The Food and Agriculture Defense Initiative is an example of congressionally
  directed funding. This initiative supports a national diagnostic network of public agricultural institutions that identify and respond to high-risk biological pathogens in the food
  and agricultural system (US Department of Agriculture, http://www.nifa.usda.gov/about
  /fed_asst.html).

Healthy Food Financing Initiative

In 2010, the Obama Administration announced the creation of an over $400 million HFFI (http://
www.acf.hhs.gov/programs/ocs/programs/community-economic-development/healthy-food
-financing), a multiyear, multiagency effort to bring grocery stores and other healthy food retailers to underserved urban and rural communities (US Department of Health and Human Services
2010). These communities, commonly referred to as *food deserts*, typically rely on fast food
outlets and convenience stores that offer little or no fresh and healthy food options. The HFFI
is a partnership between the HHS, USDA, and Department of the Treasury. Competitive grants
go to community development corporations for projects to finance grocery stores, farmers' markets, and other sources of fresh nutritious food. Such projects serve the dual purpose of creating
employment and business opportunities in low-income communities while also providing access
to healthy food options (Spar 2013). Of the 38 CED-funded projects in FY 2012, 13 were HFFI
projects. To help community leaders identify the food deserts in their area, USDA launched
the Food Environment Atlas (http://www.ers.usda.gov/FoodAtlas/). This tool provides county-
level information about grocery store, convenience store, and restaurant availability; food assistance and food insecurity; food prices and taxes; health and physical activity; and socioeconomic
characteristics.

PRIVATE SECTOR

Although at its core philanthropy represents a direct effort to help others (ideally, without expectations of getting something in return), all corporations and some individuals use charitable giving
to decrease their tax burden. The funder's motive for providing grants may be entirely charitable
(as it sometimes is for small donors), or the rationale for donating funds may be fiscal exigency
(as it always is for large donors). In either case, contributors have the right to provide funds for the
causes they value. At the same time, grant writers have the need to present funders with the most
compelling case possible to assure that their organizations benefit from the limited pool of donated
resources.

The private sector includes private foundations, corporate grant makers, grant-making public
charities, and community foundations (Box 14.4) (Foundation Center, http://www.foundationcenter
.org/getstarted/tutorials/gfr/glossary.html).

- *Private foundations*: Nongovernmental, nonprofit organization with an endowment (usually donated from a single source, such as an individual, family, or corporation) and program managed by its own trustees or directors. These are established to maintain or aid
  social, educational, religious, or other charitable activities serving the common welfare,
  primarily through the making of grants. Examples of private foundations with a history of supporting nutrition causes are the Gerber Foundation, Rockefeller Foundation,
  W.K. Kellogg Foundation (WKKF), Robert Wood Johnson Foundation (RWJF), Bill and
  Melinda Gates Foundation, and Cooper Institute.

BOX 14.4   THE FOUNDATION CENTER

Information about identifying private funders is available from the Foundation Center at
http://www.foundationcenter.org/findfunders/. Founded in 1956, the Foundation Center is an
authority on philanthropy that serves grant seekers, grant makers, researchers, policy makers,
the media, and the general public.

- *Corporate grant makers*: Company-sponsored foundations and corporate giving programs. A company-sponsored foundation (also known as a corporate foundation) is a private foundation whose assets are derived primarily from the contributions of a for-profit business. Although a company-sponsored foundation may maintain close ties with its parent company, it is an independent organization with its own endowment and, as such, is subject to the same rules and regulations as other private foundations. Corporate giving programs are grant-making programs established and administered within a for-profit business organization. Some companies make charitable contributions through both a corporate giving program and a company-sponsored foundation. Examples of corporate grant makers with a history of supporting nutrition causes are Land O'Lakes Foundation; ConAgra Foods Foundation; Johnson & Johnson; Procter & Gamble Fund; Burger King Corporation; General Mills, Inc.; and Abbott Laboratories Fund.
- *Grant-making public charity*: A public foundation is a nongovernmental public charity that operates grant programs benefiting unrelated organizations or individuals as one of its primary purposes. There is no legal or Internal Revenue Service (IRS) definition of a public foundation, but such a designation is needed to encompass the growing number of grant-making institutions that are not private foundations. Examples of grant-making public charities with a history of supporting nutrition causes are the Academy of Nutrition and Dietetics Foundation, School Nutrition Foundation, International Life Sciences Institute Research Foundation, and Share Our Strength.
- *Community foundations*: Community foundations are grant-making public charities working on behalf of a specific community or region. A community foundation is much like a private foundation; its funds, however, are derived from many donors rather than a single source, as is usually the case with private foundations. The funds available to a community foundation are usually held in an endowment that is independently administered; income earned by the endowment is then used to make grants. Community foundations invest in diverse portfolios, and management is a major aspect of each community foundation's work. All share the common goal of serving donors, nonprofit organizations, and their communities (Box 14.5).

BOX 14.5 COMMUNITY FOUNDATIONS

Community foundations make up one of the fastest-growing sectors of philanthropy in the United States. They build and strengthen communities by making it possible for a wide range of donors to create permanent, named component funds to meet critical needs. There are more than 700 community foundations in the United States, located in almost every region and state in the country, and they vary widely in asset size—as small as $100,000 to more than $1.7 billion. Community foundations accept gifts of various sizes and types from private citizens, local corporations, other foundations, and government agencies. They hold approximately $49.5 billion in assets. In 2011, community foundations received an estimated $4.5 billion in gifts and gave approximately $4.2 billion to a wide variety of nonprofit activities: the arts and education, health and human services, the environment, and disaster relief. The New York Community Trust is one of the oldest and largest community foundations in the United States. In 2011, the New York Community Trust held almost $2 billion in assets and gave $137 million in grants to support programs focused on community development and the environment; health and people with special needs; education, arts, and human justice; and children, youth, and families.

Source: Council on Foundations. Community Foundations. Available at http://www.cof.org/foundation-type/community -foundations, accessed January 29, 2015.

APPLYING FOR FUNDS

GRANT APPLICATION MECHANISMS

There are two mechanisms whereby organizations submit applications for competitive grants. Grant applications may be solicited by the funder (grant maker) or by the applicant (grant seeker); in the latter case, the applicant submits an unsolicited request for support.

Grant Maker–Initiated Requests for Proposals

Some grants are awarded in response to funder-initiated requests for proposals, such as an advertised RFA or request for proposal (RFP). Grantors may also issue a Notice of Funding Availability. This single notice contains announcements of several independent funding streams. The purpose of the notice is to assist potential applicants to better identify the programs for which they can compete and give proposals to the programs most suitable to the issues faced by the target population. It also helps eligible applicants to understand the range of issues that may be supported by various related programs and encourages collaborations among organizations that provide complementary services.

For example, each week the NIH transmits, via the NIH listserv, a table of contents (TOC) giving that week's funding announcements. The TOC contains links to each RFA, PA, and notice published for that week. Instructions for subscribing to NIH's weekly listserv are available at http://grants.nih.gov/grants/guide/listserv.htm. Proposals may be solicited in the following ways:

- PA is open for 3 years (unless otherwise stated); applications are usually accepted on standard receipt (postmarked) dates on an ongoing basis.
- RFA is a one-time solicitation, and applications must be *received at NIH* by a single receipt date specified in the announcement.
- RFP is a contract solicitation that usually has one receipt date as specified in the announcement.

Grant Seeker–Initiated Requests for Proposals

Other grants are awarded on the basis of unsolicited appeals to potential funders. In this case, the applicant takes the initiative to submit a proposal for funding within the context of the funding organization's requirements.

Examples of investigator-initiated grant mechanisms are the research project grants (R01), small research grants (R03), and exploratory/developmental research grants (R21) used by the NIH, which provide support for health-related research and development consistent with the mission of the particular NIH institute(s) to which the grant is submitted.

NIH R01

R01 grants are awarded to all types of organizations (universities, colleges, small businesses, for-profit, nonprofit, foreign and domestic, faith-based, etc.). The R01 mechanism allows an investigator to define the scientific focus or objective of the research based on a particular area of interest and competence. Almost all institutes and centers at NIH fund R01 grants. Research grant applications are assigned to an institute or center based on receipt and referral guidelines, and many applications are assigned to multiple institutes and centers as interdisciplinary and multidisciplinary research is encouraged. Each institute and center maintains a website with funding opportunities and areas of interest. Allowable costs include salary and fringe benefits for the principal investigator (PI), key personnel, and other essential personnel; equipment and supplies; consultant costs; alterations and renovations; publications and miscellaneous costs; contract services; consortium costs; facilities and administrative costs (indirect costs); and travel expenses. Modular applications are most prevalent with modules of $25,000, up to the limit of $250,000. Grants are generally awarded for 1–5 years, and applications can be renewed by competing for an additional project period. The application for an R01 follows the instructions provided in SF424 (R&R) Application Guide, available at http://grants.nih.gov/grants/funding/424/index.htm. Receipt dates for R01 grant applications are posted at http://grants.nih.gov/grants/funding/submissionschedule.htm. Only one revision of a previously reviewed R01 grant application may be submitted.

NIH R03

The small research grant (R03) offers unsolicited research support, specifically limited in time and amount, providing flexibility for initiating studies that are generally short-term or pilot projects. Furthermore, the time interval from application to funding of R03 grants is short, thus allowing new ideas to be investigated or pursued in a more expeditious manner. The common characteristic of the small research grant is the provision of limited funding for a short period of time. Examples of the types of projects that NIH institutes and centers support with R03 include the following: pilot or feasibility studies; secondary analysis of existing data; small, self-contained research projects; development of research methodology; and development of new research technology. A project period of up to 2 years and a budget for direct costs of up to two $25,000 module or one $50,000 module per year may be requested, though R03 grants cannot be renewed. One revision of a previously reviewed R03 application may be submitted.

NIH R21

The exploratory/developmental research grant (R21) offers unsolicited research support, limited in time and amount, for early and conceptual stages of project development. Examples of R21 projects include exploratory, novel studies that break new ground or extend previous discoveries toward new directions or applications; and high risk/high reward studies that may lead to a breakthrough or result in novel techniques, agents, methodologies, models, or applications that will impact future research. Projects should be distinct from those supported through R01 and R03 grants, which tend to utilize widely accepted approaches and methods. A project period of up to 2 years and a budget for direct costs of up to $275,000 (no more than $200,000 per year) may be requested, though R21 grants cannot be renewed. One revision of a previously reviewed R21 application may be submitted.

In-Kind Support

Although grant awards are usually monetary, they may also include in-kind support for (1) products, supplies, and equipment (furniture, computers, office equipment); (2) use of corporate services/facilities (financial and administrative support services, meeting space, mailing services, computer services, printing and duplicating); and (3) professional services and employee expertise (graphic arts and design, advertising, promotion marketing, advice on taxes, business and finances). Product philanthropy is a key element in many major companies' giving programs. In 2011, noncash donations made up almost one-fifth of total contributions of the largest companies in the United States (Box 14.6) (Committee Encouraging Corporate Philanthropy, http://www.corporatephilanthropy.org/pdfs/giving_in_numbers/GIN2012_finalweb.pdf).

BOX 14.6   IN-KIND SUPPORT

Good360 (http://www.good360.org, formerly Gifts in Kind International), a charity that deals in product philanthropy, maintains a network of more than 6000 retail partners that provide over 22,000 nonprofit organizations with access to millions of dollars annually in product and service donations. Since its inception in 1983, Good360 has distributed nearly $7 billion in product donations. Operating at less than 1.8% of the fair market value of products donated, it is one of the most cost-efficient charities in the world.

GRANT APPLICATIONS

In order to simplify the process of seeking support, there is a trend toward standardizing applications for grants. Many grant makers in the private sector have adopted common grant application (CGA) forms to allow grant applicants to produce a single, standardized proposal for a specific community of funders (usually in a specific geographic area, such as a state or a large city) (Box 14.7). Increasingly, electronic versions of these forms are available for grant seekers to download and enter their responses directly onto the form. In fact, many private funders of public health nutrition grants, such as the RWJF and the WKKF, require online application submission. Links to over a dozen CGA forms used in various regions of the United States are available on the Foundation Center's website at http://foundationcenter.org/findfunders/cga.html. A glossary of terms used in public health nutrition grants appears in Appendix 14.1 of this chapter.

Like many private grant funders, federal agencies require electronic grant application submission, either through Grants.gov or directly with the agency, unless otherwise specified in the RFA or RFP.

HHS, which awards more than half of all the competitive grants from the federal government, is the lead agency for Grants.gov. The "Find Grant Opportunities" feature of the website allows grant seekers to search for information on available grant opportunities using a number of criteria, including such key words as *obesity* and *schools*, or a specific agency, such as USDA or HHS. The "Apply for Grants" feature enables users to download, complete, and submit applications for grant opportunities offered by federal agencies. In sum, Grants.gov provides the following:

- A single unified platform for all federal agencies to announce their grant opportunities and for all grant applicants to find and apply for those opportunities.
- A standardized manner of locating and learning more about funding opportunities.
- A single, secure, and reliable source for applying for federal grants online.
- A simplified grant application process with reduction of paperwork.

GRANT WRITING

To write a successful application for external funding, one must start by understanding the raison d'être (reason for existence) of the prospective grantor organization. You may, for example, look at the funding agency's strategic plan, which establishes priorities and related goals and objectives to focus its investment of effort and resources over the plan period.

Consider, for example, the goals of the USDA and the NIH, two major governmental funding sources for nutrition in public health. A strategic goal of the USDA is to ensure that all American children have access to safe, nutritious, and balanced meals (http://www.ocfo.usda.gov/sp2010/sp2010 .pdf), whereas the funding philosophy of the NIH is to improve public health. These perspectives should inform your grant-writing process.

Consider also the goals of WKKF (http://www.wkkf.org) and RWJF (http://www.rwjf.org), two of the most competitive private sector funders of nutrition causes. The WKKF (http://www.wkkf .org/who-we-are/our-history.aspx) mission is to support "children, families, and communities as they strengthen and create conditions that propel vulnerable children to achieve success as individuals and as contributors to the larger community and society." The mission of RWJF is "to improve the health and healthcare of all Americans" through six broad areas of focus: child and family well-being, childhood obesity, health insurance coverage, healthy communities, health leadership, and workforce and health system improvement (Robert Wood Johnson Foundation, http://www.rwjf.org/en/about-rwjf.html).

Characteristics of the Successful Grant Application

In general, the quality of a project is the factor that determines whether it is to be funded. The organization requesting support must also demonstrate to the funding agency that it has the means to accomplish the work, which includes both expertise and resources. The funding organization must be assured that (1) the PI and his or her colleagues are qualified to do the work and (2) the institution

BOX 14.7   SAMPLE COMMON GRANT APPLICATION FORM

I. Proposal Summary
   a. Summarize the purpose of your organization.
   b. Explain why your organization is requesting this grant, the outcomes you hope to achieve, and how you will spend the funds.

II. Narrative
   a. Background.
   b. Provide a brief description of the organization's history and mission.
   c. Describe the need or problem that your organization works to address and the population served, including demographic and socioeconomic characteristics.
   d. Describe current programs and accomplishments, including recent achievements.
   e. Provide information regarding the total number of paid (full-time and part-time) and volunteer staff members.
   f. Describe your organization's relationships (formal and informal) with other organizations working to meet the same needs or providing similar services, and how you differ from these other organizations.

III. Funding Request
   a. If applying for general operating support, describe how this grant would be used.
   b. If seeking funding for a specific project, explain the project, including the following:
      i.   Statement of the project's primary purpose and the need or problem you are seeking to address
      ii. Population you plan to serve and how they will benefit from the project
      iii. Strategies you will use to implement your project
      iv. Proposed staffing pattern for the project, including the names and titles of the project directors
      v.   Anticipated length of the project
      vi. How the project contributes to your organization's overall mission

IV. Evaluation
   a. Explain how you will measure the effectiveness of your activities.
   b. Describe your criteria for a successful program and the results you expect to have achieved by the end of the funding period.

V. Attachments
   a. Financial information:
      i.   Most recent financial statement, audited if available, reflecting actual expenditures and funds received during your most recent fiscal year
      ii. Operating expense budgets for the current and most recent fiscal year
   b. List of foundation and corporate supporters and all other sources of income, with amounts, for your current and most recent fiscal year.
   c. List of other sources of funding you are soliciting and the status of each proposal.
   d. Other supporting materials:
      i.   List of board of directors, with their affiliations
      ii. Copy of your most recent IRS letter indicating your organization's tax-exempt status
      iii. One-paragraph resumes of key staff, including qualifications relevant to the request

iv. Your most recent annual report, if available

v.   No more than three articles about, or evaluations of, your organization, if
     available

Source: Adapted from Philanthropy New York and The Council of New Jersey Grantmakers. New York/New Jersey
Area Common Application Form.

has equipment and personnel to support the proposed project and will allow the PI enough time to
complete the required tasks.

Proposals succeed or fail for a number of reasons. Among these are the following:

- The strength, quality, and persuasiveness of the proposal.
- The feasibility of the proposal, including but not limited to whether the project meets a
  clear community need, suggests a unique way to solve a well-defined problem, demon-
  strates community support, has access to a workforce that can see the project through to a
  successful completion, and has a well-planned budget.
- How well the project fits the funder's mission and current funding interests.
- The reputation, track record, and financial history of the institution requesting funds.
- Competition: how many other requests the funder has received.
- Funds and timing: how much money the funder has available in this cycle.
- How well the funder knows and trusts the board and staff, if the agency requesting funds
  is a local nonprofit organization.

Parts of the Proposal

A typical proposal contains nine parts: the proposal abstract or executive summary, introduction
of the organization requesting support, the problem statement or needs assessment, project objectives, project methods or design to achieve the stated objectives, project evaluation, sustainability
or future funding, project budget, and appendices. Guidelines for writing proposals are available
online. Refer to Grants.gov for specific details concerning the preparation of grant proposals for
federal awards. Information about writing proposals for nongovernment funding is available from
the Foundation Center (http://www.foundationcenter.org). Following are brief descriptions of the
parts of a typical grant proposal: (1) abstract or executive summary, (2) introduction, (3) statement
of need, (4) goals and objectives, (5) methods, (6) evaluation, (7) logic model, (8) future funding,
(9) budget, and (10) appendices (as relevant).

Abstract or Executive Summary

Summarize the request clearly and succinctly, including brief statements about the problem or need,
project or program, funding requirements, and the grant-seeking organization and its expertise.
Like all summaries, it is written last, although it appears as the first section. It is given in proposals that are more than 15 pages long or if the funding organization requires a summary statement.

Introduction

Introduce the organization by stating its vision and mission, describe the agency's qualifications,
and establish its credibility.

Statement of Need

The purpose of this section is to present the background and significance of the project by stating
the problem(s) to be investigated or needs to be met, providing the rationale for the proposed project, indicating the current state of knowledge relevant to the proposal, and suggesting the potential
contribution of this project to the problem(s) addressed. Establish familiarity with recent research

findings and use citations both to support specific statements and also to establish familiarity with all the relevant publications and points of view.

Goals and Objectives

The goals and objectives section of the proposal describes to the potential funder what will be achieved by the project. *Goals* are broad idealistic statements with a long-term outcome in mind. (Example: "The goal of this project is to improve the nutritional value of the food served in the New York City public school system.") Most proposals do not have more than three goals. For each goal, you may develop numerous corresponding *objectives*. Objectives are specific statements that indicate to the reviewer exactly how you plan to achieve your goals. Objectives should challenge the institution to improve its functioning, expand its scope, or reach a larger target audience. They should stretch the organization's current limits to bring about significant improvements that are important to the community. Differing types of objectives may be used, such as process and outcome objectives.

- *Process objectives* may be used as intermediate markers of the organization's progress in attaining its overall goal. Process objectives measure the accomplishment of individual tasks completed as part of the implementation of a program, such as the following:

    By March 1, 2016, there will be a 50% or greater increase in the number of principals in the school district who agree to a ban on the sale of candy and sweetened soda water in school premises.

    By September 1, 2016, there will be a 50% or greater increase in the number of schools in the district that do not sell candy and sweetened soda water on school premises.
- *Outcome objectives* measure the desired outcome of the proposed program, such as the following:

    By June 1, 2016, 100% of the principals in the school district will agree to a ban on the sale of candy and sweetened soda water on school premises.

    By December 2, 2016, 100% of the schools in the district will not sell candy and sweetened soda water on school premises (Box 14.8).

BOX 14.8   SMART OBJECTIVES

Well-written objectives are SMART (specific, measurable, achievable, relevant, and time bound).

- *Specific.* Objectives state what is to be achieved. (Example: "There will be a reduction in the number of public schools in the district that sell soda and candy during regular school hours.")
- *Measurable.* Information concerning the objective can be collected, detected, or obtained from records. (Example: "There will be a 40% reduction in the number of public schools in the district that sell soda and candy during regular school hours.")
- *Achievable.* Not only is the objective possible; it is likely that the organization will be able to accomplish the task.
- *Relevant to the mission.* The objective fits into the overall mission of the funding organization as well as the mission of the organization that is applying for funding. In other words, the objective helps each organization achieve its mission.
- *Time bound.* Each objective clearly indicates how much time it would take to accomplish the desired outcome. (Example: "By January 1, 2016 there will be a 40% reduction in the number of public schools in the district that sell soda and candy during regular school hours.")

Methods

The methods section of the proposal enables the reader to visualize the implementation of the project by describing the methods and activities for addressing the identified problems and achieving the desired results. It should convince the reader that your agency knows what it is doing, thereby establishing the credibility of the agency. It is helpful to conceptualize the methods section of a proposal as addressing the time-honored questions: How? When? Why? Where? Who?

- *How*: the detailed description of what will occur from the time the project begins until it is completed. The methods used to achieve the desired outcomes should match the stated objectives. Include how the data will be collected, analyzed, and interpreted.
- *When*: the chronology of activities that must be performed to implement the project. A timetable for the project's activities presented in the form of a Gantt chart can illustrate both the order in which tasks are carried out and the length of time allotted for each activity. A Gantt chart is a bar graph that helps plan and monitor project development or resource allocation on a horizontal time scale. (See Figure 14.1 for an example.)
- *Why*: this is the place to justify chosen methods, especially if they are new or unorthodox. Cite examples of successful use of the methods in previous projects and explain why the planned work will lead to the expected outcomes; describe any new methodology and its advantage over existing methodologies, and discuss the potential difficulties and limitations of the proposed procedures and alternative approaches to achieve the aims.
- *Where*: indicate where the project will take place, which includes the location of administrative offices and areas designated for storage of sensitive documents, as well as settings for direct client contact.
- *Who*: discuss the number of staff members, their qualifications and credentials, and the specific tasks assigned to each person. Provide position descriptions for each paid staff member, indicating what percentage of time will be devoted to the project. Identify staff already employed by the organization and those to be recruited specifically for the project. (Details about individual staff members may be included here or in the appendix, depending on the length and importance of this information.) Staffing refers to volunteers and consultants, as well as to paid staff. Describe volunteer activities to underscore the value added by the volunteers as well as the cost-effectiveness of the project. Salary and

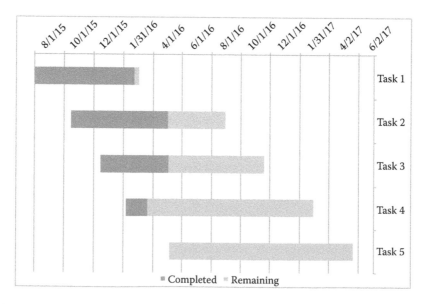

FIGURE 14.1 Sample Gantt chart.

project costs are affected by the qualifications of the staff. Indicate the practical experience required for key staff members, as well as their level of expertise and educational background. If individuals have already been selected to direct the program, summarize their credentials and include a brief biographical sketch in the appendix. A strong project director can help influence a grant decision. Describe plans for administering the project, which is especially important in a large operation or if more than one agency is collaborating on the project. Identify the staff members who are responsible for financial management, project outcomes, record keeping, and reporting.

Evaluation

Present a plan to evaluate the degree to which the project's objectives are met (outcome evaluation) and to improve the way the program works (process evaluation). Allocate 5–10% of the budget for activities related to evaluating the project. Consider budgeting for a statistician to assist with the planning and implementation of the evaluation component of the program. The value of a sound evaluation design cannot be overstated. Effective program evaluation helps to improve the program (process or formative evaluation) as well as determine the extent to which the program delivers on its promise (summative evaluation). Process evaluation provides information about the program while it is still in progress. It points to changes that might be needed to bring the project to a successful conclusion. Process evaluation focuses on program activities, outputs, and short-term outcomes. Summative evaluation, on the other hand, provides information on the project's efficacy (its ability to do what it was designed to do).

Logic Models

The WKKF supports the use of a logic model (W.K. Kellogg Foundation, http://www.wkkf.org/knowl edge-center/resources/2006/02/wk-kellogg-foundation-logic-model-development-guide.aspx) to present the working of the program. A logic model uses words and/or pictures to (1) illustrate the sequence of activities proposed to bring about change and (2) demonstrate how these activities are linked to the results the program is expected to achieve (University of Wisconsin Cooperative Extension, http://www.uwex.edu/ces/pdande/evaluation/evallogicmodel.html). A logic model can strengthen the case for investing in the proposed program as it captures in a single page what the program plans to do. Used correctly, it also helps to write the body of the proposal, clarify the services to be delivered, and streamline the evaluation process. For programs delivering primary and secondary prevention services, the logic model is a snapshot of the agency's primary services, short- and long-term goals, and intended outcomes of the services provided. It can be used as a guide to plan for new services or as the first step in planning for an evaluation of their services.

A review of current RFPs indicates that funders are requiring specificity and results, as indicated by their requests for "outcome-based evaluation," "best-practices" programs, and "sustainable organizations." The logic model was developed to meet these requests.

Figure 14.2 shows the components of a generic program logic model. Each component is linked to the next in a conditional *if–then* relationship. In this paradigm, the term *output* substitutes for

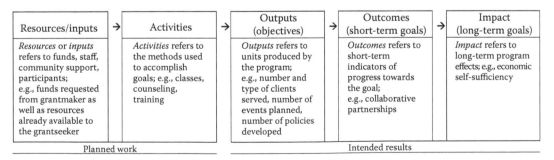

Resources/inputs →	Activities →	Outputs (objectives) →	Outcomes (short-term goals) →	Impact (long-term goals)
Resources or *inputs* refers to funds, staff, community support, participants; e.g., funds requested from grantmaker as well as resources already available to the grantseeker	*Activities* refers to the methods used to accomplish goals; e.g., classes, counseling, training	*Outputs* refers to units produced by the program; e.g., number and type of clients served, number of events planned, number of policies developed	*Outcomes* refers to short-term indicators of progress towards the goal; e.g., collaborative partnerships	*Impact* refers to long-term program effects; e.g., economic self-sufficiency
Planned work		Intended results		

FIGURE 14.2 Components of a program logic model.

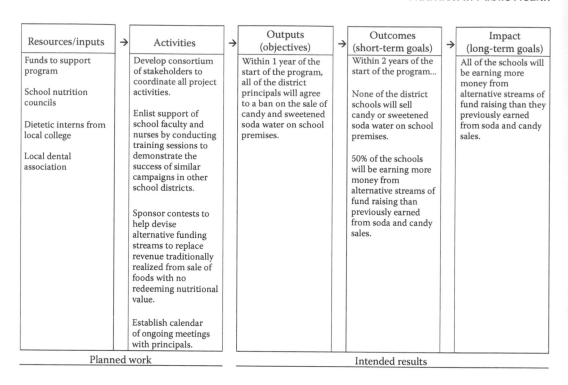

Resources/inputs →	Activities →	Outputs (objectives) →	Outcomes (short-term goals) →	Impact (long-term goals)
Funds to support program School nutrition councils Dietetic interns from local college Local dental association	Develop consortium of stakeholders to coordinate all project activities. Enlist support of school faculty and nurses by conducting training sessions to demonstrate the success of similar campaigns in other school districts. Sponsor contests to help devise alternative funding streams to replace revenue traditionally realized from sale of foods with no redeeming nutritional value. Establish calendar of ongoing meetings with principals.	Within 1 year of the start of the program, all of the district principals will agree to a ban on the sale of candy and sweetened soda water on school premises.	Within 2 years of the start of the program... None of the district schools will sell candy or sweetened soda water on school premises. 50% of the schools will be earning more money from alternative streams of fund raising than previously earned from soda and candy sales.	All of the schools will be earning more money from alternative streams of fund raising than they previously earned from soda and candy sales.

| Planned work | Intended results |

FIGURE 14.3 Sample program logic model for an initiative to eliminate the sale of foods and beverages with no redeeming nutritional value in a local school district.

objectives, *outcomes* replaces *short-term goals*, and *impact* is used instead of *long-term goals*. The components of the logic model are defined underneath each component's heading. Figure 14.3 is a sample program logic model for an initiative to eliminate the sale of foods and beverages with no redeeming nutritional value in a local school district.

Future Funding

Describe a plan for sustainability of the project. Sustainability refers to the continuation of the program even after the initial funding has ended. The Foundation Center suggests being prepared to demonstrate the long-term financial viability of the project to be funded and of the organization itself. Demonstrate that the project is *finite* (with a beginning, a middle, and an end); that it is *capacity building*, which means it will contribute to the future self-sufficiency of the organization; that it will enable the agency to expand services that might generate revenue in the future; or that it will make the organization competitive for future external funding streams (The Foundation Center, http://foundationcenter.org/getstarted/tutorials/shortcourse/index.html).

Budget

Clearly delineate costs to be met by the grant. In longer proposals, a budget narrative will be provided along with the budget work sheet.

Appendices

The appendix includes materials to elaborate on any parts of the proposal. It also contains a list of the members of the agency's board of directors, a copy of the IRS determination letter for 501(c)(3) organizations, financial documentation, and brief resumes of key staff.

Abbreviated Grant Proposals

Sometimes, a full grant proposal is not called for, either because the funder has a multistage application process or because a small amount of money is being requested. In the case of a multistage application process, funders may request concise proposals for initial review. Applicants best meeting the grant requirements are then invited to submit full-length proposals that include the parts described above (Box 14.9).

BOX 14.9 EXAMPLE SUBMISSION REQUIREMENTS OF A PRIVATE FOUNDATION GRANT

The information in this section is abstracted from a 2013 request for proposals issued by the Robert Wood Johnson Foundation (RWJF) for efforts to change public and institutional policies and environments in ways that promote improved nutrition and physical activity. Approximately $1.6 million in grants will be allocated to studies focused on improving the nutritional quality of school snacks and beverages, reducing consumption of sugary beverages, protecting children from unhealthy food and beverage marketing, and increasing access to affordable healthy foods in underserved communities.

Before selected applicants can submit a full grant proposal (up to 15 pages long accompanied by a budget and budget narrative), the RWJF requires all applicants to provide a shorter concept paper for initial review, including a project narrative (up to 3 pages long) and biosketches for key personnel. The project narrative is the most important part of the application because it is used as the primary basis for determining whether or not a project meets the minimum requirements for the grant. It should provide a clear and concise description of the project and must follow any formatting instructions provided. Proposals with narratives that do not conform to these formatting instructions will not be reviewed. The following components are required in the RWJF project narrative of the initial concept paper:

- *Project title, identification number, applicant name, and legal name of applicant organization.*
- *Project aims*: specific aims and study hypotheses.
- *Rationale*: significance and contribution of the proposed project in reducing childhood obesity, and the relevance to low-resource communities and children in lower-income and racial and ethnic minority populations at highest risk for obesity.
- *Target population, sample, and setting*: definition of the study's target population, study sample, and if applicable, the setting(s) in which the proposed study will take place (e.g., school, community, grocery store, restaurant, child-care center).
- *Research Strategy*: study design, research methods, measures, analysis plans, and intervention (if applicable).
- *Names and qualifications of the principal investigator (PI) and key project staff*: name, degree(s), title, and organization of proposed PI and key project members (e.g., co-PI and co-investigators); and description of the research qualifications and related past research or experience working with the proposed target population.

Source: Robert Wood Johnson Foundation. Healthy Eating Research: Building Evidence to Prevent Childhood Obesity. 2013 Call for Proposals. Available at http://www.rwjf.org/content/dam/files/legacy-cfp-files/overview_HER2013.pdf, accessed February 13, 2015. Robert Wood Johnson Foundation. Healthy Eating Research Round 8 Application Preview. Available at http://my.rwjf.org/viewApplication.do?cfp=2282, accessed February 13, 2015.

BOX 14.10   THE COMPONENTS OF A LETTER PROPOSAL

1. *Ask for the gift*: The letter should begin with a reference to your agency's prior contact with the funder, if any. State why you are writing and how much funding is required from the particular foundation.
2. *Describe the need*: Briefly explain why there is a need for this project, piece of equipment, or whatever is being requested.
3. *Explain what you will do*: Provide enough detail to arouse the funder's interest. Describe precisely what will take place as a result of the grant.
4. *Provide agency data*: Acquaint the funder with the organization by providing its mission statement; a brief description of programs offered; the number of people served; and staff, volunteer, and board data, as appropriate.
5. *Include appropriate budget data*: The budget appears in the letter proper or in a separate attachment. It must clearly indicate the total cost of the project.
6. *Close*: Every proposal of any length needs a strong concluding statement. Include one or two concluding paragraphs. This is a good place to call attention to the future, after the grant is completed. If appropriate, outline some of the follow-up activities that might be undertaken to begin to prepare the funders for your agency's next request. This section is also the place to make a final appeal for the proposed project. Briefly reiterate what your organization expects to accomplish and why it is important. (At this point, a bit of emotion might make the letter even more persuasive.)
7. *Attach any additional information required*: The funder may need much of the same information to back up a small request as a large one. These are a list of the members of the board of directors, a copy of the applicant agency's IRS determination letter, financial documentation, and brief resumes of key staff.

Mini-grant opportunities may be available. For example, in 2012, the Wyoming Office of Multicultural Health made available mini-grants ($100 to $1450) to provide community agencies the resources to work on local, county, and statewide projects to improve Wyoming's health disparities. Although an unsolicited opportunity for funding, the application provided very explicit instructions due to the small dollar amounts of the grants and specified that proposals cannot include requests for direct patient care, construction or renovation, fund-raising, job training for staff, political activities, clinical trials, or vocational rehabilitation (News from Wyoming Department of Health 2012).

When an unsolicited appeal is for a small amount of money (less than $1000), consider developing a solicitation letter in lieu of a full-scale proposal. A request for a contribution of $1000 or less hardly calls for more than a three- or a four-page letter. To be effective, a letter proposal will cover essentially the same points as a full proposal but in considerably less space because much less money is being requested and a much more conservative product is expected as a result of the donation (Box 14.10).

CONCLUSION

Seeking funding through grants can occupy a large part of a public health practitioner's work. Whereas many agencies at the federal level and private organizations provide funding, knowing the most appropriate agency to apply to for your particular program and needs can save a good deal of time and effort. In addition, it is extremely important to approach grant writing in an organized and deliberate, rather than a haphazard, albeit passionate, manner. Knowing exactly what you intend to do with the funds you receive—in other words, thoroughly planning before you even begin writing your grant—is very important to potential funders.

ACRONYMS

ACF	Administration for Children and Families
ACL	Administration for Community Living
AHRQ	Agency for Healthcare Research and Quality
AoA	Administration on Aging
ATSDR	Agency for Toxic Substances and Disease Registry
CACFP	Child and Adult Care Food Program
CDC	Centers for Disease Control and Prevention
CED	Community Economic Development
CFSAN	Center for Food Safety and Applied Nutrition
CGA	Common grant application
CMS	Centers for Medicare & Medicaid Services
CRISP	Computer Retrieval of Information on Scientific Projects
CSBG	Community Services Block Grant
CSFP	Commodity Supplemental Food Program
CSREES	Cooperative State Research, Education, and Extension Service
EFNEP	Expanded Food and Nutrition Education Program
FADR	Food Assistance for Disaster Relief
FDA	Food and Drug Administration
FDPIR	Food Distribution Program on Indian Reservations
FFVP	Fresh Fruit and Vegetable Program
FMNP	Farmers' Market Nutrition Program
FNS	Food and Nutrition Service
FSIS	Food Safety and Inspection Service
FY	Fiscal year
HFFI	Healthy Food Financing Initiative
HHS	Department of Health and Human Services
HIV/AIDS	Human immunodeficiency virus/acquired immunodeficiency syndrome
HRSA	Health Resources and Services Administration
IHS	Indian Health Service
IRS	Internal Revenue Service
NABG	Nutrition Assistance Block Grants
NCCDPHP	National Center for Chronic Disease Prevention and Health Promotion
NHLBI	National Heart, Lung, and Blood Institute
NIA	National Institute on Aging
NIDDK	National Institute for Diabetes and Digestive and Kidney Diseases
NIFA	National Institute of Food and Agriculture
NIH	National Institutes of Health
NORC	Nutrition and obesity research center
NSLP	National School Lunch Program
OAA	Older Americans Act
OASH	Office of the Assistant Secretary of Health
OCS	Office of Community Services
PA	Program announcement
PHHSBG	Preventive Health and Health Services Block Grant
PI	Principal investigator
RePORT	Research Portfolio Online Reporting Tools
RFA	Request for applications
RFP	Request for proposals
RWJF	Robert Wood Johnson Foundation

SAMHSA	Substance Abuse and Mental Health Services Administration
SBP	School Breakfast Program
SFMNP	Senior Farmers' Market Nutrition Program
SFSP	Summer Food Service Program
SMP	Special Milk Program
SNAP	Supplemental Nutrition Assistance Program
TANF	Temporary Assistance for Needy Families
TEFAP	The Emergency Food Assistance Program
TOC	Table of contents
USDA	United States Department of Agriculture
WIC	Special Supplemental Nutrition Program for Women, Infants, and Children
WIN	Weight-control Information Network
WKKF	W. K. Kellogg Foundation

STUDENT ASSIGNMENTS AND ACTIVITIES DESIGNED TO ENHANCE LEARNING AND STIMULATE CRITICAL THINKING

1. Using the "Awards by Location" option in the Research Portfolio Online Reporting Tools (RePORT, http://report.nih.gov), perform a search for nutrition-related projects in your state during the current fiscal year. Choose one of the projects that best addresses nutrition in public health and answer the following questions:
   - What is the name of the project?
   - Summarize the project in three to four sentences, making sure to include the project's purpose/aims, methods/activities, and expected outcomes/impact.
   - Who is the primary investigator (PI)? What is her/his title? What institution is s/he from?
   - How much funding was provided for the project?
   - What agency is funding the project? Why is this project a match for funding through this agency?
   - How long will the project take?
   - Using the "Similar Projects" tab, describe any similar projects occurring around the country. How are these projects different from the one you chose?

2. Using the federal grant program website (http://www.grants.gov), perform a search for nutrition-related grant opportunities. Choose one of the grant opportunities that best addresses nutrition in public health, click the link to additional information, and answer the following questions:
   - What is the title of the grant?
   - Summarize the purpose of this grant in two to three sentences.
   - Why is this grant being made available at this time?
   - Who can apply for this grant, and when is the application deadline?
   - How many awards will be made under this grant opportunity?
   - What is the range of funding an applicant may receive?
   - What agency is distributing the funding? Why is this grant opportunity a match for this agency?
   - Based on the information provided in the grant description, develop a project that would meet the grant's research objectives, requirements, time frame, and funding mechanism (e.g., R21 grants support exploratory studies, which should be distinct from those supported through the R01 mechanism). Discuss your project in a concept paper of up to three pages, following the format outlined in the chapter. For information pertaining to the grant-seeking organization, identify a local, state, or national organization that might submit this project for funding and is eligible to receive the

grant. Be sure to include a description of why this organization is qualified to carry out this project and work with the proposed target population.

3. Often, successful programs collaborate with local organizations, foundations, hospitals, schools, agencies, and large and small businesses. Discuss the advantages and disadvantages of collaborating with others.

4. Identify two different common grant applications (you can choose from the Foundation Center's list at http://foundationcenter.org/findfunders/cga.html or find others). Compare and contrast these applications. What are the common requirements or sections? Which requirements or sections are unique to each? Why might that be?

5. You have been asked to write a grant proposal to start a neighborhood child obesity prevention program that aims to encourage children and their caretakers to eat well and exercise regularly. This program will take place during the summer months (in between school years) and should include educational workshops and hands-on activities, such as cook shops and noncompetitive sports. Several professionals will be needed to start the program, including a medical doctor, registered dietitian, and physical activity instructor. The details and overall design of the program have been left up to you.

a. The purpose of a literature review is to document the need for your program, as well as to identify strategies for program design, implementation, and evaluation. A thorough literature review will critically examine the existing work that relates to your proposed program.

Conduct a literature review, provide a summary of the relevant literature, and show how it relates to your proposed program. Include a statement of need: Why is this program needed in your community? How will this program help neighborhood children and their families? You may want to locate information with regard to obesity and your specific population by consulting the following:

  i. Government reports of studies related to the problem itself, e.g., statistics that demonstrate the type, size, and scope of this nutrition/health-related problem on a national level; information about the at-risk population; incidence and prevalence; ages; socioeconomic status; and community assessment (include epidemiological data, mortality, morbidity, debility statistics, and surveys that have been done)

  ii. Studies that describe the characteristics and extent of the problem in your community

  iii. Evaluation of the nutritional or nutrition education needs of the at-risk population: anthropometry, biochemical assessment, clinical assessment, dietary assessment, educational needs assessment; environmental resources and challenges; etc.

  iv. Studies and reports that discuss the cause of the problem and its social and economic impact.

  v. Resources that identify specific means of prevention. What have similar programs done in the past? Were they successful? Why or why not?

b. Give your program a title. Based on your literature review, create a program logic model illustrating your design of the program. Be sure to include the resources you need, activities you will accomplish, immediate outputs of the accomplishments, program outcomes after 1 year, and program impact in 3–5 years. Before starting this logic model, review the section on grant applications, along with Figures 14.2 and 14.3.

c. List the goals and objectives of your program. Make sure your objectives are SMART (specific, measurable, achievable, relevant, and time bound).

d. Describe the program methods. (How? When? Why? Where? Who?) Also include participant eligibility criteria, other organizations involved, and any major barriers you anticipate and how your program will be able to overcome those barriers.

e. Create a Gantt chart to display the project's main activities over time.

f. Discuss how you plan to evaluate the program. What evaluation mechanism will you use and why? How will you know that you met your goals and objectives? Who are the evaluators, and who or what would be evaluated?

g. Describe a plan for sustainability of the project.

h. Create a budget work sheet, including an estimate of all costs (direct and indirect costs, salaries, etc).

i. Now that you have completed the necessary sections of a grant proposal, find a grant opportunity that would potentially fund your program. Grant opportunities can be found online through the federal grant program website (http://www.grants.gov) and the Foundation Center (http://foundationcenter.org/). Provide a brief description of the grant opportunity, including the funding organization, title and purpose of the grant, and range of possible funding.

j. Grants are usually monetary awards, but they may also include in-kind support, such as products, supplies, equipment, corporate service/facilities, professional services, and employee expertise. Refer to Good360 (http://www.good360.org). List the type of in-kind support your program could use, and where and from whom you might be able to receive this support. State how your program would benefit from the support you identified.

k. Finally, write the abstract for your grant proposal. Remember, the abstract is a brief (300 words or less) description of your proposed project.

APPENDIX 14.1 GLOSSARY OF TERMS FOR GRANTS IN PUBLIC HEALTH NUTRITION

501(c)(3)—The section of the tax code that defines nonprofit, charitable, tax-exempt organizations.

Applicant—An organization that submits a proposal for financial assistance.

Audience—Individual, group, or institution for which the organization's products and services are provided, e.g., children, adults, parents, educators, clinic visitors, or partner institutions.

Beneficiary—In philanthropic terms, the grantee receiving funds from a foundation or corporate giving program.

Benefit—Gain or payoff accruing to the project stakeholders, including target audiences, as a result of the project.

Best practices—Practices that incorporate the best objective information currently available regarding effectiveness and acceptability.

Block grant—An intergovernmental transfer of federal funds to states and local governments for broad purposes such as health, education, or community development in general. A block grant makes few requirements as to how the money is to be spent, instead offering state and local municipalities discretion, within general guidelines established by Congress and the executive branch. Annual program plans or applications are normally required.

Budget—Total estimated cost of the project, including direct costs associated with each of the project's activities, as well as indirect costs.

Budget period—The time interval into which a grant period is divided for budgetary and funding purposes.

Capacity building—Activities that assist eligible entities to improve or enhance their overall or specific capability to plan, deliver, manage, and evaluate programs efficiently and effectively to benefit low-income individuals. This may include upgrading internal financial management or computer systems, establishing new external linkages with other organizations, adding or refining a program component or replicating techniques or programs piloted in another local community, or making other cost-effective improvements.

Capital request—A planned undertaking to purchase, build, or renovate space or building or to acquire equipment.

Challenge grant—A grant that is paid only if the grant-seeking organization is able to raise additional funds from other sources.

Common grant application (CGA)—A single, standardized grant application form used by a specific community of funders (usually in a specific geographic area).

Communication strategy—Outline of the messages to be conveyed to stakeholders about the project's processes and results, the most efficient and effective channels and timing for transmitting the messages, and the means for obtaining feedback.

Community—The people living in the same district, city, state, or locale.

Community development corporation—A private nonprofit corporation that has a board of directors consisting of residents of the community and business and civic leaders, and has as a principal purpose of planning, developing, or managing low-income housing or community development activities.

Contribution—A tax-deductible gift of cash, property, equipment, or service from an individual to a nonprofit organization, often given annually.

Cost–benefit analysis—Comparison of the total cost of doing the project with the anticipated value or payoff of the project. A formal analysis involves calculating the ratio of the numerical value of the anticipated benefits to the anticipated costs.

Costs—Direct costs: personnel, material, and service expenses associated with specific project activities. Indirect costs: project expenses—such as energy, rent, and insurance—that cannot be directly tied to a specific project activity.

Data analysis—Organization, processing, and presentation of information that is collected for the purpose of making recommendations or drawing conclusions.

Desired result—Goal the project is designed to achieve for its stakeholders. It may be expressed as an outcome or an output.

Direct costs—Personnel, material, and service expenses associated with specific project activities.

Displaced worker—An individual in the labor market who has been unemployed for 6 months or longer.

Dissemination plan—Strategy for making the project's results, products, processes, or benefits accessible through acceptable communication channels so the results of the project will benefit the broader population.

Distressed community—A geographic urban neighborhood or rural community of high unemployment and pervasive poverty.

DUNS—Dun and Bradstreet Data Universal Numbering System. A nine-digit number required when applying for federal grants or cooperative agreements. Grantee organizations can verify that they have a DUNS number or take steps needed to obtain one at no cost by visiting http://fedgov.dnb.com/webform/ or by calling (866) 705-5711. The requirement for a DUNS number applies to all organizations that apply for NIH grants and cooperative agreements. Nonaffiliated individuals who apply for a grant or cooperative agreement are exempt from this requirement.

Empowerment Zone and Enterprise Community project areas (EZ/EC)—Urban neighborhoods and rural areas designated as such by the secretaries of the Department of Housing and Urban Development and Department of Agriculture.

Evaluation plan—Protocol for assessing the extent to which a project has met its goals.

Faith-based community development corporation—A community development corporation that has a religious character.

Fiscal year (FY)—A 12-month period upon which a budget is planned.

Formative evaluation—Gathering information that can be used as a management tool to improve the way a program operates while the program is in progress. It should also identify problems that occurred, how the problems were resolved, and what recommendations are needed for future implementation.

Gantt chart—Bar chart that shows graphically the duration of the project's activities (the start and end dates) as well as its milestones. It can also show the relationships between the project's activities, e.g., the finishing of one task before another begins.

General operating support—Funds, both contributions and grants, that support the ongoing services of the organization.

Goals—The broad results the project is expected to accomplish, which guide the development of the project's objectives and activities.

Grants—Usually an allocation from foundations, corporations, or government for special projects or general operating expenses. Grants may be multiyear or annual.

Hypothesis—An assumption made in order to test a theory. It should assert a cause-and-effect relationship between a program intervention and its expected result. Both the intervention and its result must be measured in order to confirm the hypothesis. The following is an example: "Eighty hours of classroom training will be sufficient for participants to prepare a week's worth of healthy meals." In this hypothesis, data would be obtained on the number of hours of training actually received by participants (the intervention) and the healthfulness of a week's worth of meals (the result) to determine the validity of the hypothesis (that 80 hours of training is sufficient to produce the result).

Implementation activities—Tasks performed to deliver the project's final products or services to the target audience.

Indian tribe—A tribe, band, or other organized group of Native American Indians recognized in the state or states in which they reside, or considered by the Secretary of the Interior to be an Indian tribe or an Indian organization.

Indicator—Measurable condition or behavior that can show that an outcome was achieved. This is usually expressed as a number or percentage of the target audience that demonstrates an observable, measurable sign or characteristic representing the intended outcome.

Indirect costs—Project expenses that cannot be directly tied to a specific project activity, e.g., energy, rent, and insurance.

In-kind support—A contribution of equipment/materials, time, and services that the donor has placed a monetary value on for tax purposes, and noncash contributions provided by nonfederal third parties. These contributions may be in the form of real property, equipment, supplies, and other expendable property.

Innovative project—One that departs from, or significantly modifies, past program practices and tests a new approach.

Intervention—Any planned activity within a project that is intended to produce changes in the target population and the environment, and that can be formally evaluated. For example, assistance in preparing a business plan is an intervention.

Job creation—New jobs, i.e., jobs not in existence prior to the start of the project. These result from new business start-ups, business expansion, development of new services industries, and other newly undertaken physical or commercial activities.

Job placement—Placing a person in an existing vacant job of a business, service, or commercial activity not related to the new development or expansion activity.

Letter of support—A letter encouraging grant or support for a project, submitted on a grant applicant's behalf by organizations with whom they partner or collaborate.

Logic model—A diagrammatic representation of a program that describes the logical linkages among program resources, conditions, strategies, short-term outcomes, and long-term impact.

Matching funds—Funds that must be supplied by the grantee in an amount equal to or a percentage of the award amount in order to receive the award. In the case of a federal grant, the matching funds must usually come from nonfederal sources.

Methodology—A sequence of activities needed to accomplish the program objectives.

Milestone—Signpost or marker that shows accomplishment of logically related activities, e.g., design and development or achievement of the project's interim or final targets.

Mission—Overall purpose of an organization. It typically identifies key broad audiences and purposes, and often broadly describes the methods by which the organization will achieve its mission.

Modular application—A type of grant application in which support is requested in specified increments without the need for detailed supporting information related to separate budget categories. When modular procedures apply, they affect not only application preparation but also review, award, and administration of the application/award.

Monitoring—Steps or processes for continual tracking of current performance in relation to a plan (e.g., schedules and budgets, number of services provided, number of participating institutions or people) and for identification of any corrective steps necessary to improve performance.

Narrative—The written portion of a grant, describing who, what, when, where, why, and how the funding will be used. Grant applications have at least two parts: the narrative and the budget.

Need—Gap between the current condition and the desired condition.

Needs assessment—Systematic process of identifying the gap between what the current state is and what the grant maker wants to achieve, and determining appropriate solutions to close the gap.

Nonprofit organization—An organization (including faith based and community based) that provides proof of nonprofit status. A nonprofit organization is qualified by the IRS as a tax-exempt organization.

Operating plan—The written plan outlining how an organization is to be operated.

Outcome-based evaluation approach—Set of principles and processes to provide information about the degree to which a project has met its goals in terms of creating benefits for individuals in the form of knowledge, skill, attitude, behavior, status, or life condition.

Outcome evaluation—An assessment of project results as measured by collected data that define the net effects of the interventions applied in the project. An outcome evaluation will produce and interpret findings related to whether the interventions produced desirable changes and their potential for being replicated. It should answer this question: Did the program work?

Outcomes—The changes in (or benefits achieved by) clients due to their participation in program activities. This may include changes to participants' knowledge, attitudes, skills, values, behavior, or status. Outcomes are often presented temporally (short term, intermediate, and long term).

Output-based evaluation approach—Set of principles and processes to provide information about the degree to which the project's products and services have achieved the desired result, e.g., the quantity or quality of services, the volume of users or participants, or the number of products that met the target audience's expectations.

Outputs—The tangible results of the major activities of the program. They are usually accounted for by their number, for example, the number of people who were screened for blood pressure, blood sugar, and cholesterol.

Performance standard—The number and percentage of clients who are expected to achieve the result. Also called *targets*, they should be set based on professional judgment, past data, research, or professional standards.

Pilot test—Dry run of a process, such as a workshop or training session, on a selected group of people in a realistic setting to obtain feedback and make necessary adjustments before delivery of the final product or service to the target audience.

Poverty Income Guidelines—Guidelines published annually by the US Department of Health and Human Services that establish the level of poverty defined as *low income* for individuals

and their families. The guideline information is posted on the Internet at http://aspe.hhs
.gov/poverty.

Principal investigator (**PI**; or program director or project director)—An individual designated by the grantee to direct the project or activity being supported by the grant who is responsible for the scientific and technical direction of a project and the day-to-day management of the project or program, and is accountable to the grantee for the proper conduct of the project or activity.

Process evaluation—The ongoing examination of the implementation of a program. It focuses on the effectiveness and efficiency of the program's activities and interventions (for example, methods of recruiting participants, quality of training activities, or usefulness of follow-up procedures). It should answer these questions: who is receiving what services, and are the services being delivered as planned?

Product—Anything created or obtained as a result of some operation or work.

Program—An organized set of services designed to achieve specific outcomes for a specified population that will continue beyond the grant period.

Program announcement (**PA**)—An announcement that a grant is open for competition.

Project—A planned undertaking or organized series of related activities that begins and ends within the grant period, and that is designed to achieve specific outcomes for its target audience. A successful project may become an ongoing program.

Project director—Main person responsible for the project; coordinates all project tasks and promotes good relationships and communications among all team members.

Project period—The total time for which a project is approved for support, including any approved extensions.

Proposal—A written document prepared to present a problem to a funding organization and to communicate to the proposal reviewers the strategy that the researcher intends to use in search of a solution to that problem. The proposal should set forth the exact nature of the matter to be investigated and a detailed account of the methods to be employed. It must answer the standard research questions: What? Why? How? When? Who? Where? To what effect?

Request for application (**RFA**)—A type of solicitation notice in which a funder announces the availability of grant monies and allows organizations to present bids on how the funding could be used. An RFA will often list the type of programs eligible for funding, expectations for use of funds, and application procedures.

Request for proposal (**RFP**)—A type of solicitation notice in which a funder announces the availability of funds for a particular project or program, and allows organizations to present bids for the project's completion. An RFP will list project specifications, application procedures, and contract terms.

Risk—Potential events or conditions that could have a positive or a negative impact on the project goals.

Risk analysis—Process of identifying risks, analyzing the likelihood that they will occur, and the degree of impact that they will have on the project goals, and selecting strategies to eliminate or manage them.

Sample—A representative subgroup of the population that is being studied.

Schedule—The start and finish dates of the project and each of the project activities. It may also include the milestones or markers showing accomplishment of logically related activities or targets, as well as relationships among the activities.

Scope—Boundary of the project described in the project plan. It includes the need that will be addressed; the target audience; the goals that will be achieved within a certain time frame; the main activities that will be performed; the project performers; and the outcome, product, or service that will result. By implication, anything that is not included in these components is "out of scope."

Self-employment—The employment status of an individual who engages in self-directed economic activities.

Self-sufficiency—A condition where an individual or family does not need, and is not eligible to receive, TANF assistance under Title I of the Personal Responsibility and Work Opportunity Reconciliation Act of 1996 (Part A of Title IV of the Social Security Act.); the economic status of a person who does not require public assistance to provide for his or her needs and that of immediate family members.

Service—Activity carried out to provide people with the use of something.

SMART—Acronym that stands for goals or targets that are specific, measurable, achievable, realistic (and relevant), and time bound.

Success story—An example that illustrates the program's positive or desired effect.

Summative evaluation—Provides information on the project's efficacy (its ability to do what it was designed to do).

Sustainability activities—Tasks performed to ensure that the project's benefits extend beyond the period of a grant or the official conclusion of the project.

Target—Measurable amount of success the proposed project should achieve within a certain time frame. When expressed as an output, it refers to the amount, quality, or volume of use the proposed project should achieve within a certain time frame. When expressed as an outcome, it refers to the measurable amount of success the proposed project should achieve with regard to the target audience's knowledge, skills, attitudes, behaviors, status, or life condition, within a certain period of time.

Target audience—Individuals, groups, or organizations that are the focus or beneficiaries of the products or services of the project. Characteristics or attributes of target audience: age, geographic location, population count, and job position of the target audience that should be considered when analyzing their needs.

Technical assistance—A problem-solving event generally using the services of a specialist. Such services may be provided on-site, by telephone, or by other communications. These services address specific problems and are intended to assist with immediate resolution of a given problem or set of problems.

Temporary Assistance for Needy Families (TANF)—The federal block grant program authorized in Title I of the Personal Responsibility and Work Opportunity Reconciliation Act of 1996 (Public Law 104–193). The TANF program transformed welfare into a system that requires work in exchange for time-limited assistance.

Third party—Any individual, organization, or business entity that is not the direct recipient of grant funds.

Third party agreement—A written agreement entered into by the grantee and an organization, individual, or business entity (including a wholly owned subsidiary) by which the grantee makes an equity investment or a loan in support of grant purposes.

Underserved area—A locality in which less than one-half of the low-income children are eligible.

Vision—Statement of what the project intends to achieve. It describes aspirations for the future without specifying the means that will be used to achieve those desired ends.

Wants—Wishes or desires of the target audience. These should be taken into consideration in determining the most appropriate solution or solutions to meet an identified need.

REFERENCES

Committee Encouraging Corporate Philanthropy. Giving in Numbers: 2012 Edition. Available at http://www.corporatephilanthropy.org/pdfs/giving_in_numbers/GIN2012_finalweb.pdf, accessed February 13, 2015.

Centers for Disease Control and Prevention. Grants. Overview. Available at http://www.cdc.gov/grants/index.html, accessed February 13, 2015.

Food and Drug Administration. Available at http://www.fda.gov/, accessed February 13, 2015.

Foundation Center. Guide to Funding Research: Glossary. Available at http://www.foundationcenter.org/get started/tutorials/gfr/glossary.html, accessed February 13, 2015.

General Services Administration. Catalog of Federal Domestic Assistance. Available at https://www.cfda.gov/, accessed February 13, 2015.

Grants.gov. Available at http://www.grants.gov/web/grants/about.html, accessed February 13, 2015.

Kaiser Family Foundation. Medicaid Moving Forward, January 2015. Available at http://kff.org/medicaid/fact -sheet/the-medicaid-program-at-a-glance-update, accessed February 13, 2015.

National Association for State Community Services Programs. Community Services Block Grant 2014 Annual Report, December 2014. Available at http://www.nascsp.org/data/files/csbg_is_survey/csbg_is_survey _fy14/2014annualreport.pdf, accessed February 13, 2015.

News from Wyoming Department of Health. Wyoming Office of Multicultural Health Announces Mini-Grants, October 15, 2012. Available at http://www.health.wyo.gov/news.aspx?NewsID=554, accessed February 13, 2015.

Nutrition Obesity Research Centers. Available at http://www.norccentral.org/home.do, accessed February 13, 2015.

Office of the Federal Register. US Government Printing Office. The United States Government Manual. Available at http://www.usgovernmentmanual.gov/, accessed February 13, 2015.

Office of Management and Budget. Prime Award Spending Data: FY2012. Available at http://www.usaspending .gov/explore, accessed February 13, 2015.

Office of Management and Budget. Prime Award Spending Data: Nutrition Grants. Available at http://www .usaspending.gov/search?form_fields={%22search_term%22%3A%22nutrition%22%2C%22spending _cat%22%3A[%22g%22]}&sort_by=dollars&per_page=25, accessed February 13, 2015.

Pitman MA. *Ask Without Fear!: A Simple Guide to Connecting Donors with What Matters to Them Most.* Mechanicsburg, PA: Executive Books, April 2008.

Robert Wood Johnson Foundation. About RWJF. Available at http://www.rwjf.org/en/about-rwjf.html, accessed February 13, 2015.

Spar K. Community Services Block Grants (CSBG): Background and Funding. Congressional Research Service Report RL32872, May 24, 2013. Available at https://www.fas.org/sgp/crs/misc/RL32872.pdf, accessed February 13, 2015.

The Foundation Center. Foundation Stats. Available at http://data.foundationcenter.org/, accessed February 13, 2015.

The Foundation Center. Proposal Writing Short Course. Available at http://foundationcenter.org/getstarted/tutori als/shortcourse/index.html, accessed February 13, 2015.

The White House. The Cabinet. Available at http://www.whitehouse.gov/administration/cabinet, accessed February 13, 2015.

University of Wisconsin Cooperative Extension. Program Development and Evaluation. Logic Model. Available at http://www.uwex.edu/ces/pdande/evaluation/evallogicmodel.html, accessed February 13, 2015.

US Department of Agriculture. Food and Nutrition Services. Programs and Services. Available at http://www .fns.usda.gov/programs-and-services, accessed February 13, 2015.

US Department of Agriculture. Food Safety and Inspection Service. Food Safety Research Priorities. Available at http://www.fsis.usda.gov/wps/portal/fsis/topics/science/food-safety-research-priorities, accessed February 13, 2015.

US Department of Agriculture. FY 2015 Budget Summary and Annual Performance Plan. Available at http:// www.obpa.usda.gov/budsum/FY15budsum.pdf, accessed February 13, 2015.

US Department of Agriculture. National Institute of Food and Agriculture. Fact Sheet. Available at http://www .nifa.usda.gov/newsroom/factsheet.pdf, accessed February 13, 2015.

US Department of Agriculture. National Institute of Food and Agriculture. Federal Assistance. Available at http://www.nifa.usda.gov/about/fed_asst.html, accessed February 13, 2015.

US Department of Agriculture. Office of the Chief Financial Officer. USDA Strategic Plan: FY 2010–2015. Available at http://www.ocfo.usda.gov/sp2010/sp2010.pdf, accessed February 13, 2015.

US Department of Health and Human Services. Administration on Aging. National Aging Network. Available at http://www.aoa.gov/AoA_Programs/OAA/Aging_Network/Index.aspx, accessed February 13, 2015.

US Department of Health and Human Services. Administration on Aging. Older Americans Act. Available at http://www.aoa.gov/AoA_programs/OAA/, accessed February 13, 2015.

US Department of Health and Human Services. Administration for Children and Families. Available at http:// www.cf.hhs.gov/, accessed February 13, 2015.

US Department of Health and Human Services. Administration for Children and Families. Office of Community Services. Community Economic Development. Available at http://www.acf.hhs.gov/programs/ocs/programs/ced, accessed February 13, 2015.

US Department of Health and Human Services. Administration for Children and Families. Office of Community Services. Community Services Block Grant. Available at http://www.acf.hhs.gov/programs/ocs/programs/csbg, accessed February 13, 2015.

US Department of Health and Human Services. Administration for Children and Families. Office of Community Services. Healthy Food Financing Initiative. Available at http://www.acf.hhs.gov/programs/ocs/programs/community-economic-development/healthy-food-financing, accessed February 13, 2015.

US Department of Health and Human Services. Administration for Community Living. Available at http://www.acl.gov, accessed February 13, 2015.

US Department of Health and Human Services. Centers for Disease Control and Prevention. Preventive Health and Health Services Block Grant. PHHS Block Grant Appropriations History. Available at http://www.cdc.gov/phhsblockgrant/history.htm, accessed February 13, 2015.

US Department of Health and Human Services. Fiscal Year 2014 Budget in Brief: Advancing the Health, Safety and Well-Being of the Nation. Available at http://www.hhs.gov/budget/fy2014/fy-2014-budget-in-brief.pdf, accessed February 13, 2015.

US Department of Health and Human Services. Historical Highlights. Available at http://www.hhs.gov/about/hhshist.html, accessed February 13, 2015.

US Department of Health and Human Services. Indian Health Service. Fact Sheet: Diabetes. Available at http://www.ihs.gov/newsroom/factsheets/diabetes, accessed February 13, 2015.

US Department of Health and Human Services. National Institutes of Health. Available at http://www.nih.gov, accessed February 13, 2015.

US Department of Health and Human Services. National Institutes of Health. Research Portfolio Online Reporting Tools (RePORT). Available at http://report.nih.gov, accessed February 13, 2015.

US Department of Health and Human Services. News Release: Obama Administration Details Healthy Food Financing Initiative, February 19, 2010. Available at http://www.usda.gov/wps/portal/usda/usdamediafb?contentid=2010/02/0077.xml&printable=true&contentidonly=truel, accessed February 13, 2015.

US Department of Health and Human Services. National Institutes of Health. Improving Diet and Physical Activity Assessment. Posted date: June 6, 2012. PA Number: PAR-12-198. Available at http://grants.nih.gov/grants/guide/pa-files/PAR-12-198.html, accessed February 13, 2015.

US Department of Health and Human Services. National Institutes of Health. National Institute of Diabetes and Digestive and Kidney Diseases. WIN. Weight-control Information Network. Available at http://win.niddk.nih.gov, accessed February 13, 2015.

US Department of Health and Human Services. National Institutes of Health. National Heart, Lung, and Blood Institute. Women's Health Initiative. Available at https://www.nhlbi.nih.gov/whi/, accessed February 13, 2015.

US Department of Health and Human Services. Office of the Assistant Secretary for Health. Available at http://www.hhs.gov/ash/, accessed February 13, 2015.

US Department of Health and Human Services. US Public Health Service Commissioned Corps. USPHS Dietitian Professional Advisory Committee. Available at http://dcp.psc.gov/osg/dietitian, accessed February 13, 2015.

W.K. Kellogg Foundation. Our History in Grantmaking. Available at http://www.wkkf.org/who-we-are/our-history.aspx, accessed February 13, 2015.

W.K. Kellogg Foundation. Logic Model Development Guide. Updated February 2006. Available at http://www.wkkf.org/knowledge-center/resources/2006/02/wk-kellogg-foundation-logic-model-development-guide.aspx, accessed February 13, 2015.

Index

Page numbers followed by f, t, and b indicate figures, tables and boxes, respectively.